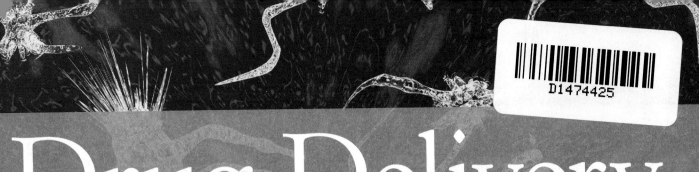

Drug Delivery

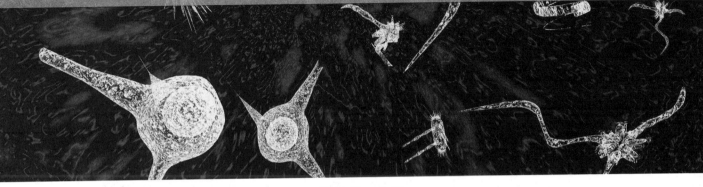

EDITED BY

Ashim K. Mitra, PhD

Chairman and Curator's
Professor, Pharmaceutical
Sciences

School of Pharmacy

University of Missouri-
Kansas City

Kansas City, Missouri

Deep Kwatra, PhD

Postdoctoral Research Fellow

School of Medicine

University of Kansas
Medical Center

Kansas City, Kansas

Aswani Dutt Vadlapudi, PhD

Scientist, Technical Services

Mylan Pharmaceuticals, Inc.

Morgantown, West Virginia

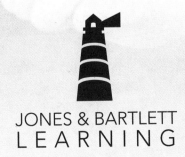

JONES & BARTLETT
LEARNING

World Headquarters
Jones & Bartlett Learning
5 Wall Street
Burlington, MA 01803
978-443-5000
info@jblearning.com
www.jblearning.com

Jones & Bartlett Learning books and products are available through most bookstores and online booksellers. To contact Jones & Bartlett Learning directly, call 800-832-0034, fax 978-443-8000, or visit our website, www.jblearning.com.

Substantial discounts on bulk quantities of Jones & Bartlett Learning publications are available to corporations, professional associations, and other qualified organizations. For details and specific discount information, contact the special sales department at Jones & Bartlett Learning via the above contact information or send an email to specialsales@jblearning.com.

Production Credits

Executive Publisher: William Brottmiller
Executive Editor: Rhonda Dearborn
Editorial Assistant: Sean Fabery
Production Editor: Louis C. Bruno, Jr.
Marketing Manager: Grace Richards
Art Development Editor: Joanna Lundeen
VP, Manufacturing and Inventory Control: Therese Connell

Composition: diacriTech
Cover Design: Michael O'Donnell
Rights and Photo Research Coordinator: Ashley Dos Santos
Cover Image: Illustration © Chronis Chamalidis/ShutterStock, Inc.; photo © photomak/ShutterStock, Inc.
Printing and Binding: Edwards Brothers Malloy
Cover Printing: Edwards Brothers Malloy

To order this product, use ISBN: 978-1-284-02568-2

Library of Congress Cataloging-in-Publication Data
Drug delivery (Mitra)
  Drug delivery / [edited by] Ashim K. Mitra, Deep Kwatra, and Aswani Dutt Vadlapudi. — First edition.
      p. ; cm.
  Includes bibliographical references.
  ISBN 978-1-4496-7425-0 (alk. paper)
  I. Mitra, Ashim K., 1954– editor. II. Kwatra, Deep, editor. III. Vadlapudi, Aswani Dutt, editor. IV. Title.
  [DNLM: 1. Drug Delivery Systems. QV 785]
  RM170
  615'.6—dc23
                                                    2014008174
6048

Printed in the United States of America
18 17 16 15 14   10 9 8 7 6 5 4 3 2 1

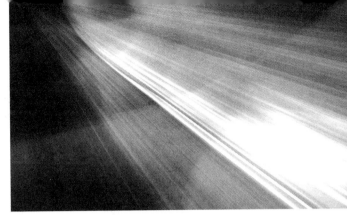
© Taewoon Lee/ShutterStock, Inc.

CONTENTS

Chapter 6   Controlled Drug Delivery   108

*Shailendra B. Tallapaka, Vamsi K. Karuturi, Sutthilug Sotthivirat,
    and Joseph A. Vetro*

Chapter 7   Polymers in Drug Delivery   129

*David Mastropietro, Srinath Muppalaneni, Young Kwon,
    Kinam Park, and Hossein Omidian*

Chapter 17　　**Peptide and Protein Drug Delivery**　　　　**405**

*Chirs Kulczar, Wyatt Roth, Stephen Carl, Olafur Gudmundsson,
and Gregory Knipp*

Chapter 18　　**Drug Metabolomics and Proteomics Analysis in Drug
Delivery and Discovery**　　　　**429**

Ravinder Earla and Ashim K. Mitra

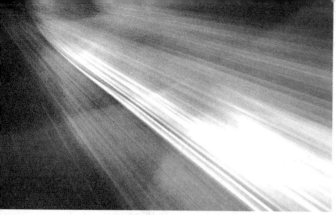

PREFACE

Drug delivery is a concept closely integrated with dosage form and route of administration. This concept is often associated with rationale-based approaches, formulation strategies, drug development technologies, and carriers for facilitating transport of a drug molecule as needed to safely achieve its desired therapeutic effect. During the past two decades, numerous drug molecules with the potential of revolutionizing the treatment of life-threatening diseases have been developed. Despite remarkable advancements, many therapeutically active pharmaceutical ingredients have been dropped from initial screening portfolios because of the lack of an efficient drug delivery method. Recent progress in the field of biotechnology, however, has encouraged researchers and scientists to develop various methods employing effective delivery systems for the administration of biologics. Numerous other technologies are also addressing ways to minimize drug toxicity and reduce adverse effects while maintaining therapeutic drug concentrations and employing suitable therapeutic regimens.

Drug delivery as a field is rapidly expanding and is of vital importance to therapeutics. There is no single text, however, that covers all areas of drug delivery at a level suitable to the needs of undergraduate, graduate, and professional students as well as peers in academia and pharmaceutical research. The majority of current texts either limit themselves to conventional technologies or focus only on a single aspect of drug delivery. This book, therefore, has been designed to thoroughly examine pertinent areas and provide a platform for developing useful concepts for drug delivery.

ORGANIZATION OF THIS TEXT

As a glance at the Contents makes clear, this book provides a very comprehensive overview of the cutting-edge research being carried out in this field with a focus on drug targeting at the molecular, cellular, and organ levels.

The first chapter, "Drug Delivery: An Evolving Concept," helps the reader understand the evolution of drug delivery concepts and recognize the factors that have an impact on drug discovery and development in pharmaceutical arenas.

Chapter 2, "Barriers to Drug Delivery," emphasizes the challenges faced by drug delivery scientists. Various barriers to drug delivery and the strategies used to overcome or evade such barriers are discussed in detail. A basic comprehension of these barriers is required to understand the concept behind the design of the delivery systems developed to overcome them.

Chapter 3, "*In Vitro* Models in Drug Discovery and Delivery," discusses various *in vitro* and *in silico* models used in the estimation of pharmacokinetic parameters of drugs and formulations with a special emphasis on cell culture models.

Chapter 4, "Routes of Drug Delivery," provides a thorough understanding of the multiple routes of administration utilized to deliver the active ingredient from common pharmaceutical dosage forms. This understanding is important as the factors that must be considered in dosage form design and selection are based not only on the patient being treated but also on the biopharmaceutically relevant advantages and disadvantages of various drug delivery routes.

The focus of Chapter 5, "Novel Drug Delivery Systems," is the wide variety of novel drug delivery systems that are currently being investigated and currently on the market.

Chapter 6, "Controlled Drug Delivery," discusses the differences between conventional and controlled drug delivery technologies. This chapter also differentiates controlled dosage forms currently available in the clinic by mechanism of release.

Chapter 7, "Polymers in Drug Delivery," describes the pharmaceutical applications of polymers in various dosage forms. This chapter allows for better understanding of polymer properties based on composition, molecular weight, and arrangement to facilitate custom design of novel delivery systems.

Chapter 8, "Multifunctional Nanocarriers for Tumor Drug Delivery and Imaging," aims to provide an overview of recent progress in the rational design of and the engineering of multifunctional systems and to illustrate the cutting-edge technology being employed in such carriers with examples of multifunctional liposomes, micelles, and nanoparticles for cancer diagnosis and treatment.

In the later part of the book, we discuss various aspects of drug delivery technologies that are utilized for various dosing routes. We also discuss how the drugs can be delivered specifically to certain organs.

Chapter 9, "Oral Delivery," provides an overview of physicochemical and biological barriers in oral delivery. Various oral dosage forms and their performance with respect to bioavailability are extensively discussed.

Chapter 10, "Ocular Drug Delivery," delves into detailed anatomy and physiology of the eye, the importance of various routes of ocular drug administration, and constraints on conventional ocular therapy. This chapter will aid in acquiring sound knowledge of various approaches to increasing ocular drug absorption. It also discusses recent progress and specific developments relating to various formulation approaches. This chapter also discusses key advances in the application of nanotechnology for gene therapy to the eye.

Chapter 11, "Transmucosal Drug Delivery," provides an overview of the importance of the transmucosal route and its advantages over traditional methods of drug delivery. This chapter describes the structure of oral mucosa, permeability barriers to drug absorption, and methods of assessing oral mucosal absorption. The chapter also details various drug delivery systems and techniques being used to optimize the delivery across oral mucosa. Commercialized formulations currently available in the market are also detailed.

Chapter 12, "Transdermal Drug Delivery," describes the anatomical and physiological factors controlling drug transport across skin. Furthermore, active transdermal technologies available to enhance percutaneous absorption and various types of transdermal patches currently available on the market are covered. This chapter also provides methods for patient counseling with regard to the proper use and precautions necessary with the application of a transdermal drug delivery system.

Chapter 13, "Pulmonary and Nasal Drug Delivery," reviews the anatomy and physiology of the respiratory tract that governs drug delivery via the nasal and pulmonary routes. This chapter allows the reader to learn pharmaceutical and physiological factors that may affect drug deposition and absorption upon nasal and pulmonary administration. Various devices used to administer drug formulations via the respiratory route are described. A detailed and comprehensive discussion of currently available dosage forms along with recent advancements in nebulizers and metered dose and dry powder inhalers are provided. This chapter will acquaint the reader with various spacer devices and their proper usage, advantages, and disadvantages. Various respiratory drug delivery devices and formulations, as well as patient counseling for inhalational devices and drug products, are also emphasized.

Chapter 14, "Vaginal Drug Delivery," offers basic understanding of anatomy and physiology of the vagina, physiological and physicochemical factors that may affect vaginal drug absorption, and characteristics of various vaginal drug delivery systems that are currently available on the market or are in the developmental stage.

Chapter 15, "Drug Delivery to the Central Nervous System: Breaking Down the Barrier," describes the structure and importance of the blood–brain barrier. This chapter offers a detailed understanding of anatomical, physiological, and pharmacological mechanisms by which the blood–brain barrier protects the central nervous system. Furthermore, current strategies for CNS drug delivery, flexibility of novel drug delivery systems, and how they can be tailor-designed to enhance CNS drug delivery are extensively discussed.

Chapter 16, "Gene Delivery: An Essential Component for Successful Gene Therapy," details the importance of gene therapy that uses a gene-coding sequence as a pharmaceutical agent. Gene therapy requires a method effective in delivering a therapeutic gene into cells and expressing proteins where treatment is needed. Several delivery systems including viral, chemical, and physical methods are discussed. Further, this chapter provides a summary on the pros and cons of each gene delivery system currently available and provides recent perspectives on remaining challenges for future development.

Chapter 17, "Peptide and Protein Drug Delivery," discusses physicochemical differences between small molecules and protein/peptide drugs. This chapter helps in understanding the challenges faced when formulating a protein/peptide drug for oral delivery and why parenteral delivery is most often needed with such drugs. An overview of the intricacies of insulin that make non-parenteral delivery challenging and the advantages and disadvantages of different alternative routes for delivering protein/peptide drugs are discussed.

Chapter 18, "Drug Metabolomics and Proteomics Analysis in Drug Delivery and Discovery," describes proteomics and mass spectrometric analysis including sample preparation, isolation, and purification techniques. This chapter also provides an overview of mass spectrometry instrumentation and ionization techniques. It describes top-down protein and bottom-up (shotgun) peptide sequencing and application of mass spectrometry in quantitative proteomics, that is, phosphorylation, glycosylation, and post-translational modifications.

FEATURES AND BENEFITS

Each chapter includes the following elements:

- *Learning Objectives* present the chapter's desired outcomes to the reader.
- *Chapter Outline* provides a preview of the material to be covered.
- *Review Questions* allow readers to apply what has been learned in the chapter and assess their understanding of the content.

INSTRUCTOR RESOURCES

Qualified instructors can receive the full suite of instructor resources, including the following:

- PowerPoint Presentations, featuring more than 350 slides
- Test Bank, containing more than 500 questions
- Instructor's Manual, including an Answer Key for the end-of-chapter Review Questions

STUDENT RESOURCES

The Navigate Companion Website features numerous study aids and learning tools to help students get the most out of their course and prepare for class, including the following:

- Chapter Quizzes
- Interactive Glossary
- Crossword Puzzles
- Interactive Flashcards
- Matching Exercises

ACKNOWLEDGMENTS

We are very grateful to all the individual authors for their excellent contributions and massive efforts in sharing their knowledge, concepts, and expertise in various aspects of drug delivery.

Finally, we would like to acknowledge the support of the publisher and thank the production team for their relentless efforts.

Ashim K. Mitra
Deep Kwatra
Aswani Dutt Vadlapudi

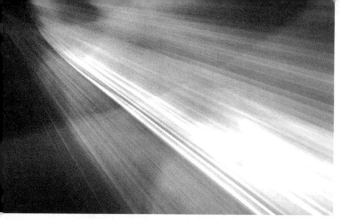

FOREWORD

Targeted and controlled drug delivery systems can have a massive impact on therapeutic efficacy and safety. These technologies enable maximum benefit from existing drugs and provide opportunities for successful transition to new drug entities. Such advancements have added an entirely new dimension to the pharmaceutical market with sales of these technologies now in the billions of dollars annually. Importantly, multidisciplinary training is needed to understand the interface of biology and chemistry to design novel drug delivery carriers and preparations that are effective and nontoxic. Within this book Dr. Ashim K. Mitra, Dr. Deep Kwatra, and Dr. Aswani Dutt Vadlapudi have done a great job assimilating large amounts of current information about this growing area, bringing together the foremost experts from their respective fields to yield a comprehensive look at drug delivery and its relevant issues.

Drug Delivery contains up-to-date material that will inform both novices as well as advanced learners in the field. A major strength of the book is its logical organization. For example, the human body provides multiple anatomical and physiological barriers to many drugs from easily reaching their target site. The book begins with detailed descriptions of the biological barriers to drug delivery and then covers drug delivery models, routes of administration, and controlled drug delivery systems, making sure the reader first grasps the basic concepts.

Critical for advancement of the field is the creation of novel polymeric materials, which is the subject of next chapter in the book. Here, the different types of polymers and their utilization to form nanoparticles and other novel drug delivery systems are described. The formation and characterization of multifunctional nanocarriers, which can be used for both controlled and targeted drug delivery, are also explained.

Next, specific issues with key routes of administration are detailed in individual chapters. For instance, parenteral, dermal, oral, ocular, pulmonary/nasal, mucosal, and vaginal drug delivery, and delivery to the central nervous system are all given specific attention.

Remarkably, this book also covers modern therapeutic modalities, including gene therapy as well as peptide and protein therapeutics such as antibodies. Delivery of these biologics via conventional carriers poses significant challenges, which are detailed, and numerous techniques are being developed to overcome these temporary hurdles. Moreover, a number of analytical tools are required to test delivery system efficiency, all of which are explained.

Taken together, this book is a very detailed and complete compilation of all the major topics in the field of drug delivery and will prove to be a handy "go-to" reference for students, teachers, and researchers in academia and the pharmaceutical industry.

W. Daniel Stamer, PhD
Joseph A. C. Wadsworth Professor of Ophthalmology
Professor of Biomedical Engineering
Duke University

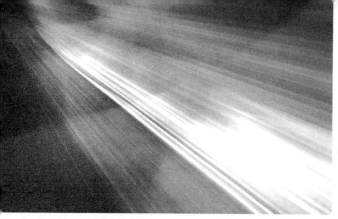

ABOUT THE EDITORS

Ashim K. Mitra

Ashim K. Mitra received his PhD in Pharmaceutical Chemistry in 1983 from the University of Kansas. He is currently a Curators' Professor of Pharmacy at the University of Missouri-Kansas City, as well as the Vice Provost for Interdisciplinary Research, Chairman of the Division of Pharmaceutical Sciences, and Co-director of the Vision Research Center at the University of Missouri-Kansas City School of Medicine. For the past three decades he has conducted extensive research in various drug delivery technologies, including ocular drug delivery. He and his research personnel have published more than 315 peer-reviewed research articles in high-impact international journals; published more than 550 abstracts at scientific meetings, including the annual conferences of the American Association of Pharmaceutical Scientists (AAPS), the Society of Toxicology, and The Association for Research in Vision and Ophthalmology (ARVO); have given more than 115 presentations to a wide audience (including several universities, pharmaceutical companies, and scientific organizations); and have been issued nine U.S. patents. Between 2013 and 2014 alone he has edited five books and contributed to more than 60 book chapters. Several of his articles have been recognized as being among the most downloaded articles in their respective journals.

Deep Kwatra

Deep Kwatra received his interdisciplinary PhD in Pharmaceutical Sciences and Molecular Biology & Biochemistry in 2011 from the University of Missouri-Kansas City. He is currently pursuing a postdoctoral fellowship at the University of Kansas Medical Center in the Department of Molecular and Integrative Physiology. He is also a pharmacist by training with a Bachelors of Pharmacy from Smriti College of Pharmaceutical Education in Indore, India. Over the past decade he has worked extensively towards development of *in vitro* cell culture models for better prediction of bioavailability of drugs and formulations. He has also developed prodrugs specifically targeted towards influx transporters on the eye for more efficient ocular drug delivery. Additionally, he has collaborated with many labs working on enhancing delivery of small molecules and biologics to the eye. He has published more than 20 peer-reviewed scientific research and review articles in high-impact international journals. He has also contributed to many books focused on different aspects of drug delivery. He has presented more than 50 abstracts at scientific meetings, including the annual American Association of Pharmaceutical Scientists (AAPS), The Association for Research in Vision and Ophthalmology (ARVO), and American Association of Cancer Research

(AACR) conferences. He was awarded the Young Investigator Award by the American Association of Indian Scientists in Cancer Research Foundation at the AACR 2012 annual meeting.

Aswani Dutt Vadlapudi

Aswani Dutt Vadlapudi received his PhD in Pharmaceutics and Drug Design in 2013 from the University of Missouri-Kansas City School of Pharmacy. He currently holds a Managerial Scientist position at Mylan Pharmaceuticals, Inc. Dr. Vadlapudi is actively engaged in improving drug delivery and drug development strategies with extensive experience in manufacturing of solid oral dosage forms, process optimization, scale-up, and investigations. His research accomplishments include transporter targeted drug delivery, prodrug development, and formulation approaches for improving oral and ocular drug absorption of both small molecules and macromolecules. He is an active member of the American Association of Pharmaceutical Scientists (AAPS) and The Association for Research in Vision and Ophthalmology (ARVO). Dr. Vadlapudi is a member of review committees and scientific boards of many international journals. He has authored and co-authored more than 25 peer-reviewed research and review articles in reputable international journals. Most of his publications are highly cited and recognized as being among the most downloaded articles in their respective journals. He has also contributed to many book chapters in the field of drug delivery and drug development.

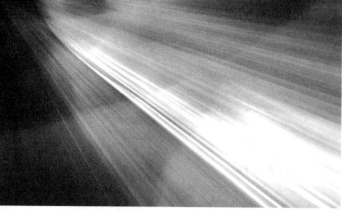

CONTRIBUTORS

Chris E. Adkins, PhD
Postdoctoral Fellow
School of Pharmacy
Texas Tech University Health Sciences Center
Amarillo, Texas
Chapter 15

Fakhrul Ahsan, PhD
Graduate Program Advisor
School of Pharmacy
Texas Tech University Health Sciences Center
Amarillo, Texas
Chapter 13

Mohammad Al Saggar, BSc
PhD Candidate
College of Pharmacy
University of Georgia
Athens, Georgia
Chapter 16

Gabriella Baki, PhD
Visiting Assistant Professor
College of Pharmacy and Pharmaceutical Sciences
The University of Toledo
Toledo, Ohio
Chapter 14

Ajay K. Banga, PhD
Professor and Department Chair
College of Pharmacy and Health Sciences
Mercer University
Atlanta, Georgia
Chapter 12

Sai H. S. Boddu, PhD
Assistant Professor
College of Pharmacy and Pharmaceutical Sciences
The University of Toledo
Toledo, Ohio
Chapters 4 and 14

Kaci A. Bohn, PhD
Assistant Professor
College of Pharmacy
Harding University
Searcy, Arkansas
Chapter 15

Stephen Carl, PhD
Associate Director of Formulation Development
Enteris BioPharma, Inc.
Fairfield, New Jersey
Chapter 17

Kishore Cholkar, MS
Research Assistant
School of Pharmacy
University of Missouri—Kansas City
Kansas City, Missouri
Chapter 10

Supriya Reddy Dasari
Research Assistant
School of Pharmacy
University of Missouri—Kansas City
Kansas City, Missouri
Chapter 10

Patrick P. DeLuca, PhD
Professor Emeritus
College of Pharmacy
University of Kentucky
Lexington, Kentucky
Chapter 5

Ravinder Earla, PhD
Research Associate
School of Pharmacy
University of Missouri-Kansas City
Kansas City, Missouri
Chapter 18

Song Gao, PhD
Research Assistant Professor
College of Pharmacy
University of Houston
Houston, Texas
Chapter 9

Ripal Gaudana, PhD
Formulation Scientist
Par Pharmaceutical Companies, Inc.
Spring Valley, New York
Chapter 4

Olafur Gudmundsson, PhD
Director
Bristol-Myers Squibb
Princeton, New Jersey
Chapter 17

Meera Gujjar, BS
PhD Candidate
College of Pharmacy and Health Sciences
Mercer University
Atlanta, Georgia
Chapter 12

Nilesh Gupta
PhD Candidate
Chair-elect, AAPS Student Chapter
School of Pharmacy
Texas Tech University Health Sciences Center
Amarillo, Texas
Chapter 13

Anushree Kishor Herwadkar, PhD
Scientist I, PRD
Teva Pharamceuticals
Pomona, New York
Chapter 12

Ming Hu, PhD
Professor
College of Pharmacy
University of Houston
Houston, Texas
Chapter 9

Bhaskara Jasti, PhD
Professor and Chairman
Thomas J. Long School of Pharmacy

University of the Pacific
Stockton, California
Chapter 11

Wen Jiang
Graduate Student
College of Pharmacy
University of Houston
Houston, Texas
Chapter 9

Vamsi K. Karuturi
Research Assistant
University of Nebraska Medical Center
Omaha, Nebraska
Chapter 6

Navdeep Kaur, PhD
Research Assistant
Thomas J. Long School of Pharmacy
University of the Pacific
Stockton, California
Chapter 11

Varun Khurana, PhD
Formulation Scientist
Insys Therapeutics, Inc.
Chandler, Arizona
Chapter 3

Gregory Knipp, PhD
Associate Professor
College of Pharmacy
Purdue University
West Lafayette, Indiana
Chapter 17

Amit Kokate, PhD
Principal Scientist
Teva Pharmaceuticals
Pomona, New York
Chapter 11

Chris Kulczar
Graduate Student
College of Pharmacy
Purdue University
West Lafayette, Indiana
Chapter 17

Young Kwon, PhD
Assistant Professor
College of Pharmacy
Nova Southeastern University
Fort Lauderdale, Florida
Chapter 7

Xiaoling Li, PhD
Associate Dean and Professor
Thomas J. Long School of Pharmacy
University of the Pacific
Stockton, California
Chapter 11

Dexi Liu, PhD
Panoz Professor of Pharmacy
College of Pharmacy
University of Georgia
Athens, Georgia
Chapter 16

Paul R. Lockman, PhD
Chair, Basic Pharmaceutical Science
School of Pharmacy
Texas Tech University Health Sciences Center
Amarillo, Texas
Chapter 15

Yong Ma, BS
Graduate Student
College of Pharmacy
University of Houston
Houston, Texas
Chapter 9

Heidi M. Mansour, PhD
Assistant Professor
College of Pharmacy
The University of Arizona—Tucson
Tucson, Arizona
Chapter 5

David Mastropietro, BPharm, RPh
Research Assistant
College of Pharmacy
Nova Southeastern University
Fort Lauderdale, Florida
Chapter 7

Samantha A. Meenach, PhD
Assistant Professor
College of Engineering

University of Rhode Island
Kingston, Rhode Island
Chapter 5

Sara Movassaghian, PhD
Postdoctoral Fellow
Center for Pharmaceutical Biotechnology and Nanomedicine
Northeastern University
Boston, Massachusetts
Chapter 8

Srinath Muppalaneni, MS
Research Assistant
College of Pharmacy
Nova Southeastern University
Fort Lauderdale, Florida
Chapter 7

Gemma Navarro, PhD
Postdoctoral Fellow
Center for Pharmaceutical Biotechnology and Nanomedicine
Northeastern University
Boston, Massachusetts
Chapter 8

Jerry Nesamony, PhD
Assistant Professor
College of Pharmacy and Pharmaceutical Sciences
The University of Toledo
Toledo, Ohio
Chapter 14

Sanko Nguyen, PhD
Postdoctoral Fellow
College of Pharmacy and Pharmaceutical Sciences
The University of Toledo
Toledo, Ohio
Chapter 14

Mohamed Ismail Nounou, PhD
Postdoctoral Fellow
School of Pharmacy
Texas Tech University Health Sciences Center
Amarillo, Texas
Chapter 15

Hossein Omidian, PhD
Assistant Professor
College of Pharmacy
Nova Southeastern University
Fort Lauderdale, Florida
Chapter 7

Chun-Woong Park, PhD
Assistant Professor
College of Pharmacy
Chungbuk National University
Cheongju, Republic of Korea
Chapter 5

Kinam Park, PhD
Showalter Distinguished Professor of Biomedical Engineering
College of Pharmacy
Purdue University
West Lafayette, Indiana
Chapter 7

Brijeshkumar Patel, PhD
Research Assistant
School of Pharmacy
Texas Tech University Health Sciences Center
Amarillo, Texas
Chapter 13

Yun-Seok Rhee, PhD
Assistant Professor
College of Pharmacy
Gyeongsang National University
Jinju, Republic of Korea
Chapter 5

Wyatt Roth, PhD
Research Scientist
Eli Lilly and Company
Indianapolis, Indiana
Chapter 17

Sujay J. Shah, BPharm
Research Assistant
School of Pharmacy
University of Missouri-Kansas City
Kansas City, Missouri
Chapter 2

Sutthilug Sotthivirat, PhD
Department of Product Value Enhancement
Merck & Company, Inc.
West Point, Pennsylvania
Chapter 6

Shailendra B. Tallapaka, BPharm
Graduate Assistant
University of Nebraska Medical Center
Omaha, Nebraska
Chapter 6

Tori B. Terrell–Hall
School of Pharmacy
Texas Tech University Health Sciences Center
Amarillo, Texas
Chapter 15

Vladimir P. Torchilin, PhD
Director
Center for Pharmaceutical Biotechnology and Nanomedicine
Northeastern University
Boston, Massachusetts
Chapter 8

Ramya Krishna Vadlapatla, PhD
Scientist, Technical Services
Mylan Pharmaceuticals, Inc.
Morgantown, West Virginia
Chapter 2

Joseph A. Vetro, PhD
Assistant Professor
College of Pharmacy
University of Nebraska Medical Center
Omaha, Nebraska
Chapter 6

Zhen Xu, PhD
Postdoctoral Fellow
School of Pharmacy
University of Maryland
Baltimore, Maryland
Chapter 5

Zhen Yang
Graduate Student
College of Pharmacy
University of Houston
Houston, Texas
Chapter 9

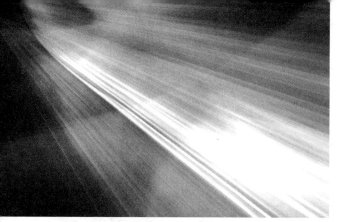

REVIEWERS

Yun Bai, PhD
Assistant Professor
School of Pharmacy
Philadelphia College of Osteopathic Medicine
Suwanee, Georgia

Mark J. Chirico, PharmD
Director, Experiential Education
College of Pharmacy
Belmont University
Nashville, Tennessee

Sarah L. Clement, EdS
Program Coordinator
Pharmacy Technology Program
Forsyth Technical Community College
Winston-Salem, North Carolina

Denise Leach, PA-C
Assistant Professor
College of Physician Assistant Studies
Alderson Broaddus University
Philippi, West Virginia

Cristobal L. Miranda, PhD, MS, DVM
Research Assistant Professor
College of Pharmacy
Oregon State University
Corvallis, Oregon

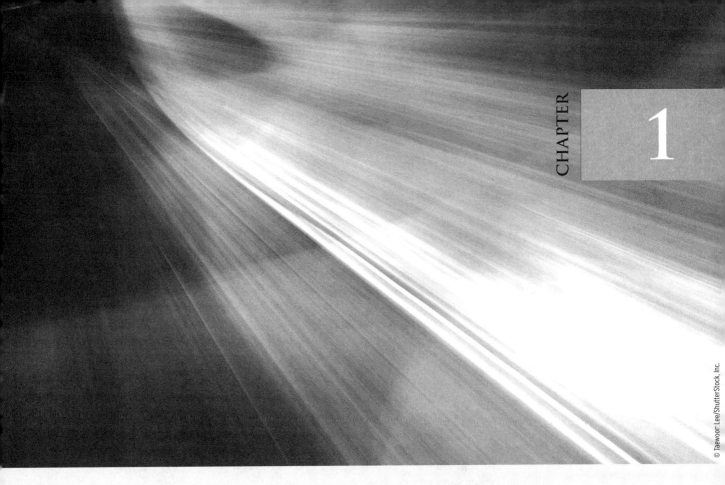

DRUG DELIVERY: AN EVOLVING CONCEPT

ASWANI DUTT VADLAPUDI, DEEP KWATRA,
AND ASHIM K. MITRA

CHAPTER OBJECTIVES

Upon completing this chapter, the reader should be able to

▶ Recognize the factors impacting drug discovery and development in pharmaceutical industry.

▶ Understand the evolution of drug delivery concept.

CHAPTER OUTLINE

Introduction

Factors in Drug Development

Commercial Goals

Chemical Limitations

In Vitro and *In Vivo* Efficacy Studies

INTRODUCTION

Drugs play a vital role in the current era of contemporary medicine. The total revenue generated from the global pharmaceuticals, biotechnology, and life sciences industry is more than $1.1 trillion in 2011, with a compounded annual growth rate of 6.7% between 2007 and 2011. Among specific segments, pharmaceuticals and biotechnology markets account for $798 and $289 billion in revenues. Interestingly, the Americas region accounts for 46% of total revenues, representing the largest share of the global market. The large market size permits pharmaceutical and biotechnology industries to invest profoundly in research and development.

Despite escalating research and development budgets, drug development is slow, with a limited number of new drugs introduced, whereas a large number of drugs are going off patent protection. The real cost of developing a new drug is considered to be greater than $800 million. Such high cost is due to the fact that many drug candidates are dropped from the preliminary screening portfolio because of their unfavorable physiochemical and biochemical properties. Drug absorption is often limited by the presence of physiological (epithelial tight junctions), biochemical (efflux transporters and enzymatic degradation), and chemical (size, lipophilicity, molecular weight, charge, etc.) barriers. Another major factor in designing and developing new drugs is the difficulty of active molecules to reach their desired and intended targets.

FACTORS IN DRUG DEVELOPMENT

Attributing to the high cost of development process, pharmaceutical companies try to create a framework in which the lead molecules with minimal ambiguity proceed further. This framework involves the study of characteristics, properties, and qualities of the lead molecules and setting of acceptable ranges for further progression of the candidate. This framework is often termed as the "developability or druggability criteria" [1]. A range of acceptable characteristics allows for molecules with properties that may not be ideal but have a high probability of success to progress. The setting of druggability and developability criteria also depends on multiple factors of commercialization and scientific feasibility, described further below.

COMMERCIAL GOALS

Because the pharmaceutical industry is a commercial entity, the lead molecule being developed as a drug needs to be profitable. Therefore, the critical and minimum acceptable properties making up the developability criteria are based on what the market desires. This process involves input from commercial, marketing, and medical professionals on Medicare needs, potential market, and existing leading products for an indication. No drug can be commercially viable if it does not meet the criteria for optimum therapeutic efficacy, good safety profile (sufficient therapeutic window), and minimal adverse effects. These factors should be the part of the developability criteria. If an agent already exists in the market with these properties, a new lead molecule may still be profitable if a large enough market exists and if the new molecule either improves the efficacy and/or the ease of delivery with a simpler therapeutic regimen.

CHEMICAL LIMITATIONS

Medicinal chemists led the early discovery of bioactive compounds during research and development. This initial process is carried out by random, high-throughput screening of compound libraries, by rational design, or both. The structures identi-fied from these methods are then further modified and optimized. After the develop-ment of a small set of related lead molecules, the initial exploratory structure–activity relationship is developed that allows for further structural changes and for selecting the most active compound. The detailed structural analysis at this stage involves more factors, such as potential stability, solubility, interaction with metabolic enzymes, and permeability, to be included in the developability criteria. Commercial aspects also may be involved, such as the novelty/patentability of the structure, scalability and the cost of industrial-scale synthesis, and the potential environmental safety issues related to production.

IN VITRO AND *IN VIVO* EFFICACY STUDIES

Initially, *in vitro* testing is carried out to narrow down the number of lead molecules based on their efficacy. Although it is a good technique for initial screening, such testing does not always result in good *in vivo* efficacy. Hence, studying the drugs in an *in vivo* animal model is essential before it is introduced into human clinical trials. For a drug to be safe and efficient in humans, it needs to be tested in an appropriate animal model that represents complex human physiology and the epidemiology of the disease. Although a molecule may be efficient *in vitro* working in a particular mechanism, it may not work in humans because of the presence of a compensatory mechanism. Thus, an *in vivo* model that has all the biochemical, cellular, and physiological complexities of human systems can truly predict the actual efficacy of the drug candidate. Another important use of *in vitro* and *in vivo* testing is the calculation of pharmacokinetic parameters that may eventually be the critical factor that decides the overall success of a compound.

PHARMACOKINETICS AND DRUG METABOLISM

Drug metabolism and pharmacokinetics (DMPK) estimations are a very critical part of the drug development process and a main reason for high attrition rates [2]. The main goal of DMPK studies is to predict the absorption, distribution, metabolism, and excre-tion of the drug candidate in humans. The dose and dosing frequency, calculated as a part of the process, provide the optimum efficacy. DMPK studies are carried out in mul-tiple animal models. However, allometric scaling and overall animal pharmacokinetics and metabolism data are applied to predict human parameters [3, 4]. A combination of *in vitro* and *in vivo* studies determines the important mechanistic parameters that regulate the pharmacokinetic profile of a drug. The lead compound with an optimized DMPK profile usually provides the highest probability of success.

Major pharmacokinetic drug parameters such as systemic bioavailability, maximum concentration achieved, time to achieve maximum concentration, and duration for which concentration is above minimum effective level are usually well correlated with the drug's efficacy and adverse effects [5]. The overall levels achieved are decided by multiple factors, such as site of administration, complexity of the dosage form, and rate at which the systemic circulation eliminates the active drug (total body clearance). Unless a rapidly acting drug is needed that has a short duration of action, usually a compound with low to moderate clearance is preferred [6].

Because oral dosing is the most common and convenient way to administer most drugs, the pharmacokinetic profile after oral dosing, including bioavailability, is a very important criterion. Additional pharmacokinetic parameters such as volume of distribution and elimination half-life are also important, and all these pharmacokinetic parameters should be calculated in different species. These results in combination with *in vitro* testing may be able to project human pharmacokinetics. Other major factors that control bioavailability and in turn the efficacy are interactions with drug-metabolizing enzymes [7, 8], efflux transporters [9, 10], and plasma proteins [11].

FINAL FORMULATION CHARACTERISTICS

Pharmacokinetic and pharmacodynamic studies should be carried out with a finished product. The crystalline state, salt form, and the presence of formulation excipients can lead to potential drug delivery and stability issues. These physiochemical properties and their eventual effects on drug delivery and pharmacokinetics should thus be a part of the drug developmental process. Aqueous solubility is one of the major drug delivery criteria, especially for orally administered drugs, because it is only the dose in the solution that can undergo the absorption process [1]. Indirectly, the crystal state of the drug is also an important factor that eventually affects both solubility and dissolution rates. The crystal state can also often determine the stability and the patentability of a molecule and hence is a critical developmental criterion. Similarly, the salt form of the molecule can also play a critical role in deciding the best solubility, dissolution rate, stability, and overall bioavailability [12].

Toxicological analysis is very important to the drug discovery and development process. The new molecules need to be tested for toxicities in both acute and chronic dosing because toxicological concerns are key factors in determining the developability of a drug and are a major cause of attrition. The factors essential for success of DMPK studies are also required for the toxicological studies, such as the selection of the appropriate animal models and suitable delivery systems and routes. Pharmacological and toxicological profiles should be studied for the active drug as well as its metabolites.

Although a single molecule in its native form may not be able to fulfill all the criteria of developability, the use of appropriate drug delivery techniques can often overcome these shortcomings. Selection of drug delivery technologies right from the early stages can lead to a more efficient and cost-effective drug development process.

DRUG DELIVERY

Since the evolution of the drug delivery concept in the 1970s, the field has advanced into an array of novel technologies that provide alternate routes of administration and/or sustained/controlled release for both novel and established pharmaceuticals. Pharmaceutical scientists increasingly depend on novel delivery technologies for successful product development and performance. Drug delivery can be defined as the method or process of administering a pharmaceutical compound to achieve a therapeutic effect in humans or animals. This process may involve utilization of several approaches, formulations, technologies, and systems to facilitate drug at the target site.

Drug delivery is a concept heavily integrated with dosage form and route of administration. The active drug needs to enter the target cells to exert its therapeutic effect. During this process, however, a number of hurdles need to be overcome. The first step in this process involves dissolution of the active agent in aqueous media (**Figure 1-1**, step A). As previously mentioned, one of the major concerns with newly developed as well as many of the existing drugs is their poor aqueous solubility. It is estimated that up to 90% of novel drug development candidates potentially display poor aqueous solubility and are classified as class II or class IV compounds based on the Biopharmaceutics Classification System [13]. Several of these compounds have solubilities in the range of 1–10 μg/mL. Such low solubility often poses significant challenges for pharmaceutical formulators and scientists to develop dosage forms that allow sufficient absorption and improved bioavailability. A drug delivery scientist can enhance the solubility of hydrophobic drugs by fabrication of nanoparticles and nanomicelles and prodrug strategies. For example, the solubility and stability of macromolecules such as proteins can be enhanced by PEGylation and microencapsulation approaches while retaining their bioactivity.

The second step in this process is to facilitate the availability of drug at the target site (Figure 1-1, step B). Once a compound is in solution, it may be delivered throughout the body. Often, the drug is required only at the physiological site of action, and hence this extensive biodistribution may cause toxicity and unwanted side effects. Active targeting strategies, therefore, direct the drug to act only at the intended target site, thereby minimizing side effects.

The last step in this process is drug uptake by cells (Figure 1-1, step C). This step plays a very crucial role in gene delivery, which can only be successful when genes are delivered at the target site and effectively enter the target cells for expression. For most therapeutics, the ultimate bioactivity is achieved only after the active molecules are taken up by cells. Each of these steps is associated with challenges at every stage.

The drug delivery technology landscape is greatly competitive and rapidly progressing. New classes of pharmaceuticals and biologics (peptides, proteins, RNA, and DNA-based therapeutics) are stimulating the rapid advancement in drug delivery technology. These new drugs typically cannot be efficiently delivered by conventional means. Controlled and sustained delivery technologies are warranted to improve drug efficacy and reduce side effects. In addition to these technologies, targetability and localized delivery would drive any system to advance from bench to bedside. Most often, delivery devices and drugs are tightly coupled. Biotech and pharmaceutical companies all over the world are currently engaged in increasing the value their combinations of drugs and delivery devices and/or systems can gain in the marketplace. Because drug development can be a very long process, advanced development and technology portfolio plans must be related to current market requirements and value propositions over a decade or more into the future.

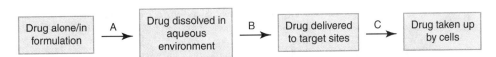

FIGURE 1-1 Fate of a drug in the body.

REVIEW QUESTIONS

1. No drug can be commercially viable unless it meets the minimum criteria of
   a. Optimum therapeutic efficacy
   b. Good safety profile (sufficient therapeutic window)
   c. Minimal adverse effects
   d. All of the above
2. The main goal of DMPK studies is to predict the _____ of the drug candidate in humans.
   a. Absorption
   b. Distribution
   c. Metabolism
   d. Excretion
   e. All of the above
3. The overall levels achieved by a drug in the body are *not* decided by which of the following factors?
   a. Site of administration
   b. Color of the formulation
   c. Complexity of the formulation
   d. Total body clearance
4. The salt form of the molecule can play a critical role in deciding the _____ of the drug.
   a. Solubility
   b. Dissolution rate
   c. Stability
   d. Bioavailability
   e. All of the above
5. Which of the following is the most common and convenient dosage form for most drugs?
   a. Intravenous
   b. Oral
   c. Topical
   d. Nasal spray
6. An ideal *in vivo* model should have all the _____ complexities of human systems.
   a. Biochemical
   b. Cellular
   c. Physiological
   d. Psychological
   e. a, b, and c
   f. All of the above

REFERENCES

1. Han C, Wang B. Factors that impact the developability of drug candidates: an overview. In: B Wang, TJ Siahaan, RA Soltero, eds. *Drug Delivery: Principles and Applications.* New York, NY: John Wiley & Sons; 2005:1–14.
2. Prentis RA, Lis Y, Walker SR. Pharmaceutical innovation by the seven UK-owned pharmaceutical companies (1964–1985). *Br J Clin Pharmacol.* 1988;25(3):387–396.
3. Mahmood I. Interspecies scaling: predicting oral clearance in humans. *Am J Ther.* 2002;9(1):35–42.

4. Mahmood I, Balian JD. The pharmacokinetic principles behind scaling from preclinical results to phase I protocols. *Clin Pharmacokinet.* 1999;36(1):1–11.

5. Woodnutt G. Pharmacodynamics to combat resistance. *J Antimicrob Chemother.* 2000;46(Suppl T1):25–31.

6. Bodor N, Buchwald P. Soft drug design: general principles and recent applications. *Med Res Rev.* 2000;20(1):58–101.

7. Lin JH. Sense and nonsense in the prediction of drug-drug interactions. *Curr Drug Metab.* 2000;1(4):305–331.

8. Rodrigues AD, Lin JH. Screening of drug candidates for their drug–drug interaction potential. *Curr Opin Chem Biol.* 2001;5(4):396–401.

9. Van Asperen J, Van Tellingen O, Beijnen JH. The pharmacological role of P-glycoprotein in the intestinal epithelium. *Pharmacol Res.* 1998;37(6):429–435.

10. Wacher VJ, Salphati L, Benet LZ. Active secretion and enterocytic drug metabolism barriers to drug absorption. *Adv Drug Deliv Rev.* 2001;46(1–3):89–102.

11. Tawara S, Matsumoto S, Kamimura T, Goto S. Effect of protein binding in serum on therapeutic efficacy of cephem antibiotics. *Antimicrob Agents Chemother.* 1992;36(1):17–24.

12. Morris KR, Fakes MG, Thakur AB, et al. An integrated approach to the selection of optimal salt form for a new drug candidate. *Int J Pharm.* 1994;105(3):209–217.

13. Dahan A, Miller JM, Amidon GL. Prediction of solubility and permeability class membership: provisional BCS classification of the world's top oral drugs. *AAPS J.* 2009;11(4):740–746.

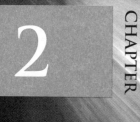

CHAPTER

2

© Taewoon Lee/ShutterStock, Inc.

BARRIERS TO DRUG DELIVERY

SUJAY J. SHAH, RAMYA KRISHNA VADLAPATLA,
AND ASHIM K. MITRA

CHAPTER OBJECTIVES

Upon completing this chapter, the reader should be able to

▸ Recognize the challenges faced by drug delivery scientists.

▸ Understand how the various types of barriers present in the human body will help understand the limitations encountered when developing a drug or its dosage form.

▸ Discuss strategies that can help overcome barriers and result in efficient delivery of drug molecules to the therapeutic site of action.

CHAPTER OUTLINE

Introduction

Physiological Barriers to Drug Delivery

    Paracellular Pathway

    Transcellular Pathway

INTRODUCTION

For decades scientists have been developing new drugs to treat various diseases, successfully bringing to the marketplace many highly potent drugs. Although these drugs are very potent, it sometimes becomes difficult to deliver the active agent to the site of action. Also, recent development of new biological products has brought newer challenges in the field of drug delivery. These challenges can be attributed to physiochemical properties of active molecules and the various barriers imposed by the body [1]. In this chapter we mainly focus on the different barriers a drug must overcome to reach its site of action at the required dose.

The human body possesses many external and internal barriers to protect itself from the environment and from substances administered by different routes. The skin is the largest barrier to topical drug delivery, whereas the epithelial layer of the gastrointestinal tract barricades the entry of drugs given orally. The blood–brain barrier (BBB) is the tightest barrier that prevents entry of drugs from the bloodstream into the central nervous system. Even when administered via the parenteral route, drugs still need to overcome many barriers, either in blood or at the site of action.

Several barriers need to be traversed to achieve therapeutic drugs concentrations at the desired site. These barriers can be categorized as physiological, biochemical, and chemical in nature. The intestinal mucosa, BBB, and the skin represent the most formidable physiological barriers. These structures inhibit entry of active medical agents, toxins, and various substances. The drugs must also overcome the biochemical barrier posed by degradation and elimination via metabolizing enzymes present in the body. Finally, it is very important for a drug to have optimum physiochemical properties to permeate across the biological barriers.

PHYSIOLOGICAL BARRIERS TO DRUG DELIVERY

Drug delivery to the desired site of action is very crucial for proper therapy. For a drug to exert its therapeutic effect, it may be crucial to cross the most important barrier—the physiological barrier. Physiological barriers may consist of a single or multiple layers of cells that control the movement of nutrients, electrolytes, and water while preventing the entry of microorganisms, toxins, and antigens. Such movement across the cellular layers is mainly through two pathways, paracellular and transcellular. The paracellular pathway controls the permeation of substances in between cells, whereas the transcellular pathway controls molecular movement through the cells (Figure 2-1). The four main physiological barriers are the intestinal epithelium, BBB, blood–ocular barrier, and skin.

PARACELLULAR PATHWAY

Drug permeation via the paracellular path represents passive transport through the spaces between the epithelial cells from the apical side to the basolateral side. This pathway allows passage of small hydrophilic molecules and is regulated by intercellular junctional complexes. The contact between epithelial cells is facilitated by three different intercellular complexes, the tight junctions, adherens junctions, and desmosomes (Figure 2-2). Tight junctions are mainly responsible for regulating paracellular transport, whereas the main roles of adherens junctions and desmosomes are to form the mechanical linkage between epithelial cells.

The tight junction is also known as *zonula occludens* and is located at the most apical portion of the epithelial cell. The name *zonula occludens* is derived from the Latin word "closing belt," which describes the functional property of this region [2]. The tight junctions span or circumscribe the cells, forming a barrier against the free movement

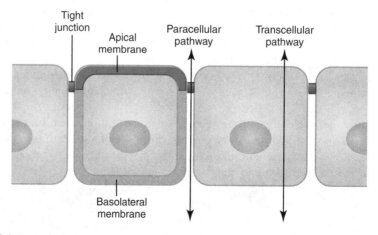

FIGURE 2-1 Paracellular and transcellular pathways.

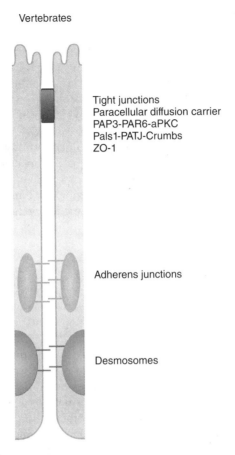

Vertebrates

Tight junctions
Paracellular diffusion carrier
PAP3-PAR6-aPKC
Pals1-PATJ-Crumbs
ZO-1

Adherens junctions

Desmosomes

FIGURE 2-2 Tight junctions.

of molecules across this layer [3]. Detailed microscopic images have revealed that tight junctions consist of a net-like array of branching fibrils. These junctions impart cell surface its polarity and control drug movement from the apical to the basolateral side. The rate and extent of permeation via paracellular pathway depends on the pore size of the tight junctions. Studies have shown that calcium plays a major role in the integrity of tight junctions. If cells are low in calcium, the tight junctions may rearrange the proteins, resulting in loss of structural integrity [4, 5]. Two other important proteins involved in tight junctions are occludin and claudin, which are responsible for the "gate" and "fence" functions. These proteins express seven domains: two extracellular, which form loops; four transmembrane, and a cytoplasmic carboxyl tail. Cell-to-cell contact is created by the extracellular domains. Three scaffolding proteins are associated with tight junctions: ZO-1, ZO-2, and ZO-3. ZO-1 is mainly responsible for interaction with occludin and claudin, thereby stabilizing junctions and cross-linking to the actin cytoskeleton [6].

Adherens junctions, also known as *zonula adherens*, are located immediately below the tight junctions and are responsible for cell–cell adhesion. Previous studies have shown that adherens junctions develop before tight junctions in this region [7]. Both of these structures work in tandem to build up the resistance across this pathway [8]. Resistance is represented as reciprocal of permeability and depends on size and charge in the paracellular pores [9]. Resistance buildup is directly proportional to the number of tight junctional strands. Within this region is the perijunctional actin–myosin II protein, which forms a ring around the epithelial cells. This ring is responsible for the permeation of solutes [8]. The main function of the adherens junction is cell–cell adhesion, which is controlled by E-cadherin, a 120-kDa glycoprotein consisting of one domain each in the extracellular, transmembrane, and cytoplasmic regions. E-cadherins are also calcium dependent and interact in a homotypic manner. The exact mechanism of E-cadherins between cells is not known. The cytoplasmic domain is also necessary for the adhesion process, and it interacts with α- and β-catenins, which form a linkage with the actin cytoskeleton [10, 11].

Desmosomes form the end region of the paracellular pathway and are located toward the basolateral side of epithelial cells [12]. They are connected to the intermediate filaments by desmoplakins. The protein known as desmoglein, a desmosomal cadherin, is responsible for the linkage between desmoplakins and the intermediate filaments [12]. Desmosomes play a less critical role in the barrier function of the paracellular pathway as compared with the other two regions.

TRANSCELLULAR PATHWAY

Movement of molecules through the lipid-rich nonporous section is known as the transcellular pathway. Passive diffusion allows the transport of molecules with appropriate physiochemical properties, primarily lipophilicity. However, hydrophilic drugs, especially large macromolecules like peptides, proteins, DNA, RNA, and their segments, have unfavorable properties to permeate through the cell membrane via the transcellular pathway. Lipid bilayers mainly consist of four regions: (1) the outermost region, mainly consisting of water molecules, responsible for interactions with other proteins and membranes; (2) polar headgroups, forming the most dense region of the bilayers, which make this region the most difficult for diffusion; (3) the nonpolar tails, responsible for limiting permeation of therapeutic agents having only a specific molecular size and shape; and (4) the innermost region, which is the most hydrophobic in nature and acts as the hydrophobic barrier [13]. Together, the apical and basolateral membranes form the rate-limiting barriers to passive diffusion of permeants [8]. Even if the drug traverses across the membrane into the cytosol, it has to overcome the metabolizing enzymes and efflux pumps, which form the biochemical barriers.

BLOOD–BRAIN BARRIER

The BBB is a protective mechanism that controls cerebral homeostasis and provides the central nervous system with unique protection against bloodborne pathogens, toxins, and chemicals [14]. It forms a complex physiological checkpoint that limits the distribution of molecules between the blood and the central nervous system [15]. The BBB prevents 98% of small molecules and 100% of large molecules from reaching the brain. It is located at the level of the capillaries between the blood and cerebral tissue and is characterized by the presence of tight intracellular junctions and polarized expression of many transport systems [16]. The BBB is located at the choroid plexus epithelium, which controls the exchange of molecules between the blood and cerebrospinal fluid.

The endothelial cells of the brain differ slightly from other tissues in that the cells lack fenestrations and express very tight junctions. These cells express membrane transporters and receptors responsible for active transport of nutrients to the brain and excretion of potentially toxic compounds from the cerebral and vascular compartments. The brain endothelium in mammals controls permeability of compounds and ions and expresses high transendothelial electrical resistance [16]. Dysfunction of the BBB causes many neurological disorders. The volume occupied by the capillaries and endothelial cells is about 1% of the total brain volume, and, as a result, the brain microvasculature has a total surface area of approximately 20 m². This highly vascularized network means that every brain cell is located approximately 20 nm from a capillary, which may allow for rapid diffusion of small molecules delivered to the brain. This possibility, however, is limited by the physiological characteristics of the BBB [16].

Astrocytes form the structural frame work of neurons and can control their biochemical environment. Astrocytes have foot processes or limbs that spread out and abut one another, encapsulating the capillaries closely associated with the blood vessels to form the BBB. Oligodendrocytes are responsible for the formation and maintenance of the myelin sheath, which surrounds axons and is essential for rapid transmission of action potentials by salutatory conduction. Microglias are mononuclear macrophages derived from the blood (Figure 2-3). The tight junctions between endothelial cells impart a very high transendothelial electrical resistance of 1500 to 2000 Ω.cm² compared with 3 to 33 Ω.cm² for other tissues. Because of this high transendothelial electrical resistance value, the aqueous pore–based paracellular diffusion in the brain is lower relative to other organs [17].

Microvessels make up an estimated 95% of the total surface area of the BBB and represent the principal route by which molecules are transferred to the brain. Compared with other organs, brain vessels are smaller in diameter and possess thinner walls. Also, the mitochondrial density in brain microvessels is higher than other capillaries, not because of more numerous or larger mitochondria but due to small dimensions of the brain microvessels and, consequently, smaller cytoplasmic area. Intercellular cleft, pinocytosis, and fenestrae are virtually nonexistent in brain capillaries. Therefore, only lipid-soluble solutes can freely diffuse through the capillary endothelial membrane.

TRANSDERMAL BARRIER

Skin, the largest organ system of the human body, performs multiple roles, ranging from protection, sensation, thermoregulation, and storage to absorption and water resistance. The transdermal form of delivery is the most successful non-oral systemic drug delivery system. The current market for transdermal medications amounts up to US$2 billion. Although there is a high demand for this route of drug delivery, very few drugs have

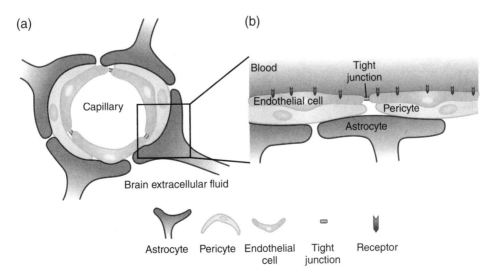

FIGURE 2-3 The blood–brain barrier.

been approved by the U.S. Food and Drug Administration to be used transdermally [18]. This can be attributed to the limitations and challenges encountered when developing a transdermal drug delivery system.

The skin has an extremely complex architecture that varies depending on the body location. The three distinct regions of the skin are the epidermis, the outermost layer, followed by the dermis and hypodermis. Remarkably, only the outermost few microns of the skin are responsible for the skin's barrier function. The stratum corneum (SC) is a compositionally and morphologically unique biomembrane. It is extremely thin (approximately one hundredth of a millimeter), the least permeable of skin layers, and the ultimate stage in the epidermal differentiation process, forming a laminate of compressed keratin-filled corneocytes (terminally differentiated keratinocytes) anchored in a lipophilic matrix. The lipids of this extracellular matrix are distinctive in many aspects: (1) this phase provides the only continuous milieu (and diffusion pathway) from the skin surface to the base of the SC; (2) the composition (ceramides, free fatty acids, and cholesterol) is unique among biomembranes and particularly noteworthy is the absence of phospholipids; (3) despite this deficit of polar bilayer–forming lipids, the SC lipids exist as multilamellar lipid-enriched extracellular matrix sheets; and (4) the predominantly saturated, long-chain hydrocarbon tails facilitate a highly ordered, interdigitated configuration and the formation of gel-phase membrane domains as opposed to the more usual (and more fluid and permeable) liquid crystalline membrane systems [19, 20]. It seems, however, that the unusual lipid matrix alone cannot explain the high resistivity of the membrane: SC architecture as a whole appears to function as a barrier for the membrane. Hence, the staggered corneocyte arrangement in a lipid continuum (similar to a brick and mortar assembly) appears to provide a highly tortuous lipoidal diffusion pathway, rendering the membrane at least a thousand times less permeable to water relative to other biomembranes.

The second layer beneath the epidermal layer is the dermis, which is much thicker than the epidermis (usually 1–4 mm). The main components of the dermis are collagen and elastic fibers. Compared with the epidermis, fewer cells and more fibers are visible in the dermis (Figure 2-4) [21]. The three major routes for the transport of molecules through the epidermis are appendageal, transcellular, and intercellular.

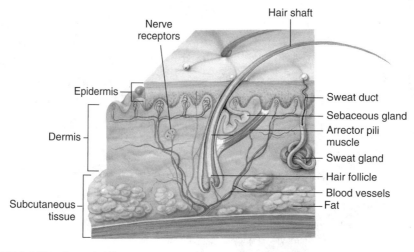

FIGURE 2-4 Structure of skin.

Appendageal transport uses hair follicles and sweat glands. Because these are breaks in the SC, they serve as a pathway for the drug molecules. Although hair follicles and sweat glands account for only 0.1% of the total skin surface, they are an important route for percutaneous absorption. For example, charged drug molecules can be internalized via hair follicles, and the flux is dramatically increased with the use of iontophoresis. The transcellular pathway consists of movement of molecules across the epithelial cells. Low-molecular-weight and lipophilic compounds can traverse across epithelial cells via passive diffusion. Hydrophobicity and molecular volume are the main properties that determine its permeability and the rate of diffusion correlates with the lipid solubility of the molecule. Finally, drugs can travel between cells via intercellular passages or channels. Intercellular lipid forms an important component of the skin barrier and is the only continuous domain in the SC [18].

BIOCHEMICAL BARRIERS TO DRUG DELIVERY

Research over the past two decades has emphasized the importance of biochemical barriers in the field of drug delivery. Apart from physicochemical barriers (i.e., stability, solubility, lipophilicity, molecular weight and size), poor bioavailability of many molecules can be attributed to the presence of biochemical barriers, including efflux pumps and metabolizing enzymes. Therapeutic efficacy of many active molecules depends largely on their ability to overcome these barriers to reach their target [22]. Here we mainly focus on the ATP-binding cassette (ABC) proteins, which play a predominant role in affecting drug transport, drug disposition, and resistance. Further emphasis is placed on the metabolizing enzymes, especially CYP3A4 (as it accounts for 50%–70% of metabolism) and its role in drug delivery.

ABC TRANSPORTERS

The ABC family includes a superfamily of membrane bound proteins involved in the translocation of various substances, including sugars, amino acids, sterols, peptides, proteins, antibiotics, toxins, and xenobiotics, in both prokaryotes and eukaryotes [23–25]. These transporters use the energy derived from hydrolysis of ATP to translocate substances across concentration gradients [26]. The human genome encodes 48 different ABC transporters, phylogenetically categorized into seven different classes (ABCA–ABCG) [27]. Fifteen different transporters have been identified to play a role in the development of multidrug resistance (MDR) [28, 29]. These transporters are usually unidirectional as opposed to several bidirectional transporters [30]. All ABC proteins function either as a single polypeptide chain or in association with homodimeric (equal) or heterodimeric (unequal) chains [31, 32]. The most important ABC transporters are P-glycoprotein (P-gp/MDR1), multidrug resistant proteins (MRPs), and breast cancer resistant protein (BCRP).

ABC transporters show at least 25% structural homology. The regions of conserved sequence motifs are the Walker A region (P-loop), Walker B region, signature C motif (LSGGQ motif), glutamine loop (Q-loop), histidine loop (H-loop), and D-loop [27, 33, 34]. Walker A and B regions help in nucleotide binding. Further, Walker A binds ATP and Walker B initiates ATP hydrolysis. The 90–120 amino acids linker between Walker A and B regions, termed as signature motif, aids in communicating transmembrane domains (TMDs) [35]. The Q- and H-loops assist in ATP hydrolysis, whereas the D-loop assists in communicating the catalytic sites [36–38].

P-GLYCOPROTEIN (P-GP/MDR1/ABCB1)

MDR1 was the first characterized ABC transporter. In 1976, Juliano and Ling [40] identified the presence of a 170-kDa protein in colchicine-resistant Chinese hamster ovary (CHO) cells. These cells also displayed cross-resistance to several amphiphilic drugs. Surface labeling studies and selective proteolysis revealed the presence of this surface glycoprotein. This protein altered the permeation of several compounds across cell membranes. Hence, the protein was designated as P-glycoprotein (in which "P" means permeability). Further work has revealed that the amount of glycoprotein present correlates with the degree of drug resistance. A similar cellular resistance phenomenon was described in 1970 by Biedler and Riehm [41]. in actinomycin resistant CHO cells. The entire structure of MDR1 was subsequently characterized by cloning and sequencing studies [42–45].

Structure

MDR1 functions as a single polypeptide transporter, consisting of two identical halves connected by the signature C motif. Each half consists of six TMDs and one nucleotide binding domain. The *MDR1* gene contains 28 exons encoding for a total of 1,280 amino acids.

Structural–Activity Relationship

TMDs 5 and 6 and 11 and 12 play a vital role in recognizing and binding the substrates. A conclusive structural–activity relationship to predict interaction of various compounds with MDR1 is not available. However, a general pattern for substrate recognition has been developed by studying the binding pattern of more than 100 known substrates [46]. A well-defined pattern of recognition elements (electron donor groups) are essential for substrate binding. These recognition elements are categorized into two types: type I and type II. Type I units exhibit two electron donor groups with a spatial separation of 2.5 ± 0.3 Å, whereas type II units show two or three electron donor groups with a spatial separation of 4.6 ± 0.6 Å. According to the strength and number of electron donor groups or hydrogen bonding acceptor groups, molecules may be classified as nonsubstrate, weak substrate, or strong substrate.

Role in Drug Delivery

Overexpression of MDR1 is implicated as one of the major mechanisms leading to the development of MDR. Accordingly, its expression has been reported in many tumor cells, including leukemia, breast, ovarian, pancreatic, gastric, and many other cancers [47–52]. Also, MDR1 is extensively localized on the apical membranes of enterocytes, brain capillary endothelial cells, brush border surface of proximal tubules, and adrenal cortex. Moderate expression is also noticed in hepatocytes, spleen, and lung, whereas prostate, ovary, and skin exhibit low expression of MDR1 [53–56]. A partial list of drug molecules effluxed by MDR1 is given in **Table 2-1**. MDR1 exhibits broad substrate specificity and is involved in effluxing many pharmacological agents such as anticancer agents, antivirals, antibiotics, steroids, immunosuppressive agents, and calcium channel blockers.

MULTIDRUG RESISTANT PROTEINS (MRPs/ABCC)

The largest branch of the ABC transporters is the ABCC subfamily. It contains 13 different proteins, including energy dependent transporters (MRP1–6/ABCC1–6, MRP7–10 /ABCC10–13), cystic fibrosis transmembrane conductance regulator (CFTR/ABCC7),

TABLE 2-1 Partial list of drug molecules effluxed by MDR (drugs that interact with MRP1)

Drugs that interact with MRP1	
Steroid molecules	Anticancer drugs
Aldosterone	Anthracenes (bisantrene)
Corticosterone	Anthracyclines (daunorubicin and doxorubicin)
Cortisol	Camptothecins (topotecan)
Dexamethasone	Epipodophyllotoxins (etoposide and teniposide)
Hydrocortisone	Taxanes (docetaxel and paclitaxel)
Progesterone	Vinca alkaloids (vinblastine and vincristine)
Protease inhibitors	Antibiotics
Indinavir	Erythromycin
Nelfinavir	Gatifloxacin
Ritonavir	Grepafloxacin
Saquinavir	Rifampin
Antihistamines	Cardiac drugs
Domperidone	Amiodarone
Fexofenadine	Digoxin
Terfenadine	Propafenone
	Quinidine
Immunosuppressive agents	3-Hydroxy-3-methylglutaryl-coenzyme A reductase inhibitors
Cyclosporine	Lovastatin
Tacrolimus (FK-506)	Simvastatin
Antihypertensive agents	Calcium channel blockers
Propanolol	Nifedipine
Reserpine	Verapamil

and sulfonylurea receptors (SUR1/ABCC8 and SUR2/ABCC9) [27, 57–59]. The founding member of the ABCC family, MRP1, was first identified by Cole et al. [60] in 1992 from doxorubicin-treated lung cancer cells (H69AR). Four years later, the second member of the ABCC family was identified. MRP2 was initially referred to as a canalicular, multispecific organic anion transporter because of its ability to transport bilirubin glucuronide in mutant rats [61, 62]. All the MRPs, except for MRP10, are ubiquitously expressed in plants, marine organisms, and several eukaryotes performing various physiological functions. The newly identified protein MRP10 encodes a functional protein only in rhesus monkey, whereas in other species it is truncated and not functionally active [63].

Structure

Computer-assisted hydropathy analyses and multiple sequence alignments studies predicted the topological structure models of MRPs (Figure 2-5). The nine functional MRPs (i.e., 1–9) were categorized into two classes based on the number of TMDs. MRPs 4, 5, 8, and 9 belong to short MRP transporters, whereas MRPs 1, 2, 3, 6, and 7 belong to the long transporters. Short MRPs resemble MDR1 with respect to structure, exhibiting 12 TMDs and 2 nucleotide-binding domains. The long transporters exhibit an additional N-terminal hydrophobic membrane spanning domain, with five TMDs of approximately 220 amino acids [64–66]. A brief overview of the genomic properties of MRPs and their localization in polarized cells is summarized in Table 2-2.

MRP4, -5, -8, -9

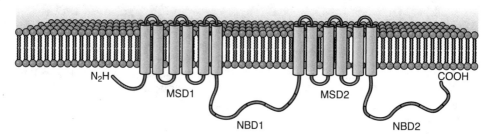

MRP1, -2, -3, -6, -7

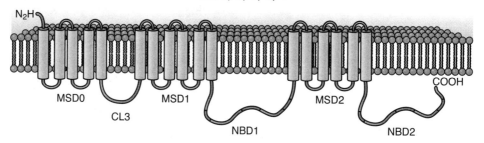

FIGURE 2-5 Predicted two-dimensional structural model of (top) MRP1 (resembling MRP2, MRP3, MRP6, and MRP7) and (bottom) MRP4 (resembling MRP5, MRP8 and MRP9) (bottom). (Data from Lage H, Dietel M. Effect of the breast-cancer resistance protein on atypical multidrug resistance. *Lancet Oncol.* Nov 2000;1:169–175.)

TABLE 2-2 Summary of structural properties and localization of MRPs 1–9

Protein	Gene Symbol	Short/ Long	Chromosomal Location	Transcript Length	Amino Acids	Localization in Polarized Cells
MRP1	ABCC1	Long	16p13.12	5927 bp	1531	Basolateral
MRP2	ABCC2 / cMOAT	Long	10q24.2	4930 bp	1545	Apical
MRP3	ABCC3 / MOAT-D	Long	17q21.33	5176 bp	1527	Basolateral
MRP4	ABCC4 / MOAT-B	Short	13q32.1	5871 bp	1325	Apical and basolateral
MRP5	ABCC5 / MOAT-C	Short	3q27.l	5851 bp	1437	Basolateral
MRP6	ABCC6 / MOAT-K	Long	16p13.12	5111 bp	1503	Basolateral
MRP7	ABCC10	Long	6p21.1	5118 bp	1492	?
MRP8	ABCC11	Short	16q12.1	4576 bp	1382	Apical and basolateral
MRP9	ABCC12	Short	16q12.1	5168 bp	1356	?

cMOAT, canalicular multispecific organic anion transporter.

Role in Drug Delivery

MRP1 is localized on the basolateral membrane of the intestine, brain, liver, and kidney, whereas MRP2 is localized on the apical membrane of the intestine, liver, kidney, and placenta [68–72]. MRP1 plays a predominant role in regulating xenobiotic detoxification, because it can transport glutathione and glucuronide conjugates. MRP2 can also regulate the transport of glutathione and glucuronide conjugates, but with relatively low affinity [73, 74]. MRP2 is functionally similar to MDR1 in terms of functionality and development of MDR [75, 76]. MRP2 also regulates hepatobiliary secretion of various drug molecules [77]. A partial list of molecules transported by both MRP1 and MRP2 is summarized in Table 2-3.

TABLE 2-3 Partial list of drug molecules effluxed by MRP1 and MRP2

Drugs That Interact With MRP1	
Protease inhibitors Ritonavir Saquinavir	Anticancer drugs Anthracyclines (doxorubicin and daunorubicin) Antifolates (methotrexate) Camptothecins (irinotecan and topotecan) Epipodophyllotoxins (etoposide and teniposide) Vinca alkaloids (vinblastine and vincristine)
Antibiotics Difloxacin Gatifloxacin Grepafloxacin	Glutathione conjugates Glutathione Leukotrienes
Glucuronide conjugates Bilirubin glucuronide Estradiol glucuronide	Tyrosine kinase inhibitors Imatinib Gefitinib
Drugs That Interact With MRP2	
Protease inhibitors Indinavir Ritonavir Saquinavir	Anticancer drugs Anthracyclines (doxorubicin) Antifolates (methotrexate) Camptothecins (irinotecan) Epipodophyllotoxins (etoposide) Vinca alkaloids (vinblastine and vincristine)
Antibiotics Erythromycin Gatifloxacin Grepafloxacin	3-Hydroxy-3-methylglutaryl-coenzyme A reductase inhibitors Pravastatin
Glutathione conjugates Glutathione Leukotrienes Oxidized glutathione N-ethylmaleimide-glutathione	Glucuronide conjugates Bilirubin glucuronide Estradiol glucuronide Ethinylestradiol-3-O-glucuronide

BREAST CANCER RESISTANT PROTEIN (BCRP/ABCG2)

BCRP is a recently identified ABC efflux transporter that plays a predominant role in acquisition of MDR [78, 79]. It was first identified in drug resistant human breast cancer cells (MCF-7/AdrVp) [80]. Although these cells lacked the existence of MDR1 and MRP1 proteins, they still conferred resistance to mitoxantrone, doxorubicin, and daunorubicin. This observation led to the identification of a new xenobiotic transporter, termed BCRP. A cDNA identical to BCRP was also cloned from human placental tissues and mitoxantrone resistant human colon carcinoma cells. Hence, this protein is also referred to as ABC-placenta and mitoxantrone resistant transporter [81, 82]. It phenotypically belongs to the G subfamily of ABC proteins. It is also designated as ABCG2 because it is the second member of the family.

Structure

A 2.4-kb messenger RNA encodes for a 75-kDa transporter. Computer-assisted topology models have predicted the structure of BCRP (**Figure 2-6**) [83, 84]. The transporter consists of a single nucleotide binding domain (residues 1–395) and a single membrane-spanning domain (residues 396–655) consisting of six TMDs [46, 80–82]. Thus, it is recognized as a half ABC transporter. To meet the functional requirement of an active ABC transporter, however, it functions as a homodimer [85–87].

Role in Drug Delivery

BCRP is highly expressed on apical membranes of small intestine, colon, placenta, bile canaliculi, colon, liver, and brain capillary endothelial cells [89–91]. It causes MDR in a variety of cancers including colon, lung, endometrial and esophageal cancers [92–94]. A partial list of drug molecules effluxed by BCRP is given in **Table 2-4**.

METABOLIZING ENZYMES

Detoxification mechanisms play a predominant role in lowering potential damage after exposure to various xenobiotics. This detoxification in the form of metabolism is broadly divided into phases I and II. Almost 70% of pharmaceuticals are metabolized by phase I enzymes, whereas remaining 30% are metabolized by phase II enzymes [95–99]. The phase I system usually involves oxidation, reduction, and hydrolysis and produces a reactive intermediate (metabolite). These metabolites are usually less active or inactive. Occasionally however, biologically more active metabolites may also be produced. These hydrophilic metabolites can be directly excreted and/or undergo phase II metabolism to produce a more soluble nontoxic conjugate via coupling with glucuronic acid, sulfuric acid, or amino acids and excreted [100–103].

CYTOCHROME P450

Cytochromes (CYPs) are heme-containing proteins that exhibit a single iron protoporphyrin IX prosthetic group. These metabolizing enzymes were first identified by their ability to bind oxygen and carbon monoxide. CYPs were named after the absorption maximum of 450 nm when bound to carbon monoxide. CYPs can catalyze oxidation, reduction, hydroxylation, and dealkylation reactions. Based on amino acid sequence homology, the superfamily of CYP enzymes is classified into families, subfamilies, and isoforms [104–106]. The human genome encodes for 18 families and

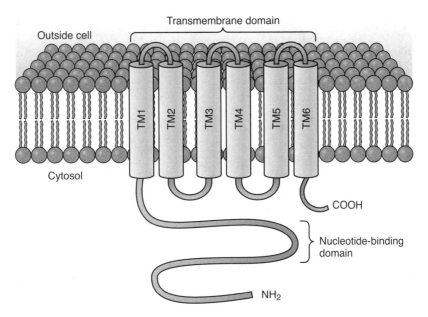

FIGURE 2-6 Predicted two-dimensional structural model of BCRP. (Data from Zaman GJ, Flens MJ, van Leusden MR, et al. The human multidrug resistance-associated protein MRP is a plasma membrane drug-efflux pump. *Proc Natl Acad Sci U S A*. Sep 13 1994;91[19]:8822–8826.)

TABLE 2-4 Partial list of drug molecules effluxed by BCRP	
3-Hydroxy-3-methylglutaryl-coenzyme A reductase inhibitors Cerivastatin Pravastatin Rosuvastatin	Anticancer drugs Anthracenes (bisantrene) Anthracyclines (daunorubicin and doxorubicin) Antifolates (methotrexate) Camptothecins (irinotecan and topotecan) Epipodophyllotoxins (etoposide and teniposide)
Tyrosine kinase inhibitors Imatinib Gefitinib	Antibiotics Ciprofloxacin Norfloxacin
Antiviral drugs Lamivudine Zidovudine	Flavonoids Genestein Quercetin

43 subfamilies of CYP genes. However, only three families, CYP1, CYP2, and CYP3, are responsible for xenobiotic metabolism in humans [107–109]. The major isoenzymes include CYP1A1, 1A2, 2A6, 2B6, 2C8, 2C9, 2C19, 2D6, 2E1, 3A4, and 3A5 [110].

Structure

This family of enzymes is the most predominant drug metabolizing enzymes representing almost 30% of hepatic CYP and 70% of intestinal CYP. Further, this family accounts for 50% to 70% of the total contribution in drug metabolism [111]. CYP3A4 is the major member of this family. A polymorphic isoform, CYP3A5 also plays a dominant role in drug metabolism. CYP enzyme is a macrocyclic porphyrin molecule with a centrally bound iron ion. The porphyrin molecule consists of four pyrrole rings connected by carbon bonds, and the pyrrolic nitrogen atoms are oriented toward the center, facilitating binding of metal ions. The heme center of CYP enzymes allows for activation and utilization of oxygen. In a monooxygenation reaction, CYP uses molecular oxygen to oxidize a substrate, whereas the other is reduced to water molecule, using electrons provided by NADPH (nicotinamide adenine dinucleotide phosphate) [112]. The basic monooxygenation reaction catalyzed by P450s is described as $R + O_2 + NADPH + H^+ = ROH + H_2O + NADP^+$.

Role in Drug Delivery

The CYP enzymes are expressed throughout the body, mainly in the liver and also in small intestine, kidneys, colon, lungs, brain, skin, and placenta [113–116]. A partial list of drug molecules metabolized by 3A4 and 3A5 is given in Table 2–5. Drugs may interact with these enzymes either as substrate or inhibitor. After chronic exposure, most substrates and inhibitors can also cause transcriptional induction.

TABLE 2-5 Partial list of drug molecules metabolized by CYP3A4

Substrates of CYP3A4 and 3A5	
HIV protease inhibitors Indinavir Lopinavir Saquinavir	Calcium channel blockers Diltiazem Felodopine Nifedipine Verapamil
Benzodiazepine Alprazolam Midazolam Triazolam	Opioid analgesic (anesthesia) Alfentanil Fentanyl Sufentanil
Antipsychotic Haloperidol Pimozide	Antitussive Codeine Dextromethorphan
Immunosuppressive agents Cyclosporin Tacrolimus (FK-506)	Steroid molecules Dexamethasone Hydrocortisone
Local anaesthetics Lignocaine Ropivacaine	Antihistamines Terfenadine Astemizole
Proton pump inhibitors Lansoprazole	Antifungals Ketoconazole
Methylxanthine Theophylline	Antibiotics Erythromycin
3-Hydroxy-3-methylglutaryl-coenzyme A reductase inhibitors Lovastatin	Anticancer drugs Taxanes (paclitaxel)
Antiemetics Granisetron	Steroid hormones Testosterone

CHEMICAL BARRIERS

The chemical structure of a compound determines its solubility and permeability profiles. In turn, the concentration at the intestinal lumen and the permeability profile of an agent are responsible for the rate and extent of absorption across the intestinal mucosa [117]. Unfavorable physiochemical properties have been a limiting factor in the absorption of small molecules and macromolecule drugs [118]. Size, structure, state, and hydrogen bonding potential are some of the properties that influence absorption of a molecule.

HYDROGEN-BINDING POTENTIAL

An important factor in the permeation of peptides and macromolecules is hydrogen-bonding potential. Studies in many *in vivo* and *in vitro* models of BBB and intestinal mucosa have shown that desolvation or hydrogen-binding potential regulates the permeation of peptides across the membranes [117, 119]. The energy needed to desolvate the polar amide bonds to allow permeation and translocation across the cell membrane is the principle behind hydrogen-bonding potential. For small molecules, the octanol-water coefficient is the best predictor of permeability with a sigmoidal relationship [119]. This is not the case with peptides; desolvation energy or hydrogen-bonding potential is a better predictor for membrane permeability of peptides.

OTHER PROPERTIES

Several other properties are also important in determining permeability via the paracellular pathway. Size, charge, and hydrophilicity play vital roles [118]. A change in the hydrophilicity may change the route by which a drug predominantly permeates across membranes. If the hydrophilicity decreases or, conversely, the lipophilicity increases, it may cause the permeant to use the transcellular route instead of the paracellular pathway. Studies have shown that permeation via the paracellular pathway is size-dependent because of the presence of tight junctions. Molecules greater than 22 Å in diameter are unable to cross the tight junctions readily [118].

STRATEGIES TO OVERCOME BARRIERS TO DRUG DELIVERY

Several strategies have been explored to overcome barriers and improve bioavailability. The most common strategy has been structural modification of molecules to change their physiochemical properties to enable them to permeate across membranes. Prodrugs and peptidomimetics are excellent examples of structurally modified drugs. Another approach used frequently is design of formulations.

PRODRUG AND STRUCTURAL MODIFICATION

Prodrugs can be defined as a pharmacologically inactive chemical derivative that need to be converted to their active form *in vivo* to exert a therapeutic response. Small molecules are good candidates for prodrug derivatization. Drugs can be modified chemically to change their physiochemical properties to render them more suitable for absorption. Once the prodrug is internalized in a cell, molecules are converted to their active form by enzymes present in the cytosol.

A targeted prodrug approach has recently gained popularity among drug delivery scientists. In this approach a moiety or ligand is chemically linked to the prodrug. This ligand is a substrate for a particular receptor/transporter expressed on the cellular membrane. The prodrug exclusively binds to this receptor/transporter complex and is taken up into the cell via an energy-dependent process. Use of peptides as prodrugs is less common. The cyclic peptide approach has shown improvement in membrane permeability. In this method, the N and C terminal of the peptide are connected via a linker/bridge. This modification to peptides renders them less susceptible to enzyme degradation and also lowers the hydrogen-bonding potential. The lipophilicity of cyclic peptides is also higher, and the transport process now predominantly adopts the transcellular pathway instead of the paracellular pathway [120]. Other chemical modifications to improve permeation are halogenations, cationization, lipidization, and conjugation to biopolymers [121].

FORMULATIONS

An optimum formulation can be very successful in increasing the permeability of drugs. Formulations are of various types and can be tailor-made depending on the type of drug, site of action, and desired route of delivery. Drugs can be entrapped in nanoparticles, micelles, liposomes, and hydrogels, which can be modified to overcome the absorption barriers.

OTHER STRATEGIES

Several other strategies have been used to cover the barriers for drug delivery. In recent years the use of surgical implants or devices for drug delivery has gained popularity. These devices or implants are surgically inserted into the target tissue or organ, which helps overcome barriers that otherwise would create a problem when the drug is administered via conventional routes. Also, with the use of surgical devices and implants, systemic toxicity and dose of therapeutic drug can be lowered significantly.

SUMMARY

Successful absorption of a drug at the site of action depends on its ability to permeate through several barriers. Drug absorption is mainly controlled via the paracellular and transcellular pathways. Depending on the location in the body, either pathway plays a predominant role in drug absorption. The tight junctions present in various parts of the body form a formidable barrier against the passage of drug molecules across the membranes. Also, metabolizing enzymes and various efflux pumps add to the problems associated with drug delivery. All these challenges need to be encountered and overcome for the development of a successful drug to treat a disease.

REVIEW QUESTIONS

1. What are the major barriers to drug delivery?
2. Comment briefly on physiological barriers.
3. Differentiate between paracellular and transcellular pathways.

4. What is the blood–brain barrier?
5. Briefly explain the structure of skin.
6. What are prodrugs?

REFERENCES

1. Kompella UB, Lee VH. Delivery systems for penetration enhancement of peptide and protein drugs: design considerations. *Adv Drug Deliv Rev.* 2001;46(1–3):211–245.
2. Lemmer HJ, Hamman JH. Paracellular drug absorption enhancement through tight junction modulation. *Expert Opin Drug Deliv.* 2013;10(1):103–114.
3. Staehelin LA. Further observations on the fine structure of freeze-cleaved tight junctions. *J Cell Sci.* 1973;13(3):763–786.
4. Gonzalez-Mariscal L, Chavez de Ramirez B, Cereijido M. Tight junction formation in cultured epithelial cells (MDCK). *J Membr Biol.* 1985;86(2):113–125.
5. Rothen-Rutishauser B, Riesen FK, Braun A, Gunthert M, Wunderli-Allenspach H. Dynamics of tight and adherens junctions under EGTA treatment. *J Membr Biol.* 2002;188(2):151–162.
6. Siahaan TJ. Chemical, biochemical and physiological barriers to oral drug delivery. In: Wang B, Siahaan TJ, Soltero RA. eds. *Drug Delivery: Principles and Applications.* Hoboken, NJ: John Wiley & Sons; 2005:15–27.
7. Mitic LL, Anderson JM. Molecular architecture of tight junctions. *Annu Rev Physiol.* 1998;60:121–142.
8. Madara JL. Regulation of the movement of solutes across tight junctions. *Annu Rev Physiol.* 1998;60:143–159.
9. Burton PS, Goodwin JT, Vidmar TJ, Amore BM. Predicting drug absorption: how nature made it a difficult problem. *J Pharmacol Exp Ther.* 2002;303(3):889–895.
10. Takeichi M. Cadherins: a molecular family important in selective cell-cell adhesion. *Annu Rev Biochem.* 1990;59:237–252.
11. Shore EM, Nelson WJ. Biosynthesis of the cell adhesion molecule uvomorulin (E-cadherin) in Madin-Darby canine kidney epithelial cells. *J Biol Chem.* 1991;266(29):19672–19680.
12. Cowin P, Burke B. Cytoskeleton-membrane interactions. *Curr Opin Cell Biol.* 1996;8(1):56–65.
13. Martinez MN, Amidon GL. A mechanistic approach to understanding the factors affecting drug absorption: a review of fundamentals. *J Clin Pharmacol.* 2002;42(6):620–643.
14. Roney C, Kulkarni P, Arora V, et al. Targeted nanoparticles for drug delivery through the blood-brain barrier for Alzheimer's disease. *J Control Release.* 2005;108(2–3):193–214.
15. Xu G, Mahajan S, Roy I, Yong KT. Theranostic quantum dots for crossing blood-brain barrier and providing therapy of HIV-associated encephalopathy. *Front Pharmacol.* 2013;4:140.
16. Weiss N, Miller F, Cazaubon S, Couraud PO. The blood-brain barrier in brain homeostasis and neurological diseases. *Biochim Biophys Acta.* 2009;1788(4):842–857.
17. Lo EH, Singhal AB, Torchilin VP, Abbott NJ. Drug delivery to damaged brain. *Brain Res Brain Res Rev.* 2001;38(1–2):140–148.
18. Naik A, Kalia YN, Guy RH. Transdermal drug delivery: overcoming the skin's barrier function. *Pharm Sci Technol Today.* 2000;3(9):318–326.
19. Gray GM, White RJ, Williams RH, Yardley HJ. Lipid composition of the superficial stratum corneum cells of pig epidermis. *Br J Dermatol.* 1982;106(1):59–63.
20. Williams ML, Elias PM. The extracellular matrix of stratum corneum: role of lipids in normal and pathological function. *Crit Rev Ther Drug Carrier Syst.* 1987;3(2):95–122.
21. Potts RO, Francoeur ML. The influence of stratum corneum morphology on water permeability. *J Invest Dermatol.* 1991;96(4):495–499.
22. Wacher VJ, Wu CY, Benet LZ. Overlapping substrate specificities and tissue distribution of cytochrome P450 3A and P-glycoprotein: implications for drug delivery and activity in cancer chemotherapy. *Mol Carcinog.* 1995;13(3):129–134.
23. Efferth T. The human ATP-binding cassette transporter genes: from the bench to the bedside. *Curr Mol Med.* 2001;1(1):45–65.
24. Rees DC, Johnson E, Lewinson O. ABC transporters: the power to change. *Nat Rev Mol Cell Biol.* 2009;10(3):218–227.
25. Locher KP. Review. Structure and mechanism of ATP-binding cassette transporters. *Philos Trans R Soc Lond B Biol Sci.* 2009;364(1514):239–245.
26. Locher KP, Borths E. ABC transporter architecture and mechanism: implications from the crystal structures of BtuCD and BtuF. *FEBS Lett.* 2004;564(3):264–268.

27. Dean M, Rzhetsky A, Allikmets R. The human ATP-binding cassette (ABC) transporter super-family. *Genome Res.* 2001;11(7):1156–1166.
28. Ambudkar SV, Kimchi-Sarfaty C, Sauna ZE, Gottesman MM. P-glycoprotein: from genomics to mechanism. *Oncogene.* 2003;22(47):7468–7485.
29. Gottesman MM. Mechanisms of cancer drug resistance. *Annu Rev Med.* 2002;53:615–627.
30. Higgins CF. ABC transporters: from microorganisms to man. *Annu Rev Cell Biol.* 1992;8:67–113.
31. Tusnady GE, Bakos E, Varadi A, Sarkadi B. Membrane topology distinguishes a subfamily of the ATP-binding cassette (ABC) transporters. *FEBS Lett.* 1997;402(1):1–3.
32. Kast C, Canfield V, Levenson R, Gros P. Membrane topology of P-glycoprotein as determined by epitope insertion: transmembrane organization of the N-terminal domain of mdr3. *Biochemistry.* 1995;34(13):4402–4411.
33. Kerr ID. Structure and association of ATP-binding cassette transporter nucleotide-binding domains. *Biochim Biophys Acta.* 2002;1561(1):47–64.
34. Linton KJ, Higgins CF. The *Escherichia coli* ATP-binding cassette (ABC) proteins. *Mol Microbiol.* 1998;28(1):5–13.
35. Hrycyna CA, Airan LE, Germann UA, Ambudkar SV, Pastan I, Gottesman MM. Structural flexibility of the linker region of human P-glycoprotein permits ATP hydrolysis and drug transport. *Biochemistry.* 1998;37(39):13660–13673.
36. Sauna ZE, Nandigama K, Ambudkar SV. Exploiting reaction intermediates of the ATPase reaction to elucidate the mechanism of transport by P-glycoprotein (ABCB1). *J Biol Chem.* 2006;281(36):26501–26511.
37. Zaitseva J, Jenewein S, Oswald C, Jumpertz T, Holland IB, Schmitt L. A molecular understanding of the catalytic cycle of the nucleotide-binding domain of the ABC transporter HlyB. *Biochem Soc Trans.* 2005;33(Pt 5):990–995.
38. Jones PM, George AM. The ABC transporter structure and mechanism: perspectives on recent research. *Cell Mol Life Sci.* 2004;61(6):682–699.
39. Moussatova A, Kandt C, O'Mara ML, Tieleman DP. ATP-binding cassette transporters in *Escherichia coli*. *Biochim Biophys Acta.* 2008;1778(9):1757–1771.
40. Juliano RL, Ling V. A surface glycoprotein modulating drug permeability in Chinese hamster ovary cell mutants. *Biochim Biophys Acta.* 1976;455(1):152–162.
41. Biedler JL, Riehm H. Cellular resistance to actinomycin D in Chinese hamster cells in vitro: cross-resistance, radioautographic, and cytogenetic studies. *Cancer Res.* 1970;30(4):1174–1184.
42. Gros P, Ben Neriah YB, Croop JM, Housman DE. Isolation and expression of a complementary DNA that confers multidrug resistance. *Nature.* 1986;323(6090):728–731.
43. Gros P, Croop J, Roninson I, Varshavsky A, Housman DE. Isolation and characterization of DNA sequences amplified in multidrug-resistant hamster cells. *Proc Natl Acad Sci USA.* 1986;83(2):337–341.
44. Ueda K, Clark DP, Chen CJ, Roninson IB, Gottesman MM, Pastan I. The human multidrug resistance (mdr1) gene. cDNA cloning and transcription initiation. *J Biol Chem.* 1987;262(2):505–508.
45. Cai J, Gros P. Overexpression, purification, and functional characterization of ATP-binding cassette transporters in the yeast, *Pichia pastoris*. *Biochim Biophys Acta.* 2003;1610(1):63–76.
46. Wang H, Lee EW, Cai X, Ni Z, Zhou L, Mao Q. Membrane topology of the human breast cancer resistance protein (BCRP/ABCG2) determined by epitope insertion and immunofluorescence. *Biochemistry.* 2008;47(52):13778–13787.
47. Campos L, Guyotat D, Archimbaud E, et al. Clinical significance of multidrug resistance P-glycoprotein expression on acute nonlymphoblastic leukemia cells at diagnosis. *Blood.* 1992;79(2):473–476.
48. Cumber PM, Jacobs A, Hoy T, et al. Expression of the multiple drug resistance gene (mdr-1) and epitope masking in chronic lymphatic leukaemia. *Br J Haematol.* 1990;76(2):226–230.
49. Verrelle P, Meissonnier F, Fonck Y, et al. Clinical relevance of immunohistochemical detection of multidrug resistance P-glycoprotein in breast carcinoma. *J Natl Cancer Inst.* 1991;83(2):111–116.
50. Marie JP, Zhou DC, Gurbuxani S, Legrand O, Zittoun R. MDR1/P-glycoprotein in haematological neoplasms. *Eur J Cancer.* 1996;32A(6):1034–1038.
51. Fojo AT, Shen DW, Mickley LA, Pastan I, Gottesman MM. Intrinsic drug resistance in human kidney cancer is associated with expression of a human multidrug-resistance gene. *J Clin Oncol.* 1987;5(12):1922–1927.
52. Fardel O, Lecureur V, Guillouzo A. The P-glycoprotein multidrug transporter. *Gen Pharmacol.* 1996;27(8):1283–1291.
53. Hunter J, Jepson MA, Tsuruo T, Simmons NL, Hirst BH. Functional expression of P-glycoprotein in apical membranes of human intestinal Caco-2 cells. Kinetics of vinblastine secretion and interaction with modulators. *J Biol Chem.* 1993;268(20):14991–14997.

54. Fojo AT, Ueda K, Slamon DJ, Poplack DG, Gottesman MM, Pastan I. Expression of a multidrug-resistance gene in human tumors and tissues. *Proc Natl Acad Sci USA.* 1987;84(1):265–269.

55. Gatmaitan ZC, Arias IM. Structure and function of P-glycoprotein in normal liver and small intestine. *Adv Pharmacol.* 1993;24:77–97.

56. Silverman JA, Schrenk D. Hepatic canalicular membrane 4: expression of the multidrug resistance genes in the liver. *FASEB J.* 1997;11(5):308–313.

57. Inagaki N, Gonoi T, Clement JPT, et al. Reconstitution of IKATP: an inward rectifier subunit plus the sulfonylurea receptor. *Science.* 1995;270(5239):1166–1170.

58. Inagaki N, Gonoi T, Clement JP, et al. A family of sulfonylurea receptors determines the pharmacological properties of ATP-sensitive K+ channels. *Neuron.* 1996;16(5):1011–1017.

59. Riordan JR, Rommens JM, Kerem B, et al. Identification of the cystic fibrosis gene: cloning and characterization of complementary DNA. *Science.* 1989;245(4922):1066–1073.

60. Cole SP, Bhardwaj G, Gerlach JH, et al. Overexpression of a transporter gene in a multidrug-resistant human lung cancer cell line. *Science.* 1992;258(5088):1650–1654.

61. Taniguchi K, Wada M, Kohno K, et al. A human canalicular multispecific organic anion transporter (cMOAT) gene is overexpressed in cisplatin-resistant human cancer cell lines with decreased drug accumulation. *Cancer Res.* 1996;56(18):4124–4129.

62. Nies AT, Keppler D. The apical conjugate efflux pump ABCC2 (MRP2). *Pflugers Arch.* 2007;453(5):643–659.

63. Annilo T, Dean M. Degeneration of an ATP-binding cassette transporter gene, ABCC13, in different mammalian lineages. *Genomics.* 2004;84(1):34–46.

64. Deeley RG, Westlake C, Cole SP. Transmembrane transport of endo- and xenobiotics by mammalian ATP-binding cassette multidrug resistance proteins. *Physiol Rev.* 2006;86(3):849–899.

65. Stride BD, Valdimarsson G, Gerlach JH, Wilson GM, Cole SP, Deeley RG. Structure and expression of the messenger RNA encoding the murine multidrug resistance protein, an ATP-binding cassette transporter. *Mol Pharmacol.* 1996;49(6):962–971.

66. Hipfner DR, Almquist KC, Stride BD, Deeley RG, Cole SP. Location of a protease-hypersensitive region in the multidrug resistance protein (MRP) by mapping of the epitope of MRP-specific monoclonal antibody QCRL-1. *Cancer Res.* 1996;56(14):3307–3314.

67. D'Iakov SI, Lebedeva IK, Lisin VV, Grishin GI. [New immunofluorescent method for the rapid determination of microbial antibiotic sensitivity]. *Antibiotiki.* 1982;27(10):761–766.

68. Zaman GJ, Flens MJ, van Leusden MR, et al. The human multidrug resistance-associated protein MRP is a plasma membrane drug-efflux pump. *Proc Natl Acad Sci USA.* 1994;91(19):8822–8826.

69. Evers R, Zaman GJ, van Deemter L, et al. Basolateral localization and export activity of the human multidrug resistance-associated protein in polarized pig kidney cells. *J Clin Invest.* 1996;97(5):1211–1218.

70. Flens MJ, Zaman GJ, van der Valk P, et al. Tissue distribution of the multidrug resistance protein. *Am J Pathol.* 1996;148(4):1237–1247.

71. Mottino AD, Hoffman T, Jennes L, Vore M. Expression and localization of multidrug resistant protein mrp2 in rat small intestine. *J Pharmacol Exp Ther.* 2000;293(3):717–723.

72. St-Pierre MV, Serrano MA, Macias RI, et al. Expression of members of the multidrug resistance protein family in human term placenta. *Am J Physiol Regul Integr Comp Physiol.* 2000;279(4):R1495–R1503.

73. Cui Y, Konig J, Buchholz JK, Spring H, Leier I, Keppler D. Drug resistance and ATP-dependent conjugate transport mediated by the apical multidrug resistance protein, MRP2, permanently expressed in human and canine cells. *Mol Pharmacol.* 1999;55(5):929–937.

74. Bodo A, Bakos E, Szeri F, Varadi A, Sarkadi B. Differential modulation of the human liver conjugate transporters MRP2 and MRP3 by bile acids and organic anions. *J Biol Chem.* 2003;278(26):23529–23537.

75. Hinoshita E, Uchiumi T, Taguchi K, et al. Increased expression of an ATP-binding cassette superfamily transporter, multidrug resistance protein 2, in human colorectal carcinomas. *Clin Cancer Res.* 2000;6(6):2401–2407.

76. Nies AT, Konig J, Pfannschmidt M, Klar E, Hofmann WJ, Keppler D. Expression of the multidrug resistance proteins MRP2 and MRP3 in human hepatocellular carcinoma. *Int J Cancer.* 2001;94(4):492–499.

77. Suzuki H, Sugiyama Y. Single nucleotide polymorphisms in multidrug resistance associated protein 2 (MRP2/ABCC2): its impact on drug disposition. *Adv Drug Deliv Rev.* 2002;54(10):1311–1331.

78. Doyle L, Ross DD. Multidrug resistance mediated by the breast cancer resistance protein BCRP (ABCG2). *Oncogene.* 2003;22(47):7340–7358.

79. Robey RW, Polgar O, Deeken J, To KW, Bates SE. ABCG2: determining its relevance in clinical drug resistance. *Cancer Metast Rev.* 2007;26(1):39–57.

80. Doyle LA, Yang W, Abruzzo LV, et al. A multidrug resistance transporter from human MCF-7 breast cancer cells. *Proc Natl Acad Sci USA*. 1998;95(26):15665–15670.

81. Allikmets R, Schriml LM, Hutchinson A, Romano-Spica V, Dean M. A human placenta-specific ATP-binding cassette gene (ABCP) on chromosome 4q22 that is involved in multidrug resistance. *Cancer Res*. 1998;58(23):5337–5339.

82. Miyake K, Mickley L, Litman T, et al. Molecular cloning of cDNAs which are highly overexpressed in mitoxantrone-resistant cells: demonstration of homology to ABC transport genes. *Cancer Res*. 1999;59(1):8–13.

83. Hazai E, Bikadi Z. Homology modeling of breast cancer resistance protein (ABCG2). *J Struct Biol*. 2008;162(1):63–74.

84. Li YF, Polgar O, Okada M, Esser L, Bates SE, Xia D. Towards understanding the mechanism of action of the multidrug resistance-linked half-ABC transporter ABCG2: a molecular modeling study. *J Mol Graph Model*. 2007;25(6):837–851.

85. Kage K, Tsukahara S, Sugiyama T, et al. Dominant-negative inhibition of breast cancer resistance protein as drug efflux pump through the inhibition of S-S dependent homodimerization. *Int J Cancer*. 2002;97(5):626–630.

86. Bhatia A, Schafer HJ, Hrycyna CA. Oligomerization of the human ABC transporter ABCG2: evaluation of the native protein and chimeric dimers. *Biochemistry*. 2005;44(32):10893–10904.

87. Xu J, Liu Y, Yang Y, Bates S, Zhang JT. Characterization of oligomeric human half-ABC transporter ATP-binding cassette G2. *J Biol Chem*. 2004;279(19):19781–19789.

88. Lage H, Dietel M. Effect of the breast-cancer resistance protein on atypical multidrug resistance. *Lancet Oncol*. 2000;1:169–175.

89. Rocchi E, Khodjakov A, Volk EL, et al. The product of the ABC half-transporter gene ABCG2 (BCRP/MXR/ABCP) is expressed in the plasma membrane. *Biochem Biophys Res Commun*. 2000;271(1):42–46.

90. Scheffer GL, Maliepaard M, Pijnenborg AC, et al. Breast cancer resistance protein is localized at the plasma membrane in mitoxantrone- and topotecan-resistant cell lines. *Cancer Res*. 2000;60(10):2589–2593.

91. Jonker JW, Smit JW, Brinkhuis RF, et al. Role of breast cancer resistance protein in the bioavailability and fetal penetration of topotecan. *J Natl Cancer Inst*. 2000;92(20):1651–1656.

92. Natarajan K, Xie Y, Baer MR, Ross DD. Role of breast cancer resistance protein (BCRP/ABCG2) in cancer drug resistance. *Biochem Pharmacol*. 2012;83(8):1084–1103.

93. Nakanishi T, Ross DD. Breast cancer resistance protein (BCRP/ABCG2): its role in multidrug resistance and regulation of its gene expression. *Chin J Cancer*. 2012;31(2):73–99.

94. Diestra JE, Scheffer GL, Catala I, et al. Frequent expression of the multi-drug resistance-associated protein BCRP/MXR/ABCP/ABCG2 in human tumours detected by the BXP-21 monoclonal antibody in paraffin-embedded material. *J Pathol*. 2002;198(2):213–219.

95. Guengerich FP. Cytochrome P450s and other enzymes in drug metabolism and toxicity. *AAPS J*. 2006;8(1):E101–111.

96. Tennant M, McRee DE. The first structure of a microsomal P450--implications for drug discovery. *Curr Opin Drug Discov Dev*. 2001;4(5):671–677.

97. Ahmad N, Mukhtar H. Cytochrome p450: a target for drug development for skin diseases. *J Invest Dermatol*. 2004;123(3):417–425.

98. Gervasini G, Carrillo JA, Benitez J. Potential role of cerebral cytochrome P450 in clinical pharmacokinetics: modulation by endogenous compounds. *Clin Pharmacokinet*. 2004;43(11):693–706.

99. Christians U. Transport proteins and intestinal metabolism: P-glycoprotein and cytochrome P4503A. *Ther Drug Monit*. 2004;26(2):104–106.

100. Cappiello M, Giuliani L, Pacifici GM. Distribution of UDP-glucuronosyltransferase and its endogenous substrate uridine 5'-diphosphoglucuronic acid in human tissues. *Eur J Clin Pharmacol*. 1991;41(4):345–350.

101. Cappiello M, Giuliani L, Rane A, Pacifici GM. Dopamine sulphotransferase is better developed than p-nitrophenol sulphotransferase in the human fetus. *Dev Pharmacol Ther*. 1991;16(2):83–88.

102. Krishna DR, Klotz U. Extrahepatic metabolism of drugs in humans. *Clin Pharmacokinet*. 1994;26(2):144–160.

103. Fisher MB, Paine MF, Strelevitz TJ, Wrighton SA. The role of hepatic and extrahepatic UDP-glucuronosyltransferases in human drug metabolism. *Drug Metab Rev*. 2001;33(3–4):273–297.

104. Kelly SL, Lamb DC, Jackson CJ, Warrilow AG, Kelly DE. The biodiversity of microbial cytochromes P450. *Adv Microb Physiol*. 2003;47:131–186.

105. Ingelman-Sundberg M. Human drug metabolising cytochrome P450 enzymes: properties and polymorphisms. *Naunyn Schmied Arch Pharmacol*. 2004;369(1):89–104.

106. Nebert DW, Nelson DR, Coon MJ, et al. The P450 superfamily: update on new sequences, gene mapping, and recommended nomenclature. *DNA Cell Biol.* 1991;10(1):1–14.

107. Nelson DR, Koymans L, Kamataki T, et al. P450 superfamily: update on new sequences, gene mapping, accession numbers and nomenclature. *Pharmacogenetics.* 1996;6(1):1–42.

108. Hukkanen J, Pelkonen O, Hakkola J, Raunio H. Expression and regulation of xenobiotic-metabolizing cytochrome P450 (CYP) enzymes in human lung. *Crit Rev Toxicol.* 2002;32(5):391–411.

109. Nelson DR. Comparison of P450s from human and fugu: 420 million years of vertebrate P450 evolution. *Arch Biochem Biophys.* 2003;409(1):18–24.

110. Slaughter RL, Edwards DJ. Recent advances: the cytochrome P450 enzymes. *Ann Pharmacother.* 1995;29(6):619–624.

111. Watkins PB, Wrighton SA, Schuetz EG, Molowa DT, Guzelian PS. Identification of glucocorticoid-inducible cytochromes P-450 in the intestinal mucosa of rats and man. *J Clin Invest.* 1987;80(4):1029–1036.

112. Williams PA, Cosme J, Vinkovic DM, et al. Crystal structures of human cytochrome P450 3A4 bound to metyrapone and progesterone. *Science.* 2004;305(5684):683–686.

113. Ding X, Kaminsky LS. Human extrahepatic cytochromes P450: function in xenobiotic metabolism and tissue-selective chemical toxicity in the respiratory and gastrointestinal tracts. *Annu Rev Pharmacol Toxicol.* 2003;43:149–173.

114. Du L, Hoffman SM, Keeney DS. Epidermal CYP2 family cytochromes P450. *Toxicol Appl Pharmacol.* 2004;195(3):278–287.

115. Liu M, Hurn PD, Alkayed NJ. Cytochrome P450 in neurological disease. *Curr Drug Metab.* 2004;5(3):225–234.

116. Zhao X, Imig JD. Kidney CYP450 enzymes: biological actions beyond drug metabolism. *Curr Drug Metab.* 2003;4(1):73–84.

117. Goodwin JT, Conradi RA, Ho NF, Burton PS. Physicochemical determinants of passive membrane permeability: role of solute hydrogen-bonding potential and volume. *J Med Chem.* 2001;44(22):3721–3729.

118. Pauletti GM, Okumu FW, Borchardt RT. Effect of size and charge on the passive diffusion of peptides across Caco-2 cell monolayers via the paracellular pathway. *Pharm Res.* 1997;14(2):164–168.

119. Burton PS, Conradi RA, Ho NF, Hilgers AR, Borchardt RT. How structural features influence the biomembrane permeability of peptides. *J Pharm Sci.* 1996;85(12):1336–1340.

120. Okumu FW, Pauletti GM, Vander Velde DG, Siahaan TJ, Borchardt RT. Effect of restricted conformational flexibility on the permeation of model hexapeptides across Caco-2 cell monolayers. *Pharm Res.* 1997;14(2):169–175.

121. Witt KA, Gillespie TJ, Huber JD, Egleton RD, Davis TP. Peptide drug modifications to enhance bioavailability and blood-brain barrier permeability. *Peptides.* 2001;22(12):2329–2343.

3 CHAPTER

IN VITRO MODELS IN DRUG DISCOVERY AND DELIVERY

Deep Kwatra, Varun Khurana, and Ashim K. Mitra

CHAPTER OBJECTIVES

Upon completing this chapter, the reader should be able to

▶ Understand the importance of *in vitro* models in drug discovery and delivery.

▶ Recognize the use of various *in vitro models* based on the barriers to conventional drug delivery.

▶ Acquire sound knowledge of various approaches to predict drug permeability and bioavailability *in vitro*.

▶ Comprehend the utility, recent progress, specific development, and issues relating to various *in vitro*, cell culture–based, and *in silico* models used in drug discovery.

▶ Understand the complexity and simplicity of various cell culture models used in intestinal drug delivery.

CHAPTER OUTLINE

INTRODUCTION

Pharmaceutical drug development frequently requires determination of drug permeability into the blood from the gastrointestinal (GI) track and then distribution into various organs that may be the site of action or elimination. Drug permeability is a key constraint that can affect the overall oral bioavailability and/or its availability at the site of action of a potential drug candidate. Advances in drug discovery techniques have led to the synthesis of more biologically active lead molecules. But many of these still fail to develop into clinically relevant drugs because of poor oral bioavailability or permeability across other biological barriers. To evaluate the absorption potential of new chemical entities, numerous *in vitro* and *in vivo* model systems have been studied.

In vitro cell culture models for studying drug permeability allow rapid screening of drugs based on their permeability across biological barriers. These provide more biological complexities than simple physicochemical techniques like parallel artificial membrane permeation assay (PAMPA), allowing for more accurate estimations. Simultaneously, *in vitro* cell culture models are also more economical and faster for screening large numbers of lead molecules when compared with *in vivo* models. *In vitro* models also allow more accurate determination of the mechanism of drug disposition (active/passive or carrier-mediated absorption, drug metabolism), which is essential in the drug delivery process. Recently, *in silico* (computational) methods to predict drug permeability have also garnered a lot of attention. Each method has its own advantages and disadvantages in determination of drug permeability; however, no single method is sufficient for proper prediction of drug absorption. A sequential use of multiple methods is required to screen, test, and identify the lead molecules with ideal pharmacokinetic properties. High-throughput methods, which are generally much less reliable, can be used for initial screening during which the identification of the number of lead molecules is very high, whereas slower yet more precise methods could be used to identify absorption parameters of the major leads.

With progress in computational techniques, combinatorial chemistry, and robotics and automation, drug companies are able to generate thousands of molecules with potential biological activity. Furthermore, the development of modern high-throughput screening has made it possible to test these compounds for their biological activity at a very rapid rate. Nevertheless, even though a large number of lead molecules are being synthesized and verified for biological activity, the attrition rate of drug molecules reaching later stages of drug development is still very high. A very low percentage of molecules going through the drug delivery process enters the market. The rate of attrition differs among different drug categories (5% for anticancer drugs versus 20% for cardiovascular), although the reasons for most failures seem to be similar. The chief reasons for failure seem to be poor physiochemical characteristics (low aqueous solubility or chemical instability) or pharmacokinetic properties (poor intestinal permeability, intestinal and or hepatic metabolism, high biliary or renal clearance). If a drug molecule does not achieve the required bioavailability, it does not go forward in the drug delivery process regardless of the bioactivity. For a drug to be clinically effective, it should be able to permeate through the initial barriers at the site of delivery to reach the plasma and to cross the barriers at the target site to achieve therapeutic levels. Thus, for most drugs that are administered orally, permeating through the GI tract acts as the first barrier. To, therefore, raise the probability of success of a lead molecule intended for oral delivery, absorption processes should be considered during its design.

Once multiple leads are produced and rapidly screened, they need to be tested for their permeability characteristics. Carrying out these studies in animals with a high number of lead molecules is not cost effective. Also, there are ethical concerns regarding the large number of animals that may be required to carry out these studies. Hence, less expensive and more reliable methods are required that can predict the permeability of drug candidates in a reproducible manner. These prediction methods need to be rapid and cost effective. Simultaneously, they need to have enough complexity to properly resemble the *in vivo* barriers they are being used to mimic. *In vitro* cell culture models provide the perfect bridge between computational methods and animal models (*in vivo* models) for the prediction of drug permeability and bioavailability.

In this chapter we discuss the various *in vitro* models used to study drug molecules for their pharmacokinetic properties, with an emphasis on orally administered drugs. To better understand the requirements for an *in vitro* model, it is important to understand the physiological characteristics of the organ you are trying to model. The small intestine acts as the major site of absorption for orally administered drugs. Hence, we need to understand the morphological characteristics of the intestine and what kind of barrier it presents to drug molecules.

MORPHOLOGY OF THE SMALL INTESTINE

The GI tract and especially the small intestine play a critical role in absorption of multiple substances. The small intestine has been naturally designed to act as a selective permeability barrier for oral absorption. For example, the intestine is designed

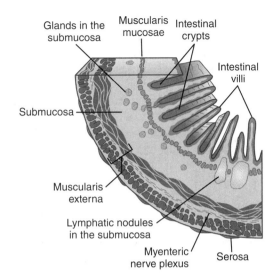

Glands in the submucosa

Muscularis mucosae

Intestinal crypts

Intestinal villi

Submucosa

Muscularis externa

Lymphatic nodules in the submucosa

Myenteric nerve plexus

Serosa

FIGURE 3-1 Anatomical layers of the small intestine.

in such a way that it allows for the absorption of essential nutrients from consumed food (carbohydrates, amino acids, peptides, lipids, and vitamins) while simultaneously excluding substances such as xenobiotics, digestive enzymes, and bacteria. This specialized and selective absorption pattern is accomplished by unique anatomical and physiological characteristics of the intestine. The presence of a mucosal layer, intercellular tight junctions, and specialized transporter systems make up the major barriers for xenobiotic transport across the intestine. An ideal model for intestinal drug transport thus should also have similar anatomical and physiological features for better predictive power (**Figure 3–1**).

BARRIERS TO INTESTINAL DRUG DELIVERY

The barriers to intestinal drug delivery can be broadly classified into physical and biochemical barriers. The physical barrier is more of an anatomical barrier that is an outcome of the tight intracellular junctions and the lipoidal nature of the cellular membrane. The biochemical barrier is the combined presence of mucosal layers, metabolic enzymes, and influx/efflux transporters. The electrical charge of the molecules and the concentration gradient generated also act as a major driving force for drug transport across the GI tract.

PHYSICAL BARRIERS

As previously mentioned, tight junctions establish the major barrier to paracellular drug transport. The cell-to-cell contact between the intestinal epithelial cells is maintained by intercellular junction complexes. These range between approximately 0.4 to 2 nm in width and have three major components: tight junctions, intermediate junctions, and spot desmosomes [2]. The tightness and density of the tight junctions vary across the length of the intestine. The tight junctions of the ileum are denser than those of the jejunum. The intermediate junctions and spot desmosomes do not serve as major barriers to drug diffusion. The tight junctional pores vary in their diameter from animals to humans, with humans having tighter junctions of about 4 to 8 Å and animals, about 10 to 15 Å [2]. Because these cellular junctions have a very small diameter and cover a very small area of the intestine (tight junctions account for less than 0.01% of the total surface area of intestine), this route is not appropriate for absorption of most dugs. Drugs with a molecular radius greater than 4 Å especially cannot pass through tight junctions [3, 4]. It has been shown, however, that during certain physiological processes and using certain chemical agents, the diameter of the tight junctions can be altered [5, 6]. Hence, studies are also being performed to deliver drugs in combination with such permeability-enhancing agents.

BIOCHEMICAL BARRIERS

The presence of drug-metabolizing enzymes, mucosa, and drug transporters (mainly efflux transporters) together form the biochemical barrier. Even though liver is the major drug metabolism site, the intestines also express enzymes such as various esterases and peptidases that can metabolize drug molecules. The cytochrome (CYP) P450 super-family members (i.e., CYP1A1, 1A2, 2D6, 3A4, 2C9, and 2C19) and enzymes such as glucuronyltransferase are also expressed in the intestine [7]. CYP3A4 is a major drug-metabolizing enzyme that accounts for 60% of all CYPs and metabolizes many clinically administered drugs [8]. Specialized membrane efflux transporters present on the intestinal lumen transport the drugs from within the cell cytoplasm back into the lumen. These transporters belong to the ATP-binding cassette (ABC) containing a superfamily of transporters called as ABC transporters. The phenomenon of limiting drug absorption through efflux transporters is also termed multidrug resistance (MDR) [9, 10]. The major members of this MDR family of transporters are P-glycoprotein (P-gp), MDR protein-2 (MRP2), and breast cancer resistance protein [11]. The expression and activity of these proteins varies significantly among various species and also in certain specific disease states. Hence, it is possible that a drug that shows reduced intestinal absorption in animal models due to its interactions with efflux transporters may have higher bioavailability in humans and vice versa, or a drug that gives sufficient bioavailability in healthy patients may have decreased bioavailability in patients with certain disease states and vice versa.

ABSORPTION PATHWAYS

As mentioned before, the tight junctions only cover 0.01% area of the total intestinal surface. The rest of the surface area consists of epithelial cell plasma membrane and its membrane proteins. The plasma membrane of the GI tract consists mainly of phospholipids and cholesterol. The drugs thus need to navigate through this lipoidal bilayer to be available in the systemic circulation. The pH across the entire GI tract is also variable, with stomach pH ranging from 1 to 3, duodenum pH from 6.0 to 6.5, and large intestine pH from 5.5 to 7.0. The ionization state of the drug molecules is decided by the pH at the absorption site. The un-ionized form is able to migrate through the lipoidal membrane much more easily when compared with the ionized form [12]. This lack of parity in drug transport based on the ionization state of the drug is explained by the pH partition hypothesis. Transport of drugs across the GI epithelia can be mediated either by active (carrier mediated) or passive processes (**Figure 3-2**). Passive transport involves simple diffusion of drug molecules in the direction of concentration gradient. The rate at which a particular compound diffuses across a membrane is governed by Fick's law:

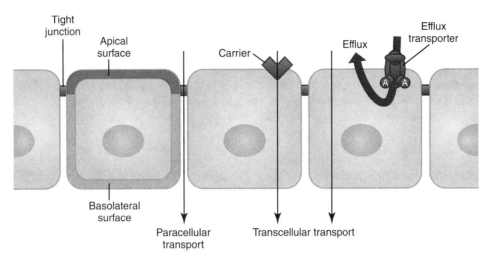

FIGURE 3-2 Factors mediating transepithelial transport.

$$\frac{dQ}{dt} = \frac{\{D * A * K(C_1 - C_2)\}}{h} \tag{1}$$

$$\frac{dQ}{dt} = \text{diffusion rate}$$

where D is the diffusion coefficient, A is the cross-sectional surface area of the membrane across which drug transfer occurs, K is the oil–water partition coefficient for the drug, h is the thickness of the membrane through which diffusion occurs, and $(C_1 - C_2)$ is the drug concentration gradient between donor and receiver compartments.

Passive Paracellular Transport

Passive transport involves the movement of drug molecules across a biological membrane without the utilization of energy or specialized carrier molecules. In paracellular transport, extracellular routes (aqueous cannels) are used for movement across the epithelium. The main driving force for passive paracellular diffusion is concentration gradient. Other electrochemical properties that may generate a potential driving force are the differences in electrical potential and hydrostatic pressure across the epithelia. Because this mode of transport occurs through the gaps between the cell junctions, the major rate-limiting factor for transport is the diameter of the tight junctions. Another major factor is the solubility of the compounds. Hence, passive paracellular transport is the preferred mode of transport for small hydrophilic molecules.

Passive Transcellular Transport

The passive transcellular mode of transport involves the movement of the drug through the cell without utilization of additional energy or carrier proteins. Hence, this pathway requires the drug to first cross the apical membrane, enter the cytoplasm, and then again cross the basolateral membrane. Because these drug molecules need to repeatedly cross the plasma membrane, which is lipoidal in nature, this route is preferred by hydrophobic compounds. As mentioned earlier, the surface area of the GI epithelia is covered mostly by cell membranes (99.9%) when compared with tight junctions. Thus, with all other factors remaining the same, drugs depending primarily on paracellular routes in theory will have low permeability profiles, whereas compounds with a preference for transcellular routes will have high rates of absorption [13]. The presence of active processes for either uptake or efflux, however, can lead to a variation from expected outcomes. For certain molecular species such as peptides and proteins, which are both large and hydrophilic molecules, specialized carriers are present. Thus, these molecules exhibit greater than expected permeability value [14, 15].

Carrier-Mediated Transport (Influx Transport)

Many nutrients like sugars, peptides, and water-soluble vitamins are hydrophilic in nature. Specialized membrane transporter proteins are expressed all along the GI tract epithelia. These transporters account for the high rate of transport for these nutrients. Along with the nutrient molecules, these transporters also transport some specific xenobiotics. Because of structural similarities between some nutrient molecules and drugs allowing for substrate recognition, transporters such as small peptides (peptide transporter 1 [PEPT1]), bile acids organic anions, nucleosides, amino acids, and mono-carboxylic acids have received significant attention [11, 14, 16]. Because these influx transporters are responsible for enhancing permeability of their substrates, these can lead to increased intestinal drug absorption. Drug molecules solubilized within the intestinal fluid interact with the transporters and get translocated across the apical membrane. PEPT1, which is physiologically responsible for the transport of di- and tripeptides, is a major influx transporter for drugs such as angiotensin-converting enzyme inhibitors, renin inhibitors, and beta-lactam antibiotics [17–19]. Because of the presence of such active transport mechanisms, these molecules show much higher intestinal absorption than observed in the absence of such transporters.

Carrier-Limited Transport (Efflux Transport)

The effect a transporter might have on overall drug bioavailability depends on the polar localization of the transporter and the direction in which it transports its substrates. Hence, influx transporters usually enhance drug permeability and efflux transporters have an opposite effect. Efflux transporters often act as drug resistance transporters and facilitate the removal of drug molecules from the cytoplasm back into the lumen. This family of efflux transporters requires energy to transport its cargo in the direction opposite to the concentration gradient. These transporters belong to the ABC superfamily of transporters and together are called the MDR proteins [10, 20, 21]. P-gp, which is the translated product of the *MDR1* gene, is the prevalent and ubiquitously expressed member of the efflux transporter family with significant expression in brain, intestine, kidney, liver, lungs, and pancreas. It has a very large substrate specificity, resulting in its ability to efflux out various classes of drugs with diverse molecular structure. All drugs within the same class, however, do not undergo the same degree of efflux. P-gp, because it is a member of the ABC transporters, has two ATP binding sites and structurally has two homologous halves each containing six transmembrane domains (**Figure 3-3**) [22–24]. Because of its location on the villus tip of enterocytes in close proximity to the lumen, it especially plays a key role in reducing the intestinal absorption of its substrate molecules [24, 25]. Mammalian P-gp displays about 60% to 65% homology with the gene expressed in other species, suggesting the role of the protein on the drug.

The multidrug resistant protein (MRP) family belongs to the *ABCC* gene family of which currently there are 13 known members [10]. These transporters have been found to be localized on the apical or basolateral membrane of hepatocytes, enterocytes, renal proximal tubule cells, and endothelial cells of the blood–brain barrier. MRPs,

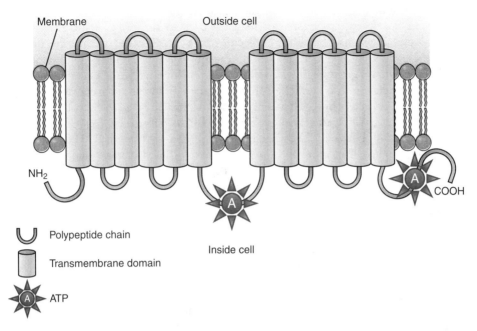

Membrane   Outside cell

NH₂

Inside cell

COOH

∪ Polypeptide chain

▯ Transmembrane domain

✴A ATP

FIGURE 3-3 Membrane topology of P-gp.

similar to P-gp, transport a structurally diverse array of substances and some metabolites (especially glutathione S-conjugates) with different substrate specificity and transport kinetics [10]. Among these proteins, four proteins play a special role in drug transport through the GI tract. MRP1, MRP2/cMOAT, and MRP3 are located in the human duodenum, whereas MRP1, MRP3, and MRP5 have been shown to be active in the colon [26]. MRP2 is the major player in intestinal efflux and is located on the apical membrane of enterocytes and colonocytes. The structure of MRP2 resembles that of P-gp and has a conserved core of 12 transmembrane domains divided into two similar halves, each half containing six helices and one ATP binding domain.

Breast cancer resistance protein was initially identified by Doyale et al. [27]. in a breast cancer cell line that strangely showed drug resistance even in the presence of verapamil, a potent P-gp inhibitor. A year later, Miyake et al. [28] also identified the same efflux pump in a mitoxantrone-resistant human colon carcinoma cell line S1-M1-80; hence, it is also known as MXR [28]. Structurally, it is different from P-gp and MRP2 in that it is a half transporter with six transmembrane helices and only one nucleotide-binding domain. Although it has some overlapping substrates with P-gp and MRP-2, it also has its own specific substrates. It is expressed in significant amounts in the small intestine and colon and hence acts as a major barrier to oral drug absorption.

Vesicular Transport

To facilitate drug permeation across the intestinal mucosa, enterocytes use specialized vesicular transport processes. The major vesicular transport processes are namely receptor-mediated endocytosis (RME), fluid-phase endocytosis (pinocytosis), and transcytosis. RME is generally used for the enhanced permeation of macromolecules but may also be involved in small molecular delivery. The macromolecular substrate attaches to the membrane receptor binding site. The receptor ligand complex then gets internalized by formation of clathrin-coated pits. After endocytosis, usually the contents of the endocytosed vacuole are delivered to the lysosome through a process called sorting.

This then results in the digestion of the ligand within the lysosome. The receptor meanwhile can be either digested or recycled back to the original site [29–31]. In fluid-phase endocytosis, the solute molecules first get dissolved within the luminal fluid. These are then internalized by bulk transport into the fluid phase of endocytic vesicles. The vesicles that form when the plasma membrane forms invaginations that pinch off are called pinosomes. The contents of these pinosomes have a fate similar to the endocytosed vesicles in RME where they are first transported to endosomes (prelysosomal vesicles), which then subsequently fuse with lysosomes [32]. The contents of the endocytosed vesicle, following fluid-phase endocytosis or RME, can bypass the lysosomes altogether and can be released across the basolateral membrane [33]. This process, known as transcytosis, is usually involved in the intestinal absorption of macromolecules that are typically unable to infiltrate the cell membranes through simple diffusion.

IN VITRO MODELS OF INTESTINAL DRUG ABSORPTION

As mentioned initially in the chapter, the orally administered drug faces multiple barriers before it crosses the intestine. Thus, an *in vitro* model for intestinal permeability should contain the appropriate complexity to accurately delineate the absorption rate and mechanism. This can be accomplished to the extent in which the permeability model incorporates the functionality of the physical and biochemical barrier components. *In vivo* models contain all the complexities required from a model and also can be used in the analysis of complex delivery systems that are difficult to be studied *in vitro*. Some disadvantages of *in vivo* studies include the need for large amounts of material, high costs, ethical constraints, time-consuming and labor-intensive nature of experiments, and complex analytical techniques required for plasma analysis. Despite the understandable complications linked to trying to reproduce all the barriers of the intestinal mucosa, multiple systems with varying degrees of relevant complexities have been developed.

IMMOBILIZED ARTIFICIAL MEMBRANE COLUMNS

These are similar to liquid chromatography columns except lipids are present instead of a polymeric stationary phase [34]. Molecules that interact strongly with the lipids get retained within the column, whereas those that do not interact are able to move freely. These lipids mimic the lipoidal environment of the cellular membrane. Because the lipid layers act as the major barriers for permeability of most solutes, it is presumed that a compound that has a long retention in the column should have good permeability across the cellular lipid bilayers. This is not the most accurate assumption because the lipid bilayer is not the only barrier, as previously mentioned. For a compound to cross the epithelial cell layer it must not only diffuse across the lipid bilayer, but it must also enter back into the aqueous environment of the cytoplasm, so it must also have some aqueous solubility. The major advantage of this technique is that it is fast and can be used for high-throughput screening. Good correlation has been shown between this technique and drug transport across Caco-2 cells, a very commonly used intestinal model. The major disadvantage of this technique lies in its premise, because it totally ignores the role of paracellular transport, carrier-mediated transport, drug metabolism, and efflux transporters on drug permeability. Because these are critical barriers to drug delivery, this technique gives an incomplete picture of drug transport.

PARALLEL ARTIFICIAL MEMBRANE PERMEATION ASSAY

PAMPA is run in a 96-well plate assay in which a standard 96-well plate is divided into two parts by a series of membrane filters. The bottom of the well is filled with buffer and the top with drug-containing solution. The filters are wetted with organic solvent and represent the cellular membrane. The rate of appearance of the drug in the bottom chamber reflects the diffusion of the drug across the lipid layer. Multiple studies have shown good correlation between fluxes measured using the PAMPA system and the bioavailability in humans for some selected compounds [35]. The major advantage of PAMPA is that it is a very simple cost-effective system, which can be used for high-throughput screening. Like the immobilized artificial membrane and most *in vitro* models lacking live cells, it ignores the role of enzymes, influx and efflux transporters, and paracellular pathways in intestinal drug absorption.

EXCISED INTESTINAL TISSUES

As the name suggests, the technique involves removal of the intestinal tissue from an animal (usually rats or mice) to study intestinal permeation. In this technique the drug solution is placed either on the mucosal side or the serosal side. Drug permeability is then determined by measuring either the disappearance or the appearance of drug from within the dosing solution. Because these tissues mostly preserve structural integrity, the permeability is determined across all the different segments. A common disadvantage is the limited viability of this type of preparation.

PERFUSED INTESTINAL TISSUES

Isolated segments of intestinal tissues are used to study drug permeability across the mucosal side, and the drug disappearance from within the solution is considered to be equal to drug absorption. This is a close enough approximation because the rate-limiting step in the intestinal absorption is the apical uptake. Because drug absorption is not the only determining factor, however, the assumption is not fully accurate. Absorption and accumulation within the mucosa without permeating across the cellular layers could lead to an overestimation of drug absorption. For example, the measurement of absorption of beta-lactam antibiotics by perfused intestinal tissues was roughly twice the true amount transported across the tissue [36].

This system has a few advantages over other models. The segmented study provides more mechanistic information about absorption and metabolism because physiological factors such as gastric emptying or intestinal transit time are absent. Similar to what was mentioned above, there are multiple disadvantages to this method. Additionally, the viability of perfused intestinal segments is limited and depends largely on the preparation technique. It has poor throughput but can be used to study absorption of drugs that are delivered using complex dosage forms.

EVERTED SACS

The everted sac is one of the oldest techniques used to study intestinal drug absorption. In this technique, a segment of the intestine is inverted inside out using a cylindrical object such as a glass rod. The two ends of the intestinal segment are tied, and the inside of the resulting sac is filled with an oxygenated buffer. This apparatus is then placed in a container with the drug to be tested. Drug permeability is calculated by measuring the drug concentration within the solution either inside or outside the sac.

The accumulation of the drug in the mucosal layer can give false readings, but studying the drug both inside and outside can additionally give the mucosal component. This technique was popular a few decades ago, but its use in recent years is limited.

INTESTINAL TISSUE MOUNTS ON USSING/DIFFUSING CHAMBERS

An Ussing chamber consists of two halves clamped together with the epithelial tissue sandwiched between them. The intestinal tissue is cut into longitudinal segments of adequate length to fit between the openings at the two ends. The preparation of the tissue for the technique varies from laboratory to laboratory. In some cases the under-lying muscle layers are left as such, but their presence does not affect the permeability because the muscle layer is not a significant barrier. The removal of this layer in some cases allows for greater longevity and better integrity of the tissue because the stripped tissue can be oxygenated at a better rate. Often, electrical measurements are made using voltage clamps. These measurements are useful in multiple ways because they allow for the determination of both the integrity of the tissue over the experiment and also the polarity of transport. The simplified model of an Ussing chamber assembly is shown in **Figure 3-4**. The determination of the transport polarity determines the involvement of transport proteins for either influx or efflux. This technique has been used with varying degrees of success with mouse intestine [37]. This instrument and the technique is also used to measure permeability across other epithelial tissues such as ocular tissues and skin and even for cells grown on permeable support.

The *in vivo* and excised tissue models (*ex vivo*) often suffer from poor correlations with human studies because of a lack of genetic similarities between animal models and humans. The expression levels and the types of drug-metabolizing enzymes and drug transporters (both efflux and influx) vary significantly between rats and humans. Because of this genetic discrepancy, *in vitro* cell culture models either from the same species or with similar protein expression profiles as humans may better reflect the permeability characteristics of a molecule [38].

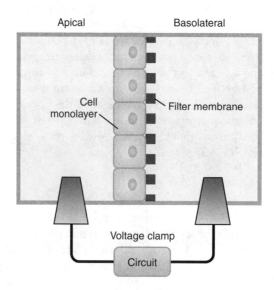

FIGURE 3-4 Simplified depiction of an Ussing chamber assembly.

ISOLATED INTESTINAL CELLS (ENTEROCYTES)

This technique involves isolating intestinal cells and growing them in culture media to study drug absorption. To prepare the cells, first the intestinal segment is cut and washed, and then the epithelial layers are exposed to either enzymes and chelating agents (alone or together) or treated with mechanical forces to dissociate the cells from the underlying tissues. This technique has very limited utility because most cells are destroyed or significantly weakened during the extraction process. Additionally, these cells when grown in culture sometimes do not settle and hence form a suspension culture, or they do not form strong enough monolayers to be useful to study transepithelial drug permeability. This technique is mainly used to study drug uptake within the cells and the metabolism of the drug by the epithelial cells.

MEMBRANE VESICLES

Brush-border membrane vesicles and basolateral membrane vesicles are the most commonly used intestinal membrane vesicles. These are generally used to study the uptake of the test molecule within them. Similar to isolated cells, these vesicles are also used to study drug uptake or metabolism by plasma membrane-bound enzymes. This system has been successfully used to study organic cation binding and PEPT1 mediated uptake of its substrates by the small intestine [39, 40]. Like the isolated cells, however, the lack of permeability characteristics make these incomplete models to mimic drug pharmacokinetics.

IN VITRO CELL CULTURE MODELS

Multiple immortalized cell lines have been derived from various organs of different species to represent the intestinal epithelia of humans. Most of these cell lines are derived from tumor tissues due to their rapid growth and ease of immortalization. Cell culture models can be used for the rapid estimation of intestinal permeability of drug candidates at a low cost, in a rapid manner, and without involving any animal or human tissues. An ideal intestinal cell culture model should have rapid cell growth, form confluent monolayers, and have similar physiological and biochemical makeup to that of differentiated intestinal epithelial cells.

Properties of an Ideal *In Vitro* Cell Culture Model

As previously mentioned, the *in vitro* model should be simple enough to be cost effective and easily reproducible yet complex enough to give an accurate estimation of the biological properties. Hence, to be considered as an effective cell culture model, it should fulfill the following requirements:

1. The cell culture model should resemble in surface morphology and topology the target organ.
2. The cells should be fast growing, have low cost of maintenance, and useful for rapid screening.
3. The cells should express all the proteins expressed by the target organ and in similar proportions to properly replicate drug–protein interactions.
4. The model should show good correlation with the mechanism of cellular permeability for compounds transported by both paracellular and transcellular routes
5. Physiochemical and pharmacokinetic characteristics of a drug may be modified based on the drug's environmental pH; thus, the model should be functional in the pH range prevailing in the target organ.
6. The model should be highly reproducible, that is, it should have low passage to passage variability.

Caucasian Colon Adenocarcinoma (Caco-2) Cells

Since they were first characterized as an intestinal permeability model in 1989, Caco-2 cells have been used as the workhorse in both industry and academia to study various aspects of intestinal permeability [41]. Although these cells were originally derived from colon carcinoma and not the small intestine, they display a lot of morphological features similar to the cells of the small intestine, such as presence of microvilli and tight intercellular junctions. One major advantage of Caco-2 cells is they express many intestinal drug-metabolizing enzymes such as the CYP family of enzymes, aminopeptidases, esterases, and sulfatases. Similarly, these cells also express many transporters present on the small intestine, such as bile acid transporters, large neutral amino acid transporter, biotin transporter, monocarboxylic acid transporter, PEPT1 and PEPT2, and various MDR transporters [42]. In the last 25 years, multiple research studies carried out across multiple countries have suggested a correlation between *in vitro* permeability values in Caco-2 cells and *in vivo* bioavailability of multiple drugs.

Encouraging *in vitro–in vivo* correlations have led to the widespread use of this model. Although the widespread use of these cells has established them as the major *in vitro* cell culture model to study drug transport, small differences in the handling of the cells in different laboratories has resulted in extensive heterogeneity within the wild-type Caco-2 cells. This gradual selection of phenotypically different cell populations of Caco-2 cells, referred to as phenotypic drift, has contributed to large variability in interlaboratory permeability measurements.

Other major problems associated with Caco-2 cells is the long culturing times of 17 to 21 days, which make these cells not ideal for high-throughput studies. These cells are also highly susceptible to bacterial contamination, which along with their long growth times makes them very difficult to maintain. Also, the long growth times combined with the frequent media requirements makes these cells more expensive to grow and maintain [42, 43].

Madin-Darby Canine Kidney Cells

The Madin-Darby canine kidney (MDCK) cell line is derived from dog renal epithelium. MDCK cells also differentiate into columnar epithelial cells and form tight junctions similar to Caco-2 cells but do it in much less time (3–5 days) when cultured on semipermeable membranes. The morphology of both Caco-2 and MDCK cells is compared in **Figure 3-5** both with low- and high-density seeding. Detailed studies have shown that permeability values for multiple drugs obtained using MDCK cells correlated well with both Caco-2 cells and human oral bioavailability. Because both MDCK and Caco-2 cells are derived from different organs of different species, the expression level of various transporters differs between the two cell lines.

The various transporters and their quantitative expression levels have been measured in both MDCK and Caco-2 cell lines [44, 45]. Expression levels of peptide transporter was found to be five times less in these cells when compared with Caco-2. Expression of monocarboxylic acid transporters on the MDCK cell line was found to correlate well with the levels found in human intestine. The presence of efflux pumps such as P-gp was also found to be comparable with Caco-2, although both cells showed less expression of these transporters when compared with human intestine.

One of the biggest advantages of MDCK cells is that these cells showed high levels of the transporter expression in 3 to 5 days post-seeding, whereas Caco-2 requires 17 to 21 days and longer (depending on the passage). Other transporters such as large neutral amino acid transporters and bile acid transporters were also expressed, albeit in insignificant amounts, and hence this cell line may not be suitable for estimating

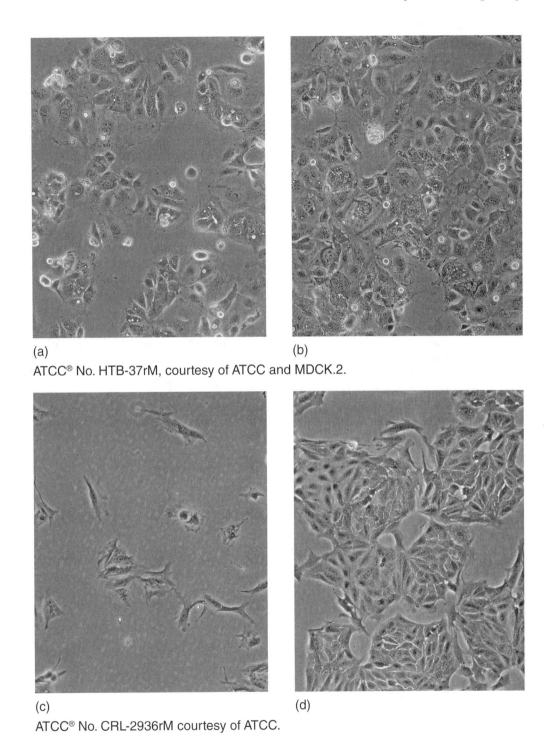

(a)   (b)

ATCC® No. HTB-37rM, courtesy of ATCC and MDCK.2.

(c)   (d)

ATCC® No. CRL-2936rM courtesy of ATCC.

FIGURE 3-5 Comparison between the morphology of Caco-2 and MDCK cells. (a) Caco-2 low density. (b) Caco-2 high density. (c) MDCK low density. (d) MDCK high density.

the effects of these transport systems on drug delivery. The faster growth and shorter differentiation time results in overall reduced costs. The MDCK cell line is a more robust cell line when compared with Caco-2 and requires less rigorous feeding over a smaller duration of time [41, 45].

Transfected MDCK Cell Lines

A number of influx and efflux transporters are present in the intestinal tract. Most of these proteins are expressed in significant quantities in Caco-2, which makes it a dominant cell line. But many transporters are not expressed at levels close to that observed in the human intestine. Thus, to overcome this shortcoming, genetically modified MDCK cell lines are being developed in which the plasmids containing genetic code for influx and efflux transporters are transfected, resulting in higher and more physiologically relevant expressions of these transporters. For example, the MDCK–MDR1 cell line in which the MDCK cells are transfected with the *MDR1* gene result in elevated expression of P-gp [46]. These monotransfected cell lines can study the contribution of a single transporter toward the bioavailability of the drug [47].

These transfected models add greatly to our knowledge and understanding of substrate specificity for a specific transporter. Information of substrate specificity can be further incorporated into computational modeling and *in silico* studies to design better substrate or inhibitor drug molecules. The transfected cell lines have already proved their utility in the field of drug interactions [48, 49]. Several compounds act as inducers or inhibitors of influx and efflux transporters. Hence, such interactions may lead to either elevation or reduction in the oral bioavailability of a coadministered drug, which shares the same transporter mechanism. These cell lines have the capability to function as high-throughput screening models for the estimation of transporter specificity. Transfected MDCK cells have been made as overexpressing transporters such as P-gp, MRPs (multiple members of the MRP family), breast cancer resistance protein, organic anion transporters, peptide transporters, and so on. Because of the interplay between efflux and metabolism in the intestine, MDCK cells with elevated expression levels of P-gp and CYP3A4 have also been developed and have been shown to be more relevant to permeability studies as compared with monotransfected cell lines [50].

2/4/A1 Cells

2/4/A1 is a fetal rat intestinal cell line reported to better represent the human small intestinal permeability when compared with Caco-2 cells, especially for passive transcellular and paracellular transport [51]. This is an immortalized cell line and forms well-differentiated monolayers with tight junctions similar to the human intestine. These cells also express multiple brush-border membrane enzymes and transporter proteins. Tight junctions in Caco-2 and MDCK cells are supposed to be higher than those observed in the small intestine. 2/4/A1 cells are proposed to be a better model to study the transport of mainly passively transported compounds through the paracellular route because of their closer correlation with intestinal tight junctions. The transport rate of poorly permeable compounds such as mannitol and creatinine across 2/4/A1 monolayers has been shown to be comparable with human jejunum, which is much faster than Caco-2 cells [52].

TC-7 Cells

TC-7 cells have been derived from Caco-2 cells as a subclone with higher expression of metabolizing enzymes. A comprehensive comparison between the permeability characteristics of TC-7 with parental Caco-2 cells has been reported [53, 54]. TC-7 clones have been reported to show similar cell morphology to Caco-2 cells. Brush-border membrane and microvilli are also present on TC-7 cells. These cells form tight junctions similar to Caco-2. The permeability values of passively and transcellularly absorbed compounds across TC-7 cells correlate well with Caco-2 cells and oral absorption in humans. The major difference between these cells and their parent cells is that these express higher levels of CYP3A4 enzyme, at levels similar to that of the human intestine. Because TC-7 cells are similar to Caco-2 cells in morphological, biochemical, and drug permeability properties, the cells appear to be a good alternative to Caco-2 cells in representing intestinal drug permeability studies, especially for those drugs highly susceptible to metabolism by CYP3A4 [55].

HT29 Cells

In the 1970s, Jørgen Fogh and coworkers developed various cell lines from human colonic carcinoma [56, 57]. Various cell types were isolated and cultured, out of which the HT29 cell line was able to undergo differentiation. This cell line also exhibited a phenotype similar to enterocytes when grown in glucose-free medium containing galactose instead [58, 59]. HT29-H cells are goblet cells that can produce mucin molecules, leading to the formation of a mucous layer similar to that present in human intestinal epithelia. At late confluence, HT29 cells appear to form a dense mucous gel with multiple mucous buds on the apical surface [53]. It was experimentally shown that the mucus produced by the human goblet cell monolayers act as a significant barrier to testosterone transport [60, 61]. This mucous layer can also act as a barrier to drug absorption because of resistance from the unstirred water layer. It can also act by stabilizing the interactions between the drug molecules being diffused and the components of the mucus. Factors affecting drug transport across the mucous barrier have been studied using this cell line. Lipophilicity was shown to be the major factor affecting transport across the mucous layer, with molecular net charge and size playing a role in limiting the transport [62, 63]. To further understand the role of mucus on drug transport, HT29-MTX, a subclone model, was developed. This cell line was derived from the parent cell line HT29 by growing cells for 6 months in a medium containing 1 μM methotrexate. This makes the cells gain the morphological and mucin-producing characteristics of goblet cells [64]. Becasue these cells still lack the expression levels of various proteins present in small intestine, Caco-2 cells have been co-cultured with HT29-MTX or HT29-H cells [65, 66].

IN SILICO METHODS

Advancements in computational technologies and improvements in our understanding of chemistry and structure activity relationships have promoted the use of *in silico* methods for determination of absorptive characteristics of the drugs. The most attractive thing about this technique is that it allows screening of compounds for absorptive efficacy even before the chemical synthesis takes place. Thus, this technique saves a lot of time and money by rapid testing of large libraries that would not be possible by any other physical or biological means. Because most molecules with less chances of going forward in the developmental process are eliminated through this process, it also reduces the ethical constraints of using a large number of animals and animal tissues for testing poor-quality drugs.

One of the major directing principles for the computational techniques is Lipinski's "rule of five," which uses some crude chemical characteristics to predict poor absorption for compounds [67]. The main parameters of the rule are that for a drug to be orally active, it should have no more than one violation of the following:

1. Molecular weight should not be greater than 500 Da.
2. H-bond donors in the molecule should not be greater than 5.

3. H-bond acceptors is the molecule should be less than 10.
4. The compound's lipophilicity, expressed as a quantity known as log *P*, should be less than 10.

These rules in their crude form have been moderately successful, and multiple exceptions to the rules exist. Over the years, many other parameters have been added or supplemented within the rule such as molecular refractivity, number of atoms within the molecule, and polar surface area [68].

In other *in silico* studies, more traditional quantitative structure–transport relationship models are used to predict cellular and tissue permeability. The advantage of quantitative structure–transport relationship models is that usually they tend to provide much more accurate determinants for success, especially when studied with small sample sizes. The major disadvantage of this technique is that it provides very little understanding of the molecular mechanisms responsible for the success or failure of a drug to permeate. Some laboratories have used a combination of the two approaches to achieve best results [69]. Currently, several models exist that claim to successfully predict human intestinal or Caco-2 permeability, but robust studies are needed to test their reliability. Unless the models are derived from diverse and reliable databases, their utility will probably remain limited to compounds that are closely related to the training sets used to initially develop them.

SUMMARY

The cost of developing a new drug entity keeps on increasing, and insufficient intestinal absorption represents a formidable impediment to the effective development of an oral drug product. Thus, knowledge of potential absorption characteristics of a compound while still in the discovery and development phase will increase the possibility of success. To achieve this goal, methods of predicting drug pharmacokinetic parameters are being applied earlier in the drug development process. In this chapter, we discussed high-throughput and high-efficiency methods for performing these screens, but currently no method fully satisfies all the criteria for an ideal model. Although high-speed assays are needed to screen large numbers of compounds in a short period of time, this should not be pursued at the expense of quality. An ideal protocol would serially eliminate more and more drugs by gradually moving to more complex systems to obtain drug molecules with the most potential for success with minimal and only necessary expenditure. Because biological activity and *in vivo* efficacy is the primary goal of all pharmaceutical scientists, if a highly efficient molecule is screened early enough for poor permeability characteristics, drug delivery scientists can further work on it to improve its shortcomings so the ultimate formulation ends in success.

REVIEW QUESTIONS

1. Which of the following mechanisms of drug transport involve the movement of the drug through the cell–cell junctions?
   a. Transcellular transport
   b. Paracellular transport
   c. Carrier mediated transport
   d. Efflux transport
2. What are the properties of an ideal *in vitro* cell culture model?

3. What are the main parameters of Lipinski's "rule of five"?
4. Which of the following cell lines produce a mucous layer?
    a. Caco-2 cells
    b. MDCK cells
    c. HT29 cells
    d. TC-7 cells
5. Which protein is over expressed in MDCK-MDR1 cells?
    a. P-glycoprotein (P-gp)
    b. Multidrug resistant protein 2 (MRP-2)
    c. Breast cancer resistance protein
    d. Oligopeptide transporter (PEPT-1)
6. Which of the following is a rat fetal cell line?
    a. HT29
    b. 2/4/A1
    c. MDCK
    d. Caco-2

REFERENCES

1. http://www.vetmed.vt.edu/education/curriculum/vm8054/Labs/Lab19/Lab19.htm
2. Madara JL. *Functional Morphology of Epithelium of the Small Intestine*, in *Comprehensive Physiology*. New York, NY: John Wiley & Sons; 2010.
3. Madara JL, Pappenheimer JR. Structural basis for physiological regulation of paracellular pathways in intestinal epithelia. *J Membr Biol*. 1987;100(2):149–164.
4. Pappenheimer JR, Reiss KZ. Contribution of solvent drag through intercellular junctions to absorption of nutrients by the small intestine of the rat. *J Membr Biol*. 1987;100(2):123–136.
5. Brayden DJ, et al. Passive transepithelial diltiazem absorption across intestinal tissue leading to tight junction openings. *J Control Rel*. 1996;38(2–3):193–203.
6. Fix JA. Strategies for delivery of peptides utilizing absorption-enhancing agents. *J Pharm Sci*. 1996;85(12):1282–1285.
7. Thelen K, Dressman JB. Cytochrome P450-mediated metabolism in the human gut wall. *J Pharm Pharmacol*. 2009;61(5):541–558.
8. Mouly S, Meune C, Bergmann JF. Mini-series: I. Basic science. Uncertainty and inaccuracy of predicting CYP-mediated in vivo drug interactions in the ICU from in vitro models: focus on CYP3A4. *Intensive Care Med*. 2009;35(3):417–429.
9. Harwood MD, et al. Absolute abundance and function of intestinal drug transporters: a prerequisite for fully mechanistic in vitro-in vivo extrapolation of oral drug absorption. *Biopharm Drug Dispos*. 2013;34(1):2–28.
10. Zhou SF, et al. Substrates and inhibitors of human multidrug resistance associated proteins and the implications in drug development. *Curr Med Chem*. 2008;15(20):1981–2039.
11. Li Y, Lu J, Paxton JW. The role of ABC and SLC transporters in the pharmacokinetics of dietary and herbal phytochemicals and their interactions with xenobiotics. *Curr Drug Metab*. 2012;13(5):624–639.
12. Kramer SD, et al. Lipid-bilayer permeation of drug-like compounds. *Chem Biodivers*. 2009;6(11):1900–1916.
13. Pade V, Stavchansky S. Estimation of the relative contribution of the transcellular and paracellular pathway to the transport of passively absorbed drugs in the Caco-2 cell culture model. *Pharm Res*. 1997;14(9):1210–1215.
14. Tsuji A, Tamai I. Carrier-mediated intestinal transport of drugs. *Pharm Res*. 1996;13(7):963–977.
15. Anderle P, Huang Y, Sadee W. Intestinal membrane transport of drugs and nutrients: genomics of membrane transporters using expression microarrays. *Eur J Pharm Sci*. 2004;21(1):17–24.
16. Dahan A, et al. Targeted prodrugs in oral drug delivery: the modern molecular biopharmaceutical approach. *Expert Opin Drug Deliv*. 2012;9(8):1001–1013.
17. Hu M, Amidon GL. Passive and carrier-mediated intestinal absorption components of captopril. *J Pharm Sci*. 1988;77(12):1007–1011.
18. Kramer W, et al. Interaction of renin inhibitors with the intestinal uptake system for oligopeptides and beta-lactam antibiotics. *Biochim Biophys Acta*. 1990;1027(1):25–30.

19. Herrera-Ruiz D, et al. Spatial expression patterns of peptide transporters in the human and rat gastrointestinal tracts, Caco-2 in vitro cell culture model, and multiple human tissues. *AAPS Pharm Sci*. 2001;3(1):E9.

20. Lorico A, et al. Disruption of the murine MRP (multidrug resistance protein) gene leads to increased sensitivity to etoposide (VP-16) and increased levels of glutathione. *Cancer Res*. 1997;57(23):5238–5242.

21. Homolya L, Varadi A, Sarkadi B. Multidrug resistance-associated proteins: export pumps for conjugates with glutathione, glucuronate or sulfate. *Biofactors*. 2003;17(1–4):103–114.

22. Desai PV, Raub TJ, Blanco MJ. How hydrogen bonds impact P-glycoprotein transport and permeability. *Bioorg Med Chem Lett*. 2012;22(21):6540–6548.

23. Ling V. Multidrug resistance: molecular mechanisms and clinical relevance. *Cancer Chemother Pharmacol*. 1997;40(Suppl.):S3–S8.

24. Sharom FJ. The P-glycoprotein multidrug transporter. *Essays Biochem*. 2011;50(1):161–178.

25. Han HK. Role of transporters in drug interactions. *Arch Pharm Res*. 2011;34(11):1865–1877.

26. Kool M, et al. Analysis of expression of cMOAT (MRP2), MRP3, MRP4, and MRP5, homologues of the multidrug resistance-associated protein gene (MRP1), in human cancer cell lines. *Cancer Res*. 1997;57(16):3537–3547.

27. Doyle LA, et al. A multidrug resistance transporter from human MCF-7 breast cancer cells. *Proc Natl Acad Sci USA*. 1998;95(26):15665–15670.

28. Miyake K, et al. Molecular cloning of cDNAs which are highly overexpressed in mitoxantrone-resistant cells: demonstration of homology to ABC transport genes. *Cancer Res*. 1999;59(1):8–13.

29. Ritchie M, Tchistiakova L, Scott N. Implications of receptor-mediated endocytosis and intracellular trafficking dynamics in the development of antibody drug conjugates. *MAbs*. 2013;5(1):13–21.

30. Shen L, Lang ML, Wade WF. The ins and outs of getting in: structures and signals that enhance BCR or Fc receptor-mediated antigen presentation. *Immunopharmacology*. 2000;49(3):227–240.

31. Kraehenbuhl JP, Campiche MA. Early stages of intestinal absorption of specific antibodies in the newborn. An ultrastructural, cytochemical, and immunological study in the pig, rat, and rabbit. *J Cell Biol*. 1969;42(2):345–365.

32. Clark SL, Jr. The ingestion of proteins and colloidal materials by columnar absorptive cells of the small intestine in suckling rats and mice. *J Biophys Biochem Cytol*. 1959;5(1):41–50.

33. Mostov KE. Transepithelial transport of immunoglobulins. *Annu Rev Immunol*. 1994;12:63–84.

34. Lazaro E, Rafols C, Roses M. Characterization of immobilized artificial membrane (IAM) and XTerra columns by means of chromatographic models. *J Chromatogr A*. 2005;1081(2):163–173.

35. Reis JM, Sinko B, Serra CH. Parallel artificial membrane permeability assay (PAMPA)—is it better than Caco-2 for human passive permeability prediction? *Mini Rev Med Chem*. 2010;10(11):1071–1076.

36. Ungell AL, et al. Membrane transport of drugs in different regions of the intestinal tract of the rat. *J Pharm Sci*. 1998;87(3):360–366.

37. Lennernas H, Nylander S, Ungell AL. Jejunal permeability: a comparison between the Ussing chamber technique and the single-pass perfusion in humans. *Pharm Res*. 1997;14(5):667–671.

38. Cao X, et al. Why is it challenging to predict intestinal drug absorption and oral bioavailability in human using rat model? *Pharm Res*. 2006;23(8):1675–1686.

39. Sugawara M, et al. Uptake of dipeptide and beta-lactam antibiotics by the basolateral membrane vesicles prepared from rat kidney. *Biochim Biophys Acta*. 2003;1609(1):39–44.

40. Dudeja PK, et al. Mechanism of thiamine uptake by human jejunal brush-border membrane vesicles. *Am J Physiol Cell Physiol*. 2001;281(3):C786–C792.

41. Volpe DA. Drug-permeability and transporter assays in Caco-2 and MDCK cell lines. *Future Med Chem*. 2011;3(16):2063–2077.

42. Sun H, et al. The Caco-2 cell monolayer: usefulness and limitations. *Expert Opin Drug Metab Toxicol*. 2008;4(4):395–411.

43. Press B, Di Grandi D. Permeability for intestinal absorption: Caco-2 assay and related issues. *Curr Drug Metab*. 2008;9(9):893–900.

44. Putnam WS, et al. Functional characterization of monocarboxylic acid, large neutral amino acid, bile acid and peptide transporters, and P-glycoprotein in MDCK and Caco-2 cells. *J Pharm Sci*. 2002;91(12):2622–2635.

45. Putnam WS, et al. Comparison of bidirectional cephalexin transport across MDCK and caco-2 cell monolayers: interactions with peptide transporters. *Pharm Res*. 2002;19(1):27–33.

46. de Souza J, et al. Comparison of bidirectional lamivudine and zidovudine transport using MDCK, MDCK-MDR1, and Caco-2 cell monolayers. *J Pharm Sci*. 2009;98(11):4413–4419.

47. Lam KCL, Rajaraman G. Assessment of P-glycoprotein substrate and inhibition potential of test compounds in MDR1-transfected MDCK cells. *Curr Prot Pharmacol*. 2012; DOI: 10.1002/0471141755.ph0713s58

48. Pal D, et al. Efflux transporters- and cytochrome P-450-mediated interactions between drugs of abuse and antiretrovirals. *Life Sci.* 2011;88(21–22):959–971.

49. Pal D, Mitra AK. MDR- and CYP3A4-mediated drug-drug interactions. *J Neuroimmune Pharmacol.* 2006;1(3):323–339.

50. Kwatra D, et al. Transfected MDCK cell line with enhanced expression of CYP3A4 and P-glycoprotein as a model to study their role in drug transport and metabolism. *Mol Pharm.* 2012;9(7):1877–1886.

51. Fagerholm U. Prediction of human pharmacokinetics—gastrointestinal absorption. *J Pharm Pharmacol.* 2007;59(7):905–916.

52. Tavelin S, et al. Prediction of the oral absorption of low-permeability drugs using small intestine-like 2/4/A1 cell monolayers. *Pharm Res.* 2003;20(3):397–405.

53. Pontier C, et al. HT29-MTX and Caco-2/TC7 monolayers as predictive models for human intestinal absorption: role of the mucus layer. *J Pharm Sci.* 2001;90(10):1608–1619.

54. Gres MC, et al. Correlation between oral drug absorption in humans, and apparent drug permeability in TC-7 cells, a human epithelial intestinal cell line: comparison with the parental Caco-2 cell line. *Pharm Res.* 1998;15(5):726–733.

55. Balimane PV, Chong S. Cell culture-based models for intestinal permeability: a critique. *Drug Discov Today.* 2005;10(5):335–343.

56. Fogh J, Sykes JA. A comparison of methods for morphological studies of cultured cells. *In Vitro.* 1972;7(4):206–227.

57. Fogh J, Trempe G. New human tumor cell lines. In: J Fogh, ed. *Human Tumor Cells In Vitro.* Heidelberg, Germany, Springer; 1975:115–159.

58. Huet C, et al. Absorptive and mucus-secreting subclones isolated from a multipotent intestinal cell line (HT-29) provide new models for cell polarity and terminal differentiation. *J Cell Biol.* 1987;105(1):345–357.

59. Zweibaum A, et al. Enterocytic differentiation of a subpopulation of the human colon tumor cell line HT-29 selected for growth in sugar-free medium and its inhibition by glucose. *J Cell Physiol.* 1985;122(1):21–29.

60. Wikman A, et al. A drug absorption model based on the mucus layer producing human intestinal goblet cell line HT29-H. *Pharm Res.* 1993;10(6):843–852.

61. Karlsson J, Wikman A, Artursson P. The mucus layer as a barrier to drug absorption in monolayers of human intestinal epithelial HT29-H goblet cells. *Int J Pharm.* 1993;99(2):209–218.

62. Larhed AW, et al. Diffusion of drugs in native and purified gastrointestinal mucus. *J Pharm Sci.* 1997;86(6):660–665.

63. Larhed AW, Artursson P, Bjork E. The influence of intestinal mucus components on the diffusion of drugs. *Pharm Res.* 1998;15(1):66–71.

64. Lesuffleur T, et al. Growth adaptation to methotrexate of HT-29 human colon carcinoma cells is associated with their ability to differentiate into columnar absorptive and mucus-secreting cells. *Cancer Res.* 1990;50(19):6334–6343.

65. Hilgendorf C, et al. Caco-2 versus caco-2/HT29-MTX co-cultured cell lines: permeabilities via diffusion, inside-and outside-directed carrier-mediated transport. *J Pharm Sci.* 2000;89(1):63–75.

66. Wikman-Larhed A, Artursson P. Co-cultures of human intestinal goblet (HT29-H) and absorptive (Caco-2) cells for studies of drug and peptide absorption. *Eur J Pharm Sci.* 1995;3(3):171–183.

67. Lipinski CA, et al. Experimental and computational approaches to estimate solubility and permeability in drug discovery and development settings. *Adv Drug Deliv Rev.* 2001;46(1-3):3–26.

68. Walters WP. Going further than Lipinski's rule in drug design. *Expert Opin Drug Discov.* 2012;7(2):99–107.

69. Chen Y, et al. Discovery of a novel acetylcholinesterase inhibitor by structure-based virtual screening techniques. *Bioorg Med Chem Lett.* 2012;22(9):3181–3187.

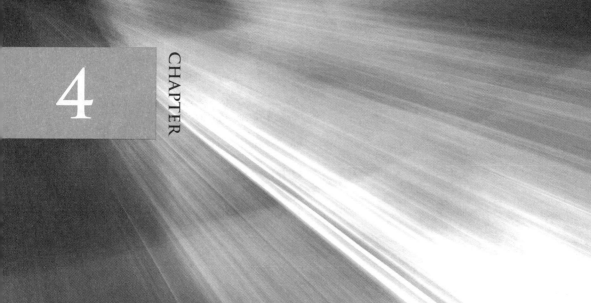

ROUTES OF DRUG DELIVERY

SAI H. S. BODDU AND RIPAL GAUDANA

CHAPTER OBJECTIVES

Upon completing this chapter, the reader should be able to

▸ Recognize common pharmaceutical dosage forms.

▸ Understand the purpose for multiple routes of administration to deliver medication.

▸ Comprehend factors that must be considered in dosage form design and selection based on the patient being treated.

▸ Describe biopharmaceutically relevant advantages and disadvantages of various drug delivery routes.

CHAPTER OUTLINE

INTRODUCTION

Drug delivery is the process of administering pharmaceutical compounds to humans or animals to achieve therapeutic benefits. Every drug has an optimum concentration that should be attained in the blood to exhibit therapeutic benefit. Any value beyond the optimum therapeutic concentration range is not desirable. The route of administration significantly affects the efficacy of drugs and is defined as the method or path by which a drug substance enters the body. For local therapy, drugs are directly applied to skin, nose, ear, or eye, depending on the disease site. Systemic effects are generally achieved by oral and parenteral administration. The pharmacokinetic parameters such as onset of action, absorption, bioavailability, time to peak serum concentration, and peak serum concentration are significantly influenced by the route of administration.

Table 4-1 shows the duration for onset of action based on routes of administration. However, other parameters such as clearance, distribution metabolism, and protein binding remain unaffected. For example, the systemic bioavailability of misoprostol (prostaglandin E_1 analogue used in treatment of peptic ulcers, medical abortion, and

TABLE 4-1 Routes of administration, along with duration for onset of action	
Route of Administration	**Duration for Onset of Action**
Intravenous	30–60 sec
Endotracheal	2–3 min
Inhalation	2–3 min
Sublingual	3–5 min
Intramuscular	10–20 min
Subcutaneous	15–30 min
Rectal	5–30 min
Ingestion	30–90 min
Transdermal	40–60 min

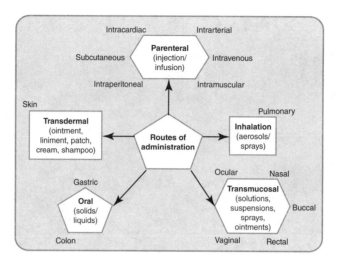

FIGURE 4-1 Routes of drug administration.

cervical priming) was studied after both vaginal and oral administrations. Results demonstrated that the area under the curve of misoprostol after vaginal administration was three times higher than it was with oral administration [1]. Increased understanding of the drug transport mechanisms resulted in identification of alternative methods of drug administration with improved ability to manage a specific problem [2].

Advances in genetic engineering and biotechnology resulted in discovery and large-scale production of therapeutic peptides and vaccines. However, development of an oral drug delivery system for macromolecules is challenging because of the presence of biological barriers (proteolysis in stomach pH, poor permeation in gastrointestinal [GI] epithelium, and membrane efflux) that restrict their absorption from the GI tract [3]. Although parenteral administration overcomes the above-mentioned disadvantages, it is associated with increased cost of therapy and patient dissatisfaction because drug administration in the form of frequent injections. In an attempt to improve patient compliance, alternative noninvasive routes such as pulmonary, nasal, rectal, and transdermal routes, among others, has gained popularity [4]. Drug delivery routes can be broadly classified under five categories (**Figure 4–1**) [5]:

1. Oral route
2. Parenteral route
3. Transmucosal route
4. Transdermal route
5. Inhalation

ORAL ROUTE

Despite advances in drug delivery, oral administration remains the most preferred route among patients and clinicians [6]. The oral drug delivery market is growing rapidly and constitutes a major market share compared with other routes of administration (**Figure 4–2**). Per os, abbreviated as PO, is a Latin term that means "by way of the mouth." Most drugs are administered in the form of tablets, capsules, powder, suspensions, and solutions (**Figure 4–3**). A tablet is a compressed form of powder that consists of a drug along with other inactive ingredients that allow proper disintegration,

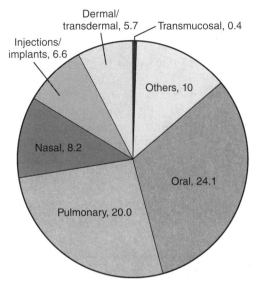

FIGURE 4-2 Market value of various pharmaceuticals depending on route of administration. (*Data* from Viswanathan S. Advances in drug delivery. *Pharmac Form Qual.* 2004;25,June/July:20–28.)

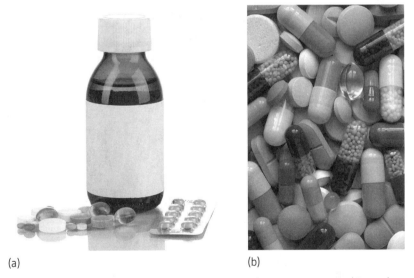

(a)   (b)

FIGURE 4-3 Commonly administered oral dosage forms. (Photo a © serezniy/iStock/Thinkstock; photo b © ajt/ShutterStock, Inc.)

dissolution, and absorption of the dosage form. Drugs are usually enclosed in a soft or hard soluble gelatin shell in capsule dosage form. Liquid dosage forms such as solutions, suspensions, and syrups are more rapidly absorbed compared with solid dosage forms, which require disintegration and dissolution before absorption. The absorption of drugs administered orally occurs partly in the mouth and stomach, and a major fraction is absorbed in the small intestine. Drugs taken orally are exposed to the harsh, acidic, and enzymatically rich environments of the stomach and duodenum. The acidic environment of the stomach (pH 2–3), along with enzymes such as proteases and lipases, alters or destroys orally administered drugs.

Epithelial cells of the GI tract form tight junctions, preventing the diffusion of most drug molecules [7, 8]. Moreover, orally administered drugs are subjected to first-pass hepatic clearance (first-pass metabolism) and GI metabolism by cytochrome P450 3A4. First-pass metabolism is mainly contributed by enzymes present in GI lumen, gut wall, and liver (**Figure 4-4**) [9]. This process can significantly reduce the amount of drug absorbed into systemic circulation. Apart from the metabolizing enzymes, efflux proteins belonging to the ATP-binding cassette transporter family, particularly ABCB1/ P-glycoprotein, present on the inner leaflet of apical membrane resist the entry of drug molecules into systemic circulation [10]. Drugs that undergo significant first-pass metabolism include buprenorphine, cimetidine, diazepam, Demerol, imipramine, lidocaine, morphine, midazolam, and propranolol.

Drugs can be protected from the harsh acidic environment of the stomach by coating tablets and capsules with acid-stable materials such as Eudragit® (poly(meth)acrylate) polymers. Amorphous solid dispersions of Eudragit 4155 F and polyvinylpyrrolidone of drug/polymer systems exhibited good stability in the stomach and are used in colon-specific delivery [11]. Mucoadhesive polymers such as chitosan increase the bioavailability of drugs by increasing the mucosal adherence of dosage forms. Chitosan is a positively charged polymer that binds to the cell membrane. It is known to increase the paracellular permeability of drugs by decreasing the transepithelial electrical resistance of cell monolayers [12].

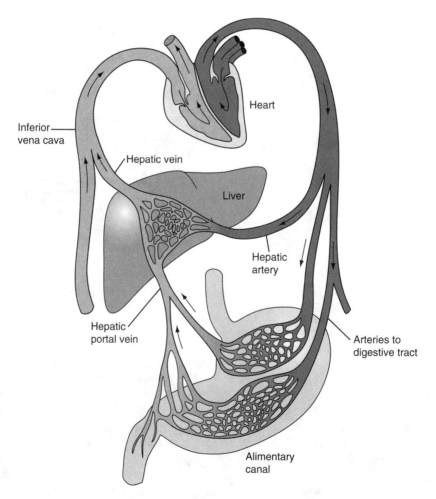

FIGURE 4-4 Hepatic portal veins responsible for first-pass metabolism.

Drug absorption is also affected by food and GI motility. The bioavailability of propranolol is higher when taken with food, griseofulvin absorption is higher after a fatty meal, and absorption is slower for tetracycline and penicillin when taken with food. Hence, patient instructions often include a direction to take on an empty stomach or with food. Nonsteroidal anti-inflammatory drugs, when taken orally on an empty stomach, can harm the stomach lining and result in the formation of ulcers.

Advantages of the oral route are:

- Most widely used route with high acceptance by patients
- Highly economical with possibility of self-medication
- Accommodates various types of dosage forms
- Does not require sterile manufacturing conditions

Disadvantages of the oral route are:

- Oral administration may not be suitable in clinical emergencies.
- Oral administration may not be suitable for children and unconscious patients.
- Drugs with bitter taste and bad odor may be associated with patient noncompliance.
- Oral administration may be associated with irritation to the gastric mucosa (e.g., salicylic acid).
- The acid content present in the stomach and digestive enzymes tend to degrade most drugs before absorption; therefore, the oral route is not preferred for protein and peptide drugs.
- The oral route is associated with hepatic first-pass metabolism, wherein the drugs are inactivated by the liver before entering systemic circulation. For example, glyceryl trinitrate is inactivated by hepatic mono-oxygenase in liver.
- Oral administration may not be suitable for drug targeting specific organs.

PARENTERAL ROUTE

In Greek/Latin language "par" means beyond and "enteral" means intestinal. Hence, the parenteral route involves the administration of drugs by a route other than the GI tract (enteron). In the parenteral route, drugs are directly introduced to systemic circulation. A recent data monitor report suggested a shift in market share away from orals to injectable drugs by the year 2014. The annual sale of injectables is expected to increase by $49 billion by 2014 due to several underlying factors such as molecular type of actives, therapeutic focus, and lifecycle stage.

This route involves the administration of drugs using a needle and syringe, which is plastic (disposable) or glass. To avoid frequent injections, the drug product can be manufactured in ways that prolong the drug release and absorption from the injection site for hours, days, or longer. The parenteral route is preferred when drug administration by the oral route fails to achieve adequate bioavailability or when rapid onset of action is required.

Advantages of parenteral administration are:

- Onset of action is fast, usually 15 to 30 seconds for intravenous and 3 to 5 minutes for intramuscular.
- Bioavailability of drugs is 100%.
- Parenteral administration can provide sustained release of drugs (days to months), for example, Depo-Provera used for birth control.
- It is a suitable alternative for drugs that are irritant to the gut.
- Intravenous infusion can deliver medication in a continuous manner (e.g., morphine for patients suffering from continuous pain).

Disadvantages of parenteral administration are:

- Patients may require assistance in administration.
- Patients may fear needles and injection, also known as belonephobia.
- There is a risk of HIV and other infectious disease transmission from needle sharing.
- Sterile preparations are required.

Generally, parenteral administration involves drug administration via the following pathways. The *intravenous route* is the administration of drugs directly into the vein using a syringe attached to a hollow needle. Drugs are administered either via direct injection with the syringe or by perfusion (**Figure 4-5**). By definition, the bioavailability of drugs after intravenous administration is 100%. The needle is introduced through the skin into a vein (an arm vein or metacarpal vein), and the contents of the syringe are injected through the needle into the bloodstream. After intravenous administration, the therapeutic effects are quickly achieved, as the initial absorption step is absent. Drug levels are accurately controlled, and it is suitable for large volumes of drugs. A peripheral IV line consists of a short catheter inserted through the skin into a peripheral vein in the hand, arm, foot, or leg. Sometimes veins in the scalp are used in infants. Central IV lines flow through a catheter attached to a tip placed in the large vein (inferior vena cava or superior vena cava or within the right atrium of the heart). Administration of drugs via central IV lines delivers them to the heart and then to the rest of the body. This is widely used for anticancer drugs that are irritating to peripheral veins due to their higher concentration and chemical composition.

Intravenous injections are also preferred for administration of high-molecular-weight compounds, especially protein and peptide drugs. However, in most cases protein formulations exhibit poor pharmacokinetic profiles because of rapid metabolism and clearance. Novel approaches such as PEGylation (covalent attachment of poly(ethylene glycol) [PEG] to protein), acylation, amino acid substitutions, and glycosylation (attaching glycans to proteins) are being used to alleviate metabolic degradation and plasma clearance. This technique also improves the safety profiles of proteins by shielding the immunogenic and antigenic epitopes. PEG is widely used in conjugation

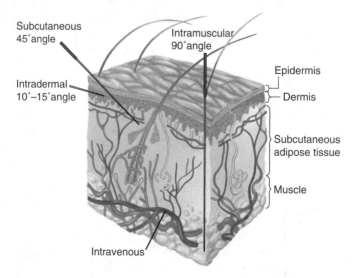

FIGURE 4-5 Subcutaneous injection of insulin.

because it is nontoxic, inexpensive, easily activated for conjugation, and commercially available with low polydispersity [13]. For example, interferon-α is absorbed rapidly (half-life of 2.3 hours) when administered subcutaneously, with an elimination half-life of 3 to 8 hours, whereas PEGylation of interferon-α with a 12-kDa linear PEG (PEG-interferon alfa-2b) and 40-kDa branched PEG (PEG-interferon alfa-2a) increases its half-life to 7 and 50 hours and elimination half-life to 4 and 11 days, respectively. The distribution of particles after intravenous injection depends on their size. Particles smaller than 0.1 µm accumulate in the bone marrow, whereas particles larger than 7 µm remain in the lungs. Particles between 0.1 and 7 µm are mostly taken up by the liver and the spleen.

Advantages of the intravenous route are:

- Provides rapid onset of action
- Possible to administer large quantities of drug
- Useful for administration of irritating or hypertonic solutions
- Provides high systemic bioavailability

Disadvantages of the intravenous route are:

- Injection leaks from veins may harm nearby tissues and result in irritation.
- The speed of drug administration should be constant.
- Reversal of drug action may not be possible.
- Oily solutions are not preferred for intravenous route.

The *subcutaneous route* involves administration of drugs into the fatty tissue below the skin (Figure 4-5). The drug slowly moves into the capillaries or reaches the bloodstream through the lymphatic vessels. This route is used most popularly for protein drugs such as insulin that are degraded in the intestine when taken orally. The absorption of drugs occurs slowly in a constant manner. The volume of fluid injected is limited, with a variable rate of resorption depending on local factors: sclerosis and circulatory state (vasodilatation and vasoconstriction) (e.g., heparin and insulin).

Advantages of the subcutaneous route are:

- Can be self-administered by the patient
- Slow and complete drug absorption

Disadvantages of the subcutaneous route are:

- This route is considered to be painful.
- Irritant drugs may result in tissue damage.
- A maximum of 2 mL can be injected.

The *intramuscular route* involves administration of drugs into muscle mass (upper arm, thigh, or buttock) (Figure 4-5). Unlike subcutaneous injection, intramuscular injection involves the use of a larger needle and administration of drugs into deeper tissues. This route is used for administering fairly large amounts of medication compared with the subcutaneous route. After intramuscular administration, drug absorption depends on physicochemical properties. Intramuscular injections are administered to vastus lateralis, dorsogluteal, ventrogluteal, and deltoid muscles (**Figure 4-6**). Upper and outer quadrants of the buttock (gluteal muscles) are used for drug administration to avoid sciatic nerve damage. Drugs administered as aqueous solutions are rapidly absorbed. For slow and constant absorption, drugs are administered in oils or other repository vehicles in a suspended form. However, the duration for onset depends on how quickly the drug is absorbed into the bloodstream from the muscle.

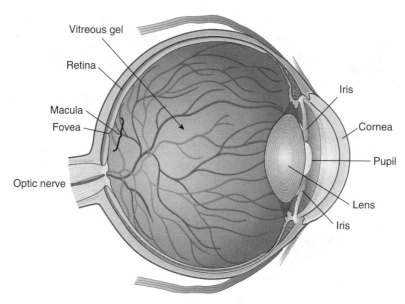

FIGURE 4-6 Structure of the eye.

Advantages of the intramuscular route are:

* Useful for suspensions and irritant solutions
* Large muscle mass available for drug administration (e.g., deltoid muscle and intragluteal)
* Offers uniform and slow drug absorption

Disadvantages of the intramuscular route are:

* A skilled person is required for drug administration.
* Careless drug administration may result in damage to nerves.
* A maximum of 10 mL may be administered by this route.

Intradermal injection is administration of drug in a small quantity beneath the skin (e.g., penicillin and BCG vaccine). The *intra-arterial route* involves administration of drugs directly into the artery and is widely used for administration of vasodilators and anesthetics (fentanyl, atropine, succinylcholine, pancuronium, and midazolam) into arteries. The intra-arterial route strictly requires the dissolution of drugs in aqueous solution.

Intrathecal injection is administration of drugs directly into the subarachnoid space of the spine or the cerebrospinal fluid to avoid the blood–brain barrier. Intrathecal injection is very painful, and hence a small amount of local anesthetic is used to numb the injection site. This route is used for producing rapid local effects on the brain, spinal cord, or meningeal layers of tissue covering them (e.g., anesthetics, antibiotics, and analgesics). Drugs administered intrathecally are readily prepared by the pharmacist or technician because they should not contain preservatives or other harmful excipients that are often present in standard injectable drug preparations. Intrathecal administration is also preferred for brain and spinal cord delivery of hydrophilic anticancer agents such as methotrexate.

Intraperitoneal injection is the injection of drugs directly into the peritoneal cavity. The intraperitoneal route is generally preferred for veterinary medicines and systemic administration of drugs in animal testing due to the ease of administration as compared with other parenteral methods. In humans, this route is widely used for replacement of blood or fluids in large amounts. Intraperitoneal administration reduces the systemic exposure of toxic chemotherapeutic agents and is particularly used in ovarian cancer treatment. After intraperitoneal administration, drugs partition inside various organs, bathing the peritoneal cavity fluids based on the physicochemical properties of drug molecules, time of exposure, and concentration administered.

Intramedullary injection is the administration of drugs directly injected into bone marrow. *Intra-articular injection* is the administration of drugs directly injected into joints. Finally, *intracavernous injection* is the injection of a drug into the base of the penis for treatment of erectile dysfunction in men. This route is preferred for the administration of vasodilators including prostaglandin, papaverine, and phentolamine.

TRANSMUCOSAL ROUTE

Mucous membranes coat the internal passages and orifices of the body with a thick fluid also called mucus. Buccal, sublingual, nasal, vaginal, and ocular mucosal linings are considered potential sites for drug administration because they offer distinct advantages over oral administration. Mucosal delivery provides noninvasive delivery to systemic circulation with a rapid onset of action. Drugs delivered through mucosa do not undergo first-pass metabolism. Transmucosal delivery requires the attachment or the retention of the drug delivery system on the mucosal surface for optimal bioavailability [14]. Mucoadhesive polymers, including polyacrylic acid, polycarbophil, sodium alginate, and chitosan, attach to the mucin surface through electrostatic or Vander Waal's force. More recently, inserts that are made of mucoadhesive polymers have been successfully used in the treatment of various diseases [15]. For example, drug-loaded polymeric microparticles are used in the controlled buccal delivery of antimicrobial, antifungal, antibiotic, local anesthetic, and antiviral drugs [14, 16].

Buccal mucosa involves the administration of drugs between the cheek and gums/gingiva. The buccal mucosa consists of leaky epithelia and has 4 to 4,000 times greater permeability than that of the skin. After buccal/sublingual administration, drugs enter the systemic circulation in 1 to 2 minutes, and peak blood levels are attained in within 10 to 15 minutes. This route is more preferable for the delivery of protein and peptide drugs. The absorption of drug is slow, and hence penetration enhancers are added to the formulation to increase the permeation rate without irritation or damage to the mucosa. These agents increase drug penetration by transiently altering the lipid bilayer or by decreasing the viscoelasticity of the mucous layer. Some of the widely used penetration enhancers include sodium EDTA, sodium dodecyl sulfate, polyoxyethylene-20-cetyl ether, benzalkonium chloride, sodium taurocholate and Azones® [14].

Delivery of drugs via the buccal route acts as a substitute for the oral route of drug administration. Buccal delivery prevents the first-pass metabolism of drugs and degradation in the harsh acidic GI environment. Drugs are administered in the form of adhesive patches, adhesive tablets, adhesive gels, and buccal films. Buccal tablets are hard and require 4 hours for disintegration. Several drug molecules such as acyclovir, salicylic acid, propranolol, dextran, α-interferon, luteinizing hormone-releasing hormone, and octreotide have been studied for buccal delivery [17].

Advantages of buccal delivery are:

- First-pass metabolism is avoided.
- The route prevents the degradation of drugs in stomach pH and enhances drug stability.
- Even though the rectal, vaginal, and ocular mucosal delivery routes offer similar advantages, they have poor patient acceptability compared with the buccal route.

Disadvantages of buccal delivery are:

- Advantages are lost if the buccal tablets are swallowed.
- Dose limit is small.
- This route of administration is potentially limited by palatability of the final formulation, and bitter drugs cannot be administered by this route due to patient noncompliance.

The *sublingual route* involves the administration of drugs under the tongue. The thin epithelial layer and large capillary network improves drug absorption and produces faster onset of action without first-pass metabolism. Once drug molecules are liberated from the dosage forms, they come in contact with the mucous membrane underneath the buccal mucosa or tongue.

The sublingual route is the most widely studied of the mucosal routes. Usually, sublingual dosage forms consist of rapidly disintegrating tablets or soft gelatin capsules filled with liquid drug. Such systems provide high drug concentrations in the sublingual region, which facilitates their absorption into systemic circulation. Sublingual mucosa is more permeable than buccal mucosa and thus provides rapid absorption and good bioavailability. Apart from the solubility of drugs in saliva, other factors including pH, molecular weight, and lipid solubility determine the bioavailability of drugs after sublingual administration. This route is also suitable for potent drugs. Being more direct and faster (requires less than 2 minutes for disintegration), drugs delivered sublingually are less prone to degradation by salivary enzymes before entering the bloodstream, whereas orally administered drugs must survive passage through stomach acid or bile and through other enzymes such as monoamine oxidase and first-pass metabolism. This route is popularly used for cardiovascular drugs, barbiturates, steroids, vitamins, and enzymes. For example, the ephedrine HCl tablet is administered by the sublingual route for asthma patients. The sublingual route is also good for nitroglycerin used in the treatment of angina (chest pain caused by an inadequate blood supply to the heart muscle) due to its rapid absorption.

Advantages of the sublingual route are:

- Onset of action is very fast and, therefore, is widely used for treatment of asthma and angina.
- Drug effects can be reversed by spitting tablet out.
- First-pass effect is avoided.

Disadvantages of the sublingual route are:

- Administration may result in toxic cardiac effects.
- Long-term administration may result in tooth discoloration and decay due to acidic or otherwise caustic drugs and fillers.
- It is difficult to place the device in the sublingual cavity, because it consists of immobile mucosa that is continuously washed by saliva.

The *sublabial* route involves the administration of drugs between the lip and the gingiva (e.g., glyceryl trinitrate in angina pectoris).

The nasal cavity is the uppermost portion of the human respiratory system, which moistens and warms the incoming air and filters out harmful particles. The nose consists of two nostrils separated by a septum. The route has been widely used for local, systemic, and central nervous system delivery. This route is more preferred by pediatric patients than the oral and buccal routes. The nasal cavity is highly vascular in nature, and hence large polar molecules (molecular weight <1,000 Da) administered in the form of solutions are rapidly absorbed. For larger molecules (molecular weight <6,000 Da), good bioavailability is achieved by use of penetration enhancers.

Over the last decade, the nasal route has been highly exploited for systemic delivery of peptides and proteins that require a rapid onset of action. Some of the marketed products of peptide drugs include buserelin from Aventis, calcitonin by Novartis, and desmopressin from Ferring [18]. The nasal cavity consists of a mucosal layer that is highly vascularized. The duration for onset of action is within 5 minutes for smaller drug molecules, and hence this route is preferred to oral administration for a faster effect. The pharmacokinetics and bioavailability of lipophilic drugs after nasal administration are similar to those of intravenous injections. Fentanyl is a good example, as the T_{max} after nasal administration is rapid (<7 minutes) with a bioavailability of 80% [19]. The bioavailability of small polar molecules and larger peptides such as insulin and calcitonin is approximately 10% and 1%, respectively. One of the major challenges is that drugs are rapidly cleared from the nasal cavity due to efficient physiological clearance mechanisms. In an attempt to increase the retention time of the drug in the nasal cavity, novel drug delivery systems such as liposomes, nanoparticles, and microparticles made of bioadhesive polymers are being investigated. Morphine is an opioid analgesic with a log P = 0.89, and bioavailability after nasal administration of simple solution is 5% to 10% with a T_{max} of 40 minutes. However, chitosan-based formulations of morphine resulted in a five- to sixfold increase of bioavailability (~60%) with a T_{max} of 15 minutes or less [20]. Several locally acting drugs such as decongestants and antiallergics and systemically acting drugs such as antimigraines and hormones have been successfully administered. Apart from the above-mentioned drugs, anesthetics and antiemetics are also administered via the nasal route.

Advantages of nasal administration are:

- Ease of administration is associated with nasal drops and sprays.
- The nasal cavity is covered by a highly vascularized and thin mucosa.
- Drug permeability of the nasal mucosa is high compared with GI mucosa and epidermis.
- Drug molecules can enter the blood circulation directly without first-pass hepatic and intestinal metabolism.
- It is the most favorable route for delivery protein and peptides.
- Rapid absorption and onset of action is quick, about 5 minutes.

Disadvantages of nasal administration are:

- This route is mainly suitable for potent drugs, as limited by volume sprayed.
- Drugs that require frequent dosing may be less suitable due to the risk of long-term side effects to the nasal epithelium.
- Nasal administration may be associated with variability in systemic drug concentrations.
- The effect of a cold or upper respiratory infection on nasal drug delivery remains unclear.

The eye is a highly protected organ, and designing an effective therapy for ocular diseases is considered a challenging task. The anterior segment is mainly protected by the eyelids, and the posterior segment is protected by the bony orbit in which the eyeball rests. The anterior segment, consisting of cornea, conjunctiva, lens, aqueous humor, and iris, is primarily responsible for the refraction of light rays (Figure 4-6). Aqueous humor occupies the spaces within the anterior segment and provides nutrients to the tissues it contacts. The posterior segment consists of sclera, choroid, retina, and optic nerve. This segment acts as a perceptive system.

Drug molecules should possess optimum lipophilicity to permeate across the cell membrane. Topically applied drugs must possess enough solubility in tear fluids, along with optimum lipophilicity, to penetrate the corneal epithelium [21]. Unfortunately, most drug molecules are either hydrophilic or lipophilic in nature.

The static and dynamic barriers result in low ocular bioavailability of drugs. Static barriers consist of impermeable corneal layers, sclera, and retina, including blood aqueous and blood–retinal barriers, whereas dynamic barriers consist of tear dilution, choroidal and conjunctival blood flow, and lymphatic clearance (**Figure 4–7**). Topical administration of drugs is the convenient and preferred delivery method. However, the ocular bioavailability of topically administered drugs is less than 5% [22]. This is attributed to several factors, including solution drainage, blinking, tear turnover, loss of drug to systemic circulation via nasolacrimal drainage, and the relatively impermeable corneal epithelium. Ocular entry of xenobiotics after systemic administration is hindered by the blood–aqueous barrier and blood–retinal barrier. After systemic administration, only 1% to 2% of the dose reaches the eye [23]. Hence, topical administration of drugs is the preferred route for the treatment of diseases affecting the anterior segment of the eye.

Topically applied drugs enter the eye either via the cornea or conjunctiva. A major fraction of drug absorbed through the cornea is distributed among the intraocular issues, whereas drug absorbed through the conjunctiva enters the systemic circulation. Ophthalmic drugs, including antimicrobials, antihistamines, mydriatics, decongestants, miotics, and cycloplegic agents, are generally administered in the form of eye drops, ointments, creams, and suspensions. To have optimum ocular bioavailability, drug molecules should remain in contact with the cornea for a prolonged period. Compared with eye drops, suspensions and ointments remain in the precorneal region for longer time periods and hence result in sustained action.

More recently, intraocular injections have gained popularity for the treatment of posterior segment diseases. Drug solutions and suspensions are administered either in the form of intravitreal or periocular injections to overcome the blood–retinal barrier. Intravitreal injections are administered directly into the vitreous cavity, whereas

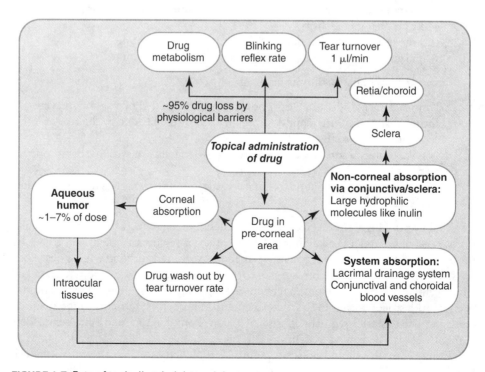

FIGURE 4-7 Fate of topically administered drug.

periocular injections are administered via subconjunctival, subtenon, retrobulbar, peribulbar, and posterior juxtascleral routes.

The *rectal mucosa* is reached by the administration of drugs into the rectum or colon via the anus in the form of suppositories and enemas (e.g., aspirin, chlorpromazine, and theophylline). Drugs administered orally can be formulated into suppositories by mixing with a waxy base that melts at rectal temperature. Unlike oral administration, a drug administered by rectal administration has a faster onset, higher bioavailability, and shorter peak and duration. The rectal wall is thin with ample blood supply, and hence drugs are readily absorbed. Suppositories are prescribed for patients suffering from nausea who have difficulty swallowing.

Rectal absorption of drugs is influenced by the following parameters: concentration of drug, time taken to liquefaction (in case of suppositories), site of administration and retention of drug at the site, lipophilicity of drug, pH of rectal contents, and presence of stool. Systemic drug levels are significantly influenced by the anatomical differences in hemorrhoidal venous drainage. Drugs placed low in the rectum are absorbed systemically by the inferior and middle rectal veins, whereas drugs placed deeper into the rectum are absorbed into the superior rectal veins and subjected to metabolism in the liver [2]. The rectal dose is usually higher than the dose administered orally. This is a more convenient route in children for administration of benzodiazepines [24].

Advantages of rectal delivery are:

- Rate of absorption is independent of food ingestion and gastric emptying time.
- First-pass metabolism of drugs is prevented.
- It results in rapid systemic effect when administered in the form of solution.
- It is a suitable route of administration in children, especially for bitter drugs.

Disadvantages of rectal delivery are:

- May result in erratic drug absorption
- Not well accepted in adults
- Interruption in drug absorption by defecation, most common with irritant drugs
- Drug degradation by microorganisms in rectum
- Less surface area for absorption compared with duodenum
- Not preferred in immunosuppressed patients in whom even a minimal trauma could lead to abscess formation

INHALATION ROUTE

The respiratory system provides an extensive surface area (>30 m^2) for drug absorption. The permeability characteristics of the respiratory tract epithelium are similar to other biological membranes, and hence lipid-soluble compounds are better absorbed compared with hydrophilic molecules. However, the pulmonary epithelium possesses high permeability for hydrophilic compounds compared with GI mucosa. Hence, drugs such as sodium cromoglicate (IX), a bischromone with a pKa of approximately 1.9, is well absorbed in the lungs. The inhalation route is successfully used in the treatment of respiratory diseases such as asthma and chronic obstructive airway disease. Inhalation therapy avoids the systemic side effects of corticosteroids such as adrenal suppression. This route provides rapid relief for asthma patients with chronic local and systemic effects.

Aerosolized administration of drugs is mostly directed to the lungs, and the absorption depends on the ability to target the particles to the sites of maximal absorption. For example, drug deposited on the alveoli is rapidly absorbed, whereas drug absorption from airways is slowly absorbed [25].

Pulmonary administration is considered a potential noninvasive route of administration for systemic delivery for many therapeutic agents. The respiratory system, mainly consisting of lungs, respiratory muscles, and airways (trachea, bronchi, bronchioles, and alveoli), provides an extremely thin (~0.1–0.2 μm) and large absorptive surface area (~70–140 m²) with good blood supply [26]. This route of administration is used for local and systemic drug delivery. Local delivery is used in the treatment of asthma, infectious diseases, and pulmonary hypertension. The pulmonary route mainly uses two techniques: intratracheal instillation and aerosol inhalation. The aerosol technique is expensive and allows uniform distribution and greater penetration into the alveolar region, whereas intratracheal instillation is less expensive and simple and has nonuniform distribution of drugs. Drug deposition after aerosol administration occurs by three mechanisms: diffusion, gravitational sedimentation, and inertial impaction. Smaller particles deposit mainly by diffusion mechanism, and larger particles are driven by gravitational force or inertial impaction. The pulmonary route has been widely used for delivery of antibiotics, muscarinic receptor antagonists, β-adrenergic mimetic, and mucolytic agents using various devices such as nebulizers, sprays, dry powder inhalers, metered dose inhalers, and pressurized atomizers. Dry powder inhalers are widely used in the delivery of small molecules and proteins to the lungs. Commercially available dry powder inhalers include Spinhaler (Fisons Pharmaceuticals, Rochester, NY) and Rotahaler (GSK, Hertfordshire, UK).

Advantages of pulmonary administration are:

* Onset of action is quick (7–10 seconds) and comparable with the intravenous route.
* Intestinal and hepatic first-pass metabolism are avoided.
* It is used for administration of heparin and insulin.
* User can alter the amount of drug or dose being administered.

Disadvantages of pulmonary administration are:

* It may be a more addictive route of administration due to faster action and instant gratification.
* Drugs administered via the inhalation route may not stay in the blood for longer durations, resulting in a need for higher dosing frequency.
* Regulating the exact dosage amount may be difficult.
* Patient may have difficulties in administration of drug via inhaler.
* It lacks reproducibility because of variation in drug deposition site.

Otologic administration is generally used for removal of wax and treatment of outer ear and ear canal infections. Wax removal ear drops consist of oil that softens waxy aggregates in the ears. They are generally used in combination with ear washes. Several drugs such as ciprofloxacin, gentamicin, hydrocortisone, dexamethasone, nystatin, and neomycin are administered in the form of ear drops.

TRANSDERMAL ROUTE

The transdermal route involves the delivery of drugs through the skin by a medicated adhesive patch. The scopolamine patch is the first transdermal patch approved by the U.S. Food and Drug Administration in 1979 for the treatment of motion sickness. Today, transdermal drug delivery is a widely accepted alternative to oral, parenteral, and transmucosal routes for delivery of hormones and pain medications [27].

This route is being examined for the delivery of antiarrhythmic drugs, antihistamines, antivirals, beta-blockers, calcium channel blockers, contraceptives, hormones, nonsteroidal anti-inflammatory drugs, insulin, α-interferon, and cancer chemotherapeutic agents. Drugs applied topically should permeate the skin, which is relatively impermeable. Epidermal layer of the skin acts as a barrier to the loss of water molecules and invasion of microorganisms [28] and mainly consists of five layers: stratum corneum, stratum lucidum, stratum granulosum, stratum spinosum, and stratum basale (**Figure 4-8**). Stratum corneum, which is composed of 10 to 30 layers of polyhedral, anucleated corneocytes, acts as an important barrier to drug molecules. Transdermal technology delivers the drug molecules to systemic circulation by overcoming the barrier properties of epidermis. Transdermal drug absorption depends on a variety of factors, including site of application, size of the molecule, hydration of skin, lipophilicity of drug, integrity and thickness of stratum corneum, and pH of the drug [2].

Transdermal patches are simple systems that release the drug in a slow and continuous manner over hours or days. Patches are useful for drugs that are quickly eliminated and require frequent administration. Examples of market patches include Nitrolingual (nitroglycerin), Transderm Scōp (scopolamine), and Catapres (clonidine). The impermeable properties of skin to large molecules forced scientists to look for alternative mechanisms such as iontophoresis and sonophoresis. Iontophoresis involves the use of small electric currents to propel drug molecules through the skin, whereas sonophoresis uses ultrasound to stimulate microvibrations that increase the penetration of drugs [29]. Recently, micron-scale needles of varying shapes and sizes have been shown to dramatically increase transdermal permeation of vaccines. Solid or hollow microneedles

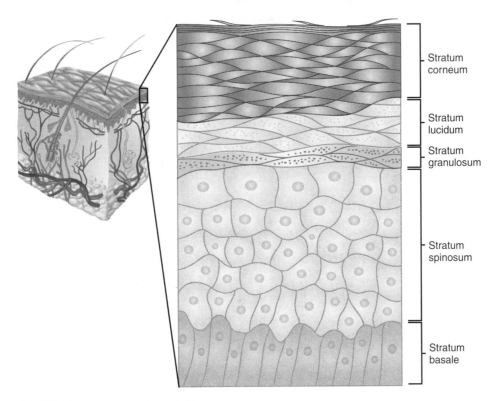

FIGURE 4-8 Layers of epidermal skin.

deliver the drugs by (1) encapsulating or coating the vaccine within or on microneedles, (2) piercing the skin using microneedles and then applying a vaccine patch, and (3) injecting the vaccine into the skin using a modified syringe or pump [30].

Advantages of transdermal drug delivery are:

- Avoids hostile GI environment and presystemic metabolism
- Drug elimination independent of gastric emptying
- Suitable for drugs with short biological half-life and narrow therapeutic window
- Increased therapeutic efficacy and decreased fluctuations
- Decreased dosing frequency and increased patient compliance
- Painless when compared with parenteral therapy
- Provides suitability of self-medication
- Most suitable for drugs with short elimination half-life that undergo extensive first-pass metabolism

Disadvantages of transdermal delivery are:

- In most cases, the effect is slow and sustained.
- Skin irritation can occur from the penetration enhancers.
- Only drugs small enough to penetrate the skin can be delivered effectively.

TRANSPORT OF DRUGS ACROSS MEMBRANES

Systemic bioavailability is often dictated by the route of administration. By definition, the bioavailability of drugs introduced into the blood is 100%. However, drugs administered by other routes need to overcome many barriers before being absorbed into systemic circulation [7].

A cell layer is composed of a phospholipid bilayer membrane (Figure 4-9) and cholesterol. Drug molecules must traverse through this lipoidal membrane before entering systemic circulation. Un-ionized drugs with low molecular weight pass easily through the lipoidal membrane compared with ionized drugs. Transport of drugs across the cell membrane is mediated by passive diffusion, active transport, and vesicle mediated transport (Figure 4-10).

Passive diffusion involves simple movement of drug molecules in the direction of the concentration gradient (Figure 4-11). The rate of drug transfer is governed by Fick's law of diffusion:

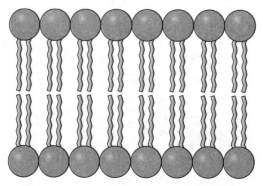

FIGURE 4-9 Schematic cross-sectional profile of a phospholipid bilayer of cell membrane.

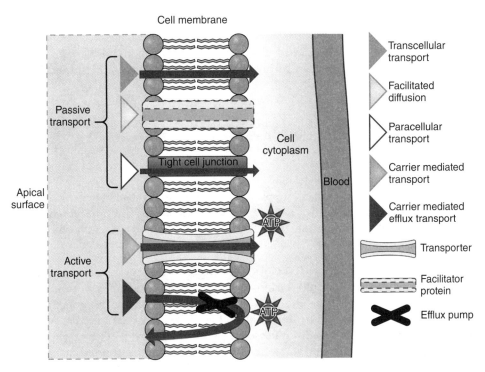

FIGURE 4-10 Intestinal drug transport mechanisms.

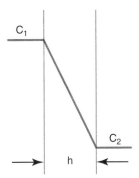

FIGURE 4-11 Passive transport of drug molecules.

$$\frac{dQ}{dt} = \frac{-DAK(C_1 - C_2)}{h} \tag{1}$$

where $\dfrac{dQ}{dt}$ is the rate of diffusion, D is the diffusion coefficient, A is the surface area of the membrane across which drug transfer occurs, K is the oil–water partition coefficient of the drug, h is the thickness of the membrane through which diffusion occurs, and $(C_1 - C_2)$ is the difference in drug concentration in areas 1 and 2, respectively.

Passive diffusion is classified into three types:

1. *Paracellular process,* in which molecules are transported via water-filled channels/pores present between the cells. Generally, low-molecular-weight hydrophilic

compounds are absorbed into systemic circulation via the paracellular route. These water-filled pores constitute only 0.01% to 0.1% of the total intestinal surface area, resulting in low absorption. Tight junctions that are present in between the apical and basolateral surface of the GI tract further reduce the penetration efficiency of hydrophilic drug molecules.

2. *Transcellular transport* involves simple diffusion of drug molecules through the plasma membrane across a cell layer. Generally, lipophilic drugs, which have more affinity for the lipoidal bilayer of the cell membrane, are primarily absorbed by this process. Many theoretical models have been developed to study transcellular transport of molecular size, charge, and lipophilicity that play an important role in determining permeability.

3. *Facilitated diffusion process* is a simple diffusion process facilitated by the transporter proteins expressed on cell membranes. Drug molecules are transported in the direction of the concentration gradient. This process does not require ATP molecules for the transport (i.e., vitamin B12 transport).

Active transport involves uptake of drug molecules by transmembrane proteins. These proteins transfer molecules against the concentration gradient (i.e., from low to high concentration) with expenditure of ATP molecules. Some transporters use the energy directly obtained from hydrolysis of ATP to drive the drug molecules, whereas others use stored energy. Na^+/K^+ ATPase, H^+/K^+ ATPase, Ca^{2+} ATPases, and ATP-binding cassette transporters belong to the category of active transporters and use the energy directly obtained from hydrolysis of ATP. Many transport systems involving peptides [31], vitamins [32], amino acids, and sugars [33] have been identified in the GI tract, which plays a vital role in transporting drug substrates. The active transport process undergoes saturation at high concentrations.

Vesicle-mediated transport involves the formation of vesicles for the transport of substances across the cell membrane. There are three types:

1. *Endocytosis* is a process that involves the formation of an inward bulge in the cell membrane that forms a vesicle. Receptor-mediated endocytosis occurs when the material to be transported binds to specific molecules in the membrane. Examples include the transport of insulin and cholesterol into animal cells.

2. *Phagocytosis* is the type of endocytosis in which white blood cells engulf invading viruses and bacteria.

3. *Pinocytosis* is a cell-drinking process that involves the uptake of fluids and particles into the cell via formation of a narrow channel in the membrane. These channels pinch off into vesicles and gradually fuse with lysosomes (consisting of enzymes) that break down contents. Pinocytosis is an energy-dependent process that requires adenosine triphosphate for the transport process.

SUMMARY

There are 111 distinct drug administration routes, as per the U.S. Food and Drug Administration. However, more than 80% of drugs available on the market are administered by oral and injectable routes. So far, oral delivery remains dominant, and the growing enthusiasm toward the targeted and local delivery of drugs for enhanced patient compliance and reduced side effects intrigues scientists to look into novel delivery routes. Over the next 5 years, the global market for nonoral drugs is expected to double from its current value of about $45 billion. Each route has unique barriers and constraints in terms of delivery. However, these obstacles and barriers could be successfully overcome through careful design of novel drug delivery systems.

REVIEW QUESTIONS

1. Define and classify the routes of administration.
2. What is first-pass metabolism? Name a few drugs that undergo first-pass metabolism.
3. Why do protein formulations exhibit poor pharmacokinetic profiles? Explain the ways to enhance the pharmacokinetic profiles of protein formulation with suitable examples.
4. What are the techniques used in administration of drugs via the pulmonary route? Explain them.
5. How can you overcome the rapid clearance of drugs from the nasal cavity?
6. Explain the static and dynamic barriers that result in low ocular bioavailability of drugs.
7. What factors govern the transdermal absorption of drugs?
8. Explain the transport process of drugs across the cell membranes.

REFERENCES

1. Zieman M, Fong SK, Benowitz NL, Banskter D, Darney PD. Absorption kinetics of misoprostol with oral or vaginal administration. *Obstet Gynecol.* 1997;90(1):88–92.
2. American Academy of Pediatrics. Committee on Drugs. Alternative routes of drug administration—advantages and disadvantages. *Pediatrics.* 1997;100(1):143–152.
3. Hamman JH, Enslin GM, Kotze AF. Oral delivery of peptide drugs: barriers and developments. BioDrugs. 2005. 19(3):165–77.
4. Andrade F, et al. Nanocarriers for pulmonary administration of peptides and therapeutic proteins. *Nanomedicine (Lond).* 2011;6(1):123–141.
5. Breitkreutz J, Boos J. Drug delivery and formulations. In: *Handb Exp Pharmacol.* 2011;205:91–107.
6. Gupta H, Bhandari D, Sharma A. Recent trends in oral drug delivery: a review. *Recent Pat Drug Deliv Formul.* 2009;3(2):162–173.
7. Friend DR. Drug delivery to the small intestine. *Curr Gastroenterol Rep.* 2004;6(5):371–376.
8. Gumbiner B. Structure, biochemistry, and assembly of epithelial tight junctions. *Am J Physiol.* 1987;253(6 Pt 1):C749–C758.
9. Chan KK, Gibaldi M. Effects of first-pass metabolism on metabolite mean residence time determination after oral administration of parent drug. *Pharm Res.* 1990;7(1):59–63.
10. Mrsny RJ. Oral drug delivery research in Europe. *J Control Release.* 2012;161(2):247–153.
11. Abu-Diak OA, Jones DS, Andrews GP. An investigation into the dissolution properties of celecoxib melt extrudates: understanding the role of polymer type and concentration in stabilizing supersaturated drug concentrations. *Mol Pharm.* 2011;8(4):1362–1371.
12. Bowman K, Leong KW. Chitosan nanoparticles for oral drug and gene delivery. *Int J Nanomed.* 2006;1(2):117–128.
13. Greenwald RB. PEG drugs: an overview. *J Control Release.* 2001;74(1–3):159–171.
14. Scholz OA, et al. Drug delivery from the oral cavity: focus on a novel mechatronic delivery device. *Drug Discov Today.* 2008;13(5–6):247–253.
15. Sudhakar Y, Kuotsu K, Bandyopadhyay AK. Buccal bioadhesive drug delivery—a promising option for orally less efficient drugs. *J Control Release.* 2006;114(1):15–40.
16. Mundargi RC, et al. Development and evaluation of novel biodegradable microspheres based on poly(d,l-lactide-co-glycolide) and poly(epsilon-caprolactone) for controlled delivery of doxycycline in the treatment of human periodontal pocket: in vitro and in vivo studies. *J Control Release.* 2007;119(1):59–68.
17. Shojaei AH. Buccal mucosa as a route for systemic drug delivery: a review. *J Pharm Pharm Sci.* 1998;1(1):15–30.

18. Illum L. Nasal drug delivery—possibilities, problems and solutions. *J Control Release*. 2003;87 (1–3):187–198.

19. Striebel HW, et al. [Pharmacokinetics of intranasal fentanyl.]. *Schmerz*. 1993;7(2):122–125.

20. Illum L, et al. Intranasal delivery of morphine. *J Pharmacol Exp Ther*. 2002;301(1):391–400.

21. Gaudana R, et al. Recent perspectives in ocular drug delivery. *Pharm Res*. 2009;26(5):1197–1216.

22. Janoria KG, et al. Novel approaches to retinal drug delivery. *Expert Opin Drug Deliv*. 2007;4(4):371–388.

23. Cunha-Vaz JG. The blood-ocular barriers: past, present, and future. *Doc Ophthalmol*. 1997;93(1-2): 149–157.

24. Graves NM, Kriel RL. Rectal administration of antiepileptic drugs in children. *Pediatr Neurol*. 1987;3(6):321–326.

25. Neale MG, et al. The pharmacokinetics of sodium cromoglycate in man after intravenous and inhalation administration. *Br J Clin Pharmacol*. 1986;22(4):373–382.

26. Patil JS, Sarasija S. Pulmonary drug delivery strategies: a concise, systematic review. *Lung India*. 2012;29(1):44–49.

27. Guy RH. Transdermal drug delivery. *Handb Exp Pharmacol*. 2010;(197):399–410.

28. Ranade VV. Drug delivery systems. 6. Transdermal drug delivery. *J Clin Pharmacol*. 1991;31(5):401–418.

29. Lavon I, Kost J. Ultrasound and transdermal drug delivery. *Drug Discov Today*. 2004;9(15):670–676.

30. Prausnitz MR, et al. Microneedle-based vaccines. *Curr Top Microbiol Immunol*. 2009;333:369–393.

31. Sugawara M, et al. Transport of valganciclovir, a ganciclovir prodrug, via peptide transporters PEPT1 and PEPT2. *J Pharm Sci*. 2000;89(6):781–789.

32. Balamurugan K, Ortiz A, Said HM. Biotin uptake by human intestinal and liver epithelial cells: role of the SMVT system. *Am J Physiol Gastrointest Liver Physiol*. 2003;285(1):G73–G77.

33. Fagerholm U, Lindahl A, Lennernas H. Regional intestinal permeability in rats of compounds with different physicochemical properties and transport mechanisms. *J Pharm Pharmacol*. 1997; 49(7):687–690.

Novel Drug Delivery Systems

Heidi M. Mansour, Zhen Xu, Samantha A. Meenach, Chun-Woong Park, Yun-Seok Rhee, and Patrick P. DeLuca

CHAPTER OBJECTIVES

Upon completing this chapter, the reader should be able to

▸ State and describe the administration routes for novel injectable depot systems.

▸ State and describe various types of sustained-release, injectable depot systems including drug types and polymer types that are used.

▸ State and describe pulmonary and nasal aerosol delivery including the different device types.

▸ Compare and contrast pulmonary and nasal aerosol delivery for local vs. systemic action.

▸ State and describe pulmonary nanomedicine including the systems used.

CHAPTER OUTLINE

INTRODUCTION

A wide variety of novel drug delivery systems are currently being investigated and currently on the market that allow for improved drug delivery and subsequent treatment of many different types of diseases. This chapter provides an overview to several types of these systems, including injectable drug depot systems (bulk and microspheres) and pulmonary aerosol systems. Such pulmonary aerosol systems include those used for local action in the lung, in the treatment of systemic diseases, nasal-specific systems, and pulmonary nanomedicine.

NOVEL INJECTABLE DEPOT DRUG DELIVERY SYSTEMS

ADMINISTRATION ROUTES

The two routes by which long-acting parenteral injections are most frequently administered are intramuscular (IM) injection and subcutaneous (SC) injection. An SC injection is given in the fatty layer of the tissue just under the skin, and an IM injection is given directly into the muscle. To determine the injectable route of administration for long-term delivery formulations, many factors should be considered, such as the safety profile, ease of administration, patient mobility, area for target injection sites, patient quality of life, and cost of therapy [1]. In many cases, the preferred route for administering a drug is by SC injection because of the greater area for target injection sites, use of shorter needles, ease of self-administration, reduced discomfort and inconvenience for patients, and a more optimal safety profile [1]. Various insulin products are given subcutaneously, and this route of administration presumably continues to represent the primary route of delivery for protein-based drugs. However, the volumes for SC injections are usually limited to no more than 1 to 2 mL, and only nonirritating substances can be injected because irritants can cause pain, necrosis, and sloughing at the site of SC injection. On the other hand, larger injection volumes (2–5 mL) can be given via the IM route. Also, mild irritants, oils, and suspensions can be injected via the IM route in large skeletal muscles (deltoid, triceps, gluteus maximus, rectus femoris, etc.) because these muscles are less richly supplied with sensory nerves and are more vascular. Therefore, a few SC injections for long-term release can be found on the market (i.e., Depo-SubQ Provera 104™, Nutropin Depot®, and Eligard®) and many long-acting IM injections are available on the market (oil-based injections, injectable drug suspensions, and injectable microspheres).

TYPES OF SUSTAINED-RELEASE INJECTABLE DEPOT SYSTEMS

Sustained-release parenteral injections can be divided into several types: oil-based injectable solutions, injectable drug suspensions, polymer-based microspheres, and polymer-based *in situ* forming systems. Oil-based injectable solutions and injectable drug suspensions control the release for weeks, whereas polymer-based microspheres and *in situ* gels can last for months. A more detailed review of each of these systems follows.

Oil-Based Injectable Solutions and Injectable Drug Suspensions

Conventional long-acting injections are usually composed of either lipophilic drugs in aqueous solvents as injectable suspensions or lipophilic drugs dissolved in vegetable oils as injectable solutions. These long-acting formulations must be administered every few weeks or so. Poorly water-soluble salt formations or prodrugs, which are synthesized by esterification of the parent drug to a long-chain fatty acid, can be used to control the dissolution rate of drug particles to prolong the absorption. Olanzapine pamoate is an example of a poorly water-soluble salt form of olanzapine, and paliperidone palmitate is an example of prodrug. Poorly water-soluble salts or fatty acid ester of drugs dissolve slowly at the injection site after IM injection because of their extremely low water solubility. The rate-limiting step of drug absorption is the dissolution of drug particles in the suspensions or in the tissue fluid surrounding the drug formulation.

A fatty acid ester of a drug is often used to prepare an oil-based parenteral solution, and the drug release rate from solution is controlled by (1) the drug partitioning between the oil vehicle and the tissue fluid and (2) the drug bioconversion rate from drug esters to the parent drug. Several other factors, however, such as injection site, injection volume, the extent of spreading of the depot at the injection site, and the fate of the oil vehicle, might affect the overall pharmacokinetic profile of the drug. Decanoic acid esters of antipsychotic drugs are widely used for these oil-based IM injections.

Polymer-Based Microspheres and *In Situ* Forming Systems

The development of polymer-based long-acting injectables is one of the most suitable strategies for the delivery of bioactive macromolecules such as peptide and protein drugs. The advantages of polymer-based formulations for the delivery of macromolecules include (1) *in vitro* and *in vivo* stabilization of the macromolecules, (2) improved systemic availability, (3) extension of the biological half-life, (4) enhanced patient convenience and compliance, and (5) reduced dosing frequency.

Among the various approaches, parenteral biodegradable microsphere systems are the most commercially successful delivery system for macromolecules. The most important factor in the design of parenteral microspheres is the selection of an appropriate biodegradable polymer. The release of the drugs from biodegradable microspheres is controlled by diffusion of the drug through the polymer matrix and/or polymer degradation. The nature of the polymer, such as the composition of copolymer ratios, polymer crystallinity, glass transition temperature, and hydrophilicity, plays a crucial role in the release process. Furthermore, the structure of the microspheres, intrinsic polymer properties, core solubility, polymer hydrophilicity, and polymer molecular weight also influence the drug release kinetics. The possible mechanisms of drug release from injected microspheres are the (1) initial release from the surface, (2) release through the microsphere pores, (3) diffusion through the intact polymer barrier, (4) diffusion through the water-swollen barrier, and (5) polymer erosion and bulk degradation. All these mechanisms together play a role in the release process [2].

One extensively studied polymeric injectable depot system is the *in situ* forming implant system. *In situ* forming implant systems are made of biodegradable products that can be injected via a syringe into the body and, once injected, congeal to form a solid biodegradable implant. This section briefly summarizes the types of *in situ* forming implants, because the topic has been intensively reviewed elsewhere [3–5].

Biodegradable injectable *in situ* forming implants are classified into five categories based on the mechanism of depot formation: thermoplastic pastes, *in situ* cross-linked polymer systems, *in situ* polymer precipitation systems, thermally induced gelling systems, and *in situ* solidifying organogels. The mechanism of depot formation of thermoplastic pastes is to form a semisolid upon cooling to body temperature after injection into the body in its molten form. Cross-linked polymer networks can be formed *in situ* in a variety of ways to form solid polymer systems or gels. Methods for *in situ* solidification of cross-linked systems include free radical reactions (usually initiated by heat or absorption of photons) or ionic interactions between small cations and polymer anions. *In situ* forming systems can also be produced by initiating polymer precipitation from a solution. In this process, a water-insoluble and biodegradable polymer is solubilized in a biocompatible organic solvent to which a drug is added that forms a solution or suspension after mixing. When this formulation is injected into the body, the water-miscible organic solvent dissipates and water penetrates into the organic phase. This leads to phase separation and precipitation of the polymer forming a depot at the site of injection. Subsequently, thermally induced gelling systems show thermoreversible sol–gel transitions and are characterized by a lower critical solution temperature. They are liquid at room temperature and produce a gel at and above the lower critical solution temperature (i.e., body temperature at 37°C). Finally, *in situ* solidifying organogels are composed of water-insoluble amphiphilic lipids, which swell in water and form various types of lyotropic liquid crystals.

TYPES OF DRUGS LOADED

Various drugs have been investigated for use in sustained-release injectable delivery systems [6]. These include small-molecular-weight drugs and protein/peptide drugs (**Figure 5-1**). Examples of drugs for sustained-release injectable delivery systems are as follows:

1. Hormone therapy (human somatropin) [7, 8]
2. Protein therapeutics such as the analogue of glucagon-like peptide-1 [9], recombinant human bone morphogenetic protein-2 [10], superoxide dismutase [11], salmon calcitonin [12, 13], and insulin [14–16]
3. Gene delivery compounds such as plasmid DNA [17–19]
4. Cancer therapeutic agents such as bleomycin [20], paclitaxel [21], cisplatin [22], and a peptide-like antineoplastic agent [23]

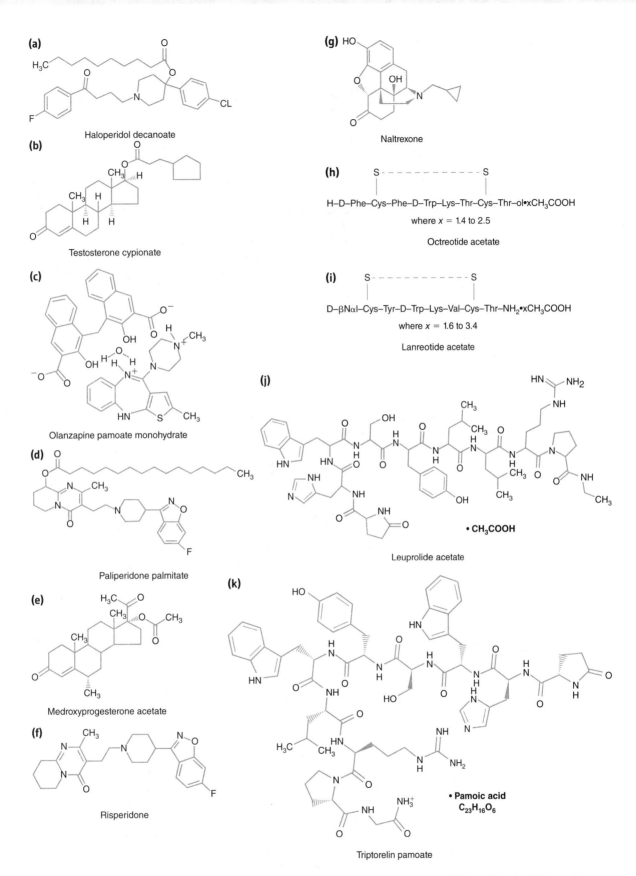

FIGURE 5-1 Examples of chemical structures of drugs for sustained-release parenteral injectables. (a, b) Drugs for oil-based injectable solutions. (c–e) Drugs for injectable drug suspensions. (f–k) Drugs for polymer-based microspheres and *in situ* forming systems.

5. Postoperative pain therapeutic agents such as ketorolac tromethamine [24]
6. Schizophrenia drugs such as aripiprazole [25] or olanzapine [26]
7. Contraceptive peptide vaccines [27]
8. Drugs to treat alcohol dependence such as naltrexone [28]
9. Immunosuppressive drugs such as rapamycin [29]

Despite a number of parenteral depot studies using a variety of these drugs, only drugs in limited therapeutic areas are available on the market. For example, antipsychotic drugs and hormones have been used for more than five decades in the field of schizophrenia and hormone replacement therapy. Since the first launching of the microsphere formulation Lupron Depot® for the palliative treatment of advanced prostate cancer in 1989, several microsphere formulations and *in situ* forming implants have been released on the U.S. market. The therapeutic indications and drugs of commercialized products include those used for the palliative treatment of advanced prostate cancer (leuprolide acetate, triptorelin pamoate), the treatment of acromegaly (octreotide acetate, lanreotide acetate), the long-term treatment of growth failure (somatropin-rDNA origin), the treatment of schizophrenia (risperidone), and the treatment of alcohol dependence (naltrexone).

TYPES OF POLYMERS USED TO FORM INJECTABLE SYSTEMS

Many microsphere research reports have demonstrated the usefulness of biodegradable polymers such as poly(lactide-co-glycolic acid) (PLGA) [30–37], polycaprolactone (PCL) [38], polyanhydride [39], polyorthoesters [40], and polyalkylcyanoacrylate microspheres [41, 42]. Examples of biodegradable polymer structures for sustained-release parenteral injectables are shown in **Figure 5-2**. Examples of the use of some of these systems follows.

The Atrigel® technology that is used in the Eligard® system (containing leuprolide acetate and PLGA) was the first successful once-monthly *in situ* forming implant produced for the palliative treatment of advanced prostate cancer. In addition, many reports have been published on novel biodegradable *in situ* forming polymers such as multiblock poly(ether ester urethanes) consisting of poly-[(R)-3-hydroxybutyrate], polyethylene glycol (PEG), polypropylene glycol polymer [43], PEG grafted chitosan polymer (Chitosan–PEG) [44], methoxypoly(ethylene glycol)–poly(sebacic acid–D, L–lactic acid)–methoxy poly(ethylene glycol) triblock copolymer (mPEG–poly(SA–LA)–mPEG) [45], PCL–PEG–PCL triblock copolymer [46], and PLGA–PEG–PLGA triblock copolymer [47].

INTRODUCTION: PULMONARY AEROSOLS

Inhalation aerosol delivery may be divided into the upper respiratory tract (i.e., nasal, throat) and the lower respiratory tract (i.e., pulmonary/lung). Pulmonary delivery is most often achieved via three principal devices: nebulizers, pressurized metered dose inhalers (pMDIs), and dry powder inhalers (DPIs) [48]. Nasal delivery systems include nonpressurized metered dose sprays, pressurized metered dose sprays, atomized (nonmetered squeeze) pumps, nasal DPIs, and nebulizers. Various strategies such as aerodynamic particle size optimization, deaggregation mechanisms, and inhalation mode are being applied to efficiently deposit aerosol drugs to the desired respiratory regions. Pulmonary and nasal cavities are targets for small-molecule delivery and also for biological macromolecule absorption. They offer an important alternative and noninvasive route of administration. To cover the scope of novel inhalation aerosolsystems for local and systemic therapies, this section is

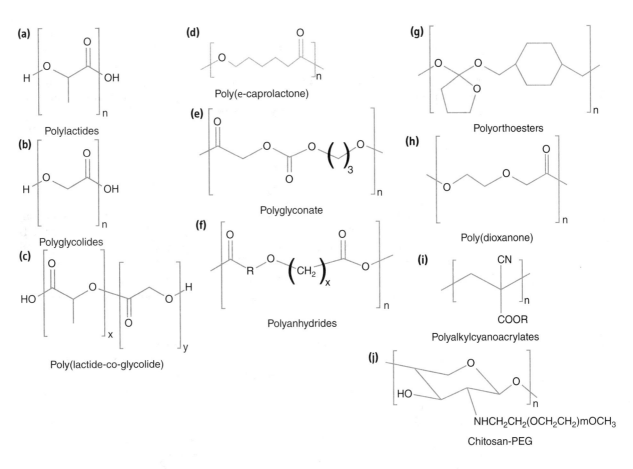

FIGURE 5-2 Examples of biodegradable polymer structures for sustained-release parenteral injectables.

subdivided into pulmonary delivery using pMDIs or DPIs, nasal delivery, and delivery via pulmonary nanomedicine.

PULMONARY AEROSOL DELIVERY FOR LOCAL ACTION

Pulmonary aerosols that directly deliver microgram quantities of drugs are mainly used for local treatments, typically the treatment of asthma and chronic obstructive pulmonary disease (COPD). The pMDI and DPI, both of which emerged since 1950s, have become the major devices used for treating these diseases because of their portability, convenience, ease of use, and robustness. The nebulizer, which is intended for continuous drug delivery in contrast to the bolus delivery, is not discussed here. With these devices, drugs are delivered directly to the pulmonary tract to treat the cause and symptoms of these diseases. Locally acting inhaled therapies include but are not limited to antibacterials and antivirals for the treatment of cystic fibrosis and other pulmonary-related infections [49,50], anticancer drugs for lung cancer therapies [51], and gene therapies using viral vectors (e.g., α_1-antitrypsin) for the treatment of diseases such as emphysema [52].

The drugs used for treating asthma or COPD fall mainly into the classifications of β_2-adrenergic agonists, anticholinergics, corticosteroids, and mast cell stabilizers. Once the pharmacological targets for these diseases are identified, delivering the drugs to the site of action should consider the pharmacological aspects in the airways, which may influence therapeutic effectiveness and unwanted aerosol exposure. For instance, the distribution of receptors in incorrect pulmonary regions could result in ineffective treatment. Adrenergic receptors are more localized in the lung periphery, and cholinergic receptors are more centrally located in the lung [53]. This should help to guide the deposition of respirable drugs for β_2-adrenergic agonists such as albuterol or anticholinergics such as ipratropium. Corticosteroids are intended for whole lung delivery to treat inflammation, the underlying cause of these diseases [54]. Once these drugs are dispersed as aerosol drugs, the deposition of the aerosols in the respiratory tract involves several mechanisms, including inertial impaction, gravitational settling, Brownian motion, interception, and electrostatic interaction. These mechanisms have been discussed in several books [55–57].

Pressurized Metered Dose Inhalers

The pMDI comprises several components, including the propellant, drug formulation, pressurized container, metering valve, and actuator [58, 59]. Drugs from pMDIs are initially prepared as suspensions or solutions in a propellant, typically a liquefied compressed gas such as chlorofluorocarbons (CFCs) and hydrofluoroalkanes (HFAs) [60]. The suspension systems contain micronized drug dispersed in propellant with or without a small number of surfactants. Because drugs are often poorly soluble in the propellant, the solutions often require the addition of cosolvents. The metering chamber precisely fills one dose (typically 25–100 µL) [58] by means of a metering valve. The respirable aerosols are formed when the propellant containing the drug suspension is forced out of the container through a narrow atomization nozzle in the actuator, which causes shear thinning, droplet formation, and, concurrently, propellant evaporation. The selection of propellants, drug formulation, and device design can affect the aerosol performance.

Historically, the initial pMDIs used CFC propellants 11, 114, and 12 with satisfactory physicochemical (nonflammability, drug compatibility) and thermodynamic properties (vapor pressure stability) [59, 61]. They maintained a constant vapor pressure whenever the inhaler was full or nearly empty at a given temperature, which ensured reproducible spray characteristics and dosing [62]. In the last few decades, the pMDI design has undergone revolutionary reformulation after several international agreements, such as the 1987 Montreal protocol [63], which initially limited the use of CFC propellants because of its ozone-depleting effects and eventually phased out their use by 2009 in the United States [64–66]. The HFA family compounds currently used for pMDI propellants include HFA 134a (1,1,1,2-tetrafluoroethane) and HFA 227 (1,1,1,2,3,3,3-heptafluoropropane) [61]. The reformulation with HFA propellants to achieve product bioequivalence to the CFC-based pMDIs has caused many challenges due to the differences in propellant vapor pressure, drug solvency, and formulation stability. The characteristic physicochemical properties of CFC and HFA propellants used in pMDIs have been discussed elsewhere [67]. For both systems the spray velocity after actuation is a result in the difference between the propellant vapor pressure and atmospheric pressure [59]. The vapor pressures of HFAs are generally higher than that of CFCs so the defining characteristics of HFA pMDI sprays such as droplet size and velocity are much different from those of CFC-based pMDIs. Additionally, HFA propellants are more polar than CFCs, represented by the much higher dielectric constants [64]. Consequently, the solubility characteristics of the drug, surfactant, and water in liquefied HFA propellants are all altered when compared with CFCs [68]. For example, a small number of U.S. Food and Drug Administration (FDA)-approved surfactants such as oleic acid and lecithin are insoluble in HFAs, and require the addition of a cosolvent, typically ethanol [65]. The increased solubility of HFAs in water may affect the formulation stability due to moisture ingress, crystallinity changes, and Ostwald ripening (particle growth) in the suspension formulation [69].

In the current market, suspension pMDI formulations are more common, but a few solution formulation products such as QVAR® (beclomethasone dipropionate and HFA 134) have been developed. Solution formulations have the potential of achieving higher fine particle dose and, with ethanol as a cosolvent, a lower spray velocity [58, 68]. For suspension formulations, the drugs must be formulated to result in an aerodynamic size range of 1 to 5 µm for suitable deep-lung deposition [70]. Those larger than 10 µm are generally deposited in the oropharyngeal region, whereas droplets and particles smaller than 1 µm are likely to be exhaled [70]. A variety of technologies exists for manufacturing microparticles intended for either pMDI and DPI formulations, including spray drying [71] and jet milling [72]. Many supercritical fluid technologies have also been exploited for generating pulmonary drug particles that contain well-defined morphology and size characteristics [73, 74].

The vapor pressure inside a pMDI ranges between 90 and 600 kPa [58]. The pMDI container components include the canister and valve stem, which must be able to withstand these pressures. Most containers marketed use aluminum alloy or glass containers with polymeric coatings. The former is preferred compared with glass because it is lighter, more durable, and light-proof. For either container type, coating with various fluorocarbon polymers may be useful to prevent drug adhesion to the container wall, which can help ensure more consistent dosing [75]. The metering chamber and valve stem are usually made of stainless steel or polymer. pMDIs are multidose inhalers and are typically designed to contain 100 to 200 doses. The entire pMDI container is fitted upside down into a plastic actuator equipped with an atomization nozzle with a diameter between 0.14 and 0.6 mm [58]. Theoretical approaches have been used to predict the droplet formation from a pMDI followed by experimental validation [76, 77]. Empirically, Equation (1) has been derived to predict the fine particle dose as a function of actuator nozzle diameter (A, mm), the metered volume size (V, µL), and the HFA 134 content (C_{134}, %) [78]:

$$\text{Fine-particle dose (\%)} = 2.1 \times 10^{-5} \times A^{-1.5} \times V^{-0.25} \times C_{134}{}^{3} \qquad \text{Eq. (1)}$$

Equation (1) indicates that the fine-particle dose is reduced when cosolvents or other excipients are added in the formulation and that this may be overcome by narrowing the nozzle diameter [78].

The successful delivery using a pMDI product requires using the correct inhalation technique, which can be improved via patient instruction and training. A key point in the effective use of a pMDI is the coordination of actuation and patient inspiration. It is generally accepted that the correct technique for using a pMDI involves the actuation of the pMDI at the onset of a slow but deep inspiration followed by the patient holding his or her breath for a few seconds after inspiration [67]. Slow inhalation can reduce the inertial impaction of large particles to the back of the throat and facilitate propellant evaporation. Breath holding allows drug particles that enter the lungs to sediment in the airway under gravity. Many efforts have been made to improve patient compliance and to overcome the inadequate use of pMDIs. For patients who cannot easily coordinate inhaler actuation and inspiration, several novel pMDIs have been developed to incorporate user-friendly features or add-on devices. These include breath-actuated pMDIs such as the Autohaler®, which triggers actuation at certain flow rate [58]; velocity-modifying devices such as the Tempo® inhaler, which reduces the spray velocity by a vortex mechanism [58]; and valved-holding chambers such as the OptiChamber®, which allows delivery via tidal breathing [79]. These devices reduce human coordination errors and make pMDIs easier to use. Furthermore, in 2003 the FDA issued guidance to the effect that new pMDIs must be equipped with a dose counter that indicates the number of doses, further assisting patients in their use of these devices [80].

Dry Powder Inhalers

Dry powder inhalers (DPIs) involve the dispersion of powder formulations for the delivery of therapeutics to treat pulmonary diseases. DPIs have become an important alternative to pMDIs and have gone through a number of evolutionary changes over the last few decades [81]. DPIs are predicted to eventually supersede pMDI as the most popular devices as powder technology and device design advance [81, 82]. Unlike pMDIs, passive DPIs can be actuated by a patient's inspiratory flow, requiring no inhalation coordination. In addition, propellant-free dosage forms offer advantages such as formulation stability and low environmental impact. DPI systems themselves are composed of three key components: the dry powder/drug formulation, inhalation device, and dose-metering system/component [48]. The formulation, device, and inspiratory maneuver of the patient determine the efficiency of the drugs reaching the site of action and eventually the clinical outcome of the product [70]. The goals of device innovation include design of efficient aerosolization mechanisms, reproducible dose metering, high drug loading, reduced dependence on inspiratory flow rates, and user friendliness.

As mentioned previously, respirable drug particles smaller than 5 μm are often cohesive during delivery due to interparticulate interactions. The interparticulate forces between drug–drug, drug–carrier, and carrier–carrier are well documented and consist primarily of van der Waals, capillary, electrostatic, and frictional forces and mechanical interlocking [70, 83]. A myriad of factors are known to influence these forces, including particle size, size distribution, particle morphology, surface roughness, crystalline state, drug loading, and external environment [84]. The involvement of these forces at the solid–solid interface of the powder can lead to particle aggregation [85]. Among them, van der Waals forces are dominant in uncharged DPI formulations [85]. Capillary forces arise from capillary condensation and liquid-bridge formation at high relative humidity [83]. Electrostatic forces are mainly generated in drug pharmaceutical powder processing [86]. These adhesive forces need to be overcome for drugs to effectively disperse into aerosols. This can be achieved by both the powder formulation and processing as well as through the effective design in the specific DPI used. Many efforts have been made to manipulate these interparticulate forces. As one example, low-density (porous or hollow) particles have been generated by spray drying, rapid expansion of supercritical fluids, and other particle engineering methods [87, 88]. Because of their particle size and reduced number of surface contact points, interparticulate cohesive forces are reduced, allowing for more effective dispersion.

The classical approaches to prepare dry powder formulations involve systems with respirable drug alone (carrier free) or drug with larger carrier particles (carrier based), the most common carrier being α-lactose monohydrate. Carrier-free formulations generally require well-controlled processes to form loose drug-loaded microparticle aggregates of different sizes. These types of systems are used in commercial DPIs such as Pulmicort® [89] and Bricanyl® [90]. The carrier particles in the more widely used carrier-based formulations, typically ranging in size from 50 to 150 μm, function primarily to increase powder flow and to facilitate drug aerosol dispersion when actuated. They also act as excipients for uniform capsule filling and to modify pulmonary drug release [72, 91–93]. Other sugar or sugar alcohols such as glucose, trehalose, mannitol, and sorbitol have also been used or explored for use as carriers [91, 94]. Ternary blends have been prepared in which small particle excipients (e.g., sugars, L-leucine, etc.) are introduced to carrier-based formulations to aid in powder dispersion [95, 96].

The design of the DPI device can provide fluid dynamic pathways for the inspiratory flow to entrain and aerosolize respirable drugs from a static powder bed. The powder aerosolization may be considered in terms of static powder, dilation, fluidization, and deaggregation [81, 97]. In passive DPIs, the only source of energy comes from the patient inspiration maneuver. Currently, dozens of passive DPI devices are available on the market and appear quite dissimilar from one another [72, 98]. Each type of DPI device has unique airflow paths and internal geometry, which caters to distinct airflow parameters designed to disperse a specific dry powder formulation. The devices are usually compact with tortuous pathways that facilitate a variety of fluidization and deaggregation mechanisms such as impaction, turbulence, or fluid shear [81]. An intrinsic parameter, the specific resistance R_D, is dependent on the internal dimensions and geometry of the airflow path of the DPI device and is independent of the airflow [99, 100]. DPI devices with higher R_D are expected to generate greater turbulence at a given airflow rate, resulting in more effective powder dispersion and delivery. However, the rate of effort necessary to operate devices requiring a higher R_D may exceed the patient's capability and compromise the powder dispersion [101].

The ideal formulation should disperse the drug efficiently and reproducibly at varied rates of inhalation. From the patient's perspective, the use of passive DPIs depends on the strength of the patient's inspiration. The inhalation technique of one DPI differs from another as a result of the different specific resistances used for drug dispersion in each type of inhaler. The inhalation technique of DPIs differs greatly from that of pMDIs. Generally, a relatively high peak inhaled flow rate (e.g., >50 L/min) is needed for efficient drug dispersion [102]. Training and adequate instruction are necessary because different DPIs require different device handling and inhalation techniques [103, 104]. Some passive DPIs are triggered by breath when the peak inhaled flow rate reaches a threshold (e.g., Prohaler®), aiding in the coordination and actuation of these devices and allowing for more effective use by the patient.

The metering of DPIs is closely linked to the device itself and may involve either single-dose or multidose formulations [105]. Single-dose formulations refer to the premetered individual capsule, whereas multidose formulations involve different forms and can be further classified as multiple premetered blisters, strips, capsules, or multidose reservoirs [106]. Single-dose products (e.g., Rotahaler® and Spinhaler®) have to a large extent been superseded by multidose products (e.g., Diskus® and Turbuhaler®). These multidose devices typically contain 60 to 200 doses and are in this sense the powder equivalent of pMDIs.

Overall, many design components factor into the effective delivery of drug powders via DPIs including the drug/powder formulation itself, design of the DPI device, and method of patient actuation and use. Despite the seemingly complex nature of these devices, they offer a very attractive alternative to conventional pMDIs because of their ability to deliver many types of drugs and formulations that are difficult to deliver otherwise.

Active Dry Powder Inhalers

As described in the previous section, most DPIs achieve aerosol dispersion solely by the patient's inhalation maneuver. Therefore, the pulmonary dose depends on the strength and length of the patient's inhalation, which may vary from breath to breath and person to person. This is acceptable when delivering respirable drugs such as β_2-agonists. However, more accurate dosing is crucial for systemic drugs or drugs with narrow therapeutic windows such as inhaled corticosteroids. Active systems have become an expanding area of interest since the 1990s, and quite a few of these systems are in the development stages or have been launched on the market (Table 5-1). An advantage of these active systems is they are user-friendly, which may potentially reduce patient variability in regards to device actuation [107].

Active DPIs impart self-containing electrical or mechanical energy that facilitates drug aerosolization. Several active DPIs such as the Nektar pulmonary inhaler (Exubera® device) uses a bolus of compressed air manually generated through an onboard pump to disperse the powder [108]. In this system, a vortex dispersion chamber collects the dispersed powder and allows the drug to be delivered at a low flow rate. In the inhaler developed by Oriel, the input of vibrational (piezoelectric) energy with powder specific frequencies is used to facilitate aerosol dispersion and improve dosing reproducibility [109]. Other devices such as the Spiros® DPI applies a twin-blade impeller that can be triggered to disperse the drug at low flow rates [110], whereas the Taper® DPI applies a spring-loaded hammer to release a dose as the patient inhales [107].

Unfortunately, active DPIs are usually more complex because of these additional features. Also, they are costly for both development and manufacturing, which has become an obstacle in the successful commercialization of many active DPIs. An example is the Exubera® delivery system: Although the system overall was effective in dispersing powder formulations and received approval both in Europe and the United States in March 2006, its expense and putative side effects caused Pfizer to withdraw the system from the market a year later [111, 112]. Overall, however, active DPIs may be the most viable option for patients whose condition does not allow for effective actuation of the more popular passive DPIs.

TABLE 5-1 Active DPIs under development or launched on the market			
Device	**Company**	**Dispersion Mechanism**	**Reference**
Exubera	Nektar Therapeutics-Pfizer	Compressed air	Harper et al. [108]
Taper	3M	Hammer impact	Schultz et al. [107]
Un-named	AirPharma	Compressed air	Young et al. [276]
Aspirair	Vectura	Compressed air	Tobyn et al. [277]
Spiros	Dura Pharmaceuticals	Battery-powered impeller	Mecikalski et al. [110]
Oriel	Oriel Therapeutics	Piezoelectric vibration	Crowder & Hickey [109]
Airmax	Norton Healthcare	Compressed air	Keating [278]
MicroDose	MicroDose Tech.	Piezoelectric vibration	Fleming [279]
ActiSpire	AirPharma	Compressed air	Young et al. [280]
Un-named	Univ. of Western Ontario	Compressed air	Zhu et al. [281]

Data from: Newman SP, Peart J. Dry powder inhalers. In: Newman SP, ed. *Respiratory Drug Delivery: Essential Theory and Practice.* Richmond, VA: Respiratory drug delivery online/VCU; 2009:257-307.

Antibacterials

The respiratory tract is a port of entry for many bacteria and viruses that cause local pulmonary or systemic infectious diseases [113]. Pathogens such as *Pseudomonas aeruginosa* and *Staphylococcus aureus* are often acquired by inhalation and colonize in the airways. Aerosolized antibacterial and antiviral agents are often administered to reverse or control local respiratory or systemic infections as a replacement or alternative to oral or intravenous administrations. These aerosolized antibacterial drugs are mainly used for several clinical conditions, including cystic fibrosis and pneumonias. Inhaled drugs have the advantage of delivering high local concentrations directly to the site of infection, often resulting in a reduction of systemic toxicity. This is exemplified in two marketed antibacterial drugs, tobramycin (TOBI®, Novatis Pharmaceutical Corp.) and aztreonam (Cayston®, Gilead Science Inc.) for the treatment cystic fibrosis patients infected with *P. aeruginosa* [49, 114]. The success of these antibiotics spurred the interest in the development of other drugs to be used in this capacity. Several pulmonary antibiotics in aerosol formulations are undergoing clinical trials, including levofloxacin (phase III), ciprofloxacin (BAY Q3939, Bayer, phase I), amikacin (Arikace, Transave Inc., phase III), and moxifloxacin (BAY 12 8039, phase III) [49]. Clinical trials are also investigating the potential in using these drugs during acute exacerbation and for the prevention or delay in the onset of the infection.

For effective and safe aerosol delivery of antibacterials, their inhalation safety profiles still need to be established through rigorous testing. For example, the optimal dosing of the drugs currently being investigated in this capacity still need to be determined, which will require more clinical data support. Furthermore, there have been concerns that inhaled antibacterials may increase the appearance of resistant bacteria. In one study, resistant *Pseudomonas* species were reported with prolonged treatment of inhaled tobramycin [115]. Recent studies of inhaled antibacterials for nosocomial pneumonia, however, did not support such concern [116].

Antivirals

Similar to the pulmonary antibacterials, pulmonary antivirals have been developed for the treatment of viral infections in the respiratory tract. Ribavirin (Virazole®), a synthetic antiviral agent, was approved in 1985 for the treatment of severe lower respiratory infections due to the respiratory syncytial virus [117]. Although the successful treatment of respiratory syncytial virus with inhaled ribavirin was reported in several case studies [118], its efficacy is somewhat controversial [119]. Because of its hemolytic anemia side effect, as well as the shift of focus toward development of live attenuated vaccines, ribavirin therapy is not currently used routinely [119]. Zanamivir (Relenza®, GlaxoSmithKline), a neuraminidase inhibitor, is a relatively new antiviral drug approved in the United States since 1999 for the prophylaxis and treatment of influenza A and B virus. It is formulated in dry powder form and delivered via the Diskhaler® device [120]. A new DPI drug in the same neuraminidase inhibitor family, laninamivir octanoate (Inavir®, Daiichi Sankyo), has been marketed in Japan since 2010 but is not yet available in the United States [121].

The role of aerosol therapy has certainly expanded beyond the focus on the treatment of asthma and local infections. Pulmonary delivery of therapeutic proteins, vaccines, and other biological macromolecules for systemic action has been gaining great interest in recent years [122]. The targeting sites for systemic action are generally believed to be in the lower airways, particularly the alveolar region [123]. The huge alveolar surface area (about 150 m^2) with ultrathin epithelial cell linings (0.1 to 0.5 μm in thickness) and high vascularization allows for quick absorption of inhaled macromolecules through the lung epithelium. The duration of action for systemic delivery is generally limited by intrinsic clearance of the lungs [124]. In this sense, the development of sustained or extended-release systems for pulmonary aerosols is less investigated despite the fact the effectively designed systems capable of avoiding lung clearance could be easily used.

Three major classes of systemically acting drugs are being developed for pulmonary delivery: peptides and proteins, vaccines, and analgesics [125]. The first two classes of aerosol drugs are highlighted below. Although analgesics have the advantage for quick action through the pulmonary route, they are not covered here because they have been more thoroughly reviewed elsewhere [126–128]. It is worth mentioning that even if many small molecule drugs for local actions are delivered by pMDIs, aerosol macromolecules for systemic delivery are mainly formulated using aqueous nebulizers and solid dosage form DPIs. The main reason is that the propellant and other formulation ingredients in pMDIs are not compatible with the drug in use (e.g., for example, vaccines) [129]. Dry powder formulations are potentially advantageous in this application because they have greater stability than aqueous formulations and do not require reconstitution or refrigeration.

Pulmonary Delivery of Peptides and Proteins

Needle-free pulmonary delivery opens up an alternative route for peptide and protein therapies that are usually administered parenterally (Table 5-2). Because of the advances in recombinant DNA technology, many commercial quantities of bioengineered proteins and peptides such as hormones, growth factors, monoclonal antibodies, and cytokines have been launched onto the market or are under clinical investigation for systemic applications [130, 131]. There is no clear-cut distinction between peptides and proteins, but in general polypeptide molecules larger than 30 to 35 amino acids, often with interchain bonding, are categorized as proteins. Some pulmonary delivered proteins and peptides used for systemic actions, including insulin (51 amino acids) [132, 133] and leuprolide (9 amino acids) [132, 134], have been studied extensively. One inhaled insulin formulation in dry powder form, Exubera®, was marketed from August 2006 to October 2007 for the treatment of type 1 and type 2 diabetes. Before the advent of the inhaled insulin, patients generally receive multiple daily injections for treatment of their disease, including long-acting insulin once or twice a day and short-acting insulin before meals. Inhaled insulin replaces short-acting insulin and eliminates as many as four injections per day [132, 133]. The peptide leuprolide has been investigated for the treatment of prostate cancer, endometriosis, and uterine fibroids and has a long history in animal and clinical studies [132, 134]. The pulmonary route offers the portal of delivering a much wider range of protein and peptide-based drugs for systemic action, as seen in Table 5-3.

Other systemically targeted peptides and proteins currently under different stages of investigation include interferon-α, interferon-γ, α$_1$-antitrypsin, parathyroid hormone, growth hormone, glucagon-like peptide 1, and granulocyte-macrophage colony-stimulating factors. Inhaled administration produces different pharmacokinetic profiles in comparison with therapeutics given parenterally. It is generally accepted that the molecular weight for acceptable rates of absorption for peptides and proteins ranges from 5 to 20 kDa, primarily because of the relatively tight junctions between alveolar epithelial cells [70]. As would be expected in insulin delivery, rapid absorption through the lung epithelium into the lung is desirable. Time-action profiles have shown that inhaled

Table 5-2 Comparison of advantages and disadvantages for pulmonary and parenteral delivery of systemically acting drugs

Advantages	Disadvantages
Parenteral route	
Barriers to drug absorption: major barrier stratum corneum is easy to avoid; other barriers lipid matrix excreted by cells, endothelial cells of the capillary vasculature, metabolic enzymes	Less convenient, formulation reconstitution required, sterility and pyrogen-free conditions required in-hospital treatment
Precision in dosing	Needle injection required (SC, IM, intravenous), more invasive, less patient compliance
No hepatic first-pass effect, high bioavailability, cost-effective	Less safe, potential for infection or embolism
Controlled release formulation possible	Absorption variability, difficult to reverse toxicity
Pulmonary route	
Major barrier thin alveolar epithelium is easy to penetrate; large alveolar surface area and vascularization for quick drug absorption; other barriers macrophage, mucocilliary clearance, metabolic enzymes on the type II alveoli	Dosing variability caused by formulation, device, and patient inhalation
Portable devices, needle-free delivery, safer	Require appropriate inhalation techniques
Rapid onset of action compared with SC; lung surfactant aids in dissolution and absorption	Low effective dose with respect to the nominal dose
No hepatic first-pass effect	More difficult to manufacture, costly device and formulation

insulin reaches maximal insulin concentration more rapidly than both regular insulin [135] and SC insulin [136]. For equivalent dosing, the exposure time was shorter with inhaled insulin than SC administration, suggesting the risk of delayed hypoglycemia may be less with inhaled insulin administration [137]. The most recent published studies showed a new promising dry powder formulation of inhaled insulin, Technosphere® (Afrezza®, MannKind), which is in phase III clinical trials [138, 139]. For this formulation, studies showed both rapid systemic uptake of insulin (T_{max} = 12–14 minutes) and fast onset of drug action [136]. The FDA requested more study data of Afrezza® in early 2011 [140]. Another drug, the glucagon–like peptide 1 and its PEGylated conjugates, are also under evaluation in their ability to treat diabetes and obesity via the pulmonary route where therapeutics in this application delivered via the SC route suffer from too short of a circulating half–life (~2 minutes) [141].

Many innovations in formulation and device technologies have been applied for the delivery of inhaled peptides and proteins. For example, cospray drying with carbohydrates has been used to improve stability in lyophilized insulin (PulmoSol®, Nektar Therapeutics) [142]. Particle engineering has produced low–density porous particles

TABLE 5-3 Examples of investigated pulmonary delivery of proteins and peptides for systemic actions

Proteins and Peptides	Molecular Weight (Da)	Systemic Application	Reference
Lysine-vasopressin	1056	Diabetes insipidus	Martin & Mathew [282]
Leuprolide acetate	1209	Prostate cancer, endometriosis, uterine fibroids	Adjei et al. [134,283,284] Patton [132]
Calcitonin	3455	Osteoporosis, hypercalcemia	Komada et al. [285] Patton [286]
Glucagon-like peptide 1	4111	Diabetes, obesity	Leone et al. [141]
Parathyroid hormone	ca. 9400	Osteoporosis	Codron et al. [287]
Insulin	ca. 5800	Type 1 and type 2 diabetes	Gansslen [288] Patton et al. [289] Laube [133]
Granulocyte-macrophage colony-stimulating factor	ca. 14,400	Idiopathic alveolar proteinosis, neutropenia	Tazawa et al. [290]
Interferon-α	ca. 19,000	Hepatitis C, melanoma, bronchioalveolar carcinoma	Kinnula et al. [291]
α_1-Antitrypsin	ca. 44,324	α_1-Antitrypsin deficiency	Griese et al. [292]
Human growth hormone	ca. 22,000	Growth hormone deficiency, cachexia	Walvoord et al. [293]
Human immunoglobulin G	ca. 150,000	Prophylaxis	Bot et al. [294]

containing rifampicin with high uniformity (PulmoSpheres®, Alliance Pharmaceutical) that enhance alveolar deposition and bioavailability [122]. Devices have been tailored for the delivery of proteins or peptides via liquid mists (e.g., Aerogen® device, Aeroneb) or dry powder aerosols (e.g., Medtone® device, MannKind or AIR® device, Alkermes) [122].

Several critical aspects, however, still need to be addressed to ensure the success of inhalation peptides and proteins therapies, such as ensuring the dosing accuracy, increasing bioavailability, and cost-effectiveness. As an example, insulin has a relatively narrow therapeutic window and ensuring the dosing accuracy is critical to avoid side effects such as hypoglycemia. The bioavailability of inhaled insulin is typically around 10% to 15%, presumably because of enzymatic degradation in the alveoli and mucociliary clearance of the delivered drug [143, 144]. Factors such as cellular transporters and surfactants may also affect drug uptake and bioavailability [144]. Because of high cost and supply issues, only a few protein and peptide pulmonary therapeutics have progressed through to clinical trials. More research is also warranted to evaluate the impact of patient characteristics on the inhalation delivery of peptide and protein drugs. For example, the different durations of breath holding after one inspiration of insulin have been investigated using the AERx® (Aradigm) delivery system [145].

Pulmonary Delivery of Vaccines

Aerosol vaccination provides a noninvasive, cost-effective, yet powerful route to fight against infectious diseases [146]. Needle-free delivery avoids potential hazards such as transmission of bloodborne diseases like HIV when dealing with needles. Its ease of administration may also help to facilitate mass vaccination campaigns [146, 147].

Below the pulmonary epithelium are a host of immune cells, including local antigen-presenting cells (dendritic cells and alveolar macrophages [148]) that continuously sample inhaled antigens and present them to T cells and bronchoalveolar lymphoid tissue [146, 149]. The inhalation route has an advantage in triggering an immune response that is initiated at the port of entry for many airborne pathogens and as a result should be particularly effective in the prevention or elimination of respiratory infections caused by bacteria such as tuberculosis and viruses such as influenza and measles [113, 150]. The delivery of vaccine antigens to the pulmonary mucosa can induce immune responses both locally and systemically [151, 152]. The inhalation route may also be used to vaccinate children whose immunological response cannot be induced subcutaneously due to the interference of maternally derived antibodies [122].

A host of bacterial and viral pathogens that cause pulmonary diseases and the corresponding vaccines and adjuvants have been reviewed elsewhere [113, 146]. Many pulmonary vaccines are in the preclinical stages for protection against tuberculosis [146, 153], influenza [151, 154, 155], measles [156, 157], hepatitis B [158–160], and diphtheria [161, 162]. A few pioneer clinical studies of pulmonary vaccines, including those for measles [163–166], tuberculosis [167], and human papillomavirus [168], have been carried out, some of them in large populations. Several pulmonary vaccine candidates are also being explored for the prophylactic vaccination of airborne pathogens such as *Bacillus anthracis* and *Francisella tularensis*, which are deadly pathogens that could be intentionally released in a bioterrorist attack [169, 170].

Successful pulmonary vaccination depends on inducing one specific or multiple immune responses in the airway mucosa and systemic immune system. Vaccine antigens can be presented in a variety of forms, including live attenuated, inactivated, subunit or recombinant proteins, toxoid, and DNA vaccines [113]. Adjuvants (immunostimulators) may be added to the formulations to enhance immunogenicity. In addition to the effectiveness of inhaled vaccines themselves, the selection of the appropriate aerosol formulation and the correct inhaler device are essential. Vaccines should retain their potency upon pharmaceutical processing such as spray drying and upon formulation reconstitution [171, 172]. Most pulmonary vaccinations use aqueous formulations, dry powder formulations reconstituted upon use, and dry powder aerosol formulations [122]. These formulations should be well dispersed into respirable particles when aerosolized.

To evaluate the effectiveness of an aerosolized measles vaccine, several modern nebulizers such as those developed by Omron, Trudell, and Aerogen have been evaluated in clinical trials [122]. Subsequently, dry powder formulations delivered by DPIs have several advantages. As described previously, these solid-state powders result in improved formulation stability and offer the advantage of being free of cold-chain storage complications associated with liquid-based vaccines. The particulate nature of dry powder vaccines may also enhance immunogenicity because antigen-presenting cells in the lungs tend to uptake dry particles, which elicits an additional immune response [173]. Several specially designed DPIs are being used for the evaluation of inhaled vaccinations. For example, the PuffHaler® (Aktiv-Dry) and the BD Solovent® (BD Technologies) are being evaluated in the delivery of dry powder inhaled measles vaccines

[157]. Vaccine-containing dry powder aerosols are generated by manually compressed air. Pulmonary delivery can be achieved in two steps when the aerosols are first contained in a plastic bag and then are inhaled orally or in a single step when masks (Puff-mask and Sol-mask) are connected [157]. The delivery using these devices can also be achieved intranasally (discussed below) if nasal prongs such as Puff-nasal® and Sol-nasal® are attached to the devices [157]. Further reading into the development of dry powder formulations for pulmonary vaccine delivery can be found elsewhere [174].

NASAL AEROSOL DELIVERY

Local and systemic nasal aerosol delivery has been in practice for a long time [175]. Several types of nasal aerosol delivery systems are available, including nonpressurized metered dose sprays, pressurized metered dose sprays, atomized (nonmetered squeeze) pumps, nasal DPIs, and nebulizers. Other intranasal delivery systems, which are not nasal aerosols, such as the nose drop, saturated cotton pledget, and insufflators, are not discussed here [175, 176]. A wide variety of nasal aerosol formulations has been developed that include solutions, suspensions, and dry powders. Nasal sprays with aqueous solutions have been the most frequently used in the treatment of local conditions such as rhinitis, sinusitis, and nasal congestions. Examples of a number of currently marketed nasal aerosol products for local delivery are listed in **Table 5-4**.

TABLE 5-4 Examples of marketed nasal aerosol products used for local action					
Product	**Drug**	**Device Type**	**Mechanism of Action**	**Treatment**	**Company**
Nasonex®	Mometasone furoate monohydrate	Nonpressurized metered dose spray	Anti-inflammatory corticosteroid	Allergic rhinitis, sinusitis	Merck
Afrin®	Oxymetazoline hydrochloride	Nonpressurized metered dose spray	α-Adrenergic agonist	Sinus congestion	Schering-Plough
Rhinolast®	Azelastine hydrochloride	Nonpressurized metered dose spray	Antihistamine	Allergic rhinitis	Meda Pharmaceutical
Rhinocort® Turbuhaler®	Budesonide	Nasal dry powder (device metered)	Anti-inflammatory corticosteroid	Immotile cilia syndrome, rhinitis	AstraZeneca
Nasacort®	Triamcinolone acetonide	Pressurized metered dose nasal spray	Anti-inflammatory corticosteroid	Allergic rhinitis	Sanofi Aventis Pharmaceutical
Qnasl®	Beclomethasone dipropionate	Pressurized metered dose nasal spray	Anti-inflammatory corticosteroid	Allergic rhinitis	Teva Respiratory
Aeroneb Solo®	Diagnostic agent	Nasal mesh nebulizer			Aerogen

Similar to the pulmonary route for systemic delivery, the highly vascularized nasal cavity allows for rapid drug transport into the bloodstream without undergoing first-pass hepatic metabolism. This provides yet another convenient and noninvasive alternative to parenteral and transdermal delivery pathways. Nasal delivery is also a safe route for patients who cannot easily breathe orally, such as pediatric patients. Nasal aerosols for systemic delivery can be categorized according to their corresponding drug types: proteins and peptides for a variety of treatments, vaccines to induce mucosal and/or systemic immune responses, and opioids for pain relief. The delivery of proteins and peptides can be exemplified as the intranasal administration of calcitonin and insulin, which have been studied the most extensively [177, 178]. Nasal vaccination against smallpox infection appeared more than 1,000 years ago [179]. Currently, nasal flu vaccines have become reliable and routine methods of prophylaxis against influenza infections.

A unique feature of the nasal cavity is that the olfactory tissue is in close contact with the central nervous systems (CNS), which is particularly useful for delivering drugs to this part of the body. Nasal formulations have been used to deliver opioids such as fentanyl for pain control and cocaine for drug abuse. Examples of nasal aerosols for systemic applications include but are not limited to migraine drugs such as sumatriptan (Imitrex®, Sun Pharmaceuticals), zolmitriptan (Zomig®, AstraZeneca), therapeutic proteins and peptides such as calcitonin (Miacalsin®, Novartis), insulin, hormones such as estradiol hemihydrate and progesterone, analgesics such as butorphanol tartrate (Stadol®, Cigna), morphine, nasal vaccines for the treatment of influenza (FluMist®, MedImmune), and measles. Successfully marketed nasal aerosol products are listed in Table 5-5.

TABLE 5-5 Examples of marketed nasal aerosol products for systemic action

Product	Drug	Device Type	Mechanism of Action	Treatment	Company
Imitrex®	Sumatriptan	Nonpressurized metered dose spray	Serotonin agonist	Migraine headaches	GlaxoSmithKline
Zomig®	Zolmitriptan	Nonpressurized metered dose spray	Serotonin agonist	Migraine headaches	Impax Pharmaceuticals
Aerodiol®	Estradiol hemihydrate	Nonpressurized metered dose spray	Estrogen replacement	Postmenopausal hormone replacement therapy	Servier Laboratories
Miacalcin®	Salmon calcitonin	Nonpressurized metered dose spray	Inhibition of bone resorptive process	Postmenopausal osteoporosis	Novartis
Stadol®	Butorphanol tartrate	Nonpressurized metered dose spray	Opiate antagonist	Pain relief	Cigna
FluMist®	Influenza vaccine live	Single-dose spray	Mucosa vaccination	Influenza immunization	MedImmune

The nasal cavity incorporates multiple features such as breathing, smell sensing, and mucociliary clearance. Optimal nasal drug targeting differs for local, systemic, and CNS delivery.

Nasal Aerosols for Local Action

Locally acting nasal aerosols are commonly used in the treatment of rhinitis, sinusitis, nasal congestion, and nasal polyps. The classes of nasal drugs for these conditions include anti-inflammatory corticosteroids (e.g., mometasone furoate) [180], antihistamines (e.g., azelastine hydrochloride) [181, 182], and α-adrenergic agonists (e.g., oxymetazoline hydrochloride) (Table 5-4). The efficacies of combined therapies using two nasal drugs with distinct mechanisms of action, for example, both corticosteroids and antihistamine [183, 184] or α-adrenergic agonist combined with a corticosteroid [185, 186], have been evaluated. The combined therapy is expected to enhance the effectiveness of single-drug therapy for the treatment of conditions such as severe allergic rhinitis or persistent nasal congestion.

The distribution of drugs in the nasal cavity depends on the types of delivery system and the techniques of administration [176]. Most approved nasal aerosol products (e.g., Nasonex®, Merck) are aqueous formulations used for local action as nonpressurized metered dose sprays. Similar to pulmonary pMDIs, nasal pMDIs using ozone-depleting CFC propellants were prohibited in the United States since 2006. New formulations using the propellants HFA 134a and bechlomethasone dipropionate (e.g., Qnasl®, Teva Respiratory) have recently entered the market for the treatment of persistent allergic rhinitis [187]. DPIs (e.g., Turbuhaler®, AstraZeneca) loaded with nasal formulations (e.g., Rhinolast®, AstraZeneca) have been marketed for the treatment of allergic rhinitis [188]. For chronic sinusitis, delivery of drug to the middle and superior meatuses (sinus openings) is desirable. Furthermore, lung deposition is deemed an unwanted side effect for nasal delivery [189], and respirable particles below 9 μm have an increased chance to deposit in the lung when inhaled nasally [189].

Several new nasal delivery technologies have been developed to optimize nasal targeting and avoid lung deposition [190]. A new nasal delivery system using breath-powered Bi-Directional™ technology is currently in phase III clinical trials [176, 191]. This system contains a connected nosepiece and mouthpiece. When the user exhales through the mouthpiece into the nosepiece that is inserted and sealed in one nostril, the soft palate is automatically elevated to isolate the nasal cavity from the rest of the respiratory tract because of the positive oropharyngeal pressure. This creates an open loop for the airflow with drugs to enter one nostril, pass entirely around the nasal septum, and exit through the other nostril [191]. This technology circumvents the lung deposition and is suitable for delivering both liquid and powder formulations [191]. Nasal devices for local actions are mainly multidose products and are well suited for drugs to be administered over a prolonged period of time.

Nasal Delivery of Proteins and Peptides

With the development of recombinant technology, dozens of therapeutically active proteins and peptides have been produced and evaluated for nasal aerosol delivery [175, 192]. Similar to the pulmonary route, nasal delivery offers much lower protein and peptide degradation than the oral route [193]. A good example of the nasal aerosol delivery of calcitonin-salmon (Miacalcin®, Novartis). Calcitonin is a linear polypeptide made of 32 amino acids that participates in the calcium homeostasis by lowering blood calcium ion concentration and inhibiting bone resorption [194]. Miacalcin® is used in the treatment of postmenopausal osteoporosis and is administered as a nonpressurized metered dose nasal spray. The intranasal delivery of insulin and insulin analogues, however, have been shown to not alter blood insulin and glucose levels. Surprisingly, these therapeutics rapidly gain access to the cerebrospinal fluid after nasal administration [195] (see Intranasal CNS Delivery, below). Intranasal insulin is now being investigated for the treatment of Alzheimer's disease [196]. Several other therapeutic proteins can also be delivered intranasally (see Intranasal CNS Delivery, below).

One of the key issues for the nasal aerosol delivery of proteins and peptides is drug absorption, which may greatly influence the systemic bioavailability of the drugs. Similar to pulmonary airways, the highly vascularized mucosa lining of the turbinates and conchae in the nasal cavity provide good drug absorption by means of paracellular or transcellular mechanisms [175]. The absorption of drugs follows either paracellular or transcellular pathways and is influenced by multiple factors, including the physicochemical properties of the formulations, drug distribution in the nasal cavity, and mucociliary clearance [175]. The surface area available for drug absorption in the nasal cavity, however, is only about 180 cm^2, which is much smaller than that in the lungs.

Larger or hydrophilic protein or peptide molecules often show poor bioavailability because they are less likely to pass through the nasal epithelial cell layer [175]. In addition, the osmolarity and pH of the formulation may influence both drug deposition in the nasal cavity and transport pathways [175]. Absorption enhancers such as cyclodextrins, phospholipids, and chitosan are often used to increase the absorption and bioavailability of protein and peptide drugs [197]. It should be noted, however, that some absorption enhancers for nasal aerosol delivery are also nasal irritants that may inflict damage to the nasal membrane [197]. For example, chitosan enhances drug absorption by opening tight junctions between epithelial cells [197, 198]. The development of safer absorption enhancers may encourage patient compliance and acceptance of these types of nasal aerosol products in the clinical trials. Sustained-release formulations using bioadhesive polymers and biodegradable microspheres are known to increase the residence time and enhance the absorption to aid in drug availability [199]. In general, a broad distribution of nasal drugs on mucosal surfaces is desirable for systemic drug absorption [176]. Delivery of drugs to the posterior turbinate region may benefit from higher drug permeability and shorter residence time, which is suitable for drugs intended for rapid uptake and quick onset of action, such as zolmitriptan for the treatment of migraine headache [200]. Furthermore, slower mucociliary clearance increases drug residence time and may enhance drug absorption [201], and the rate of mucociliary clearance can be influenced by several factors such as the diseased state of the nasal passage and resulting formulations [201].

Nasal Aerosol Vaccines

The first nasal aerosol vaccination dated back more than 1,000 years ago from an anecdotal report that the Chinese blew pulverized smallpox scabs into the nostrils of others to immunize them to the disease [179]. Today, nasal aerosols provide a safe, needle-free, efficacious vaccination against seasonal and pandemic influenza [202]. It is generally known that vaccination via the nasal route is relevant in pulmonary vaccination because nasal-associated lymphoid tissue, which bears some similarities with the Peyer's patches of the intestine, is one of the mucosal-associated lymphoid tissue components [203]. The nasal-associated lymphoid tissue is situated under the nasal epithelium with specialized epithelial cells called microfold (M) cells. Phagocytosis of antigens by M cells and dendritic cells stimulates the recruitment of helper T cells and induces mucosal immune responses similar to those seen in pulmonary immunization [204].

The topic of nasal influenza vaccination has been extensively reviewed in recent years [203, 205–208]. Compared with conventional IM or SC vaccination, the nasal route induces the immune response at the site of pathogen entry and results in a better cellular immune response [205, 206]. The commercial product FluMist® (MedImmune) uses a live attenuated influenza vaccine that induces an immune response similar to those induced by natural influenza infection, and this is a perfect example of "infect to protect" [209]. FluMist® is approved in several countries, including the United States, Europena Union, and Canada, and has been in use for individuals aged between 2 and 49 years since the 2007–2008 influenza season [208, 209]. Many other nasal aerosol vaccines with increased immunogenicity and less adverse effect are in development, including the measles vaccine [157], tuberculosis vaccine [153, 210], human papillomavirus vaccine [211], smallpox vaccine [212], and anthrax vaccine [213, 214]. Devices used for nasal influenza vaccines are mainly single- or dual-dose spray products that are intended for single-dose regimens. For example, a prefilled device (Accuspray™, Becton Dickinson Technologies) is used to deliver FluMist® [176].

Intranasal CNS Delivery

The targeting of therapeutic agents, especially large biomolecules to the CNS, is challenging because most are unable to cross the blood–brain barrier from systemic blood circulation. In general, the blood–brain barrier only allows a few small (<500 Da) and lipophilic molecules to enter the CNS via the bloodstream [215]. Sufficient evidence, however, has shown that intranasal administration of many therapeutic agents can rapidly gain access to the cerebrospinal fluid or different regions of the CNS. Clinical or animal studies have shown that a broad spectrum of therapeutic agents, including small lipophilic molecules such as cocaine [216] and morphine [217]; large protein molecules such as insulin (5.8 kDa) [195], leptin (16 kDa) [218], and nerve growth factor (27.5 kDa) [219]; a selected oligonucleotide [220]; and plasmid DNA (3.5–14.2 kb) [221], have been successfully delivered to the CNS after intranasal administration. It should be noted that those large biomolecules fall into the nanoparticle size range and can be categorized as nanomedicine, discussed in Pulmonary Nanomedicine, below.

There are four proposed pathways for the transport of molecules from the nasal cavity to the CNS [222]. The major pathway that allows therapeutics to directly enter the CNS is the olfactory nerve pathway. The olfactory region is located in the superior portion of the nasal cavity in an area of approximately 370 mm² [223]. The olfactory nerves are connected with the trigeminal nervous system between the brain and external environment. This pathway provides a shortcut that allows intranasally applied drug to be transported to the CNS within minutes [224]. Drug concentrations in the olfactory bulbs are generally among the highest in CNS concentration [222, 225]. The second pathway is the trigeminal nerve pathway. The trigeminal nerve innervates the respiratory and olfactory epithelium of the nasal passages. The evidence showing that significant drug distribution to the trigeminal nerve and caudal brain areas such as the brainstem and cerebellum after intranasal delivery suggests that the trigeminal nerves are involved [222, 226]. For small and lipophilic drugs, there is also a good chance that intranasal administration to the CNS follows the vascular pathway because of the highly vascularized nasal mucosa [222]. Drugs delivered to the cerebrospinal fluid and the lymphatic drainage provides the fourth pathway for intranasal CNS delivery [222].

The development of intranasal CNS delivery is still in its infancy [227]. The elucidation of the underlying delivery pathways, the implications of the formulation factors, and pharmacokinetic and pharmacodynamic relationships are essential to improve the treatment of neurological diseases by the intranasal route [227, 228]. The capability of intranasal CNS delivery also raises safety issues, because of the possibility of exposing the CNS to undesired substances when drugs are delivered in the nasal cavity.

PULMONARY NANOMEDICINE

Nanomedicine is the application of nanotechnology to medicine, in particular, in diagnostic testing and drug delivery systems [229]. In pharmaceutical and drug delivery literature, nanoparticles are generally expressed between 1 and 1000 nm in either dimension [230, 231]. Particles in this submicron size range often demonstrate biological relevant characteristics such as enhanced permeability and absorption and distinct physicochemical properties from microparticles such as increased aggregation, altered deposition profiles as a function of particle size and breathing pattern, and enhanced solubility. Various drugs investigated for local or pulmonary delivery have been described in the sections above. A more detailed list of pulmonary drugs prepared for nanoparticle delivery has been reviewed previously [229]. Nanoparticulate systems in pulmonary delivery offer many advantages, including (1) the potential to achieve uniform distribution and deep lung deposition; (2) enhanced drug dissolution rates and solubility; (3) faster and high uptake by the pulmonary epithelial cell, therefore enhancing systemic absorption and bioavailability; (4) the avoidance of the lung's normal clearance mechanisms (e.g., alveolar macrophage uptake); (5) the capability of being formulated into rapid or sustained release dosage forms; (6) protection of encapsulated or absorbed drugs from degradation; and (7) improving drug targeting and subsequently reducing systemic toxicity [232, 233].

Nanoparticles have a high surface area to volume ratio. Because of their strong tendency to agglomerate, resistance to flow during pharmaceutical processing, and tendency to be exhaled during inhalation, the use of neat nanoparticle drugs for pulmonary delivery is limited. Although a few review articles and book chapters have extensively covered a variety of nanoparticle drug delivery systems including liposomes, polymeric nanocarriers, polymeric micelles, solid lipid nanoparticles (SLNs), microemulsions, nanogels, and submicron lipid emulsions [229, 233–239], this section briefly touches on several classes of drug-loaded nanocarrier systems and nanodrug particle aggregates for pulmonary delivery, because they appear most frequently in the literature. These include encapsulation of pulmonary drugs into nanoparticulate carrier systems (polymers and dendrimers), encapsulation of drugs in lipid self-assembly systems (liposomes) and SLNs, and nanodrug particle aggregates.

Polymeric Nanoparticulate Systems

Polymeric nanoparticles have been extensively studied in drug delivery systems for both parenteral and pulmonary routes [229, 236]. The main roles of polymeric nanoparticles are to act as carriers, to protect the drug from degradation, and to control drug release [240]. Several biodegradable or biocompatible polymers, including PLGA, polylactic acid, PCL, alginic acid, gelatin, or chitosan, are often used to encapsulate therapeutic agents intended for pulmonary delivery into polymeric (colloidal carrier) systems [241, 242]. Polymeric nanoparticle sizes range from 1 to 1000 nm [243]. A more detailed list of these polymeric nanoparticulate systems has been reviewed previously [229]. Because of their biocompatibility and surface modification capability, polymeric nanoparticles have been extensively evaluated for the sustained release of pulmonary drugs. For example, surface-modified PLGA nanoparticles with chitosan have been used to improve the pulmonary delivery of calcitonin via nebulization [244]. Enhanced drug absorption was attributed to sustained drug release in the bronchial mucus and lung tissue due to the absorption enhancing effect of the modified PLGA nanoparticles [244]. The use of modified cationic polymers such as polyethyleneimine is another example that shows the versatility of these nanocarriers used in pulmonary gene delivery [245]. Details of pulmonary gene delivery using cationic polymer have been reviewed elsewhere [246].

One special class of polymeric nanoparticulate systems is dendrimer-based nanoparticles. Dendrimers are monodispersed nanoparticles that contain repeated and hyperbranched structures around a core molecule. Their sizes typically range from 1 to 10 nm depending on the generation. Dendrimers have been widely used to encapsulate a variety of small molecular drugs such as heparin for the prevention of thrombosis [247] and macromolecules such as small interfering (si)RNA and plasmid DNA for gene and antisense therapy [248]. They encapsulate drugs by covalent conjugation, ionic interaction (e.g., dendrimer–DNA complex), or acting as a unimolecular micelle [249]. Advantages of using dendrimers as nanocarrier systems in pulmonary delivery include their monodispersity, high water solubility, and highly functionalizable surface moieties. Several studies have been published regarding pulmonary applications of dendrimers as systemic delivery carriers for macromolecules [245, 247, 250, 251].

The study of polymeric and dendrimer nanoparticles for pulmonary delivery is mainly in the preclinical stage. In contrast to other means of systemic administrations, the controlled release properties of inhaled nanoparticles for systemic administration are not well explored. Data for sufficient drug loading and desired drug release kinetics for pulmonary delivery are still absent. The biodegradability and toxicity profiles using these systems over repeated dosing and the long-term influences of these systems to the lung surfactants should also be closely examined.

Liposomes and Solid Lipid Nanoparticulate Systems

Both liposomes and SLNs are colloidal lipid-based systems. Liposomes are self-assembled phospholipid vesicles that resemble cell bilayers, with sizes ranging from 50 to above 1000 nm. Liposomes are one of the most extensively investigated nanoparticle systems for controlled pulmonary delivery [130, 252–256]. Liposomes can be prepared from synthetic phospholipids or surfactants endogenous to the lungs such as dipalmitoylphosphatidylcholine and the commercial lung surfactant Alveofact® (Dr. Karl Thomae GmbH, Biberach, Germany). This suggests that when delivered, they can enter the surfactant pool in the lung without eliciting an immune response.

Many pulmonary drugs have been encapsulated into liposomes for the treatment of lung cancer, tuberculosis, cystic fibrosis, lung infection, asthma, and COPD [256]. Among them, the use of liposomes as nonviral vectors for gene therapy has seen great attention in recent years [257–260]. DNA, siRNA, and antisense oligodeoxynucleotide are gene molecules that silence disease-causing genes. Anionic–cationic electrostatic interactions allow for these materials to complex with cationic liposomes to form polyplex nanoparticles. Their stability increases greatly compared with naked gene molecules used in gene delivery. For example, the self-assembled formation of liposome-polycation-DNA nanoparticles has been achieved by stepwise electrostatic interactions. By incorporating the anisamide targeting ligand, these liposomal nanoparticles can provide the selective delivery of antisense oligodeoxynucleotide and siRNA to treat lung cancer [257].

Drug targeting can also be achieved using liposomes coupled with targeting ligands or by using PEGylation. Although liposomes prepared in solution can be administered using a nebulizer, an alternative way is to prepare liposomal dry powders for DPI administration. Liposomal dry powder formulations can be prepared by reverse-phase evaporation followed by spray drying or spray freeze-drying [261]. Liposomal dry powder systems avoid the stability issues often seen with nebulized liposomal solutions, and they have been used to encapsulate a variety of pulmonary drugs, including bronchodilators, anti-inflammatories, antimicrobials, immunomodulators, and chemotherapeutics [130, 253, 254, 256].

SLNs are lipid matrices that are solid at body temperature. The advantages of using SLN systems in pulmonary delivery include the successful encapsulation and immobilization of drugs in the solid matrix, controlled release profiles, the possibility of high drug loading and production efficiency, and faster *in vivo* degradation and lower toxicity compared with polymeric nanoparticles. Similar to liposomal systems, solution SLN formulations for nebulizers or dry powder SLN formulations for DPIs can be prepared for pulmonary delivery [262]. SLNs have been investigated for the treatment of tuberculosis using encapsulated rifampicin, isoniazid, and pyrazinamide by emulsion solvent diffusion techniques [263]. Nebulized SLN formulations greatly increase the mean residence time and drug bioavailability compared with oral doses [263]. SLNs have also been used to encapsulate macromolecules such as DNA for gene delivery [264]. and insulin in therapeutic protein delivery [265].

Microparticle Aggregates of Nanodrug Particulates

Instead of using simple nanocarrier systems, a variety of novel technologies and formulation approaches has been used for the preparation of drug particles in nanosize ranges. Because of the strong adhesive forces between nanoparticles, they tend to form low-density microparticle aggregates that often exhibit improved aerodynamic behavior for efficient pulmonary delivery. In nature, microparticles such as spores from fungi or molds can be easily aerosolized. They contain underlying nanostructures that aggregate into microparticles. Other advantages of these nanoparticle-aggregated microparticles are increased solubility of poorly soluble drugs, enhanced penetration of cell barriers, and avoidance of alveolar macrophage uptake.

Methods of nanoparticle production often begin with the preparation of a nanosuspension. Nanosuspensions have been prepared using a variety of techniques, including reactive high gravity controlled precipitation [266], antisolvent precipitation [267], and microemulsions [268, 269]. Nanoparticle suspensions of one drug in the solution of another have been explored for combination therapies. For example, an anticancer paclitaxel nanoparticle suspension was introduced into a cisplatin solution [270]. An antiasthmatic drug fluticasone propionate nanosuspension (about 400 nm) was added to an albuterol sulfate solution [271]. After the solution is formed, the resulting colloidal suspensions are then flocculated using a compound such as L-leucine to disrupt the electrostatic repulsion between nanoparticles. The nanoparticles are then aggregated into a more favorable microparticle system by means of carefully controlled spray drying [266, 267, 269], spray freeze drying, lypholization [270], or supercritical fluid technology [272] to create nanoparticle-aggregated microparticles in the desired respirable size. It should be noted that the nanoparticle-aggregated microparticles are typically low-density aggregates with favorable aerodynamic properties [239].

In recent years, a few novel nanoparticle technologies have been developed. For example, the Technosphere® developed by MannKind uses crystalline fumaryl diketopiperazine as substrate plates, and drug nanoparticles are adsorbed onto these plates for effective delivery of calcitonin (Miacalsin®, Novartis), parathyroid hormone, and insulin for systemic actions [273]. Nonaggregated albuterol sulfate nanoparticles were prepared by coating drug particles with sublimated L-leucine in an aerosol flow reactor. Albuterol sulfate nanoparticles, about 65 nm in diameter, were generated by atomizing a precursor solution, and the L-leucine coating was achieved simultaneously [274].

SUMMARY

Sustained-release injectable depot systems are possible through the formation of a depot or reservoir at the site of injection after drug administration. As a result, the injectable depot system is one of the most effective systems for long-term drug delivery. Because of the enhanced quality of life and cost of therapy supported by the advances in drug formulation and polymer science, more sophisticated injectable depot systems will be developed and commercialized in the near future.

Aerosol drug delivery is yet to be a mature route of administration after several decades of unremitting scientific innovation in devices and formulations. Many new DPI devices that are more efficient in drug dispersion and user-friendly have been developed. More efficient and environmental friendly formulations have been developed. The delivery of inhaled aerosols directly to the airways offers many advantages for both local and systemic therapy. For local action, the prominent therapeutic category of interest is asthma and COPD. Drugs intended for the maintenance treatment of these diseases, such as inhaled bronchodilators and corticosteroids, when they are inhaled, offer clinical advantages, including rapid onset of drug action, low dosage, and decreased incidence of side effects.

The airway is the portal of pathogen entry for pulmonary infection. In this sense, the pulmonary delivery of antibacterial and antiviral agents can offer the advantage of high local concentrations of drug targeting at the origin of the infection. For systemic action, the large surface area of thin alveolar epithelium and lung surfactant lining allow for fast onset of action and improved drug absorption, especially for macromolecular delivery such as peptides and proteins. Systemic delivery via the pulmonary route may also circumvent drug inactivation caused by hepatic first-pass effect. A large number of systemic diseases have been investigated, including but not limited to diabetes, osteoporosis, growth hormone deficiency, and pain management.

Both pulmonary and nasal routes offer advantages for vaccine delivery, as pulmonary, nasal, and oral immune systems contribute to almost 80% of all immunocytes that accumulate in or transit between various mucosal-associated lymphoid tissues, which form the first line of defense against pathogens. Noninvasive, easy to administer, and cost-effective, inhaled vaccinations have shown great potential for mass vaccination campaigns. Furthermore, a unique feature of nasal aerosol delivery is the capability for CNS delivery through the olfactory trigeminal nervous system that circumvents the blood–brain barrier.

Although most of the effort in the last decades focused on the microparticulate systems for pulmonary delivery, the exploration of nanomedicines for pulmonary delivery has gained great attention recently. The large surface area to volume ratio of nanoparticles enables further opportunities for innovations of drug targeting and sustained release therapies.

REVIEW QUESTIONS

1. Which of the following prescription nasal products are used for systemic drug delivery by the nasal aerosol delivery route?
   a. Zomig®, Imitrex®, Miacalcin®
   b. Rhinocort®, Zomig®, Flonase®
   c. Flumist®, Nasalcrom®, Zomig®
   d. Zomig®, Veramyst®, Flumist®
   e. Miacalcin®, Nasonex®, Imitrex®

2. Which statement is correct regarding the advantages of pulmonary inhalation aerosol delivery?
   a. Requires a high dose and has a fast onset of action
   b. Requires a low dose and has a slow onset of drug action
   c. Requires a high dose and has a slow onset of action
   d. Requires a low dose and has a fast onset of action
   e. None of the above

3. True or False: Pulmicort® Turbuhaler® DPI does not contain lactose carrier particles.
   a. True
   b. False

4. PLGA is which polymer type?
   a. A diblock copolymer from the natural-origin polymer class
   b. A diblock copolymer from the synthetic polyester-based polymer class
   c. A triblock copolymer from the synthetic polyester-based polymer class
   d. A triblock copolymer from the natural-origin polymer class

5. Which of the following statements is correct regarding immediate drug release versus controlled drug release?
   a. Immediate release is zero-order and controlled release is first-order.
   b. Immediate release is first-order and controlled release is second-order.
   c. Immediate release is zero order and controlled release is super zero-order.
   d. Immediate release is first-order and controlled release is zero-order.

6. Which statement is correct regarding inhalation aerosol vaccine delivery?
   a. FluMist® contains an antiviral drug.
   b. FluMist® Diskhaler® contains a live attenuated virus and an antiviral drug.
   c. FluMist® contains a live attenuated virus.

REFERENCES

1. Prettyman J. Subcutaneous or intramuscular? Confronting a parenteral administration dilemma. *Medsurg Nurs.* 2005;14(2):93–98; quiz 99.

2. Sinha VR, Trehan A. Biodegradable microspheres for protein delivery. *J Control Release.* 2003;90(3):261–280.

3. Hatefi A, Amsden B. Biodegradable injectable in situ forming drug delivery systems. *J Control Release.* 2002;80(1–3):9–28.

4. Packhaeuser CB, Schnieders J, Oster CG, Kissel T. In situ forming parenteral drug delivery systems: an overview. *Eur J Pharm Biopharm.* 2004;58(2):445–455.

5. Chitkara D, Shikanov A, Kumar N, Domb AJ. Biodegradable injectable in situ depot-forming drug delivery systems. *Macromol Biosci.* 2006;6(12):977–990.

6. Mansour HM, Sohn M, Al-Ghananeem A, DeLuca PP. Materials for pharmaceutical dosage forms: molecular pharmaceutics and controlled release drug delivery aspects. An invited review. *Int. J. Mol. Sci.* 2010:11:3298–3322.

7. Jostel A, Shalet SM. Prospects for the development of long-acting formulations of human somatropin. *Treat Endocrinol.* 2006;5(3):139–145.

8. Capan Y, Jiang G, Giovagnoli S, Na KH, DeLuca PP. Preparation and characterization of poly(D, L-lactide-co-glycolide) microspheres for controlled release of human growth hormone. *AAPS Pharmscitech.* 2003;4(2):E28.

9. Gao ZH, Tang Y, Chen JQ, et al. A novel DPP-IV-resistant analog of glucagon-like peptide-1 (GLP-1): KGLP-1 alone or in combination with long-acting PLGA microspheres. *Peptides.* 2009;30(10):1874–1881.

10. Woo BH, Fink BF, Page R, et al. Enhancement of bone growth by sustained delivery of recombinant human bone morphogenetic protein-2 in a polymeric matrix. *Pharm Res.* 2001;18(12):1747–1753.

11. Giovagnoli S, Blasi P, Ricci M, Rossi C. Biodegradable microspheres as carriers for native superoxide dismutase and catalase delivery. *AAPS Pharmscitech.* 2004;5(4):1–9.

12. Dani BA, DeLuca PP. Preparation, characterization, and in vivo evaluation of salmon calcitonin microspheres. *AAPS Pharmscitech.* 2001;2(4):22.

13. Dani BA, Raiche AT, Puleo DA, DeLuca PP. A study of the antiresorptive activity of salmon calcitonin microspheres using cultured osteoclastic cells. *AAPS Pharmscitech.* 2002;3(3):E21.

14. Naha PC, Kanchan V, Panda AK. Evaluation of parenteral depot insulin formulation using PLGA and PLA microparticles. *J Biomater Appl.* 2009;24(4):309–325.

15. Shenoy DB, D'Souza RJ, Tiwari SB, Udupa N. Potential applications of polymeric microsphere suspension as subcutaneous depot for insulin. *Drug Dev Ind Pharm.* 2003;29(5):555–563.

16. Jiang G, Qiu W, DeLuca PP. Preparation and in vitro/in vivo evaluation of insulin-loaded poly(acryloyl-hydroxyethyl starch)-PLGA composite microspheres. *Pharm Res.* 2003;20(3):452–459.

17. Capan Y, Woo BH, Gebrekidan S, Ahmed S, DeLuca PP. Influence of formulation parameters on the characteristics of poly(D, L-lactide-co-glycolide) microspheres containing poly(L-lysine) complexed plasmid DNA. *J Control Release.* 1999;60(2–3):279–286.

18. Capan Y, Woo BH, Gebrekidan S, Ahmed S, DeLuca PP. Preparation and characterization of poly (D,L-lactide-co-glycolide) microspheres for controlled release of poly(L-lysine) complexed plasmid DNA. *Pharm Res.* 1999;16(4):509–513.

19. Gebrekidan S, Woo BH, DeLuca PP. Formulation and in vitro transfection efficiency of poly (D, L-lactide-co-glycolide) microspheres containing plasmid DNA for gene delivery. *AAPS Pharmscitech.* 2000;1(4):E28.

20. D'Souza R, Mutalik S, Udupa N. In vitro and in vivo preparation evaluations of bleomycin implants and microspheres prepared with DL-poly (lactide-co-glycolide). *Drug Dev Ind Pharm.* 2006;32(2):175–184.

21. Lee JY, Kim KS, Kang YM, et al. In vivo efficacy of paclitaxel-loaded injectable in situ-forming gel against subcutaneous tumor growth. *Int J Pharm.* 2010;392(1–2):51–56.

22. Lee YS, Lowe JP, Gilby E, Perera S, Rigby SP. The initial release of cisplatin from poly(lactide-co-glycolide) microspheres. *Int J Pharm.* 2010;383(1–2):244–254.

23. Shenoy DB, D'Souza RJ, Udupa N. Poly(DL-lactide-co-glycolide) microporous microsphere-based depot formulation of a peptide-like antineoplastic agent. *J Microencapsul.* 2002;19(4):523–535.

24. Sinha VR, Trehan A. Development, characterization, and evaluation of ketorolac tromethamine-loaded biodegradable microspheres as a depot system for parenteral delivery. *Drug Deliv.* 2008;15(6):365–372.

25. Nahata T, Saini TR. D-optimal designing and optimization of long acting microsphere-based injectable formulation of aripiprazole. *Drug Dev Ind Pharm.* 2008;34(7):668–675.

26. Nahata T, Saini TR. Optimization of formulation variables for the development of long acting microsphere based depot injection of olanzapine. *J Microencapsul.* 2008;25(6):426–433.

27. Cui C, Stevens VC, Schwendeman SP. Injectable polymer microspheres enhance immunogenicity of a contraceptive peptide vaccine. *Vaccine.* 2007;25(3):500–509.

28. Liu YD, Sunderland VB, Liu YD, O'Neil AG. In vitro and in vivo release of naltrexone from biodegradable depot systems. *Drug Dev Ind Pharm.* 2006;32(1):85–94.

29. Jhunjhunwala S, Raimondi G, Thomson AW, Little SR. Delivery of rapamycin to dendritic cells using degradable microparticles. *J Control Release.* 2009;133(3):191–197.

30. Dai C, Wang B, Zhao H. Microencapsulation peptide and protein drugs delivery system. *Coll Surf B Biointerf.* 2005;41(2–3):117–120.

31. Shameem M, Lee H, DeLuca PP. A short term (accelerated release) approach to evaluate peptide release from PLGA depot-formulations. *AAPS PharmSci.* 1999;1(3):E7.

32. Burton KW, Shameem M, Thanoo BC, DeLuca PP. Extended release peptide delivery systems through the use of PLGA microsphere combinations. *J Biomater Sci Polym Ed.* 2000;11(7):715–729.

33. Kostanski JW, Dani BA, Reynolds GA, Bowers CY, DeLuca PP. Evaluation of orntide microspheres in a rat animal model and correlation to in vitro release profiles. *AAPS Pharmscitech.* 2000;1(4):E27.

34. Kostanski JW, Thanoo BC, DeLuca PP. Preparation, characterization, and in vitro evaluation of 1- and 4-month controlled release orntide PLA and PLGA microspheres. *Pharm Dev Technol.* 2000;5(4):585–596.

35. Ravivarapu HB, Burton K, DeLuca PP. Polymer and microsphere blending to alter the release of a peptide from PLGA microspheres. *Eur J Pharm Biopharm.* 2000;50(2):263–270.

36. Woo BH, Jiang G, Jo YW, DeLuca PP. Preparation and characterization of a composite PLGA and poly(acryloyl hydroxyethyl starch) microsphere system for protein delivery. *Pharm Res.* 2001;18(11):1600–1606.

37. Jiang G, Woo BH, Kang F, Singh J, DeLuca PP. Assessment of protein release kinetics, stability and protein polymer interaction of lysozyme encapsulated poly(D,L-lactide-co-glycolide) microspheres. *J Control Release.* 2002;79(1–3):137–145.

38. Karatas A, Sonakin O, Kilicarslan M, Baykara T. Poly (epsilon-caprolactone) microparticles containing levobunolol HCl prepared by a multiple emulsion (W/O/W) solvent evaporation technique: effects of some formulation parameters on microparticle characteristics. *J Microencapsul.* 2009;26(1):63–74.

39. Sun L, Zhou S, Wang W, Su Q, Li X, Weng J. Preparation and characterization of protein-loaded polyanhydride microspheres. *J Mater Sci Mater Med.* 2009;20(10):2035–2042.

40. Deng JS, Li L, Tian YQ, Ginsburg E, Widman M, Myers A. In vitro characterization of polyorthoester microparticles containing bupivacaine. *Pharm Dev Technol.* 2003;8(1):31–38.

41. Gao H, Wang JY, Shen XZ, Deng YH, Zhang W. Preparation of magnetic polybutylcyanoacrylate nanospheres encapsulated with aclacinomycin A and its effect on gastric tumor. *World J Gastroenterol.* 2004;10(14):2010–2013.

42. Lherm C, Müller RH, Puisieux F, Couvreur P. Alkylcyanoacrylate drug carriers. II. Cytotoxicity of cyanoacrylate nanoparticles with different alkyl chain length. *Int J Pharm.* 1992;84(1):13–22.

43. Loh XJ, Goh SH, Li J. New biodegradable thermogelling copolymers having very low gelation concentrations. *Biomacromolecules.* 2007;8(2):585–593.

44. Bhattarai N, Ramay HR, Gunn J, Matsen FA, Zhang M. PEG-grafted chitosan as an injectable thermosensitive hydrogel for sustained protein release. *J Control Release.* 2005;103(3):609–624.

45. Zhai Y, Deng L, Xing J, Liu Y, Zhang Q, Dong A. A new injectable thermogelling material: methoxy poly(ethylene glycol)-poly(sebacic acid-D,L-lactic acid)-methoxy poly(ethylene glycol) triblock co-polymer. *J Biomater Sci Polym Ed.* 2009;20(7–8):923–934.

46. Liu CB, Gong CY, Huang MJ, et al. Thermoreversible gel–sol behavior of biodegradable PCL-PEG-PCL triblock copolymer in aqueous solutions. *J Biomed Mater Res Part B Appl Biomater.* 2008;84B(1):165–175.

47. Chen S, Pieper R, Webster DC, Singh J. Triblock copolymers: synthesis, characterization, and delivery of a model protein. *Int J Pharm.* 2005;288(2):207–218.

48. Hickey AJ, ed. *Pharmaceutical Inhalation Aerosol Technology* (2nd ed.). New York, NY: Marcel Dekker; 2004.

49. Park CW, Hayes DJ, Mansour HM. Pulmonary inhalation aerosols for targeted antibiotics drug delivery. Invited paper. *Eur Pharmac Rev.* 2011;16.(1):32–36.

50. Garcia-Contreras L, Hickey AJ. Pharmaceutical and biotechnological aerosols for cystic fibrosis therapy. *Adv Drug Deliv Rev.* 2002;54:1491–1504.

51. Schreier H, Gonzalez-Rothi RJ, Stecenko AA. Pulmonary delivery of liposomes. *J Control Release.* 1993;24:209–223.

52. Eljamal, Inventor. Method and apparatus for pulmonary administration of dry powder alpha1-antitrypsin. US Patent 5,993,783. 1999.

53. Gardenhire DS. Airway pharmacology. In: Wilkins RL, Stoller JK, Kacmarek RM, eds. *Egan's Fundamentals of Respiratory Care* (9th ed.). St. Louis, MO: Mosby; 2009:667–692.

54. Bennett WD, Brown JS, Zeman KL, Hu S-C, Scheuch G, Sommerer K. Targeting delivery of aerosols to different lung regions. *J Aeros Med.* 2002;15(2):178–188.

55. Gonda I. Targeting by deposition. In: Hickey AJ, ed. *Pharmaceutical Inhalation Aerosol Technology* (2nd ed.). New York, NY: Marcel Dekkar; 2004:65–88.

56. Wang C. Behavior of aerosol particles. *Inhaled Particles* (vol. 1). London: Elsevier; 2005:55–78.

57. Hinds WC. *Aerosol Technology: Properties, Behavior, and Measurement of Airborne Particles* (2nd ed.). New York, NY: John Wiley & Sons; 1999.

58. Newman SP. Principles of metered-dose inhaler design. *Respir Care.* 2005;50(9):1177–1190.

59. Purewal TS, Grant DJ, eds. *Metered Dose Inhaler Technology*. Boca Raton, FL: CRC Press; 1997.

60. Purewal TS. Metered dose inhaler (MDI) systems. *Int J Pharm.* 1999;186(1):1–2.

61. Noakes TJ. CFCs, their replacements, and the ozone layer. *J Aeros Med.* 1995;8(1):S-3–S-7.

62. Sanders P. *Principles of Aerosol Technology*. New York, NY: Van Nostrand Reinhold; 1970.

63. Handbook for the Montreal Protocol 1987. Montreal protocol on substances that deplete the ozone layers 26 ILM 1541. http://infohouse.p2ric.org/ref/17/16875.pdf. 1987.

64. Bowman PA, Greenleaf D. Non-CFC metered dose inhalers: the patent landscape. *Int J Pharm.* 1999;186(1):91–94.

65. Purewal TS. Alternative propellants for metered dose inhalers. *Aerosol Spray Rep.* 1998;37(11/12):20–25.

66. U.S. Food and Drug Administration. Use of ozone-depleting substances; removal of essential-use designation. http://www.fda.gov/OHRMS/DOCKETS/98fr/03p-0029-nfr0001.pdf. Accessed 2005.

67. Newman SP, Peart J. Pressurized metered dose inhalers. In: Newman SP, ed. *Respiratory Drug Delivery: Essential Theory & Practice*. Richmond, VA: Respiratory Drug Delivery Online/Virginia Commonwealth University; 2009:177–215.

68. Vervaet C, Byron PR. Drug surfactant propellant interactions in HFA formulations. *Int J Pharm.* 1999;186(Sep 10):13–30.

69. Purewal TS. Formulation of metered dose inhalers. In: Purewal TS, Grant DJW, eds. *Metered Dose Inhaler Technology.* Buffalo Grove, IL: Interpharm; 1998.

70. Hickey AJ, Mansour HM. Delivery of drugs by the pulmonary route. In: Florence AT, Siepmann J, eds. *Modern Pharmaceutics* (vol. 2, 5th ed.). New York, NY: Taylor and Francis; 2009:191–219.

71. Seville PC, Li HY, Learoyd TP. Spray-dried powders for pulmonary drug delivery. *Crit Rev Therap Drug Carrier Syst.* 2007;24(4):307–360.

72. Hickey AJ, Mansour HM. Formulation challenges of powders for the delivery of small molecular weight molecules as aerosols. In: Rathbone MJ, Hadgraft J, Roberts MS, Lane M, eds. *Modified-Release Drug Delivery Technology* (vol. 2, 2nd ed.). New York, NY: Informa Healthcare; 2008:573–602.

73. Van Oort MM, Sacchetti M. Spray-drying and supercritical fluid particle generation techniques. In: Hickey AJ, ed. *Inhalation Aerosols: Physical and Biological Basis for Therapy* (vol. 221, 2nd ed.). New York, NY: Informa Healthcare; 2007:307–346.

74. Chow AHL, Tong HHY, Chattopadhyay P, Shekunov BY. Particle engineering for pulmonary drug delivery. *Pharm Res.* 2007;24(3):411–437.

75. Smyth HD. The influence of formulation variables on the performance of alternative propellant-driven metered dose inhalers. *Adv Drug Deliv Rev.* 2003;55(7):807–828.

76. Dunbar CA, Watkins AP, Miller JF. An experimental investigation of the spray issued from a pMDI using laser diagnostic techniques. *J Aerosol Med.* 1997;10(4):351–368.

77. Dunbar CA, Watkins AP, Miller JF. A theoretical investigation of the spray issued from a pMDI. *Atom Spray.* 1997;7:417–436.

78. Lewis DA, Ganderton D, Meakin BJ, Brambilla G. Theory and practice with solution systems. *Respir Drug Deliv IX.* 2004;1:109–115.

79. Newman SP. Additional technology for pressurized metered dose inhalers. In: Newman SP, ed. *Respiratory Drug Delivery: Essential Theory & Practice.* Richmond, VA: Respiratory drug delivery online/VCU; 2009:217–256.

80. U.S. Food and Drug Administration. *Guidance for Industry: Integration of Dose Counting Mechanisms into MDI Drug Products.* Rockville, MD: USFDA; 2003.

81. Dunbar C, Hickey AJ, Holzner P. Dispersion and characterization of pharmaceutical dry powder aerosols. *KONA Powd Part.* 1998;16:7–45.

82. Chan HK. Inhalation drug delivery devices and emerging technologies. *Exp Opin Ther Pat.* 2003;13(9):1333–1343.

83. Israelachvili JN. *Intermolecular and Surface Forces: With Applications to Colloidal and Biological Systems* (2nd ed.). London, UK: Academic Press; 1992.

84. Xu Z, Mansour HM, Hickey AJ. Particle interactions in dry powder inhaler unit processes. *J Adhes Sci Technol Spec Iss Adhes Asp Pharm Sci.* 2011;25 (4/5):451–482.

85. Visser J. van der Waals and other cohesive forces affecting powder fluidization. *Powd Technol.* 1989;58(1 (May):1–10.

86. Matsusaka S, Masuda H. Electrostatics of particles. *Adv Powd Technol.* 2003;14(2):143–166.

87. Clark AR, York P. SCF-Pulmonary Pharmaceuticals: the uncoated truth. Paper presented at *Resp Drug Deliv X.*. 2006(1):317–326.

88. Edwards DA, Hanes J, Caponetti G, et al. Large porous particles for pulmonary drug delivery. *Science.* 1997;276(5320):1868–1871.

89. Wetterlin K. Turbuhaler: a new powder inhaler for administration of drugs to the airways. *Pharm Res.* 1988;5:506–508.

90. Martin GP, MacRitchie HB, Marriott C, Zeng XM. Characterisation of a carrier-free dry powder aerosol formulation using inertial impaction and laser diffraction. *Pharm Res.* 2006;23(9):2210–2219.

91. Smyth H. Excipients for pulmonary formulations. In: Katdare A, Chaubal MV, eds. *Excipient Development for Pharmaceutical, Biotechnology, and Drug Delivery Systems.* New York, NY: Informa Healthcare USA; 2006:225–249.

92. Smyth H, Hickey AJ. Carriers in drug powder delivery: implications for inhalation system design. *Am J Drug Deliv.* 2005;3:117–132.

93. Sheth P, Myrdal P. Excipients utilized for modifying pulmonary drug release. In: Smyth H, Hickey AJ, eds. *Controlled Pulmonary Drug Delivery*: New York, NY: Springer; 2011:237–263.

94. Zeng XM, MacRitchie HB, Marriott C, Martin GP. Humidity-induced changes of the aerodynamic properties of dry powder aerosol formulations containing different carriers. *Int J Pharm.* 2007;333(1–2):45–55.

95. Jones MD, Price R. The influence of fine excipient particles on the performance of carrier-based dry powder inhalation formulations. *Pharm Res.* 2006;23(8 (August):1665–1674.

96. Adi H, Larson I, Chiou H, Young P, Traini D, Stewart P. Role of agglomeration in the dispersion of salmeterol xinafoate from mixtures for inhalation with differing drug to fine lactose ratios. *J Pharm Sci.* 2008;97(8):3140–3152.

97. Crowder TM, Hickey AJ, Louey MD, Orr N. *A Guide to Pharmaceutical Particulate Science* (1st ed.). Boca Raton, FL: Interpharm Press/CRC; 2003.

98. Islam N, Gladki E. Dry powder inhalers (DPIs)—a review of device reliability and innovation. *Int J Pharm.* 2008;360(1–2):1–11.

99. Clark AR, Hollingworth AM. the relationship between powder inhaler resistance and peak inspiratory conditions in healthy volunteers—implications for in vitro testing. *J Aeros Med.* 1993;6:99–110.

100. Louey MD, Van Oort M, Hickey AJ. Standardized entrainment tubes for the evaluation of pharmaceutical dry powder dispersion. *J Aeros Sci.* 2006;37 (11):1520–1531

101. Dunbar CA, Morgan B, VanOort M, Hickey AJ. A comparison of dry powder inhaler dose delivery characteristics using power. *PDA J Pharm Sci Technol.* 2000;54(6):478–484.

102. Hickey AJ. *Inhalation Aerosols: The Physiological Basis for Therapy* (vol. 221, 2nd ed.). New York, NY: Informa Healthcare, USA; 2007.

103. Lavorini F, Magnan A, Dubus JC, et al. Effect of incorrect use of dry powder inhalers on management of patients with asthma and COPD. *Respir Med.* 2008;102(4):593–604.

104. Wilson DS, Gillion MS, Rees PJ. Use of dry powder inhalers in COPD. *Int J Clin Pract.* 2007;61(12):2005–2008.

105. Crowder TM. Precision powder metering utilizing fundamental powder flow characteristics *Powd Technol.* 2007;173(3):217–223.

106. Hickey AJ, Crowder TM, Inventors. Dry powder inhaler devices: multidose dry powder drug packages, controlled systems, and associated methods. U.S. patent US6971383B2 on December 6, 2005.

107. Schultz RK, Miller NC, Smith DK. Powder aerosols with auxiliary means of dispersion. *J Biopharm Sci.* 1992;3:115–121.

108. Harper NJ, Gray, De Groot J, et al. The design and performance of the Exubera pulmonary insulin delivery system. *Diabetes Technol Ther.* 2007;9(Suppl 1):S16–S27.

109. Crowder, TM, Hickey AJ. Powder specific active dispersion for generation of pharmaceutical aerosols. *Int J Pharm.* 2006;327(1–2):65–72.

110. Mecikalski MB, Williams DR, Thueson O, Inventors. Dry powder inhaler. San Diego, CA: Dura Pharmaceuticals; 1996.

111. Black C, Cummins E, Royle P, Philip S, Waugh N. The clinical effectiveness and cost-effectiveness of inhaled insulin in diabetes mellitus: a systematic review and economic evaluation. *Health Technol Assess* 2007;11(33):1–126.

112. Heinemann L. New ways of insulin delivery. *Int J Clin Pract Suppl.* 2011;(170):31–46.

113. Tonnis WF, Kersten GF, Frijlink HWet al. Pulmonary vaccine delivery: a realistic approach? *J Aeros Med Pulm Drug Deliv.* 2012;25(5):249–260.

114. Newhouse MT, Hirst PH, Duddu SP, et al. Inhalation of a dry powder tobramycin pulmosphere formulation in healthy volunteers. *Chest.* 2006;124:360–366.

115. Smith AL, Ramsey BW, Hedges DL, et al. Safety of aerosol tobramycin administration for 3 months to patients with cystic fibrosis. *Pediatr Pulm.* 1989;7(4):265–271.

116. Karvouniaris M, Makris D, Triantaris A, Zakynthinos E. Inhaled antibiotics for nosocomial pneumonia. *Inflamm Allerg Drug Targets.* 2012;11(2):116–123.

117. Eggleston M. Clinical review of ribavirin. *Infect Control.* 1987;8(5):215–218.

118. Luo YH, Huang CY, Yang KY, Lee YC. Inhaled ribavirin therapy in adult respiratory syncytial virus-induced acute respiratory distress syndrome. *Arch Bronconeumol.* 2011;47(6):315–317.

119. Vujovic O, Mills J. Preventive and therapeutic strategies for respiratory syncytial virus infection. *Curr Opin Pharmacol.* 2001;1(5):497–503.

120. Cao B, Wang DY, Yu XM, et al. An uncontrolled open-label, multicenter study to monitor the antiviral activity and safety of inhaled zanamivir (as Rotadisk via Diskhaler device) among Chinese adolescents and adults with influenza-like illness. *Chin Med J.* 2012;125(17):3002–3007.

121. Katsumi Y, Otabe O, Matsui F, et al. Effect of a single inhalation of laninamivir octanoate in children with influenza. *Pediatrics.* 2012:129(6):e1431–1436.

122. Laube BL. The expanding role of aerosols in systemic drug delivery, gene therapy, and vaccination. *Respir Care.* 2005;50(9):1161–1176.

123. Agu RU, Ugwoke MI, Armand M, et al. The lung as a route for systemic delivery of therapeutic proteins and peptides. *Respir Res.* 2001;2(4):198–209.

124. Niven RW. Delivery of biotherapeutics by inhalation aerosol. *Crit Rev Ther Drug Carrier Syst.* 1995;12(2–3):151–231.

125. Anderson P, Newman SP. Drugs for topical and systemic delivery by the pulmonary route. In: Newman SP, ed. *Respiratory Drug Delivery: Essential Theory & Practice.* Richmond, VA: Respiratory drug delivery online/VCU; 2009:337–382.

126. Ward ME, Mather LE, Farr SJ, et al. Morphine pharmacokinetics after pulmonary administration from a novel aerosol delivery system. *Clin Pharmacol Ther.* 1997;62(6):596–609.

127. Coyne PJ, Smith TJ. Nebulized fentanyl citrate improves patients' perception of breathing, respiratory rate, and oxygen saturation in dyspnea. *J Pain Symptom Manage.* 2002;23(2):157–160.

128. Farr SJ, Otulana BA. Pulmonary delivery of opioids as pain therapeutics. *Adv Drug Deliv Rev.* 2006;58(9–10):1076–1088.

129. Hickey AJ. Summary of common approaches to pharmaceutical aerosol administration. In: Hickey AJ, ed. *Pharmaceutical Inhalation Aerosol Technology* (2nd ed.). New York, NY: Marcel Dekker; 2004:385–421.

130. Misra A, Jinturkar K, Patel D, Lalani J, Chougule M. Recent advances in liposomal dry powder formulations: preparation and evaluation. *Exp Opin Drug Deliv.* 2009;6(1):71–89.

131. Adjei AL. *Inhalation Delivery of Therapeutic Peptides and Proteins* (vol. 107, 1st ed.). New York, NY: Informa Healthcare; 1997.

132. Patton JS. Deep-lung delivery of therapeutic proteins. *Chem Tech.* 1997;27(12):34–38.

133. Laube B. Treating diabetes with aerosolized insulin. *Chest.* 2001;120(3 Suppl):99S–106S.

134. Adjei A, Hui J, Finley R, et al. Pulmonary bioavailability of leuprolide acetate following multiple dosing to beagle dogs: some pharmacokinetic and preclinical issues. *Int J Pharm.* 1994;107 (Jun 20):57–66.

135. Rave KM, Nosek L, et al. Dose response of inhaled dry-powder insulin and dose equivalence to subcutaneous insulin lispro. *Diabetes Care.* 2005;28(10):2400–2405.

136. Richardson PC, Boss AH. Technosphere insulin technology. *Diabetes Technol Ther.* 2007;9(Suppl 1): S65–S72.

137. Rave KM, Heise T, Pfutzner A, Boss AH. Coverage of postprandial blood glucose excursions with inhaled technosphere insulin in comparison to subcutaneously injected regular human insulin in subjects with type 2 diabetes. *Diabetes Care.* 2007;30(9):2307–2308.

138. Cassidy JP, Amin N, et al. Insulin lung deposition and clearance following Technosphere(R) insulin inhalation powder administration. *Pharm Res.* 2011;28(9):2157–2164.

139. Neumiller JJ, Campbell RK, Wood LD. A review of inhaled technosphere insulin. *Ann Pharmacother.* 2010;44(7–8):1231–1239.

140. Afrezza. http://afresa.blogspot.com/2010/05/all-about-technosphere-technology.html. Accessed December, 10, 2012.

141. Leone B, Grant, Greene, et al. Evaluation of novel particles as an inhalation system for GLP-1. *Diabetes Obes Metab.* 2009;11(11):1050–1059.

142. White S, Bennett DB, Cheu S, et al. Exubera: pharmaceutical development of a novel product for pulmonary delivery of insulin. *Diabetes Technol Ther.* 2005;7(6):896–906.

143. Patton J, Trinchero P. Bioavailability of pulmonary delivered peptides and proteins: alpha-interferon, calcitonins and parathyroid hormone. *J Control Release.* 1994;28:79–85.

144. Byron PR. Determinants of drug and polypeptide bioavailability from aerosols delivered to the lung. *Adv Drug Deliv Rev.* 1990;5(1–2):107–132.

145. An B, Reinhardt RR. Effects of different durations of breath holding after inhalation of insulin using the AERx insulin diabetes management system. *Clin Ther.* 2003;25(8):2233–2244.

146. Lu D, Hickey AJ. Pulmonary vaccine delivery. *Exp Rev Vaccines.* 2007;6(2):213–226.

147. Garcia-Contreras L, Kazantseva M, Hickey AJ. Evaluation of anti-tubercular aerosols in infected guinea pigs. Paper presented at World Congress of Tuberculosis, June 3–5, 2002, Washington, DC.

148. Garcia-Contreras L, Jones LD, Hickey AJ. Alevolar macrophages: a target for drug delivery. *Respiratory Drug Delivery IX*, 2004:1:33–40.

149. Tschernig T, Pabst R. Bronchus-associated lymphoid tissue (BALT) is not present in the normal adult lung but in different diseases. *Pathobiology.* 2000;68(1):1–8.

150. Blank F, Stumbles P, von Garnier C. Opportunities and challenges of the pulmonary route for vaccination. *Exp Opin Drug Deliv.* 2011;8(5):547–563.

151. Lau YF, Wright AR, Subbarao K. The contribution of systemic and pulmonary immune effectors to vaccine-induced protection from H5N1 influenza virus infection. *J Virol.* 2012;86(9):5089–5098.

152. Song K, Bolton DL, et al. Genetic immunization in the lung induces potent local and systemic immune responses. *Proc Natl Acad Sci USA.* 2010;107(51):22213–22218.

153. Garcia-Contreras L, Awashthi S, Hanif S, Hickey AJ. Inhaled vaccines for the prevention of tuberculosis. *J Mycobac Dis.* 2012;S1:002.

154. Amorij JP, Saluja, et al. Pulmonary delivery of an insulin-stabilized influenza subunit vaccine prepared by spray-freeze drying induces systemic, mucosal humoral as well as cell-mediated immune responses in BALB/c mice. *Vaccine.* 2007;25(52):8707–8717.

155. Smith DJ, Bot S, Dellamary L, Bot A. Evaluation of novel aerosol formulations designed for mucosal vaccination against influenza virus. *Vaccine.* 2003;21(21–22):2805–2812.

156. de Swart RL, LiCalsi C, Quirk AV, et al. Measles vaccination of macaques by dry powder inhalation. *Vaccine*. 2007;25(7):1183–1190.

157. Lin WH, Griffin DE, Rota PA, et al. Successful respiratory immunization with dry powder live-attenuated measles virus vaccine in rhesus macaques. *Proc Natl Acad Sci USA*. 2011;108(7):2987–2992.

158. Thomas C, Gupta V, Ahsan F. Particle size influences the immune response produced by hepatitis B vaccine formulated in inhalable particles. *Pharm Res*. 2010;27(5):905–919.

159. Thomas C, Rawat A, Hope-Weeks L, Ahsan F. Aerosolized PLA and PLGA nanoparticles enhance humoral, mucosal and cytokine responses to hepatitis B vaccine. *Mol Pharm*. 2011;8(2):405–415.

160. Muttil P, Prego C, Garcia-Conteras L, et al. Immunization of guinea pigs with novel hepatitis B antigen as nanoparticle aggregate powders administered by the pulmonary route. *AAPS J*. 2010:12(3):330–337.

161. Muromtsev, SN, Borodiiuk, NA. [The importance of dosage of diphtheria anatoxin in primary inhalation immunization and reimmunization in experiments on animals]. *Zhurn Mikrob Epidemiol Immunobiol*. 1962;33:19–23.

162. Amidi M, Pellikaan HC, et al. Diphtheria toxoid-containing microparticulate powder formulations for pulmonary vaccination: preparation, characterization and evaluation in guinea pigs. *Vaccine*. 2007;25(37–38):6818–6829.

163. Cutts FT, Clements CJ, Bennett JV. Alternative routes of measles immunization: a review. *Biologicals*. 1997;25(3):323–338.

164. Dilraj A, Cutts FT, et al. Response to different measles vaccine strains given by aerosol and subcutaneous routes to schoolchildren: a randomised trial. *Lancet*. 2000;355(9206):798–803.

165. Dilraj A, Sukhoo R, Cutts FT, Bennett JV. Aerosol and subcutaneous measles vaccine: measles antibody responses 6 years after re-vaccination. *Vaccine*. 2007;25(21):4170–4174.

166. Wong C, Rm, Islas R, et al. Immunogenicity of aerosol measles vaccine given as the primary measles immunization to nine month old Mexican children. *Vaccine*. 2006;24(5):683–690.

167. Rosenthal SR, McEnery JT, Raisys. Aerogenic BCG vaccination against tuberculosis in animal and human subjects. *J Asthma Res*. 1968;5(4):309–323.

168. Nardelli H, Lurati F, Wirthner D, et al. Immune responses induced by lower airway mucosal immunisation with a human papillomavirus type 16 virus-like particle vaccine. *Vaccine*. 2005;23(28):3634–3641.

169. Mikszta JA, Sullivan VJ, et al. Protective immunization against inhalational anthrax: a comparison of minimally invasive delivery platforms. *J Infect Dis*. 2005;191(2):278–288.

170. Wayne Conlan J, Shen H, Kuolee R, Zhao X, Chen W. Aerosol-, but not intradermal-immunization with the live vaccine strain of *Francisella tularensis* protects mice against subsequent aerosol challenge with a highly virulent type A strain of the pathogen by an alphabeta T cell- and interferon gamma- dependent mechanism. *Vaccine*. 2005;23(19):2477–2485.

171. Burger JL, Cape SP, et al. Stabilizing formulations for inhalable powders of live-attenuated measles virus vaccine. *J Aeros Med Pulm Drug Deliv*. 2008;21(1):25–34.

172. LiCalsi C, Maniaci MJ, Christensen T, Phillips E, Ward GH, Witham C. A powder formulation of measles vaccine for aerosol delivery. *Vaccine*. 2001;19(17–19):2629–2636.

173. Raychaudhuri, Rock KL. Fully mobilizing host defense: building better vaccines. *Nature Biotechnol*. 1998;16(11):1025–1031.

174. Sou T, Meeusen EN, de Veer M, Morton DA, Kaminskas LM, McIntosh MP. New developments in dry powder pulmonary vaccine delivery. *Trends Biotechnol*. 2011;29(4):191–198.

175. Chien YW, Su KSE, Chang SF. *Nasal Systemic Drug Delivery* (vol. 39). New York, NY: Marcel Dekker; 1989.

176. Djupesland PG. Nasal drug delivery devices: characteristics and performance in a clinical perspective—a review. *Drug Deliv Transl Res*. 2013:3(1):42–62.

177. Moses AC, Gordon GS, et al. Insulin administered intranasally as an insulin-bile salt aerosol. Effectiveness and reproducibility in normal and diabetic subjects. *Diabetes*. 1983;32(11):1040–1047.

178. Salzman R, Manson JE, et al. Intranasal aerosolized insulin. Mixed-meal studies and long-term use in type I diabetes. *N Engl J Med*. 1985;312(17):1078–1084.

179. Early Chinese inoculation. http://www.historyofvaccines.org/content/timelines/smallpox. Accessed December 15, 2012.

180. Karaki M, Akiyama K, Mori N. Efficacy of intranasal steroid spray (mometasone furoate) on treatment of patients with seasonal allergic rhinitis: comparison with oral corticosteroids. *Auris Nasus Larynx*. 2012:40(3):277–281.

181. Horak F, Zieglmayer, UP. Azelastine nasal spray for the treatment of allergic and nonallergic rhinitis. *Exp Rev Clin Immunol*. 2009;5(6):659–669.

182. Bernstein JA. Azelastine hydrochloride: a review of pharmacology, pharmacokinetics, clinical efficacy and tolerability. *Curr Med Res Opin*. 2007;23(10):2441–2452.

183. Carr W, Bernstein J, Lieberman P, et al. A novel intranasal therapy of azelastine with fluticasone for the treatment of allergic rhinitis. *J Allerg Clin Immunol*. 2012;129(5):1282–1289.

184. Hampel FC, Ratner PH, et al. Double-blind, placebo-controlled study of azelastine and fluticasone in a single nasal spray delivery device. *Ann Allerg Asthma Immunol*. 2012;105(2):168–173.

185. Rael EL, Ramey J, Lockey RF. Oxymetazoline hydrochloride combined with mometasone nasal spray for persistent nasal congestion (pilot study). *World Allerg Org J*. 2011;4(3):65–67.

186. Baroody FM, Brown, et al. Oxymetazoline adds to the effectiveness of fluticasone furoate in the treatment of perennial allergic rhinitis. *J Allerg Clin Immunol*. 2011;127(4):927–934.

187. Meltzer EO, Jacobs RL, et al. Safety and efficacy of once-daily treatment with beclomethasone dipropionate nasal aerosol in subjects with perennial allergic rhinitis. *Allerg Asthma Proc*. 2012;33(3):249–257.

188. Andersson M, Lindqvist N, Svensson C, Ek L, Pipkorn U. Dry powder inhalation of budesonide in allergic rhinitis. *Clin Otolaryngol Allied Sci*. 1993;18(1):30–33.

189. U.S. Department of Health and Human Services, Food and Drug Administration (FDA), Center for Drug Evaluation and Research. *Guidance for Industry: Bioavailability and Bioequivalence Studies for Nasal Aerosols and Nasal Sprays*. Bethesda, MD: U.S. FDA, CDER; 2003.

190. Albu S. Novel drug-delivery systems for patients with chronic rhinosinusitis. *Drug Design Dev Ther* 2012;6:125–132.

191. Djupesland PG, Skretting, Winderen, Holand. Bi-directional nasal delivery of aerosols can prevent lung deposition. *J Aeros Med*. 2004;17(3):249–259.

192. Illum L. The nasal delivery of peptides and proteins. *Trends Biotechnol*. 1991;9(8):284–289.

193. Hoyer H, Perera G, Bernkop-Schnürch A. Noninvasive delivery systems for peptides and proteins in osteoporosis therapy: a retroperspective. *Drug Dev Industr Pharm*. 2010;36(1):31–44.

194. Halkin V, Reginster JY. Efficacy and tolerability of calcitonin in the prevention and treatment of osteoporosis. *BioDrugs*. 1998;10(4):295–300.

195. Born J, Lange T, Kern W, et al. Sniffing neuropeptides: a transnasal approach to the human brain. *Nat Neurosci*. 2002;5(6):514–516.

196. Benedict C, Hallschmid M, Schultes B, Born J, Kern W. Intranasal insulin improves memory in humans. *Psychoneuroendocrinology*. 2004;29(10):1326–1334.

197. Davis SS, Illum L. Absorption enhancers for nasal drug delivery. *Clin Pharmacokinet*. 2003;42(13):1107–1128.

198. Tengamnuay P, Sahamethapat A, Sailasuta A, Mitra AK. Chitosans as nasal absorption enhancers of peptides: comparison between free amine chitosans and soluble salts. *Int J Pharm*. 2000;197(1–2):53–67.

199. Ritthidej GC. Nasal delivery of peptides and proteins with chitosan and related mucoadhesive polymers. In: van der Walle CF, ed. *Peptide and Protein Delivery* (1st ed.). San Diego, CA: Academic Press; 2011:47–68.

200. Rapoport AM, Bigal ME, et al. Zolmitriptan (Zomig). *Exp Rev Neurother*. 2004;4(1):33–41.

201. Merkus FW, Verhoef JC, et al. Nasal mucociliary clearance as a factor in nasal drug delivery. *Adv Drug Deliv Rev*. 1998;29(1–2):13–38.

202. Wong JP, Christopher ME, et al. Aerosol and nasal delivery of vaccines and antiviral drugs against seasonal and pandemic influenza. *Exp Rev Respir Med*. 2010;4(2):171–177.

203. Almeida AJ, Alpar HO. Nasal delivery of vaccines. *J Drug Target*. 1996;3(6):455–467.

204. Tamura S, Asanuma H, Ito Y, et al. Formulation of inactivated influenza vaccines for providing effective cross-protection by intranasal vaccination in mice. *Vaccine*. 1994;12:310–316.

205. Amorij JP, Hinrichs WLI, et al. Needle-free influenza vaccination. *Lancet Infect Dis*. 2010;10(10):699–711.

206. Dlugonska H, Grzybowski M. Mucosal vaccination—an old but still vital strategy. *Ann Parasitol*. 2012;58(1):1–8.

207. Esposito S, Montinaro V, Groppali E, Tenconi R, Semino M, Principi N. Live attenuated intranasal influenza vaccine. *Hum Vaccines Immunother*. 2012;8(1):76–80.

208. Carter NJ, Curran MP. Live attenuated influenza vaccine (FluMist(R); Fluenz): a review of its use in the prevention of seasonal influenza in children and adults. *Drugs*. 2011;71(12):1591–1622.

209. Ambrose CS, Luke C, Coelingh K. Current status of live attenuated influenza vaccine in the United States for seasonal and pandemic influenza. *Influenza Other Respir Viruses*. 2008;2(6):193–202.

210. Xing Z, McFarland CT, et al. Intranasal mucosal boosting with an adenovirus-vectored vaccine markedly enhances the protection of BCG-primed guinea pigs against pulmonary tuberculosis. *PloS one*. 2009;4(6):e5856.

211. Nieto K, Kern A, Leuchs B et al. Combined prophylactic and therapeutic intranasal vaccination against human papillomavirus type-16 using different adeno-associated virus serotype vectors. *Antiviral Ther*. 2009;14(8):1125–1137.

212. Bielinska AU, Chepurnov AA, et al. A novel, killed-virus nasal vaccinia virus vaccine. *Clin Vaccine Immunol.* 2008;15(2):348–358.

213. Sloat BR, Cui Z. Nasal immunization with a dual antigen anthrax vaccine induced strong mucosal and systemic immune responses against toxins and bacilli. *Vaccine.* 2006;24(40–41):6405–6413.

214. Wang SH, Kirwan SM, et al. Stable dry powder formulation for nasal delivery of anthrax vaccine. *J Pharm Sci.* 2012;101(1):31–47.

215. Pardridge WM. Preparation of Trojan horse liposomes (THLs) for gene transfer across the blood-brain barrier. *Cold Spring Harbor Prot.* 2010 Apr;2010(4):pdb.prot5407. doi: 10.1101/pdb.prot5407.

216. Chow HS, Chen Z, Matsuura GT. Direct transport of cocaine from the nasal cavity to the brain following intranasal cocaine administration in rats. *J Pharm Sci.* 1999;88(8):754–758.

217. Westin U, Piras E, Jansson B, et al. Transfer of morphine along the olfactory pathway to the central nervous system after nasal administration to rodents. *Eur J Pharm Sci* 2005;24(5):565–573.

218. Schulz C, Paulus K, Lehnert H. Central nervous and metabolic effects of intranasally applied leptin. *Endocrinology.* 2004;145(6):2696–2701.

219. Chen XQ, Fawcett JR, et al. Delivery of nerve growth factor to the brain via the olfactory pathway. *J Alzheim Dis.* 1998;1(1):35–44.

220. Hashizume R, Ozawa T, Gryaznov SM, et al. New therapeutic approach for brain tumors: intranasal delivery of telomerase inhibitor GRN163. *Neuro-Oncol.* 2008;10(2):112–120.

221. Han IK, Kim MY, et al. Enhanced brain targeting efficiency of intranasally administered plasmid DNA: an alternative route for brain gene therapy. *J Mol Med.* 2007;85(1):75–83.

222. Dhuria SV, Hanson LR, et al. Intranasal delivery to the central nervous system: mechanisms and experimental considerations. *J Pharm Sci.* 2010;99(4):1654–1673.

223. Jones N. The nose and paranasal sinuses physiology and anatomy. *Adv Drug Deliv Rev.* 2001;51(1–3):5–19.

224. Wen MM. Olfactory targeting through intranasal delivery of biopharmaceutical drugs to the brain: current development. *Discov Med.* 2011;11(61):497–503.

225. Dhuria SV, Hanson LR, et al. Novel vasoconstrictor formulation to enhance intranasal targeting of neuropeptide therapeutics to the central nervous system. *J Pharm Exp Ther.* 2009;328(1):312–320.

226. Banks WA, During MJ, Niehoff ML. Brain uptake of the glucagon-like peptide-1 antagonist exendin(9–39) after intranasal administration. *J Pharm Exp Ther.* 2004;309(2):469–475.

227. Landis MS, Boyden T, Pegg S. Nasal-to-CNS drug delivery: where are we now and where are we heading? An industrial perspective. *Ther Deliv.* 2012;3(2):195–208.

228. Misra A, Kher G. Drug delivery systems from nose to brain. *Curr Pharm Biotechnol.* 2012;13(12):2355–2379.

229. Mansour HM, Rhee YS, Wu X. Nanomedicine in pulmonary delivery. *Int J Nanomed.* 2009;4(December):299–319.

230. Sung JC, Pulliam BL, Edwards DA. Nanoparticles for drug delivery to the lungs. *Trends Biotechnol.* 2007;25(12):563–570.

231. Gupta RB, Kompella UB. *Nanoparticle Technology for Drug Delivery.* New York, NY: Taylor & Francis; 2006.

232. Beck-Broichsitter M, Schmehl T, Seeger W, Gessler T. Evaluating the controlled release properties of inhaled nanoparticles using isolated, perfused, and ventilated lung models. *J Nanomater.* 2011;1–16.

233. Rhee YS, Mansour HM. Nanopharmaceuticals I: nanocarrier systems in drug delivery. Invited paper. *Int J Nanotechnol Spec Iss Nanopharm.* 2011;8(1/2):84–114.

234. Wu X, Mansour HM. Nanopharmaceuticals II: application of nanoparticles and nanocarrier systems in pharmaceutics and nanomedicine. Invited paper. *Int J Nanotechnol Spec Iss Nanopharm.* 2011;8(1/2):115–145.

235. Mansour HM, Park CW. Therapeutic and clinical aspects of nanomedicines and nanopharmaceutical products. In: Brenner S, ed. *The Nanomedicine Handbook for Clinicians* (vol. 1). London, UK: CRC Press; 2011.

236. Mansour HM, Park CW. Nanoparticle lung delivery and inhalation aerosols for targeted pulmonary nanomedicine. In: Kumar A, Mansour HM, Friedman A, Blough E, eds. *Nanomedicine in Drug Delivery* (vol. 1). London, UK: CRC Press/Taylor & Francis; 2012.

237. Mansour HM, Park CW, Bawa R. Design and development of approved nanopharmaceutical products. In: Bawa R, ed. *Clinical Nanomedicine: From Bench to Bedside. Series of Nanomedicine* (vol. 1). London, UK: Pan Stanford Publishing/CRC Press; 2011:1–27.

238. Mansour HM, Rhee YS, Park CW, DeLuca PP. Lipid nanoparticulate drug delivery and nanomedicine. In: Moghis A, ed. *Lipids in Nanotechnology* (1st ed.). Urbana, IL: American Oil Chemists Society Press; 2011:221–268.

239. Watts AB, Williams III RO. Nanoparticles for pulmonary delivery. In: Smyth HDC, Hickey AJ, eds. *Controlled Pulmonary Drug Delivery*. New York, NY: Springer; 2011.

240. Almeida AJ, Souto. Solid lipid nanoparticles as a drug delivery system for peptides and proteins. *Adv Drug Deliv Rev.* 2007;59(6):478–490.

241. Vij N. Synthesis and evaluation of airway targeted PLGA nanoparticles for drug delivery in obstructive lung diseases. *Methods Mol Biol.* 2012;906:303–310.

242. El-Baseir MM, Phipps MA, Kellaway IW. Preparation and subsequent degradation of poly (L-lactic acid) microspheres suitable for aerosolization: a physico-chemical study. *Int J Pharm.* 1997;151:145–153.

243. Tiwari SB, Amiji MM. A review of nanocarrier-based CNS delivery systems. *Curr Drug Deliv.* 2006;3(2):219–232.

244. Yamamoto H, Kuno Y, Sugimoto S, Takeuchi H, Kawashima Y. Surface-modified PLGA nanosphere with chitosan improved pulmonary delivery of calcitonin by mucoadhesion and opening of the intercellular tight junctions. *J Control Release.* 2005;102(2):373–381.

245. Rudolph, Schillinger, Plank, et al. Nonviral gene delivery to the lung with copolymer-protected and transferrin-modified polyethylenimine. *Biochim Biophys Acta.* 2002;1573(1):75–83.

246. Densmore CL. Advances in noninvasive pulmonary gene therapy. *Curr Drug Deliv.* 2006;3(1):55–63.

247. Bai S, Ahsan F. Synthesis and evaluation of pegylated dendrimeric nanocarrier for pulmonary delivery of low molecular weight heparin. *Pharm Res.* 2009;26(3):539–548.

248. Boas U, Heegaard PM. Dendrimers in drug research. *Chem Soc Rev.* 2004;33(1):43–63.

249. Tekade RK, Dutta T, Gajbhiye V, Jain NK. Exploring dendrimer towards dual drug delivery: pH responsive simultaneous drug-release kinetics. *J Microencaps.* 2009;26(4):287–296.

250. Bai S, Thomas C, Ahsan F. Dendrimers as a carrier for pulmonary delivery of enoxaparin, a low-molecular weight heparin. *J Pharm Sci.* 2007;96(8):2090–2106.

251. Kukowska L, Raczka E, et al. Intravascular and endobronchial DNA delivery to murine lung tissue using a novel, nonviral vector. *Hum Gene Ther.* 2000;11(10):1385–1395.

252. Zeng XM. The controlled delivery of drugs to the lung. *Int J Pharm.* 1995;124:149–164.

253. Chougule MB, Padhi BK, Misra A. Nano-liposomal dry powder inhaler of amiloride hydrochloride. *J Nanosci Nanotechnol.* 2006;6(9–10):3001–3009.

254. Chougule MB, Padhi BK, Misra A. Nano-liposomal dry powder inhaler of tacrolimus: preparation, characterization, and pulmonary pharmacokinetics. *Int J Nanomed.* 2007;2(4):675–688.

255. Joshi M, Misra AN. Pulmonary disposition of budesonide from liposomal dry powder inhaler. *Methods Find Exp Clin Pharmacol.* 2001;23(10):531–536.

256. Willis L, Hayes DJ, Mansour HM. Therapeutic liposomal dry powder inhalation aerosols for targeted lung delivery. *Lung.* 2012;190(3):251–262..

257. Li SD, Huang L. Targeted delivery of antisense oligodeoxynucleotide and small interference RNA into lung cancer cells. *Mol Pharm.* 2006;3(5):579–588.

258. Eliyahu H, Joseph A, Schillemans JP, et al. Characterization and in vivo performance of dextran-spermine polyplexes and DOTAP/cholesterol lipoplexes administered locally and systemically. *Biomaterials.* 2007;28(14):2339–2349.

259. Griesenbach U, Geddes DM, Alton EW. Gene therapy progress and prospects: cystic fibrosis. *Gene Ther.* 2006;13(14):1061–1067.

260. Schwarz LA, Johnson JL, et al. Delivery of DNA-cationic liposome complexes by small-particle aerosol. *Hum Gene Ther.* 1996;7(6):731–741.

261. Bi R, Shao W, Wang Q, Zhang N. Spray-freeze-dried dry powder inhalation of insulin-loaded liposomes for enhanced pulmonary delivery. *J Drug Target.* 2008;16(9):639–648.

262. Muller RH, Mader K, Gohla S. Solid lipid nanoparticles (SLN) for controlled drug delivery—a review of the state of the art. *Eur J Pharm Biopharm.* 2000;50(1):161–177.

263. Pandey R, Khuller GK. Solid lipid particle-based inhalable sustained drug delivery system against experimental tuberculosis. *Tuberculosis.* 2005;85(4):227–234.

264. Rudolph C, Schillinger U, Ortiz A, et al. Application of novel solid lipid nanoparticle (SLN)-gene vector formulations based on a dimeric HIV-1 TAT-peptide in vitro and in vivo. *Pharm Res.* 2004;21(9):1662–1669.

265. Liu J, Gong T, Fu H, et al. Solid lipid nanoparticles for pulmonary delivery of insulin. *Int J Pharm.* 2008;356(1–2):333–344.

266. Hu T, Chiou H, Chan HK, et al. Preparation of inhalable salbutamol sulphate using reactive high gravity controlled precipitation. *J Pharm Sci.* 2008;97(2):944–949.

267. Bhavna, Ahmad FJ, et al. Nano-salbutamol dry powder inhalation: a new approach for treating broncho-constrictive conditions. *Eur J Pharm Biopharm.* 2009;71(2):282–291.

268. Dickinson PA, Howells SW, Kellaway IW. Novel nanoparticles for pulmonary drug administration. *J Drug Target.* 2001;9(4):295–302.

269. Li HY, Zhang F. Preparation of nanoparticles by spray-drying and their use for efficient pulmonary drug delivery. *Methods Mol Biol.* 2012;906:295–301.

270. El-Gendy N, Berkland C. Combination chemotherapeutic dry powder aerosols via controlled nanoparticle agglomeration. *Pharm Res.* 2009;26(7):1752–1763.

271. El-Gendy N, Pornputtapitak W, Berkland C. Nanoparticle agglomerates of fluticasone propionate in combination with albuterol sulfate as dry powder aerosols. *Eur J Pharm Sci.* 2011;44(4):522–533.

272. Shekunov BY, Chattopadhyay P, Seitzinger J, Huff R. Nanoparticles of poorly water-soluble drugs prepared by supercritical fluid extraction of emulsions. *Pharm Res.* 2006;23:196–204.

273. leone-Bay A, Grant M. Technosphere technology: a platform for inhaled protein therapeutics. *ON Drug Deliv.* 2006:8–11.

274. Lahde A, Raula J, Kauppinen EI. Simultaneous synthesis and coating of salbutamol sulphate nanoparticles with L-leucine in the gas phase. *Int J Pharm.* 2008;358(1–2):256–262.

275. Newman SP, Peart J. Dry powder inhalers. In: Newman SP, ed. *Respiratory Drug Delivery: Essential Theory & Practice.* Richmond, VA: Respiratory drug delivery online/VCU; 2009:257–307.

276. Young P, Thompson J, Woodcock D, Aydin M, Price R. The development of a novel high-dose pressurized aerosol dry-powder device (PADD) for the delivery of pumactant for inhalation therapy. *J Aeros Med.* 2004;17(2):123–128.

277. Tobyn M, Staniforth JN, et al. Active and intelligent inhaler device development. *Int J Pharm.* 2004;277(1–2):31–37.

278. Keating GM, Faulds D. Airmax: a multi-dose dry powder inhaler. *Drugs.* 2002;62(13):1887–1895; discussion 1896–1887.

279. Fleming FS. The MicroDose DPI, a true platform inhaler. *ON Drug Deliv.* 2007:26–29.

280. Young PM, Thompson, Woodcock, Aydin, Price. The development of a novel high-dose pressurized aerosol dry-powder device (PADD) for the delivery of pumactant for inhalation therapy. *J Aerosol Med.* 2004;17(2):123–128.

281. Zhu J, Wen J, Zhang H. Dry powder inhaler. London, Ontario, Canada: The University of Western Ontario; 2011.

282. Martin FI, Mathew TH. The treatment of diabetes insipidus with synthetic lysine-vasopressin by inhalation. *Med J Australia.* 1964;2:984–986.

283. Adjei A, Doyle R, Pratt M, Finley R, Johnson E. Bioavailability of leuprolide following intratracheal administration to beagle dogs. *Int J Pharm.* 1990;61(Jun 11):135–144.

284. Adjei A, Garren J. Pulmonary delivery of peptide drugs: effect of particle size on bioavailability of leuprolide acetate in healthy male volunteers. *Pharm Res.* 1990;7:565–569.

285. Komada, Iwakawa, Yamamoto, Sakakibara, Okumura. Intratracheal delivery of peptide and protein agents: absorption from solution and dry powder by rat lung. *J Pharm Sci.* 1994;83(6):863–867.

286. Patton J. Pulmonary delivery of drugs for bone disorders. *Adv Drug Deliv Rev.* 2000;42:239–248.

287. Codrons V, Vanderbist F, Verbeeck RK, et al. Systemic delivery of parathyroid hormone (1–34) using inhalation dry powders in rats. *J Pharm Sci.* 2003;92(5):938–950.

288. Gansslen M. About inhalation of insulin [abstract]. *Klin Wochenschr.* 1925;4:71.

289. Patton JS, Bukar J, Nagarajan S. Inhaled insulin. *Adv Drug Deliv Rev.* 1999;35(2–3):235–247.

290. Tazawa R, Nakata K, Inoue Y, Nukiwa T. Granulocyte-macrophage colony-stimulating factor inhalation therapy for patients with idiopathic pulmonary alveolar proteinosis: a pilot study; and long-term treatment with aerosolized granulocyte-macrophage colony-stimulating factor: a case report. *Respirology.* 2006;11(Suppl):S61–S64.

291. Kinnula V, Cantell K, Mattson K. Effect of inhaled natural interferon-alpha on diffuse bronchioalveolar carcinoma. *Eur J Cancer.* 1990;26(6):740–741.

292. Griese M, Latzin P, Kappler M, et al. Alpha1-antitrypsin inhalation reduces airway inflammation in cystic fibrosis patients. *Eur Respir J.* 2007;29(2):240–250.

293. Walvoord EC, et al. Inhaled growth hormone (GH) compared with subcutaneous GH in children with GH deficiency: pharmacokinetics, pharmacodynamics, and safety. *J Clin Endocrinol Metab.* 2009;94(6):2052–2059.

294. Bot AI, Tarara TE, et al. Novel lipid-based hollow-porous microparticles as a platform for immunoglobulin delivery to the respiratory tract. *Pharm Res.* 2000;17(3):275–283.

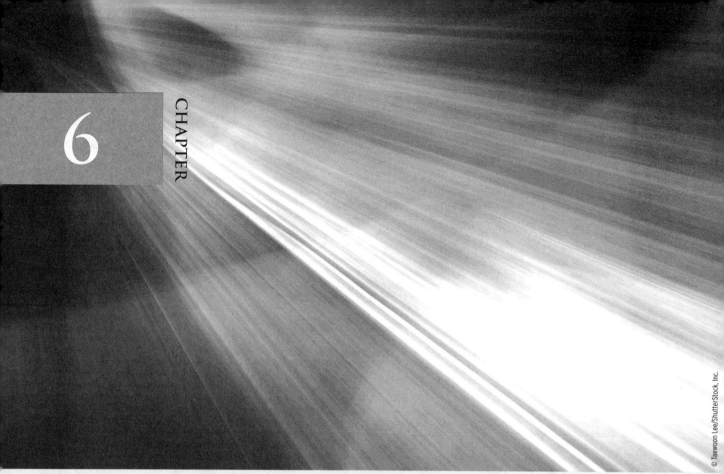

CHAPTER 6

CONTROLLED DRUG DELIVERY

SHAILENDRA B. TALLAPAKA, VAMSI K. KARUTURI,
SUTTHILUG SOTTHIVIRAT, AND JOSEPH A. VETRO

CHAPTER OBJECTIVES

Upon completing this chapter, the reader should be able to

▸ Define pharmacotherapy.

▸ Name the major types of therapeutic outcomes.

▸ Understand the basics of pharmacokinetics.

▸ Know the differences between conventional and controlled drug delivery.

▸ Differentiate between controlled delivery dosage forms currently available in the clinic by their mechanism of drug release.

CHAPTER OUTLINE

Introduction

Conventional Drug Delivery

INTRODUCTION

Pharmacotherapy, the most common form of therapy, is the use of drugs that produce effects on or within the body that are beneficial in the treatment of a given medical condition (i.e., produce therapeutic effects). Depending on the nature of the medical condition and capabilities of existing drugs, the ultimate goal of pharmacotherapy is to achieve one or more desired therapeutic outcomes, ranging from preventing the medical condition (*prophylactic therapy*), reducing or eliminating clinical signs/symptoms of the medical condition (*symptomatic therapy*), slowing or stopping the progression of the medical condition (*abortive therapy*), and/or curing the medical condition (*curative therapy*) (Table 6-1) [1].

To increase the likelihood of achieving the desired therapeutic outcome, the therapeutic effect of the drug must be maintained for a duration that is sufficient for the specific medical condition with minimal or acceptable side effects during or after treatment [1]. As such, the drug must be administered to the patient such that the concentration of drug at its site of action within the body (C_S) is maintained at levels that produce the therapeutic effect (i.e., therapeutic concentrations) but do not produce unacceptable adverse effects over the required duration of therapy. This is accomplished by administering the drug in a dosage form that is safe for the desired administration route (Table 6-2) at a dose and dose frequency that maintains therapeutic concentrations of C_S that do not produce unacceptable adverse effects in the target or peripheral tissues.

TABLE 6-1 Examples of Desired Therapeutic Outcomes for Specific Medical Conditions

Medical Condition	Desired Therapeutic Outcome	Type of Therapy	Indicated Drug Class	Therapeutic Effect
Hypertension	Prevent sequelae of hypertension: heart disease, stroke, blindness	Prophylactic therapy	Antihypertensive	Lower blood pressure
Allergy	Minimize symptoms: drainage, itchiness	Symptomatic therapy	Antihistamine	Decrease drainage
Migraine	Decrease severity and duration of attacks	Abortive therapy	Serotonin receptor agonist	Constrict blood vessels in the brain
Sinus infection	Eliminate infection	Curative therapy	Antibiotics	Kill bacteria in the sinuses

If the site of drug action is easily identified and localized to a specific, accessible region of the body, the drug can be directly administered at or near its site of action (local drug delivery). The site of action for most drugs, however, is diffuse throughout the body and not directly accessible. As such, these drugs must be administered directly (intravenous) or indirectly (extravascular) into the bloodstream and carried to the site of action by the plasma (systemic drug delivery) (**Figure 6-1**) [2].

Extravascular routes are most commonly used for systemic drug delivery (**Table 6-3**). These routes require that the drug is dissolved in local biological fluids and *absorbed* into the bloodstream through available absorption sites where it is then simultaneously *distributed*

TABLE 6-2 Routes of Administration and Safe Dosage Forms	
Route of Administration	**Dosage Forms**
Intraocular	Solutions Suspensions Implants
Intranasal	Solutions Sprays Ointments
Inhalational	Aerosols Inhalers Nebulizers Smoking Vaporizer
Oral	Tablets Capsules Solutions Elixirs Emulsions Suspensions Syrups Powders Pastes Ointments Gels Chewing gums
Rectal	Suppositories Enemas Ointments Solutions Gels Hydrogels Murphy drip
Vaginal	Vaginal rings Ointments Pessaries Douches Sponges Emulsions Tablets

Continues

Route of Administration	Dosage Forms
Topical	Ointments
	Liniments
	Pastes
	Films
	Hydrogels
	Liposomes
	Creams
	Lotions
	Lip balm
	Medicated shampoos
	Dermal patches
	Transdermal patches
	Transdermal sprays
	Powders
Intravenous	Solutions
	Suspensions
	Liposomes
Intramuscular	Solutions
	Suspensions
Subcutaneous	Solutions
	Suspensions
	Liposomes
	Microspheres
	Insulin pumps
	Implants

TABLE 6-2 Routes of Administration and Safe Dosage Forms (*Continued*)

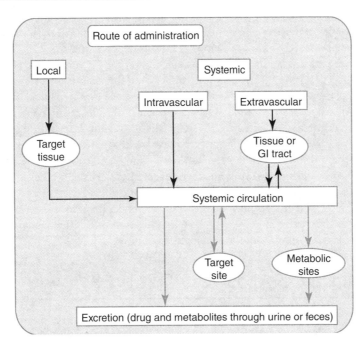

FIGURE 6-1 Schematic of drug absorption, distribution, metabolism, and elimination processes for different routes of administration.

TABLE 6-3 Some Common Extravascular Routes of Administration

Route of Administration	Example
Enteral	Oral Sublingual Nasogastric
Parenteral	Intramuscular Subcutaneous

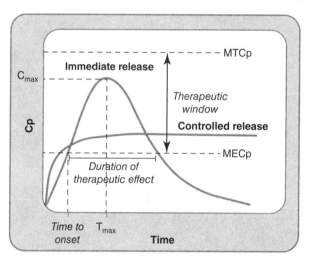

FIGURE 6-2 Plasma concentration versus time profiles of immediate and controlled-release formulations.

throughout the body, *metabolized*, and *excreted*. Given that blood plasma is in equilibrium with the active site of the drug, C_s is then assumed to be proportional to the concentration of drug in the plasma (C_p) [3]. This allows the time–dependent change in C_s to be indirectly monitored after systemic delivery by determining the C_p versus time (**Figure 6-2**). The rate of drug absorption, time until the onset of the therapeutic effect, and magnitude and duration of the therapeutic effect can then be roughly determined by relating the C_p to therapeutic and toxic effects. The C_p where the therapeutic effect is first observed is called the minimum effective concentration (**MEC$_p$**), the C_p where dose–limiting toxic effects are first observed is called the minimum toxic concentration (**MTC$_p$**), and the range of drug concentrations in the plasma between MEC$_p$ and MTC$_p$ is called the **therapeutic window**. The rate of drug absorption is then reflected as the time it takes to reach maximal C_p (T_{max}), the time until the onset of the therapeutic effect is the time required for C_p to reach the MEC$_p$, the magnitude of the therapeutic effect (to a certain extent depending on the drug) is the maximal C_p (C_{max}), and the duration of the therapeutic effect is the total time the C_p remains within the therapeutic window.

CONVENTIONAL DRUG DELIVERY

The rates of absorption and elimination for most drugs follow first-order kinetics. As such, the rate of absorption into the bloodstream is proportional to the concentration of drug in biological fluids at the absorption site and the rate of elimination from the plasma is proportional to the C_p. This means that increasing the concentration of drug at the absorption site or in the plasma increases the rate of drug absorption or elimination, respectively. The change in C_p over time is then the difference between the rate the drug is absorbed into the bloodstream versus the rate that drug is eliminated from the plasma.

Drugs administered by extravascular routes must be released from the dosage form and dissolved in available biological fluids before they can be absorbed into the bloodstream. The rate of systemic absorption from these routes consequently involves a series of two kinetic processes: (1) the rate the drug is released from the dosage form followed by (2) the rate the drug is absorbed [2]. The slowest step is then the rate-limiting step and ultimately determines the overall rate of drug absorption.

Conventional dosage forms release the entire dose of drug into available biological fluids immediately after administration (i.e., immediate release). As such, the rate-limiting step is the rate of drug absorption into the bloodstream. Given that the concentration of drug at the site of absorption is initially higher than in the plasma, the rate of drug absorption is faster than the rate of drug elimination and causes an initial increase in the C_p over time (Figure 6-2). The rate of drug absorption then decreases over time as the concentration of drug at the absorption site decreases due to absorption (and level of drug metabolism for the given extravascular route), whereas the rate of elimination increases over time due to the increase in the C_p. When the rates of drug absorption and elimination eventually become equal, the C_p reaches a steady-state maximum (C_{max}). After this point, the rate of drug elimination becomes faster than the rate of drug absorption and the C_p decreases until the drug is completely eliminated from the body. This results in a classic "bell-shaped" C_p versus T profile that is characteristic of drugs administered in conventional dosage forms (Figure 6-2). The therapeutic effect using conventional dosage forms is then maintained for the required duration by dosing at a frequency that maintains the C_p versus T profile as a series of bell-shaped curves that remain within the therapeutic window.

Conventional dosage forms, although frequently used, have potential disadvantages. The biggest disadvantage is that the fluctuating C_p results in an uneven therapeutic effect and increases the potential for adverse side effects. Another disadvantage is the potential for decreased patient compliance, because the need for multiple dosing throughout the day can be a major inconvenience, especially for patients with chronic medical conditions that require pharmacotherapy for the remainder of their lives.

CONTROLLED DRUG DELIVERY

Controlled-release dosage forms, unlike conventional dosage forms, release the total dose of drug into available biological fluids at a slower, more constant rate after administration (i.e., controlled release). As such, the rate-limiting step for drug absorption is the rate the drug is released from the dosage form. Once the rate of drug release from the dosage form equals the rate of drug absorption, the steady-state concentration of drug at the site of absorption remains constant and leads to a constant rate of drug absorption. Given that the steady-state concentration of drug at the site of absorption is initially greater than in the plasma, the rate of absorption is faster than the rate of elimination and causes an initial increase in the C_p over time (Figure 6-2). The C_p then steadily increases until the rate of drug absorption equals the rate of elimination. Given that the rate of drug absorption is constant, however, the rates of drug absorption and elimination remain equal over time and result in a flat C_p versus T profile (Figure 6-2) that persists until the dose of drug is completely released from the dosage form.

Controlled-release formulations offer several advantages over conventional dosage forms, such as increased patient safety through the ability to maintain a constant C_p and improved patient compliance by decreasing the dosing frequency through an increase in the therapeutic duration for a given dose of drug. Many controlled-release dosage forms are currently available in the clinic for a variety of drugs and can be categorized based on the mechanisms used to control the rate of drug release. These mechanisms can be adapted to achieve controlled drug delivery for both local and systemic drug delivery.

MECHANISMS OF DRUG RELEASE

The rate at which a drug is released from the dosage form is a function of many physical, chemical, and biological processes that depend on drug properties (solubility, polarity, size, etc.), type of excipients (e.g., polymers, binding agents), methods used in preparing the dosage form, and route of administration (this determines the environment in which the dosage form will be present, e.g., gastrointestinal tract for oral administration, respiratory tract for intranasal administration) [4]. Some of the processes include diffusion of active and inactive components of the dosage form, hydration of the dosage form, swelling of polymers in the dosage form, polymer degradation, drug degradation, change in the pH of microenvironment because of drug or polymer degradation, dissolution of drug or polymer, phagocytosis of the dosage form (e.g., microparticles, liposomes, etc.) by the mononuclear phagocyte system, and gastric emptying. Many of these processes simultaneously affect drug release kinetics and make it difficult to design a formulation that controls all these processes. In most cases, these processes occur in a sequence where one process is significantly slower than the others. This slowest step is the rate-determining step and, consequently, determines the overall rate of drug release.

A controlled-release formulation is optimized based on one or more rate-determining processes involved in drug release. In this section, drug release mechanisms used to achieve zero-order release (i.e., a constant rate of drug release regardless of the concentration of drug remaining in the dosage form) in the clinic are discussed along with specific examples of drugs that take advantage of these controlled-release dosage forms.

DIFFUSION-CONTROLLED SYSTEMS

Diffusion is a mass transport phenomenon in which the molecules of a substance travel from a region of high concentration to a region of low concentration through Brownian motion. Diffusion occurs in most drug delivery systems; in controlled drug delivery systems, polymers are often used to control the diffusion of drug into the surrounding medium. Generally, the drug is either uniformly dispersed in a polymer matrix (monolithic systems) or is present in the core of the formulation that is covered by a rate-determining polymeric membrane (reservoir systems) [4]. In these systems the molecules of different substances like water, drug, polymer, their degradation products, and components of the surrounding medium diffuse in and out of the dosage form at the same time. The net movement of a substance is driven by the concentration gradient and can be explained by Fick's laws of diffusion [4]. As the drug outside the dosage form is cleared immediately (sink conditions), it can be assumed that the concentration of drug is always higher inside the dosage form. Therefore, the drug diffuses out of the formulation until the entire dose is completely released, and the rate at which the drug diffuses out can be controlled by the polymer and type of system (monolithic or reservoir).

Monolithic Systems

In monolithic systems, drugs are uniformly dispersed and completely or partially dissolved in a water-insoluble polymer matrix and released from the system through simple diffusion. In the case of polymers that do not swell, dissolve, or degrade with time in the presence of water, drug release under sink conditions follows nonlinear kinetics where the rate of drug release is inversely proportional to the square root of time (i.e., the drug release rate is initially very fast and decreases gradually over time). This is because water molecules immediately diffuse into the system once the dosage form comes into contact with an aqueous medium and the drug simultaneously diffuses out. This creates a drug-free region within the polymer matrix called the "depletion zone" through which remaining drug molecules must travel before reaching the water layer. The thickness of the depletion zone and subsequent diffusion path of the drug increases with time as more drug leaves the dosage form. This causes a decrease in the release rate as the remaining dose of drug must travel farther and farther before it reaches the water layer [5]. This is similar to a reservoir system in which the membrane thickness increases with time. In some formulations the matrix contains an additional polymer that dissolves quickly once it comes into contact with water and leaves behind a porous matrix. In these systems the drug release is affected by the solubility of the drug in surrounding media, relative size of drug molecules, and diameter and shape of the pores.

Although it is difficult to achieve zero-order kinetics with monolithic systems, they are easy to prepare and cost-effective [5]. They also have the added advantage of not dumping the entire dose of drug if the matrix is faulty. As such, they can be formulated so the patient can break the formulation in half to reduce the dose without significantly affecting the kinetics of drug release.

Examples of monolithic systems in the clinic are Nitro-Dur® and the Exelon® patch. Nitro-Dur® is a transdermal patch designed to deliver nitroglycerin over 24 hours to prevent angina pectoris in patients suffering from coronary artery disease (see www.merck.com/product/usa/pi_circulars/n/nitro-dur/nitrodur_pi.pdf). In this system, the drug is homogenously dispersed in a gel-like matrix composed of an acrylate polymer with a resinous cross-linking agent. The drug-containing polymer matrix, which also acts as the patch adhesive, is covered by an impermeable backing on one side and a removable protective liner on the other side. The system is designed to release 0.02 mg nitroglycerine per hour per cm^2 of applied area. It is available as 0.1-, 0.2-, 0.3-, 0.4-, 0.6-, and 0.8-mg/h patches [6–8]. The Exelon® patch is a matrix type transdermal system containing rivastigmine, a reversible cholinesterase inhibitor indicated for the treatment of mild to moderate dementia associated with Alzheimer's and Parkinson's diseases (see www.exelonpatch.com). The patch consists of four layers: a backing layer, a drug-containing acrylic matrix, a silicone adhesive matrix, and a release liner. It is available as 4.6-, 9.5-, and 13.3-mg/day patches [9].

Reservoir Systems

In reservoir systems, the drug is present as a reservoir that is surrounded by a rate-controlling polymer membrane. The rate-controlling membrane is usually composed of a water-insoluble polymer with or without solvent-filled pores. In the case of a homogenous nonporous membrane, the drug diffuses out of the dosage form after dissolving in the polymer matrix, and the rate of drug diffusion depends on the solubility of the drug in the polymer matrix [10]. In the case of a porous membrane, the pores are immediately filled with the solvent (usually water) upon administration and the drug diffuses out of the pores. The drug release rate depends on the porosity and tortuosity of the rate-controlling membrane [5]. The overall drug release kinetics depend on the relative amount of drug loaded in the dosage form. When the amount of loaded drug is less than its solubility in the surrounding media, the entire drug dissolves immediately after media (e.g., water) diffuses into the system. The concentration of drug inside the dosage form then decreases continuously with time, and drug release follows first-order kinetics (i.e., decreases over time as the concentration of drug decreases in the dosage form) if the membrane's properties do not change with time. If the amount of loaded drug is higher than its solubility in the surrounding media, the drug will not be completely dissolved once the media diffuses into the dosage form. As long as undissolved drug is present, the drug concentration of media inside the dosage form remains constant and the drug release rate will follow zero-order kinetics [11] (i.e., the rate of drug release will be constant regardless of the amount of drug remaining in the dosage form). Once undissolved drug is exhausted, however, the drug release rate will follow first-order kinetics (i.e., decreases as the concentration of drug remaining in the dosage form decreases).

Unlike monolithic systems, reservoir systems are capable of achieving zero-order release kinetics and can also sustain drug release for a very long time. They often require complicated manufacturing processes, however, and potentially cause severe side effects if the rate-controlling membrane is defective or becomes compromised and releases the entire dose of drug immediately upon administration.

There are several examples of reservoir systems in the clinic. Retisert® (Figure 6-3, [13]) is a nonerodible polymer ocular implant for the treatment of chronic noninfectious uveitis affecting the posterior segment of the eye (see www.retisert.com). The implant consists of a 0.59-mg pellet of fluocinolone acetonide coated with a layer of polyvinyl alcohol that acts as a rate-controlling membrane and is itself partially covered with a layer of water-impermeable silicone elastomer. The pellet is affixed to a polyvinyl alcohol suture strut using a silicone adhesive. Drug diffuses through the polyvinyl alcohol layer in the region not covered by the silicone elastomer. Retisert® is surgically implanted into the posterior segment of the affected eye and releases fluocinolone acetonide at an initial rate of 0.6 µg/day that decreases over the first month to a steady state between 0.3 and 0.4 µg/day over 30 months [12]. The same technology is used for the Vitrasert® ocular implant.

Mirena® is a hormonal intrauterine device used as a reversible contraceptive (see http://www.mirena-us.com). It is a soft, flexible, 32-mm long 'T'-shaped device containing 52 mg of levonorgestrel [14]. The drug is contained in a cylindrical reservoir that is wrapped around the stem of the device and covered by a nonporous polydimethylsiloxane membrane. The device is designed to release the drug within the uterine cavity at a rate of 20 µg/day. It is effective for 5 years, after which the drug release rate decreases by ~50%. A monofilament brown polyethylene thread is attached to a loop at the bottom of the T-shaped body for removal [14].

Duragesic® is a reservoir transdermal patch that delivers fentanyl as an analgesic through the skin for 3 days (Figure 6-4, [17]). The system consists of an impermeable backing, a rate-controlling membrane, and an amine-resistant contact adhesive layer covered by a strippable backing. The drug, dissolved in a gel made of ethanol, water, and gelling agent (hydroxyethylcellulose, hydroxypropylcellulose, and hydroxypropylmethylcellulose), is incorporated in a reservoir that is formed between the impermeable

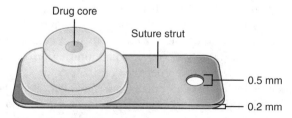

FIGURE 6-3 Schematic of Retisert.

backing and the rate-controlling membrane. The system is designed to release the drug at a constant rate that is linearly dependent on the applied area (i.e., drug release rate increases with an increase in the area of the applied area). Duragesic® is available in five strengths (12, 25, 50, 75, and 100 μg/h) that are accomplished by increasing the size of the patch [15, 16].

Hybrid Systems

In hybrid systems, a monolithic polymer matrix that contains the drug is surrounded by a rate-controlling membrane. Using a monolithic polymer matrix as the drug reservoir allows these systems to achieve zero-order drug release kinetics without dose dumping.

   Examples of hybrid systems in the clinic are Cypher® sirolimus-eluting coronary stent and Catapres-TTS®. Cypher® is a drug-eluting stent used in the treatment of atherosclerosis (**Figure 6-5**, [20]). It is the combination of a bare metal stent to open up coronary arteries partially occluded by atherosclerosis and a controlled-release formulation of sirolimus to slow the formation of atherosclerotic plaques within the lumen of the stent (see www.cordislabeling.com). The stent, a mesh of electropolished stainless steel (316L), is coated with the sirolimus formulation on luminal and abluminal surfaces. The coating consists of three layers: a base coat of parylene C followed by the main coat made up of polyethylene-covinyl acetate and poly-n-butylmethacrylate (67%:33%) mixed with sirolimus, and a top coat of poly-n-butylmethacrylate to control the drug release. The drug is slowly released into the arterial wall to prevent restenosis with about 80% of the dose released over 30 days and the entire dose released after 90 days [18, 19].

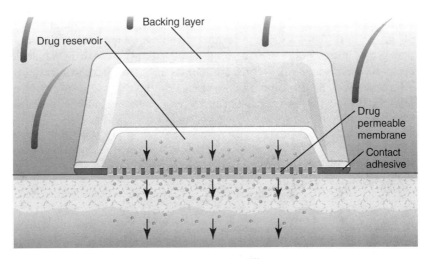

FIGURE 6-4 Schematic of a transdermal patch showing its different components.

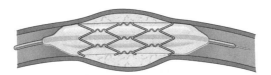

FIGURE 6-5 Illustration of a drug-eluting stent.

Catapres-TTS® is a transdermal therapeutic system of clonidine for the treatment of hypertension. It is a 0.2-mm-thick multilayered film consisting of a backing layer of pigmented polyester and an aluminum film; a drug reservoir of clonidine, mineral oil, polyisobutylene, and colloidal silicon dioxide; a microporous polypropylene membrane that acts as the rate-controlling membrane; and an adhesive formulation of clonidine, mineral oil, polyisobutylene, and colloidal silicon dioxide. Clonidine in the adhesive layer quickly saturates the site of application after which the drug diffuses at a constant rate through the rate-controlling layer for 7 days. Steady-state plasma levels of clonidine are achieved after 3 days of application and persist for 8 hours after removal of the patch. Catapres-TTS® is available in three strengths to deliver clonidine at 0.1, 0.2, or 0.3 mg/day [21].

EROSION-CONTROLLED SYSTEMS

Polymer erosion, defined as the loss of mass from a degrading polymer matrix, is a complex process that is a result of simultaneous degradation and diffusion of the polymer chains. In erosion-controlled systems, drug molecules are either entrapped or encapsulated within the polymeric matrix through many techniques, including emulsification–solvent evaporation, spray drying, precipitation, coacervation, coextrusion, and self-assembly. The rate of drug release is controlled by polymer matrix erosion, which depends on the physicochemical properties of the polymer, like reactive functional groups, swellability, crystallinity, hydrophobicity, chain length, and water diffusivity.

Erosion of the polymer matrix can be of two types: bulk erosion or surface erosion. In systems that undergo bulk erosion, water rapidly penetrates the entire dosage form and polymer degradation occurs throughout the matrix. The rate of drug release from bulk-eroding systems varies with time and can be differentiated into three phases (**Figure 6-6**). Shortly after administration, water penetrates into the polymer matrix and forms pores; surface-bound and encapsulated drug molecules that have access to these water-filled pores are quickly released into the surrounding medium ("burst phase"). At the same time, the penetrated water begins to hydrolyze the polymer into degradation products. The dissolved polymer degradation products affect the

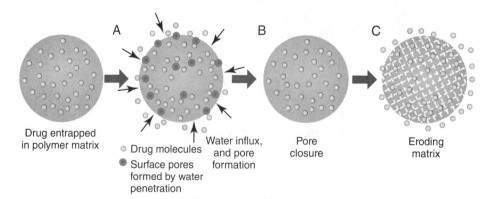

FIGURE 6-6 Schematic of drug release mechanism from a bulk-eroding matrix. In the "burst" phase (A), drug diffuses through the surface pores formed during water penetration. There is limited amount of drug release in the lag phase (B) during which surface pores close due to polymer relaxation. The final phase (C) is characterized by rapid release of drug due to disintegration of eroded matrix after polymer degradation.

polymer matrix by catalyzing hydrolysis, increasing osmolality, and, possibly, crystallizing and plasticizing the polymer [22]. The plasticizing effect of degradation products and water decreases the glass transition temperature to cause polymer relaxation and increase chain mobility. Polymer chain relaxation and rearrangement leads to pore-closure ("self-healing"). Self-healing is followed by a steep decline in drug release rate called the "lag phase." The existence of fewer pores and slower drug diffusion through the dense polymer network limits drug release during this phase. After the lag phase, the erosion of polymer matrix occurs to form pores through the dissolution of polymer degradation products. As erosion proceeds, the pores grow in size and drug molecules rapidly diffuse through these pores into the surrounding medium to begin what is sometimes called the "second burst phase" (**Figure 6-7**). The high porosity that results from the eroding matrix also provides higher surface area for dissolution. The rate of drug release during this phase depends on the rate of polymer erosion and drug diffusion.

In surface erosion, the erosion of the polymer matrix begins at the outer surface of the dosage form and gradually moves inward, resulting in drug release and a decrease in the device dimensions (**Figure 6-8**). Drug release occurs sequentially from the eroding

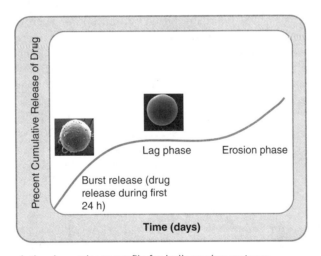

FIGURE 6-7 Cumulative drug release profile for bulk erosion systems.

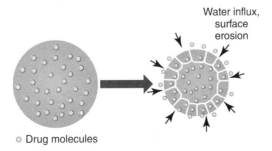

FIGURE 6-8 Schematic depicting the drug release mechanism of a surface-eroding matrix. The drug entrapped in the outer surface is released as polymer erosion proceeds from outer layers to inner layers. The size of the matrix decreases as erosion proceeds inwards with time.

surface of the dosage form, and the rate of polymer erosion is directly proportional to the external surface area and remains constant throughout the process [23]. The erosion rate can be adjusted by changing the size and shape of the dosage form. Surface erosion is ideal for controlling the rate of drug release and protecting encapsulated drug against degradation *in vivo*. Surface erosion, however, is tough to achieve because water penetrates into the polymer matrix before surface erosion can occur [24]. Most polymers used for erosion-controlled systems such as polyanhydrides and polyorthoesters undergo bulk erosion.

There are several examples of erosion-controlled systems in the clinic. Lupron depot® is a depot suspension of leuprolide acetate for the palliative treatment of advanced prostate cancer. It is available as a 1-, 3-, 4-, or 6-month release system that is prepared as a prefilled dual-chamber syringe of lyophilized sterile microspheres and diluent that are combined just before intramuscular administration. Leuprolide acetate incorporated in biodegradable lactide/glycolide copolymer is released through bulk erosion of the polymer matrix. A single administration of Lupron Depot® (7.5 mg) produces mean plasma leuprolide concentrations of 20 ng/mL at 4 hours and 0.36 ng/mL at 4 weeks. In clinical studies, administration of Lupron Depot® 7.5 mg to patients with stage D2 prostate adenocarcinoma once every 4 weeks for 24 weeks increased serum testosterone levels by 50% above baseline during first week of treatment. Serum testosterone levels were reduced to chemical castration range within 4 weeks of initial depot administration in 94% of patients (51 out of 54) [25].

Gliadel® wafer is a U.S. Food and Drug Administration–approved biodegradable disc implanted under the skull for the treatment of high-grade malignant glioma and recurrent gliobastoma multiforme. It can also be used as an adjunct to surgery and radiation. Carmustine [1,3-bis(2-chloroethyl)-1-nitrosourea, or BCNU], a nitrosourea oncolytic agent, is homogeneously distributed in biodegradable polyanhydride copolymer, polifeprosan 20 (poly[bis(p-carboxyphenoxy) propane: sebacic acid; 20:80) for controlled local delivery. The release of carmustine from Gliadel® is a combination of drug diffusion and erosion of the polymer matrix. About 70% of the copolymer degrades within 3 weeks, and the monomers carboxyphenoxypropane and sebacic acid are eliminated by kidney and liver metabolism, respectively. Gliadel® increases median overall survival of patients by 33% (32 weeks) compared with placebo (24 weeks). Six-month survival rates of patients suffering from glioblastoma increased from 36% (26/73) with placebo to 56% (40/72) with Gliadel® wafer [26].

Zoladex® is an injectable sustained-release 3.6-mg depot of goserelin acetate, a gonadotropin-releasing hormone superagonist used for the treatment of prostate and breast cancers. Goserelin acetate is dispersed in biodegradable polymer, poly(lactide-co-glycolide) matrix. Subcutaneous injection of Zoladex® provides continuous release of goserelin over a 28-day period that is initially slow for 8 days followed by a rapid, continuous release for the remaining 20 days. Zoladex® decreases serum levels of testosterone in men to levels observed after surgical castration and decreases serum estradiol in women to levels observed in postmenopausal women 2 to 4 weeks after therapy [27].

SWELLING-CONTROLLED SYSTEMS

Swelling can be defined as the increase in the volume of a system caused by the absorption of a liquid or vapor. This is the characteristic property of drug delivery systems that contain hydrophilic polymers that change from a glassy (hard) state to a rubbery state upon hydration. This is because the absorption of water reduces the glass transition temperature of the polymer and causes the polymer chains to relax (the end to end distance of the polymer chain increases) [28, 29]. As a result there is an increase in the volume of the system and the mobility of the polymer chains.

In swelling-controlled drug delivery systems, the drug is homogenously mixed with a glassy polymer and compressed. When the monolithic device is dry, the polymer remains glassy and impermeable for the drug. When it is exposed to an aqueous environment (like the gastrointestinal tract), however, water penetrates into the system and causes the polymer matrix to swell [28]. Swelling begins at the outer layer and moves radially inward as water penetrates into the system; the moving boundary that separates the swollen matrix from the nonswollen matrix is known as the "swelling front" [28, 29]. The polymer matrix becomes softer with increasing water content and turns into a gel. Polymer chains in the gel layer are not only longer but also more mobile. This causes the polymer chains to disentangle and move away from each other and, consequently, erode the gel layer. The outermost layer that separates the polymer matrix from the aqueous media is known as the "erosion front." Inside the swollen matrix the region closer to the swelling front contains both dissolved and undissolved drug, whereas the region near the erosion front contains only dissolved drug. The boundary that separates these two regions is known as the "diffusion front" (**Figure 6-9**) [28]. The drug concentration in between the swelling and diffusion fronts depends on the solubility of the drug and remains constant as long as there is undissolved drug present. Once undissolved drug is exhausted, however, the concentration of drug in between the swelling and diffusion decreases.

In swelling-controlled systems, the drug has to diffuse from the swelling front to the erosion front once it is released from the nonswollen matrix (i.e., through the gel layer in undissolved and dissolved forms) before it can enter into the surrounding aqueous media. The rate at which drug diffuses through the system depends on the drug concentration gradient within the gel layer. The drug concentration gradient is determined by the drug solubility in the gel layer and its thickness. The gel layer thickness varies with time and depends on the rate at which the matrix swells and erodes. In the beginning, the rate of swelling is greater than the rate of erosion, and the gel layer thickness

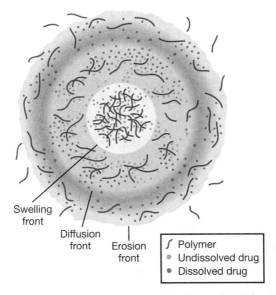

Swelling front

Diffusion front   Erosion front

| ∫ Polymer |
| ∘ Undissolved drug |
| • Dissolved drug |

FIGURE 6-9 The upper base of a hydroxypropylmethylcellulose (HPMC) cylindrical matrix containing 60% w/w of buflomedil pyridoxalphosphate, placed in between two transparent discs after 1 hour of swelling–release. (Data from Colombo P, Bettini R, Santi P, Peppas NA. Swellable matrices for controlled drug delivery: gel-layer behaviour, mechanisms and optimal performance. *Pharma Sci Technol To.* Jun 2000;3(6):198-204.)

increases quickly because of rapid water penetration. In this phase, drug release kinetics follows Fickian and non-Fickian kinetics. After some time, the rate of water penetration decreases because of an increase in the diffusional distance and, consequently, slows the rate of swelling. When the rates of swelling and erosion become equal, the gel layer thickness becomes constant and drug release follows zero-order kinetics (i.e., drug release rate becomes constant regardless of the concentration of drug remaining in the dosage form). Once the entire polymer is swollen, however, the gel layer thickness decreases and drug release follows first-order kinetics (i.e., drug release rate decreases as the concentration of drug remaining in the dosage form decreases) [28].

Although drug release kinetics for most swelling-based systems can be broadly explained by the thickness of the gel layer, drug release kinetics are different for cross-linked and non–cross-linked polymer matrices. The kinetics for these two types of matrices are better explained by the movements of the various fronts, but that is beyond the scope of this chapter.

Examples of swelling-controlled systems in the clinic are Dilacor XR® and Glumetza®. Dilacor XR® is a capsule containing multiple units of 60-mg extended-release dilitiazem HCl tablets for the treatment of hypertension [30] that is based on Geomatrix™ technology (Skyepharma, Muttenz, Switzerland). Each dilitiazem HCl unit is a trilayered tablet consisting of a swellable hydrophilic core containing the drug sandwiched between two support layers that are less hydrophilic than the core (**Figure 6-10**). Drug release occurs from the regions of hydrophilic core exposed to water. The rate of drug release is consequently controlled by the support layers, which restrict the hydration of the core and determine the surface area of hydrophilic core available for drug release (**Figure 6-11**) [31]. Dilacor XR® capsules are designed to release the entire dose of drug over 24 hours and are available in 120-, 180-, and 240-mg strengths.

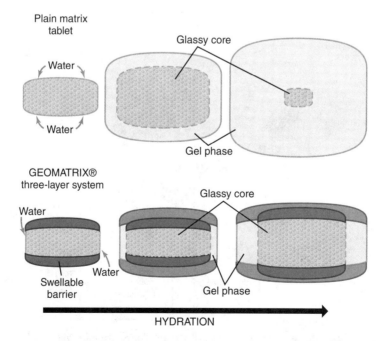

FIGURE 6-10 A schematic depicting the swelling behavior of a plain hydrophilic matrix tablet and Geomatrix™ trilayered tablet upon hydration. The plain matrix tablet swells in all directions, whereas the swelling of Geomatrix™ tablet is restricted by the support layers.

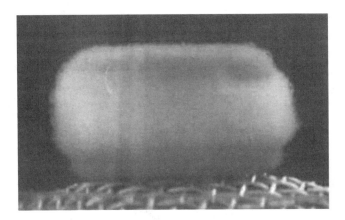

FIGURE 6-11 Photograph taken after 2 hours of dissolution of a Geomatrix™ tablet with a hydroxypropylmethylcellulose swellable barrier. (Reproduced from Conte U, Maggi L, Colombo P, La Manna A. Multi-layered hydrophilic matrices as constant release devices [GeomatrixTM Systems]. *Journal of Controlled Release.* 1993;26[1]:39–47, with permission from Elsevier.)

Glumetza® is a swelling-based gastroretentive formulation of metformin hydrochloride for the treatment of type 2 diabetes. The drug is embedded in a hydrophilic polymeric matrix that swells to 150% of its original size 15 minutes after oral administration. The swollen tablet is retained in the stomach for 8 to 9 hours due to its increased size where the entire dose of drug diffuses out of the system. The tablet has to be administered with food to maximize gastric retention and drug bioavailability. Glumetza® is marketed in 500- and 1000-mg strengths [34–36].

OSMOSIS-CONTROLLED SYSTEMS

Osmosis can be defined as the diffusion of solvent molecules from a region of low-solute concentration to a region of high-solute concentration that are separated by a semipermeable membrane (a membrane that allows solvent molecules to pass but not the solute molecules). Osmosis is similar to diffusion where solute molecules move from a region of high concentration to a region of low concentration. The difference is that osmosis involves the movement of the solvent (e.g., water) across a semipermeable membrane between the two regions and not the solute molecules. As such, the only way to achieve equilibrium is for the solvent molecules to move from one region to the other. This process can be used in drug delivery systems to create an osmotic pump, which can push the drug out of the dosage form independent of the drug concentration and physiological conditions. In such delivery systems, osmotic pressure between the dosage form and the surrounding environment is the rate-determining phenomenon that can be controlled by using different types of semipermeable membranes and pharmaceutical excipients to control the osmotic pressure. Osmosis-driven delivery systems are very versatile and can be easily configured to achieve different drug release rates depending on the requirements. Osmotic drug delivery devices are currently available as orally administered tablets and implantable devices. These devices use different types of osmotic pumps, described below.

Oral Osmotic Pump

Oral osmotic pumps have been developed to control the drug release in gastrointestinal tract independent of the physiological factors. Many types of oral osmotic pumps are reported in the literature and are available commercially. They can be broadly classified into single- and multi-compartment pumps [37].

Single-Compartment Pump

Also known as an elementary osmotic pump, the single-compartment pump is the simplest form of osmotic system available in the market. This system, first developed by Alza Corporation in the 1970s as OROS® (Osmotic Release Oral Systems), consists of a solid drug core surrounded by a rigid semipermeable membrane that acts as the osmotic pump [37, 38]. A small orifice is laser drilled into the membrane to provide a channel for drug release. When the tablet is orally administered, water from the gastric fluid enters through the semipermeable membrane and dissolves the drug. The dissolved drug is then pushed out of the orifice because of the increase in pressure caused by the diffused water (**Figure 6-12**). Drug is released at a constant rate as long as the concentration of drug in the core remains saturated. The rate of release is controlled by the osmotic pressure, which depends on the drug solubility in water and the semipermeable membrane used. Although this device has the advantage of having pH independent release, its usage is limited to drugs that are highly soluble in water. Other water-soluble excipients can also be incorporated into the core to increase the osmotic pressure. Variations of this type of pump include controlled porosity pump, osmotic bursting pump, and enteric-coated elementary osmotic pump [37].

Multiple-Compartment Pump

Multiple-compartment pumps are multilayered tablets that contain separate compartments for the drug and osmotic excipients. The simplest form of multiple compartment pump is the push-pull osmotic pump developed in the 1980s. This system consists of two layers: one layer that contains the drug and the other layer known as the push compartment that contains osmotic agents and a swellable polymer. Both layers are covered by a semipermeable membrane with a laser-drilled orifice near the drug compartment to control the water influx. Upon exposure to the gastrointestinal tract, water from the gastric fluid enters both layers at the same time. Water influx into the system causes the

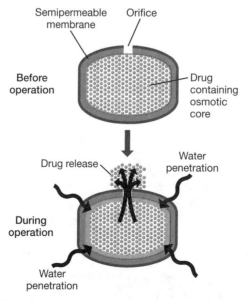

FIGURE 6-12 Schematic depicting the drug release mechanism of an elementary osmotic pump.

polymer in the push compartment to swell and push dissolved drug out of the drug compartment (**Figure 6-13**). In these systems, the drug release rate is independent of drug solubility and the pH of the gastric media. These systems can also be used to deliver drugs that do not have high solubility in water and are not compatible with commonly used osmotic excipients. Other multiple-compartment pumps include sandwiched osmotic tablets and longitudinally compressed tablets [37].

Implantable Osmotic Pump

Implantable osmotic pump drug delivery systems were developed to provide long-term treatment (up to 12 months) for chronic conditions. Although the first implantable osmotic pump was developed in 1955 by Rose and Nelson, it was used only for research in animal models until 2000 when the Duros® system (developed by Alza Corporation) was approved for human use. The implant consists of a 44-mm titanium alloy cylinder with a rate-controlling polyurethane semipermeable membrane at one end and a diffusion moderator with an orifice at the other end. Inside the cylinder the osmotic engine compartment and drug reservoir are separated by a piston (**Figure 6-14**). When the system is subcutaneously implanted, water in surrounding tissue diffuses through the semipermeable membrane into the osmotic engine compartment, which contains sodium chloride. The water influx expands the engine compartment and extends

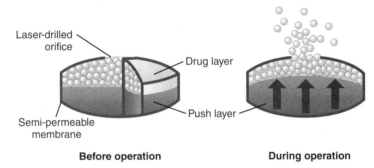

FIGURE 6-13 Schematic depicting the drug release mechanism of a push–pull system.

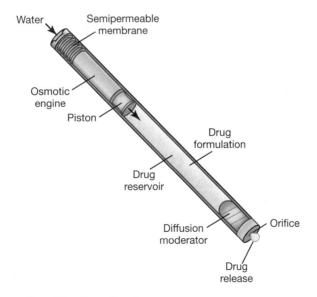

FIGURE 6-14 Cross-section of the Duros® system.

pressure on the piston, resulting in its movement. The movement of the piston pushes dissolved drug inside the reservoir out of the system through the orifice [41]. The rate of drug release is equal to the rate of water influx into the engine, which is controlled by the semipermeable membrane and sodium chloride concentration in the engine. The engine contains excess NaCl so the osmotic pressure and subsequent drug release rate remain constant. The system is designed so that excess undissolved NaCl is present even after the entire drug is released [42]. The semipermeable membrane and the NaCl content in the engine compartment can be modified to achieve different release rates.

The Duros® system achieves precise control over the release rate independent of the environment in which it operates. Given that the drug release rate is relatively slow, it can be used to deliver both small- and large-molecular drugs in both aqueous and non-aqueous vehicles [41]. The device can also be modified for site-specific drug delivery by attaching a catheter to the orifice to direct the flow of drug to the target tissue.

Examples of Osmosis-Controlled Systems in the Clinic

Fortamet® is a once-daily extended-release formulation of metformin hydrochloride for the treatment of hyperglycemia related to type 2 diabetes. It uses the patented single-composition osmotic technology, or SCOT™, to control the rate of drug release. It is an elementary osmotic pump consisting of an osmotically active core containing a mixture of the drug and small quantities of excipients. It is surrounded by a semipermeable membrane with two laser-drilled holes on either side of the tablet for drug release. The rate of drug release is zero-order as long as there is undissolved drug, after which it follows first-order kinetics. The membrane remains intact during the gastrointestinal transit, after which it is excreted in the feces [43].

Glucotrol XL is an oral extended-release formulation of glipizide for the treatment of hyperglycemia related to type 2 diabetes. It uses the Oros™ push–pull technology developed by Alza Corporation to control the rate of drug release. It consists of a push layer with high-molecular-weight polyethylene oxide as the swelling polymer and sodium chloride as the osmogen. The semipermeable membrane is a mixture of water-insoluble ethylcellulose and water-soluble polyethyleneglycol. The presence of polyethyleneglycol increases the membrane porosity and subsequent water permeability and release rate of the drug. The rate of drug release remains constant as long as there is an osmotic gradient. Water-insoluble components of the formulation pass through the gastrointestinal tract and are excreted in feces. Glucotrol XL® is marketed as a once-daily oral tablet designed to deliver 2.5, 5, or 10 mg of glipizide [44].

Viadur® is a Duros™-based osmotic implant designed to deliver leuprolide acetate for 12 months and is used in the palliative treatment of advanced prostate cancer. The implant is composed of a polyurethane rate-controlling membrane, an elastomeric piston, a polyethylene diffusion moderator, and an osmotic engine that contains sodium chloride, sodium carboxymethyl cellulose, povidone, magnesium stearate, and sterile water for injection. Viadur® contains 72 mg of leuprolide acetate dissolved in 104 mg of dimethyl sulfoxide that is released at the rate of 120 μg/day. Viadur® is surgically implanted under the skin in the inner region of the upper arm [45].

SUMMARY

Controlled drug delivery is any approach that increases the duration of a drug's therapeutic effect by controlling the rate that the dose of drug is administered to the patient. The extravascular administration of dosage forms that release the dose of drug at a constant rate is the most common form of controlled drug delivery in the clinic. This offers one or more potential advantages, including an increase in the duration of the therapeutic effect for a given dose of drug and a decrease in drug toxicity, drug dose, and dosing frequency.

REVIEW QUESTIONS

1. What is the rate-limiting step for drug absorption in controlled drug delivery systems?
2. Explain the mechanism of drug release from monolithic systems.
3. What are the major factors that govern the drug release from reservoir systems?
4. What is an implantable osmotic pump? Briefly explain the release mechanism in osmosis-controlled systems with examples.
5. Briefly explain what happens during the lag phase of release in a bulk-eroding system.
6. Why is surface erosion tough to achieve in erosion-controlled systems?

REFERENCES

1. Cipolle RJ, Strand L, Morley P. *Pharmaceutical Care Practice: The Patient-Centered Approach to Medication Management,* 3rd ed. McGraw-Hill Medical; 2012.
2. Shargel L,Wu-Pong S, Yu A. *Applied Biopharmaceutics and Phamacokinetics*, 6th ed. New York: McGraw-Hill; 2012.
3. DiPiro JT, Spruill WJ, Wade WE, Blouin RA, Pruemer JM. *Concepts in Clinical Pharmacokinetics,* 4th ed. American Society of Health-System Pharmacists; 2005.
4. Siepmann J, Siepmann F. The modified drug delivery landscape: academic viewpoint. In: Rathbone MJ, Hadgraft J, Roberts MS, Lane ME, eds. *Modified-Release Drug Delivery Technology,* vol. 2. New York: Informa Health Care; 2008. pp. 17–34.
5. Heller J. Use of polymers in controlled release of active agents. In: Robinson JR, Lee VH, eds. *Controlled Drug Delivery: Fundamentals and Applications.* New York: Marcel Dekker; 1987.
6. Nitro-Dur prescribing information. Available at: http://www.merck.com/product/usa/pi_circulars/n/nitro-dur/nitrodur_pi.pdf. Accessed January 21, 2013.
7. Hadgraft J. Pharmaceutical aspects of transdermal nitroglycerin. *Int J Pharm.* 1996;135(1–2):1–11.
8. Gale R, Hunt J, Prevo ME. Transdermal drug delivery, passive. In: Mathiowitz E, ed. *Encyclopedia of Controlled Drug Delivery*, vol. 2. New York: John Wiley & Sons; 1999.
9. Exelon patch prescribing information. Available at: http://www.accessdata.fda.gov/drugsatfda_docs/label/2012/022083s016lbl.pdf. Accessed January 21, 2013.
10. Park K. *Controlled Drug Delivery Challenges and Strategies.* Washington, DC: American Chemical Society; 1997.
11. Procan Sr (procainamide) drug information. Available at: http://www.rxlist.com/procan-sr-drug.htm. Accessed January, 16, 2013.
12. Retisert prescribing information. Available at: http://www.bausch.com/en/ECP/Our-Products/Rx-Pharmaceuticals/Rx-Pharmaceuticals-ECP/~/media/Files/Downloads/ECP/pharma/retisert-prescribing-information.ashx. Accessed January 21, 2013.
13. Nicholson BP, Singh RP, Sears JE, Lowder CY, Kaiser PK. Evaluation of fluocinolone acetonide sustained release implant (Retisert) dissociation during implant removal and exchange surgery. *Am J Ophthalmol.* 2012;154(6):969–973.
14. Mirena prescribing information. Available at: http://labeling.bayerhealthcare.com/html/products/pi/Mirena_PI.pdf. Accessed January 21, 2013.
15. Duragesic prescribing information. Available at: http://www.duragesic.com/sites/default/files/pdf/duragesic_0.pdf. Accessed January 21, 2013.
16. Gale RM, Lee ES, Taskovich LT, Yum SI, Inventors; Alza Corporation, assignee. Transdermal administration of fentanyl and device therefor. U.S. patent 458858005/13/1986.
17. Alexander A, Dwivedi S, Ajazuddin, et al. Approaches for breaking the barriers of drug permeation through transdermal drug delivery. *J Control Release.* 2012;164(1):26–40.

18. Instructions for use Cypher™ sirolimus-eluting coronary stent on Raptor™ over-the-wire delivery system. Available at: http://www.accessdata.fda.gov/cdrh_docs/pdf2/P020026c.pdf. Accessed January 21, 2013.

19. Drug-eluting stent design. Available at: http://www.news-medical.net/health/Drug-Eluting-Stent-Design.aspx. Accessed January 21, 2013.

20. Mishra S, Waksman R. Procedural results and clinical outcomes after full metal jacket drug-eluting stent implantation in single coronary lesions. *Cardiovasc Revasc Med.* 2006;7(2):82.

21. Catapres-TTS prescribing information. Available at: http://www.accessdata.fda.gov/drugsatfda_docs/label/2012/018891s028lbl.pdf. Accessed January 21, 2013.

22. Fredenberg S, Wahlgren M, Reslow M, Axelsson A. The mechanisms of drug release in poly(lactic-co-glycolic acid)-based drug delivery systems—a review. *Int J Pharm.* 2011;415(1–2):34–52.

23. Tamada JA, Langer R. Erosion kinetics of hydrolytically degradable polymers. *Proc Natl Acad Sci USA.* 1993;90(2):552–556.

24. von Burkersroda F, Schedl L, Gopferich A. Why degradable polymers undergo surface erosion or bulk erosion. *Biomaterials.* 2002;23(21):4221–4231.

25. Lupron Depot® label information. Available at: http://www.accessdata.fda.gov/drugsatfda_docs/label/2012/019732s038lbl.pdf. Accessed January 21, 2013.

26. Gliadel® wafer label information. Available at: http://www.accessdata.fda.gov/drugsatfda_docs/label/2003/020637s016lbl.pdf. Accessed January 21, 2013.

27. Zoladex label information. Available at: http://www.accessdata.fda.gov/drugsatfda_docs/label/2011/019726s054lbl.pdf. Accessed January 21, 2013.

28. Colombo P, Bettini R, Santi P, Peppas NA. Swellable matrices for controlled drug delivery: gel-layer behaviour, mechanisms and optimal performance. *Pharm Sci Technol Today.* 2000;3(6):198–204.

29. Colombo P. Swelling-controlled release in hydrogel matrices for oral route. *Adv Drug Deliv Rev.* 1993;11(1–2):37–57.

30. Dilacor XR prescribing information. Available at: http://www.accessdata.fda.gov/drugsatfda_docs/label/2011/020092s017lbl.pdf. Accessed January 21, 2013.

31. Wilding IR, Davis SS, Sparrow RA, Ziemniak JA, Heald DL. Pharmacoscintigraphic evaluation of a modified release (Geomatrix®) diltiazem formulation. *J Control Release.* 1995;33(1):89–97.

32. Conte U, Maggi L. A flexible technology for the linear, pulsatile and delayed release of drugs, allowing for easy accommodation of difficult in vitro targets. *J Control Release.* 2000;64(1–3):263–268.

33. Conte U, Maggi L, Colombo P, La Manna A. Multi-layered hydrophilic matrices as constant release devices (GeomatrixTM Systems). *J Control Release.* 1993;26(1):39–47.

34. Glumetza prescribing information. Available at: http://www.glumetzaxr.com/assets/pdfs/current_PI_PW2.pdf. Accessed January 21, 2013.

35. Gusler GM HS, Connor AL, Wilding IR, Berner B. Pharmacoscintigraphic evaluation of metformin ER in healthy volunteers. Paper presented at AAPS annual meeting, Salt Lake City, Utah, October 26–30, 2003.

36. Lalloo AK, McConnell EL, Jin L, Elkes R, Seiler C, Wu Y. Decoupling the role of image size and calorie intake on gastric retention of swelling-based gastric retentive formulations: pre-screening in the dog model. *Int J Pharm.* 2012;431(1–2):90–100.

37. Gupta BP, Thakur N, Jain NP, Banweer J, Jain S. Osmotically controlled drug delivery system with associated drugs. *J Pharm Pharmac Sci.* 2010;13(4):571–588.

38. Verma RK, Krishna DM, Garg S. Formulation aspects in the development of osmotically controlled oral drug delivery systems. *J Control Release.* 2002;79(1–3):7–27.

39. Shokri J, Ahmadi P, Rashidi P, Shahsavari M, Rajabi-Siahboomi A, Nokhodchi A. Swellable elementary osmotic pump (SEOP): an effective device for delivery of poorly water-soluble drugs. *Eur J Pharm Biopharm.* 2008;68(2):289–297.

40. Malaterre V, Ogorka J, Loggia N, Gurny R. Approach to design push-pull osmotic pumps. *Int J Pharm.* 2009;376(1–2):56–62.

41. Wright JC, Culwell J. Long-term controlled delivery of therapeutic agents by the osmotically driven Duros implant. In: Rathbone MJ, Hadgraft J, Roberts MS, Lane ME, eds. *Modified-Release Drug Delivery Technology,* vol. 2. New York: Informa Health Care; 2008:143–149.

42. Wright JC, Tao Leonard S, Stevenson CL, et al. An in vivo/in vitro comparison with a leuprolide osmotic implant for the treatment of prostate cancer. *J Control Release.* 2001;75(1–2):1–10.

43. Fortamet extended-release tablets prescribing information. Available at: http://www.fortamet.com/pdf/Fortamet_PI.pdf. Accessed January 21, 2013.

44. Glipizide extended release tablets prescribing information. Available at: http://www.pfizer.com/files/products/uspi_glipizide.pdf. Accessed January 21, 2013.

45. Viadur® (leuprolide acetate implant) prescribing information. Available at: http://www.accessdata.fda.gov/drugsatfda_docs/label/2011/021088s025lbl.pdf. Accessed January 21, 2013.

POLYMERS IN DRUG DELIVERY

DAVID MASTROPIETRO, SRINATH MUPPALANENI,
YOUNG KWON, KINAM PARK, AND HOSSEIN OMIDIAN

CHAPTER OBJECTIVES

Upon completing this chapter, the reader should be able to

▶ Discuss the pharmaceutical applications of polymers in various dosage forms.

▶ Be familiar with common pharmaceutical polymer classes and identify their common applications in pharmacy and pharmaceutical dosage forms.

▶ Understand how properties of polymers can change based on composition, molecular weight, and arrangement.

▶ Examine how different polymer characteristics can be used to custom-design novel delivery systems.

▶ Understand the importance of safety and quality of polymers used in pharmaceutical medications.

▶ Present the utility of polymers to optimize drug formulation development by using examples of approved drug products.

CHAPTER OUTLINE

INTRODUCTION

Almost all dosage forms (e.g., tablets, capsules, suppositories, liquids, etc.) are made by mixing pure drug with other inactive components, called excipients. These inactive ingredients are often used to make the product easier to manufacture and to provide stability throughout its shelf life. In addition, excipients are used to make medicinal products more acceptable to patients by masking the taste of drugs, decreasing side effects, or requiring less frequent dosing by controlling drug release over time. A large majority of pharmaceutical excipients are natural or synthetic polymers. Those polymers that occur in nature from plant and animal sources, such as cellulose, pectin, and chitosan, are considered natural, whereas synthetic polymers, such as polyvinylpyrrolidone and poly(vinyl alcohol), are commercially made.

Historically, polymers have been used in the pharmaceutical industry to solve issues related to drug delivery and manufacturing. By using polymers with varying solubility, swellabililty, and other functional properties, many applications for their use have been found. For example, drugs that are unstable in the low pH of the stomach or that are irritating to the gastric mucosa have used polymers to delay drug release until the intestines are reached. Suspensions have used water-soluble polymers for viscosity modification to thicken the aqueous phase and to allow drug particles to remain suspended for accurate dosing. Polymers that are insoluble in saliva have been used to mask the unpleasant taste of certain drugs. Gel-forming polymers have been used orally to extend the release of drugs in solid dosage forms and topically in the form of nongreasy and cosmetically appealing preparations. In tablet manufacturing alone, polymers have been used as diluents, binders, lubricants, film coatings, antiadherents, and disintegrants in a variety of formulations.

Perhaps one of the largest areas in pharmaceutics using polymers is controlled drug delivery applications. With the use of polymers, drug release can be adjusted to provide a constant or varying type of drug release over a prolonged period of time. Because oral drug delivery systems (e.g., tablets, capsules, and liquids) are the most common type of dosage form, polymers are extensively used in these formulations. Oral medications are also the type most practically encountered in the clinical setting. Therefore, we have chosen to emphasize polymer examples in the first section that are relevant to oral delivery systems and to medications that may be commonly encountered in clinical practice. Because the use of polymers throughout all aspects of pharmacy is extensive, however, this chapter also highlights other uses and familiarizes the reader with important properties and roles that polymers play as novel drug delivery platforms.

POLYMER BASICS

Polymers [1] are large, high-molecular-weight substances composed of a large number of repeating units. These macromolecules are synthesized as smaller repeating units (or monomers) that become attached covalently into a chain-like structure. As the number of repeating units increases, so does the molecular weight of the polymer, which alters its associated physical and chemical properties. When a polymer is composed of only a single repeated monomer unit, it can best be described as a homopolymer. If the material is a polymer chain containing two different monomer units, it is known as a copolymer. The formation of copolymers is useful when each monomer has a desirable property that, when combined, form a custom polymer having exactly the right properties for a job. Although more than two different monomers or polymers can be attached in a polymer structure, pharmaceutical polymers are most often homopolymers, copolymers, and two-polymer blends. A polymer blend is formed by physically mixing two or more differing polymers to form a material with altered properties. **Figure 7-1** shows these different polymer compositions.

As implied above, the final property of a polymer largely depends on the monomer(s) making up the polymer and also on how the chains bond and interact with one another. For copolymers, the arrangement of the monomer units in the polymer chain is also important. At the micromolecular level, monomers A and B can be attached to one another in the form of ABAB (alternate copolymer), ABBA (random copolymer), AABB (block copolymer), or B grafted onto a backbone AAAA structure (graft copolymer). On the other hand, from a macromolecular perspective, a polymer chain can be seen as linear, branched, or cross-linked. In linear polymers, the monomers are joined together end-to-end, making single chains that are flexible and can easily interact with each other. Branched polymers have side-branch chains that extend out from the central structure and reduce the ability of the polymer chains to pack together. In cross-linked polymers, adjacent chains are bonded to one another at various locations and in all directions along their length, forming a three-dimensional network. Cross-linking typically forms rigid polymers and makes hydrophilic polymers swell instead of dissolve when placed in aqueous solutions. All these factors make it possible for the same polymer to have different properties by creating it in different forms, as shown in **Figure 7–2**. By using different monomers, it also makes it possible to create tailor-made polymers having a desired property. The properties of these customized macromolecules can be further altered by producing polymers of different molecular weight. For example, the viscosity of an aqueous solution of methylcellulose (2%) having a molecular weight of 10,000 can be increased 20-fold if methylcellulose with a molecular weight of 26,000 is used [2].

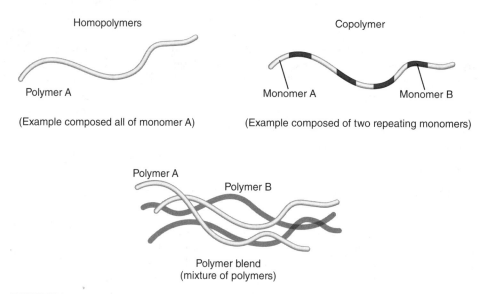

FIGURE 7-1 Various polymer systems: homopolymers, copolymers, and polymer blends.

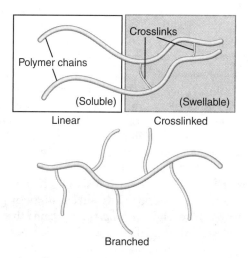

FIGURE 7-2 Polymer topology: linear, branched, and cross-linked structures.

QUALITY AND SAFETY ISSUES

During drug development, emphasis is usually placed on the safety and efficacy of the active drug component and less on inactive ingredients, which are assumed to be safe and inert. More recently, the safety of excipients in drug product is gaining more attention, particularly in children and pediatric populations [3]. For pharmaceutical applications, the quality and safety of polymers must be demonstrated to regulatory bodies before initial approval. It must be shown that polymers used as excipients will not cause harm or adverse effects from short-, intermediate-, or long-term use [4]. Although a polymer may be approved in one product, its use in another product at a different concentration or different route of administration requires new safety data.

When taken orally, most pharmaceutical polymers are not degraded or metabolized in the gastrointestinal (GI) tract or systemically absorbed. Often, they are of such high molecular weight that absorption is considered insignificant to have any pronounced physiological action. For this reason, they are generally considered nontoxic and safe for oral consumption and topical routes of administration. Although rare, patients can experience severe allergic reactions to polymers, particularly when given parenterally. For example, serious anaphylactic reactions have been reported in patients receiving intra-articular corticosteroid injections that were later found to be caused solely by the suspending agent (carboxymethylcellulose sodium) used in the formulation [5, 6].

Biocompatibility and biodegradability are also important safety aspects to consider when using pharmaceutical polymers to deliver drugs to the site of action. Biocompatibility is important when a polymer surface interacts with a biological environment [7]. Biocompatibility can refer to materials that do not cause injury, damage, or adversely affects biological function when exposed to the tissues of a biological system. Biocompatibility is important for polymers that are intended to remain in the body for extend periods and should, therefore, elicit minimal to no immune response. Biodegradable polymers break down from their original structure in biological environments. For drug delivery, biodegradable polymers release drugs as they become degraded in biological fluids to nontoxic byproducts. They are particularly advantageous when used as implants because the need for surgical removal of a nonbiodegradable implant is eliminated. Biodegradation of polymers generally occurs through hydrolysis reactions that shorten the polymer chain length as water enters the bulk polymer structure [8]. Additionally, some polymers degrade by enzymes of microorganisms through hydrolytic or oxidative degradation [9].

PHARMACEUTICAL POLYMERS

Many different types of polymers are used in pharmacy and in pharmaceutical formulations. They make up the plastic bottles used to store various medications, adhesives used to label medications, as bags and tubing for intravenous administration, and as excipients in almost all dosage forms. There is no uniform classification system for this vast array of polymeric materials. However, they can be categorized in different ways depending on what polymer properties and characteristics are most important to the field of interest. Pharmaceutical polymers are often categorized based on their origin, chemical structure, water solubility, pharmaceutical application, or biodegradability. We have listed below some important pharmaceutical polymers and classified them as cellulose derivatives, hydrocolloids, and synthetically derived.

CELLULOSE DERIVATIVES

Cellulose is an abundant natural resource from plants that is composed of glucose monomers attached together to form long and tightly packed chains. Despite being hydrophilic, cellulose is water insoluble due to extensive intra- and intermolecular hydrogen bonding. Over time, semisynthetic derivatives of cellulose were made to enhance solubility in both organic and aqueous liquids. Chemical modification of cellulose involves replacing some or all of the hydroxyl (–OH) groups found in each glucose residue of the cellulose chain. The degree of substitution represents the amount of substituent groups replacing hydroxyl groups and, therefore, affects the final product properties. Methyl substitutions on the cellulose structure produces methylcellulose, a water-soluble cellulose derivative. Further substitution with hydroxypropyl groups produces hydroxypropyl methylcellulose, a mixture of methyl and hydroxypropyl substitutions. Examples of these derivatives and other cellulose ethers used in a broad range of pharmaceutical applications can be seen in **Figure 7-3**. Other substitution modifications can be made to the cellulose structure (i.e., esterification) including cross-linking between cellulose chains. Cellulose derivatives have become a very large and important class of polymers to the pharmaceutical industry [10]. Cellulose and its derivatives have been used to modify the viscosity of liquid preparations and as suspending agents to help stabilize suspensions. In solid dosage forms, cellulose derivatives are used as fillers, bulking agents, binders, disintegrants, glidants, and as a component in matrix tablets [11].

Methylcellulose

Methylcellulose is used as a binder and film coating for tablet formulations and as a thickener, emulsifier, and stabilizer in liquid and semisolid dosage forms. It is found commercially in such products as Menest® and Premphase® oral tablets, Carafate® and Gantrisin® oral suspensions, Lac-Hydrin® topical lotion, and Phisohex® topical emulsion.

To solubilize methylcellulose, it should be dispersed in cold water where it will hydrate and produce a clear viscous material with pseudo-plastic flow properties. Although soluble in glacial acetic acid, it is insoluble or practically insoluble in ethanol, saturated salt solutions, glycols, and hot water. Because it is more soluble in cold water

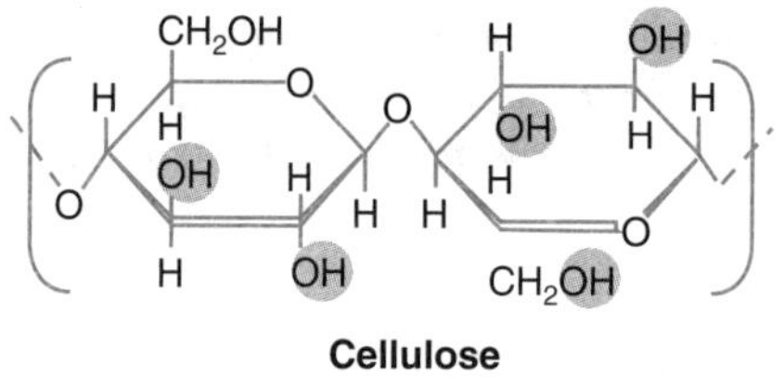

Cellulose

Possible substitution sites on each glucose residue are highlighted

Methyl cellulose	Hydroxypropyl methylcellulose	Carboxymethylcellulose
–CH$_3$	–CH$_3$	–CH$_2$COOH
	–CH$_2$CH(CH$_3$)OH	

Ethyl cellulose	Hydroxypropyl cellulose	Hydroxyethyl cellulose
–CH$_2$CH$_3$	–CH$_2$CH(CH$_3$)OH	–CH$_2$CH$_2$OH

FIGURE 7-3 Pharmaceutically available cellulosics or cellulose derivatives.

Sol-gel transition temperature

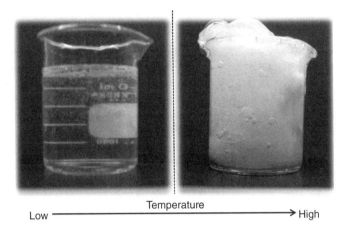

Low ——————— Temperature ——————→ High

FIGURE 7-4 Sol–gel transition in reverse thermosensitive hydrogels (5 wt% methyl cellulose solution aq).

than hot water, it displays different properties at low and high temperatures and is referred to as a thermogelling polymer. This unique feature of methylcellulose can be shown when an aqueous solution is seen as a free-flowing liquid at low temperature but becomes a semisolid gel as the temperature increases and then returns to a solution upon cooling. Figure 7-4 shows this transition from a liquid solution to a gel. Methylcellulose has applications in pharmaceutical dosage forms as a thickener, binder, film-former, and an emulsifier and stabilizer in liquid and semisolid preparations [10]. Because it is nonionic, its viscosity is stable over the large pH range of 3 to 11. For example, sucralfate suspension, useful for the treatment of duodenal ulcers, uses methylcellulose (0.25%) as a suspending agent [12]. Methylcellulose helps to form a more stable and homogeneous suspension of sucralfate compared with that formed with deionized water only [13]. Suspending agents such as methylcellulose increase viscosity of the solution and may help decrease interparticle attraction by forming a film around the insoluble suspended particles. These properties help prevent rapid sedimentation of the drug particles and prevent caking and aggregation of settled particles upon standing. However, the thixotropic nature of methylcellulose solutions allows the viscosity of the suspension to be reduced upon agitation (shaking the bottle) so a patient can easily pour the proper dose from the dispensed container.

Therapeutically, methylcellulose itself is used orally as a bulk-forming laxative. It can absorb and swell in intestinal fluid to form an emollient gel in the bowels. This increases stool weight, stimulates peristalsis, and helps facilitate the passage of intestinal contents. Although marketed as a laxative, the water absorptive properties of methylcellulose can also be used to manage diarrhea and help change the consistency of the stools. It is available commercially as a powder that is mixed in cold water or juice before administration. Because methylcellulose is not soluble in hot water, patients must be instructed that hot beverages should not be used to mix the product because it will not properly dissolve and may result in improper dosing. Manufacturers also suggest that unlike other soluble fibers that ferment in the large intestine, methylcellulose does not breakdown and is, therefore, associated with less discomfort from gas and bloating [14].

Hydroxypropyl Methylcellulose

Often referred to as hypromellose, hydroxypropyl methylcellulose is a hydrophilic polymer found in a large array of pharmaceutical application. It is commonly used as a binder, film-coating agent, suspending agent, and emulsifier. It can also slow drug release when included in solid oral dosage forms. Additionally, capsule shells made out of hydroxypropyl methylcellulose have been developed as an alternative to animal-derived gelatin forms. Hydroxypropyl methylcellulose is found in many ophthalmic preparations and is used as an artificial tears solution for patients with reduced tear production to relieve ocular dryness and irritation. It is used in other ophthalmic medications, such as Maxitrol® and Omnipred® suspensions, and other products, such as Striant® mucoadhesive buccal system, Astelin® nasal spray, Suboxone® sublingual films, and Hyzaar® or Lipitor® oral tablets.

Carboxymethyl Cellulose

Carboxymethyl cellulose is formed by carboxymethylating cellulose and is typically found as a sodium or calcium salt. These forms are used as diluents, binders, coatings, and suspending agents. They also swell in aqueous solutions and can, therefore, be used as disintegrants in tablet formulations. The sodium salt of carboxymethyl cellulose is found as an excipient in products such as Vibramycin® and Dilantin® oral suspensions, Kenalog-10® and Lupron Depot® injectable suspensions, Viadur® implant, and Aphthasol® oral paste. The calcium salt is used in prescription products such as Atacand® and Nolvadex® tablets and Omnicef® oral capsules. Therapeutically, carboxymethyl cellulose sodium is used as a long-acting ophthalmic solution for ocular lubrication. For example, the product Refresh Tears® uses 0.5% carboxymethyl cellulose sodium to moisturize dry eyes and a higher 1% concentration (Refresh Liquigel®) that provides extended relief due to a higher viscosity and longer retention on the eye [15]. The cross-linked form of carboxymethylcellulose sodium is found in products such as the Levoxyl® and Relpax® oral tablets, Sustiva® and Onglyza® film-coated tablets, and Abilify Discmelt® orally disintegrating tablets.

Ethyl Cellulose

Ethyl cellulose is a cellulose derivative having ethyl group substitutions attached on the cellulose backbone structure. It is unique in that it is water insoluble and can be used as a barrier for drug release, a viscosity-modifying agent, a binder, a filler, a granulation aid, and a coating material in a wide range of pharmaceutical dosage forms. Incorporating ethyl cellulose into matrix tablets can help control drug release [16, 17]. Because it is hydrophobic and water insoluble, it can be used as a coating to mask the taste of unpleasant drugs in oral dosage forms. Ethyl cellulose can be found in many extended- and controlled-release tablets and capsules such as Wellbutrin XL®, Ultram ER®, Detrol LA®, Effexor XR®, and the extended-release Tussionex® suspension.

Other Common Cellulose Derivatives

Many other cellulose derivatives exist that have applications in a variety of different dosage forms. A very popular type of cellulose is the microcrystalline form, produced by reducing the chain length of cellulose under an acid hydrolysis reaction and leaving the stronger crystalline regions behind. Examples of drug products having microcrystalline cellulose include Nasonex® and Flonase® nasal suspensions, Prevacid® and Pepcid® oral suspensions, Ambien® and Topamax® (oral tablets), and Singulair® chewable tablets.

Hydroxyethyl cellulose is a water-soluble excipient used in Covera HS® and Invega ER® tablets, Duragesic® transdermal patches, and otic suspensions of Ciprodex® and Tobradex®. *Hydroxypropyl cellulose* is a nonionic cellulose derivative that can be used as an active ingredient, for example, in the ophthalmic insert product Lacrisert®. It can also be used to gel alcohol-based drug reservoirs of transdermal patches such as Estraderm® and Testoderm TTS®. The buccal soluble film Onsolis® also uses hydroxypropyl cellulose. *Cellulose acetate* is a very common cellulose derivate used to delay drug release, such as in the products Procardia XL® and Glucotrol XL® tablets. *Cellulose acetate phthalate* is a cellulose derivative that is not soluble in the gastric pH. For this reason, it is commonly seen as an enteric coating for drugs, such as on Azulfidine En-tabs® and Dulcolax® tablets.

HYDROCOLLOIDS

Hydrocolloids are high-molecular-weight polysaccharides from natural origins. They are extracts from seaweeds and plants or can be microbial polysaccharides produced by bacteria. Typically, they are used to modify product rheology and are added to a formulation as a thickener, gelling agent, emulsifier, stabilizer, or suspending agent. These polysaccharide gums are generally hydrophilic, where some display excellent thickening properties and others show gelling properties. Because they are derived from natural sources, they are considered nontoxic and biodegradable.

Alginic Acid

Alginic acid and its salts (e.g., sodium or calcium alginate) are collectively called alginates. Alginic acid is a polysaccharide extracted from brown seaweed. It is a copolymer comprised of two sugar acids, mannuronic and guluronic acids. The rheological property of the alginate is determined by the distribution of these two sugars. Alginates richer in guluronic segments form stronger gels, especially in the presence of divalent ions such as calcium. Alginates can thicken gel solutions and act as a film-former and stabilizing agent. Alginic acid can be used as a tablet binder and emulsifying agent and the sodium salt used for thickening and emulsifying purposes. The sodium salt of alginic acid dissolves in water to form a viscous solution. This solution can rapidly transform from a liquid to a gel state when in contact with a divalent cations such as calcium (Ca^{2+}). **Figure 7-5** demonstrates how small beads of sodium alginate rapidly form when the alginate solution is added dropwise into a calcium chloride solution.

Gaviscon® is an over-the-counter medication that takes advantage of alginate to treat heartburn and acid reflux. The product combines alginic acid with a mixture of antacids to neutralize gastric acidity and prevent gastric contents from refluxing into the esophagus by forming a floating viscous barrier, called raft [18]. The alginic acid precipitates in the low pH of the stomach to form a gel that traps carbon dioxide gas released from the antacid component reacting with the gastric acid [19]. The entrapped air causes the gelatinous mass to rise on top of the gastric contents and act as a barrier to the acidic contents refluxing up into the esophagus. Because of its floating mechanism of action, patients should be instructed that it will work best when not taken before meals and that tablets should be chewed and swallowed, not dissolved in the mouth, so the floating barrier is formed all at once in the stomach [20].

Carrageenan

Carrageenan is a natural ingredient obtained from red seaweed. Three types, iota, kappa, and lambda, are of interest for industrial use and differ in their chemical structure, water solubility, and gelling properties. Iota carrageenan is soluble in hot water and forms a

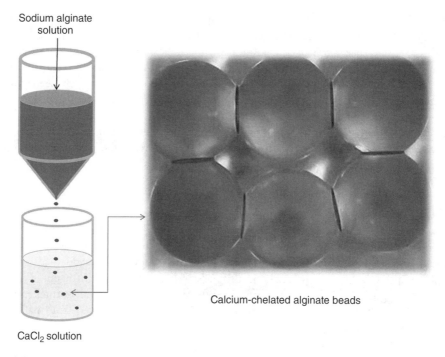

Sodium alginate
solution

Calcium-chelated alginate beads

CaCl$_2$ solution

FIGURE 7-5 Ionotropic gelation of sodium alginate in the presence of calcium ion.

strong gel in the presence of calcium. Kappa carrageenan is also soluble in hot water but gels strongly in the presence of potassium. Lambda carrageenan is soluble in cold water and does not gel, but rather forms highly viscous solutions that can be used in formulations as a thickening agent. Prescription products such as Dexilant® and Pradaxa® use capsule shells that are made from a mixture of hydroxypropyl methylcellulose, potassium chloride, and kappa carrageenan. The addition of carrageenan as the gel network former and potassium as the gelation promoter to solutions of hydroxypropyl methylcellulose allows the capsules to form at room temperature [21, 22]. Carrageenans can also act synergistically with other hydrocolloids, such as kappa carrageenan and locust bean gum. Carrageenans are used as a suspending and viscosity-enhancing agent for liquids and are found in tablets, capsules, and suppositories [23].

Pectin

Pectin is a natural anionic heteropolysaccharide prevalently found in fruit cell walls. It is largely made up of galacturonic acid residues. Pectins can interact with oppositely charged polymers or calcium and other divalent cations to form a cross-linked gel network [24]. Pectins have traditionally been used in pharmaceutical products as a gelling agent, are considered to be nontoxic, and have been used to deliver drugs by the oral, nasal, and topical routes [25]. A fentanyl nasal spray called Lazanda® uses a pectin-based formulation (PecSys) that turns from an aqueous solution into a gel when applied to the mucosal surfaces of the nose. The gel transition provides controlled absorption of fentanyl without the formulation running down the back of the nose and unintentionally swallowed, thus losing a portion of the dose [26]. Pectin is more recently gaining attention for its use in colon-specific drug delivery applications because it is selectively digested by colonic bacteria.

Xanthan Gum

Another high-molecular-weight natural polymer, produced by microbial fermentation, is xanthan gum. It is a heteropolysaccharide that can be used as a thickening agent and as a suspending and emulsifying agent for water-based products. In pharmaceutical applications, xanthan gum is found in barium sulfate suspensions that are given orally as a contrast agent for use in certain diagnostic procedures. Xanthan gum gives the suspension excellent coating abilities in the intestinal tract and allows a smaller dose of barium sulfate to be used [27]. This eliminates the problems associated with using a thick and highly concentrated contrast medium that cannot move along the entire GI tract for proper imaging. Xanthan gum can also be used to make controlled-release tablets. In this capacity, fluid easily penetrates the tablet surface and hydrates the outermost layer, forming a thick gel that impedes rapid drug release from the lower layer. The product Opana ER® (oxymorphone hydrochloride extended release) uses TIMERx® technology consisting of xanthan gum with locust bean gum to create an oral extended-release tablet of oxymorphone [28]. The two gums create a barrier upon swelling, which slows the diffusion of the drug out of the inner core. Xanthan gum can also be found in products that are specially formulated for dysphagic patients and allows them the ability to safely consume liquid beverages [29].

Chitosan

Chitosan is a cationic polymer obtained from the very abundant natural source of chitin. Chitin is isolated from the exoskeleton of crustaceans such as crabs and shrimp and turned into chitosan through a partial deacetylation process. Chitosan can be used in pharmaceutical preparations as a coating agent, tablet binder, gel former, and mucoadhesive polymer to enhance drug permeation and bioavailability. It is a biocompatible and biodegradable polymer that has been studied for use in various drug delivery applications including the oral, buccal, nasal, transdermal, parenteral, vaginal, and rectal routes [30]. Currently, no commercially available product uses chitosan; however, in the future it is expected to play a major role in drug delivery as its use is being evaluated in many new formulations undergoing clinical trials [31].

SYNTHETIC POLYMERS

Synthetic polymers can be found in many aspects of drug delivery and offer some advantages over natural polymers, a significant one being that they can be reproduced in a controlled way to provide consistent polymer properties. This is opposed to natural polymers that may differ in consistency and quality based on variables such as weather and geographical location. Synthetic polymers can be custom made and used to formulate medications that lower the frequency of administration, lessen side effects, hide unpleasant tastes and odors, protect the active ingredient, and bring the active drug directly to the site of action or absorption.

Methacrylic Acid Ester Copolymers

Methacrylic acid ester copolymers are a common type of pharmaceutical excipient used for coating applications (e.g., enteric, protective, taste masking) and as a component to achieve controlled drug release. When used externally, they may also give solid oral dosage forms a smooth and glossy appearance that can facilitate ease of administration. By using monomers with different functional groups, properties such as solubility can be altered to produce polymers for specific applications. For example, a polymer having acidic groups (e.g., carboxylic acid) attached would have pH-dependent solubility and behave differently in the stomach versus the small intestine depending on its ionization state. Alternatively, if monomers having neutral and pH-independent substituent groups were used, the polymer would remain insoluble but still permeable to drug release. These various copolymers are available under the trade name Eudragit® and may be seen listed as different types of methacrylic acid and methacrylate copolymers under inactive ingredient for many prescription drug products. For example, the extended-release drug product Kadian® lists methacrylic acid copolymer as an inactive ingredient in all different products strengths [32]. This copolymer has methacrylic acid as a component giving it pH-dependent solubility. Inside Kadian capsules are small pellets of morphine coated with insoluble ethyl cellulose, soluble polyethylene glycol, and the pH-soluble methacrylic acid copolymer. Once the pellets are released from the capsule shell in the stomach, polyethylene glycol quickly dissolves and forms pores in the pellets that GI fluid can enter into and allow morphine to diffuse out. As the pellets enter the higher pH regions of the intestines, the methacrylic acid copolymer becomes soluble and increases the size and number of pores on the pellet surface, allowing greater amounts of morphine to be released [33]. Although not mentioned in the product labeling, care should be taken when patients are concurrently taking antacids or gastric acid–blocking agents that may increase the pH of the stomach and prematurely release a larger amount of morphine. Other drugs having pH-sensitive polymer coats that may dissolve at a high pH such as enteric coatings are likely to have similar issues with early dissolutions.

Polyvinyl Alcohol

Polyvinyl alcohol is produced from polyvinyl acetate, where the acetate groups are partially hydrolyzed and replaced with hydroxyl groups. The degree to which this hydrolysis occurs creates polyvinyl alcohol polymers that are soluble and insoluble in water. Cross-linked forms of polyvinyl alcohol are insoluble but swellable in water. This hydrophilic polymer has approved uses in transdermal patches; jellies that dry on the skin; immediate-, sustained-, and controlled-release formulations; and in artificial tear drop solutions [34].

Polyvinylpyrrolidone

Polyvinylpyrrolidone is a synthetic neutral homopolymer that comes in many different grades. The soluble grade, commonly referred to as povidone, is widely used in the pharmaceutical industry. Some of its pharmaceutical uses include film former, binder, taste masker, stabilizer, and solubilizer. Perhaps the most well-known use of this polymer is its complexation with iodine to form the disinfectant solution povidone-iodine. This 10% aqueous solution sold under such names as Betadine® can be used as a fast-acting antiseptic for minor cuts and scrapes and for preoperative skin preparations.

Crospovidone is the insoluble cross-linked form of polyvinylpyrrolidone. Due to cross-linking, the polymer swells in aqueous solutions and is used as a superdisintegrant in tablet formulations. It is also an ideal disintegrant for wet granulation in tablet manufacturing because its disintegrating properties are maintained even after being dried. Commercially available crospovidone with a small particle size (~30 μm) is ideally suited for oral disintegrating tablet dosage forms because it has a smooth mouth feel, provides good physical strength, and still provides rapid disintegration [35].

Carbomers

A carbomer is the general name given to any of a specific group of high-molecular-weight cross-linked polymers of acrylic acid known commercially as Carbopol® polymers. These polymers are chemically cross-linked to form copolymers that are not

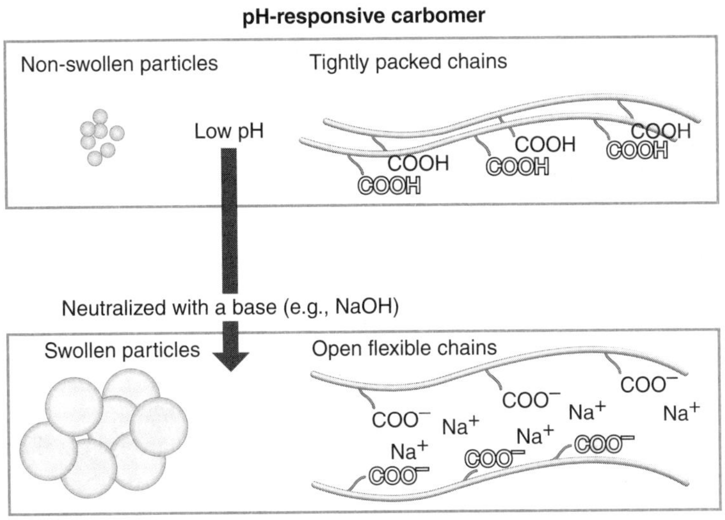

FIGURE 7-6 pH-Dependent swelling of carbomer, a cross-linked poly(acrylic acid).

soluble but swellable in water. They form acidic aqueous solutions that can transform to a more viscous gel state when in alkaline environments where the pH rises to above the pKa. This pH change is achieved by neutralizing the polymer with a basic substance, which creates negative charges along the chain. The internal repulsion forces of this ionization helps to uncoil and open the polymer chains, resulting in a more viscous solution (**Figure 7-6**). Carbopols have applications in suspensions; creams; buccal, rectal, and nasal formulations as a gel matrix; and in tablets as a matrix material or coating material for controlling drug release [36]. Carbomers are also beneficial as emulsifying and suspending agents. Their use is very popular among topical gels formulations. For example, the topical testosterone gel product Androgel® 1.62% contains carbopol 980, which is most likely used in the formulation as the gelling agent because it can form a hydroalcoholic gel with the ethyl alcohol component also found in the product.

Polyethylene Glycol

Polyethylene glycol (PEG) is a synthetic polymer formed by an addition reaction of ethylene oxide and water with a general formula of $H(OCH_2CH_2)_nOH$, where n represents the number of ethylene oxide repeating units [37]. Each PEG is labeled with a number indicating the average molecular weight of the polymer, ranging from 200 to 8000. PEGs having molecular weights below 600 are liquids at room temperature and those above are soft or waxy solids. PEG use in pharmaceutical preparations include its application as an ointment and suppository base, viscosifying agent, lubricant, and solvent in oral, rectal, topical, ophthalmic, and parenteral dosage forms [23]. PEG 3350 is a very popular over-the-counter laxative found in Miralax® and in various prescription bowel-cleaning products for use before colonoscopy. PEG 3350 is soluble but nonabsorbable and creates an osmotic effect that brings water into the bowels, softens the stool, and facilitates a bowel movement.

Poloxamers

Poloxamers (also called Pluronics®) are triblock copolymers based on ethylene oxide and propylene oxide. Different forms that have altered physical properties are commercially made and differ in terms of molecular weight and the proportion of each monomer.

Because of the hydrophilic and hydrophobic character of the blocks, the poloxamers form micelles in an aqueous medium and gels at higher concentrations and temperatures [38]. When the temperature that causes gelation is close to that of body, the poloxamer can be administered as a solution and then gel *in situ* to provide extended drug release. The uses of poloxamers in pharmaceutical products include emulsifier, solubilizing agent, binder, and suspending agent.

Ion Exchange Resins

Ion exchange resins (IERs) are insoluble high-molecular-weight polymers that have been used in the pharmaceutical industry since the late 1950s [39]. The main property that makes them appealing for drug delivery is their ability to reversibly interchange ions in an aqueous environment, such as in the GI tract. The ions exchanged can be simple inorganic ions (e.g., Na^+, Ca^{+2}, Cl^-) or larger organic ions such as an ionized drug. The exchange of ions is made possible by basic or acidic functional groups that line the polymer backbone. These polymer chains are also cross-linked, making them insoluble in water and other aqueous environments. The high molecular weight of these compounds makes them nonabsorbable in the GI tract and, therefore, considered safe for oral consumption with no systemic side effects.

In pharmaceutical applications, the most common IERs are cross-linked polystyrene or cross-linked polymethacrylate polymers. Polystyrenic resins, such as cholestyramine, are made from styrene monomers that are cross-linked with divinyl benzene [40]. Polymethacrylate resins use salts or esters of methacrylic acid as monomers and are commonly cross-linked using divinyl benzene. For example, Amberlite IRP64 is an insoluble porous copolymer derived from methacrylic acid and divinyl benzene [41].

After polymerization, further chemical reactions are used to attach acidic or basic functional groups at repeating positions along the base structure of the resin. These functional groups are attached covalently to the polymer backbone and can impart either a negative or a positive charge that then determines the type of ions they exchange. IER are named based on the charge of the ions they can exchange. The four types of IERs and the commonly attached functional groups are as follows:

1. Strong cation exchange resins having $-SO_3H$ functional groups
2. Weak cation exchange resins having $-COOH$ or $-COOK$ functional groups
3. Strong anion exchange resins having $-NR_3$ functional groups
4. Weak anion exchange resins having $-NR_2$ or $-NRH$ functional groups

where R may be any organic group.

IERs can act as carriers for drug molecules and help increase the physical and chemical stability of the therapeutic agent they hold. The binding of a drug to an exchange resin functional group occurs through weak ionic interactions where the attached drug is often more stable than free drug. For example, nicotine quickly discolors when exposed to air and light, but the drug-resinate form used in nicotine chewing gum and lozenges makes the products much more stable. Once a drug is loaded onto an IER, its release can be triggered by the exchange of a counter-ion. This exchange of drug for counterions can be used to preferentially release a drug from a resin when a specific delivery site is reached in the GI tract where only high counter-ions exist.

Pharmaceutical scientists have found many applications for IERs that go beyond just acting as a drug carrier, such as modifying drug release, masking taste, increasing dissolution, and acting as disintegrants. Nicotine gum used for smoking cessation is again an example of a pharmaceutical product using IERs to modify drug release. When a patient chews on the gum a small number of times, the nicotine that is bound to the sorbitol-based resin is released. The patient then "parks" the gum in the cheek region, and only when another small dose of nicotine is needed does the patient chew the gum again. Another IER example is Tussionex® suspension that uses the Pennkinetic™ system. This suspension system contains small beads of sulfonated styrene-divinyl benzene copolymer complexed with the drugs hydrocodone and chlorpheniramine. The polymer matrix regulates drug release by using PEG to control swelling rate and coating the hydrocodone resinates with ethyl cellulose to act as a rate-limiting permeable coating. Polacrillin potassium is an example of a popular and very effective tablet-disintegrating agent [42]. The product is the salt of methacrylic acid and divinyl benzene and can swell to about 150%, which makes it effective for breaking up a tablet after ingestion. IERs in ocular delivery can be useful for drugs that are irritating to the eye and cause a stinging or burning sensation upon administration. The most notable example for this type of use is a novel suspension of betaxolol called Betoptic S® in which an IER in a polymer structured vehicle resulted in less ocular irritation and dose reduction of one-half compared with the original solution formulation [43].

Although traditionally thought of as an excipient or drug carrier, unloaded ion exchange polymer can be given as a therapeutic agent. The first approved use of an IER in this way was cholestyramine, used to sequester bile acids in the GI tract as a means to lower hypercholesterolemia. Once bound to the resin, the bile acids–resin is eventually removed from the GI tract and excreted in the stools. This forces the liver to draw up cholesterol from the systemic circulation to produce more bile salts, thus lowering blood cholesterol levels. The original powder-mix formulation of the product was not well received by patients due to the large amount of powder needed per dose and side effects such as constipation, abdominal discomfort, and flatulence. New technologies later allowed the development of a high-capacity bile acid-binding resin that could be given in tablet form with less GI side effects [44]. Eventually, a similar therapeutic resin was developed that reduced phosphate levels in patients having end-stage renal disease. This product, Sevelamer® (Renagel®), is a nonabsorbable phosphate-binding polymer that also exhibits some degree of bile acid binding.

The use of sodium polystyrene sulfonate as an IER to treat hyperkalemia was first approved in 1958 under the trade name Kayexalate® [45]. When the kidneys can no longer remove potassium due to kidney failure, removal of excess potassium can be achieved by artificial means in the GI tract. In the colon, the polystyrene sulfonate salt works by exchanging sodium for potassium ions. The potassium bound to the resin cannot be absorbed and helps in lowering systemic potassium levels as the potassium bound resinate travels along the GI tract and is eliminated in the stools.

POLYMERS IN PHARMACEUTICAL DOSAGE FORMS

As described above, pharmaceutical polymers provide unique physiochemical properties that make them ideally suited for incorporation into a variety of different dosage forms. In this section, we highlight some of the major roles polymers have played as a formulation excipient.

POLYMERIC COATINGS

Polymer coatings for solid oral dosage forms serve many different functions:

- Protection of sensitive drugs from light, air, moisture, and gastric fluids
- Masking the tastes and odors of unpleasant drugs
- Providing control over drug release, making it delayed or sustained

- Site-specific drug delivery (e.g., colon targeting)
- Improve product appearance and ease of administration

The type of polymer coating used on the dosage form depends on the service it is intended to perform, some of which are briefly discussed below.

Controlled Release

In general, polymers that are insoluble in GI fluids can be used as coatings to provide sustained release. Ideally, these polymers act as diffusion-controlled barriers to drug release and are not affected by pH. Insoluble polymers that are permeable to water such as ethyl cellulose are popular for this type of application [46]. Additionally, certain methacrylic acid copolymers (Eudragit® RL and Eudragit® RS) that are water insoluble and have pH–independent swelling are used to manufacture prolonged–action dosage forms.

Products that have significantly reduced the number of daily dosages a patient needs to take by using these types of polymers have likely helped to improve patient compliance for many drug regimens. For example, the once-daily product Procardia XL® is composed of a bilayer tablet having an osmotically active drug core of nifedipine that is completely coated with a semipermeable membrane of cellulose acetate, a water-insoluble polymer. Delivery of the drug out of the tablet is controlled by the rate at which solvent crosses the cellulose acetate membrane into the tablet and then carrying the drug out through a laser-formed hole through the coating [47].

pH-Sensitive Coatings

These types of coatings are sensitive to pH and can act as barriers that delay drug release until certain areas of the GI tract are reached. They are useful to protect sensitive drugs from the harsh pH of the stomach, protect the stomach from drugs that cause gastric irritation, and mask the taste and odor of medicinal products. They are also useful to deliver drugs directly to the site of action at the further ends of the GI tract such as the colon.

A dosage form encounters considerable change in pH as it is placed in the mouth and moves along the GI tract. In the mouth, saliva pH typically ranges from 6.0 to 7.4 [48]. The pH then drops to between 1 and 2 in the stomach (to 4 during digestion), and then increases in the small intestine to about 6 and 7 and up to 7 and 8 in the distal ileum [49]. These very different pH ranges must be considered on how they can affect a drugs stability, dissolution, and absorption when orally administered.

Enteric Coatings

Enteric coatings are polymers designed to remain intact in the acidic environment of the stomach and then dissolve after passing into the alkaline environment of the small intestine. Enteric coatings are commonly anionic polymers that contain ionizable carboxylic groups such as methacrylic acid. In the stomach, the methacrylic group is unionized and the coating is hence insoluble, but at higher pHs of the small intestine, the functional groups become ionized and the polymer coating becomes soluble. The enteric coating may be used on an oral product to help minimize drug irritation to the stomach or esophageal lining, prevent drug degradation at low pH, and improve absorption and effectiveness.

Certain medications that affect the stomach mucosa and are not well tolerated when immediately released in the stomach can be enterically coated. For example, bisacodyl is a stimulant laxative that uses an enteric coating (cellulose acetate phthalate) to prevent stomach upset and achieve greater effect by targeting release of the drug to the large intestine.

The stability of various medications are susceptible to the harsh pH of the stomach. For example, Prevacid® (lansoprazole) is susceptible to fast decomposition in the gastric pH [50]. Prevacid is, therefore, formulated as a delayed-release capsule filled with enteric-coated drug granules. The enteric coating is a suspension containing a pH-sensitive methacrylic acid copolymer. Patients must be instructed to never crush or chew enteric-coated medications as undesirable side effects and therapeutic failure may result.

Although not considered a side effect, another use for enteric coating has been to decrease the "fishy burp" or after taste that can occur when taking fish oil supplements [51]. These products are available from a number of manufacturers and typically use either synthetic methacrylic acid copolymers or alginate and cellulose derivatives under the name "food glaze" as enteric-type coatings.

Safe Delivery

At times, products contain drugs that may pose a danger to those that may handle or be exposed to them during dispensing or during administration to others. For example, the product Proscar® contains the antiandrogen drug finasteride that is a potential risk for a male fetus. Therefore, women who are pregnant or may potentially become pregnant should not directly come in contact with the active drug. The manufacturer has, therefore, placed a protective film that entirely coats the tablet to prevent contact during normal handling [52]. Based on the inactive ingredients, the film is likely a mixture of the water-soluble components hydroxypropyl cellulose LF and hydroxypropyl methylcellulose. It is imperative that patients and caregivers be educated that crushed or broken pieces of the tablet are not handled by women of childbearing age.

Site-Specific Delivery

Dosage forms that can travel with a medication through the upper GI tract and delay drug release until the colon is reached are desirable to treat certain diseases of the colon (e.g., Crohn's disease, ulcerative colitis, colon cancer). Site-specific delivery of drugs to the colon can also minimize possible local and systemic side effects that would result from a drug being released and absorbed in the stomach or small intestine. Multiple layers of a pH-sensitive coating is one of the easiest methods to target drug delivery to the colon; this dosage form will not disintegrate in the stomach or small intestine but preferentially in the neutral to alkaline pH at the small and large intestine junction [49]. The drug product Asacol®, used to treat ulcerative colitis, is produced as an enteric-coated delayed-release tablet containing the anti-inflammatory drug mesalamine for colon-targeted drug delivery. Delayed release of mesalamine to the terminal ileum is achieved by using a methacrylic acid copolymer (Eudragit S) that dissolves above pH 7 or greater [53]. Another marketed product, Entocort EC®, indicated for the treatment of Crohn's disease, uses a pH-based system to deliver the corticosteroid budesonide to the ileum and ascending colon. The Entocort EC formulation contains microgranules of sugar surrounded by budesonide in ethyl cellulose and an outer core of a methacrylic acid copolymer (Eudragit L 100–55) that dissolves at a pH of 5.5 or higher [54].

Taste and Odor Masking

Polymer films can be used to mask the unpleasant taste or smell of drugs by forming a sealed barrier that limits contact of the offensive substance with the taste buds. This barrier, however, must not prevent the drug from being properly released once swallowed. A good tasting product is pleasing to the patient and may lead to greater compliance, better therapeutic treatment, and more business for the company [55].

The application of polymer coating to drug products is an easy method to mask taste and odor of various drugs. Cationic polymers that are pH sensitive such as Eudragit E 100 are ideal coating polymers for this purpose. Eudragit E100 is soluble up to pH 5 and, therefore, should remain insoluble as a coating in the oral cavity yet quickly dissolve once in the acidic environment of the stomach.

Orapred ODT® tablets are an example of a drug product that uses a taste masking technique to reduce the unpleasant taste of prednisolone beyond what the natural flavoring and sweetening agents in the product already do. Taste masking is achieved using a coating combination of various cellulose derivatives (e.g., hypromellose) and methacrylate copolymers that can moderate dissolution both independent and dependent of pH, respectively [56].

POLYMERS AS RHEOLOGY MODIFIER

The flow behavior of solutions, suspensions, emulsions, and semisolids can be adjusted and controlled using polymers. Viscosity can influence flow behavior and is, therefore, an important characteristic in pharmaceutical formulations. Viscosity can be viewed as a measure of the resistance of a fluid to flow under an applied force. Polymer molecules can interact with water and form a network that interferes with the flow of molecules to move past each other. In the dry state, polymer chains are coiled and bound up but assume an extended conformation when dissolved or allowed to swell in an aqueous solution, by which the viscosity of the system will show an increase. When the solvent is water, gums are a good excipient for increasing viscosity because they are hydrophilic and have large molecular weights [1]. For example, the antibiotic suspension Omnicef®, which is made by reconstituting a powder, contains a mixture of guar and xanthan gum to enhance viscosity [57]. Synthetic polymers are also useful for increasing viscosity of various pharmaceutical products. The ophthalmic suspension Azopt® uses the highly cross-linked synthetic polymer carbomer 974P as a suspending agent [58]. This bioadhesive carbomer forms highly viscous gels and can increase the bioavailability of ophthalmic preparations.

TRANSDERMAL DELIVERY

A transdermal patch may contain a number of polymers each designed to serve a different purpose that helps deliver the contained medication through the skin surfaces over an extended time. A typical passive transdermal patch is multilayered with polymers starting with the outer backing and ending with the release liner. For reservoir type patches, the drug is sandwiched between the backing layer and a rate-controlling membrane. The drug reservoir may use polymers to gel a drug solution or act as a solid polymer–drug matrix. The adhesive layer is also a polymeric component and may simply act to adhere the patch to the skin, or for drug-in-adhesive systems, the drug can be dispersed in this layer. Examples of polymers used to form matrices for transdermal applications include cross-linked PEG, methacrylic acid copolymers (e.g., Eudragit S-100, Eudragit E-100), ethyl cellulose, polyvinylpyrrolidone, and hydroxypropyl methylcellulose [59].

In transdermal patches where the drug is in a reservoir compartment, rate-controlling polymeric membranes are used. The drug may diffuse either through the membrane or through micropores in the structure to reach the skin. Ethylene vinyl acetate copolymer is a popular rate-controlling membrane in transdermal patches. For example, the nitroglycerin reservoir patch Transderm-Nitro® uses an ethylene vinyl acetate copolymer as the semipermeable membrane to control nitroglycerin release [60]. Pressure-sensitive adhesives such as polyisobutylene and polyacrylates [61], backing films such as polyurethane and polyethylene, and polyester film release liners are other polymers that can be found in transdermal delivery devices [62].

EXTEMPORANEOUS COMPOUNDING

At times, it may be appropriate for a pharmacist to compound a prescription medication using an active drug(s) mixed with other initial components, such as when a drug is not commercially available in the desired strength or dosage form or a patient has allergies and sensitivities to components in the marketed formulations. Pharmaceutical polymers are often used as vehicles for the active drug in compounded formulations.

For example, some ointment bases used to compound semisolid preparations are pharmaceutical polymers, including a water-soluble base made by mixing PEGs and aqueous hydroalcoholic or alcoholic gel bases made from various carbomers [23]. PEG polymers can also be used as a base for making suppositories [63]. Certain mixtures of PEGs can be made that dissolve at temperatures close to that of the body, making them ideal for this route of administration.

Polymers can also be used to compound oral suspensions and emulsions. When a liquid form of a medication is not available, a suspension can be made using crushed tablets of the commercial product. Premade oral suspending vehicles can be used to make uniform and physically stable suspensions this way by using products such as Ora-Plus® (Paddock Laboratories) that contain mixtures of cellulose derivatives, xanthan gum, and carrageenan [64]. Emulsions can also be compounded in the pharmacy using certain emulsifying agents. For example, acacia can be used as an emulsifying agent to make a primary oil-in-water emulsion using a mortar and pestle, although vigorous trituration is needed.

POLYMERS FOR ADVANCED DRUG DELIVERY APPLICATIONS

To maximize drug absorption, many drugs are administered either extravascularly or directly into the bloodstream through intravascular injection. These parenteral routes, however, can be associated with large fluctuations in drug concentrations and the development of toxic side effects. Therefore, frequent injections and close monitoring of adverse effects may be required for an effective treatment. To overcome such shortcomings of conventional drug therapy, polymeric drug delivery systems have been widely studied for decades. The versatility of polymeric materials has allowed novel designs that could potentially meet several criteria for successful drug delivery. When compared with traditional therapy, polymeric delivery systems are designed to achieve increased or equivalent efficacy, reduced side effects and toxicity, and improved patient compliance.

Delivery of therapeutic agents is challenging because many drugs have very short half-lives in the blood and are susceptible to physical or chemical degradation. This is especially the case for macromolecular proteins, peptides, and nucleic acid–based agents, where their delivery is mainly possible using polymeric systems. Although many therapeutic proteins, peptides, or DNA-based drugs are available with the advent of biotechnology, these drugs tend to be too large to be absorbed via nonparenteral routes and, therefore, require frequent and costly injections to achieve therapeutic concentrations over time, causing poor patient compliance due to pain, adverse reactions at the injection sites, and potential side effects. To overcome these limitations, controlled- and sustained-release polymeric systems have been extensively studied. These systems can also protect biological macromolecules against degradation by enzymes or changes in pH.

Polymeric systems can be classified as diffusion controlled, such as monolithic (matrix) and reservoir, and chemically controlled, such as biodegradable and polymer drug conjugates that use pendant chains with degradable spacers. The sections below highlight some important applications where polymers are being used as drug delivery systems. A more detailed review of polymeric systems for drug delivery can be found elsewhere [65].

IMPLANTABLE POLYMERS

When either synthetic or natural polymeric materials are implanted into a tissue by surgery, biocompatibility is the key concern. If the implantable polymeric delivery system is biodegradable, the implant is expected to remain at the site of implantation and produce no toxic byproducts during biodegradation. Poly(lactic acid), poly(glycolic acid), or their copolymers (i.e., poly(lactide-co-glycolide) [PLGA]); polycaprolactone; polyanhydrides; poly(phosphazines); and polyorthoesters are main examples of biodegradable implantable polymers. Notable examples of nonbiodegradable implantable polymers are silicones, polyurethanes, and poly(2-hydroxyethyl methacrylate). More information regarding biomedical polymers can be found elsewhere [66].

INJECTABLE POLYMERS

Biodegradable polymers can be designed into injectable systems for the purpose of sustained drug delivery. The ability to design injectable drug delivery systems eliminates the surgical procedures necessary with implants. Although a few of the aforementioned pharmaceutical and biomedical polymers are not water soluble, methods have been developed to design them into injectable systems. One method is to fabricate those polymers into microparticles small enough (20–200 μm) to pass through an 18- to 20-gauge needle. There has been extensive research on peptide/protein delivery using biodegradable polymer microspheres during the last three decades. Despite challenges, Lupron Depot® (leuprorelin acetate-loaded PLGA microspheres [Takeda/Abbott]) has been successfully marketed for the treatment of prostate cancer.

An alternative approach in injectable drug delivery systems with biodegradable polymers is to use the concept of *in situ* forming devices. Using organic solvents at concentrations acceptable by U.S. Food and Drug Administration guidelines, Eliaz and Kost [67] designed *in situ*–forming injectable system with PLGA and glycofurol, a water-miscible solvent. When injected into subcutaneous tissues, the solvent diffuses out to the blood and the injection mixture forms a hardened matrix from which the drug can be released over time [67]. Polyorthoester injectable semisolid formulations were proposed by van de Weert et al. [68] for safe delivery of peptides and proteins due to mild formulation conditions.

Finally, temperature-sensitive polymers have been developed and studied by many researchers in which their aqueous solution property is temperature dependent [69]. Such polymers are balanced in terms of hydrophilicity and hydrophobicity, and with the drug in an aqueous solution, they form an *in situ* hydrogel upon injection into subcutaneous tissues because of higher body temperature [70, 71]. Similarly, intratumoral injection of OncoGel™ (Protherics, Inc.), an injectable formulation of PLGA-PEG-PLGA and paclitaxel, an anticancer drug, demonstrated efficient drug solubilization and retention of paclitaxel from injection site (i.e., no burst effect) with minimal distribution into other organs [69]. Phase I (superficial solid tumor lesions) [72] and phase II (inoperable esophageal cancer) [73] clinical trials have been completed.

THERMOSENSITIVE BIODEGRADABLE POLYMERS

In situ injectable systems for sustained and controlled drug delivery are more attractive than implantable systems (which require surgery) or microsphere systems (which require multistep fabrication processes). When it comes to encapsulating labile drugs, such as proteins and peptides, microencapsulation processes tend to be harsh to many such agents. Therefore, *in situ*–forming, aqueous-based devices offer injectable systems with mild processing conditions for drug encapsulation.

Jeong and coworkers [70] synthesized block copolymers consisting of PEG and poly(lactic acid) or PLGA blocks, an injectable solution at or above 45°C. The solution becomes gel at 37°C body temperature. This was the first injectable, biodegradable *in situ* matrix for sustained drug release using a thermosensitive polymer [70]. Furthermore, triblock copolymers of PEG-PLGA-PEG were developed with a delicate hydrophilichydrophobic balance, displaying sol-to-gel (lower transition) and gel-to-sol (upper transition) transitions with increasing temperature 74]. The lower transition means the system is soluble at below a body temperature of 37°C and becomes gel once injected. The mechanism of this transition originates from the amphiphilic nature of the block copolymer and is dictated by thermodynamics, as the polymer can be viewed as polymeric surfactants forming micelles (core–shell self-assembly). Upon further increase in polymer concentration, the micelles are believed to be packed and interact with each other, hence forming a hydrogel. Increases in temperature beyond a certain point will cause the polymer to repel water and collapse, which is called syneresis [74]. The polymer structure is manipulated to keep the body temperature well within these two transitions.

Jeong and coworkers [71] demonstrated the *in vivo* degradation and stability of the hydrogel in rats. Initially, a transparent gel was formed upon subcutaneous injection of PEG-PLGA-PEG in rats. With gel hydrolysis and subsequent loss of PEG-rich segments (where PEG is more water soluble and is preferentially lost during hydrolysis), the gel becomes more opaque. Overall, the gel could maintain the mechanical integrity for 1 month at the injection site [71]. These authors also studied drug release from the hydrogel with ketoprofen (a model hydrophilic drug) and spironolactone (a model lipophilic drug). Ketoprofen exhibited first-order release kinetics over 2 weeks, whereas spironolactone exhibited a prolonged release over 2 months. The data were fitted by mathematical models and were best explained by taking into account diffusion, degradation, and the assumption of the microdomain structure of the hydrogel (i.e., hydrophilic and lipophilic domains dispersed across the gel matrix) [75].

A similar polymer with the reverse block sequence, PLGA-PEG-PLGA, has also exhibited thermogelling properties with a similar biodegradability and biocompatibility [69, 76]. Again, the aqueous solution of PLGA-PEG-PLGA demonstrated increased viscosity by 10,000 times upon temperature-induced sol–gel transition, as confirmed by dynamic mechanical analysis. Because of the surfactant nature of the block copolymer, a poorly water-soluble drug, such as paclitaxel, could be solubilized 400- to 2000-fold above its water solubility and released continuously over 50 days [69]. The release of poorly water-soluble drugs exhibited an inverse "S"-shaped pattern from the triblock copolymer hydrogels, because the initial diffusion follows a first-order kinetic until the rate reaches a plateau, followed by acceleration of drug release as the matrix starts degrading. Paclitaxel-loaded PLGA-PEG-PLGA (OncoGel™) has undergone phase I and II clinical trials. The OncoGel™ system demonstrated equivalent efficacy with 10-fold lower doses compared with the maximum tolerated dose of the drug [69]. This *in situ*–forming hydrogel may be an attractive candidate system for protein and peptide agents for sustained release. Careful optimization of loading conditions of insulin (model protein drug) and glucagon-like peptide-1 (GLP-1, an insulinotropic peptide with the molecular weight of 3500) exhibited continuous release with reduced initial burst effect. In the case of insulin, its self-association states were controlled by adding stoichiometric amount of zinc ions. Subcutaneous injection of insulin-loaded PLGA-PEG-PLGA mixture in male Sprague-Dawley rats resulted in continuous *in vivo* release up to 2 weeks, which has the potential to meet basal insulin requirements [77].

GLP-1 is a therapeutic peptide that stimulates insulin secretion in type 2 diabetes. The release of this peptide from the PLGA-PEG-PLGA system was studied both *in vitro* and *in vivo* [78]. GLP-1 has binding sites for zinc, and the self-association behavior of GLP-1 upon addition of zinc is controlled before loading. The *in vitro* release at 37°C demonstrated nearly zero-order release for over 2 weeks. Further study was performed *in vivo* with Zucker diabetic fatty rats as a type 2 diabetes animal model, where mildly elevated blood glucose was induced by continuous feeding of a high-fat diet and obesity. A single subcutaneous injection of GLP-1–loaded polymer helped control the blood glucose for 2 weeks [78].

POLYMERS AS EXTRACELLULAR MATRIX

Poly(*N*-isopropylacrylamide) (poly(NIPAAm)) has drawn much interest because its lower critical solution temperature (LCST) at about 32°C falls in the range of ambient to body temperatures. Above its LCST, this polymer loses water, becomes insoluble, and precipitates (collapses), a process known as entropy-triggered dehydration [79]. The LCST of poly(NIPAAm) can be modulated by incorporating comonomers with different hydrophobicities [79, 80]. If a hydrophilic (or ionic) monomer such as acrylic acid is incorporated into poly(NIPAAm), the copolymer becomes a hydrogel instead of being precipitated above its LCST [80]. This makes the hydrogel system an attractive candidate for tissue engineering application as an extracellular matrix. One example is to entrap insulin-secreting cells (pancreatic islet cells) in the hydrogel, ultimately for the treatment of type 1 diabetes, where patients struggle with producing insulin and controlling blood sugar [81].

Vernon and coworkers [81] encapsulated the islets of Langerhans, isolated from the pancreases of Sprague-Dawley rats, into poly(NIPAAm-co-acrylic acid) copolymer solution in water. The sol-to-gel transition for this polymer occurs over 30 to 34°C, which is below body temperature. The encapsulated islet cells were viable for 4 weeks and maintained functional insulin secretion *in vitro* for 1 month [81]. Upon successful proof of concept, this system will be the key content of a biohybrid *rechargeable* artificial pancreas. Conceptually, due to the temperature sensitivity of the matrix, the extracellular matrix loaded with the cell can be replaced by fresh ones by changing the temperature [81].

In the past three decades, temperature-responsive polymers have been extensively studied for biomedical use [79, 82, 83]. The application of poly(NIPAAm) in tissue engineering has expanded to a new area termed "cell sheet engineering," which was pioneered by Dr. Teruo Okano. The concept is based on the cell culture surface grafted with poly(NIPAAm). Above LCST, at 37°C, the grafted polymer collapses and the surface becomes hydrophobic, which provides a condition for cell attachment and growth. Upon growth of a monolayer (i.e., a cell sheet), the temperature is brought to lower than LCST, and the surface fully hydrates and allows easy detachment of the cell layer. This method is different from the conventional cell detachment method using trypsin and does not damage the cells. This technique can be used to "build" a tissue layer by layer and has a great potential in repairing damaged organs [84].

Pharmacokinetically Modified Actives

Many therapeutic macromolecules (e.g., proteins) have extremely short plasma half-lives when administered by injection. This rapid elimination tends to be largely hepatic, and the elimination process is initiated by protein–protein interaction (e.g., opsonization). The pharmacokinetic profile of a biotechnology drug can be dramatically changed through chemical modification of the agent with water-soluble polymers. In particular, PEG has shown to be effective in extending plasma half-lives of biological macromolecules through covalent "PEGylation." Because of the bulky nature of PEG chains, the pegylated therapeutic protein is protected from other macromolecules inactivating them. This effect is based on the so-called stealth phenomenon, which signifies steric repulsion between large molecules. Examples include pegylated insulin with improved physical stability and increased plasma half-life [85]. More recently, PEG-interferon alfa-2a (Pegasys® [Genentech]) has been marketed for the treatment of chronic hepatitis C in adults [86].

Targetable Polymeric Systems

A polymer–drug conjugate is a polymeric drug carrier with adjustable side chains (i.e., pendant chains). A polymer with controllable molecular weight and sufficient water solubility can be conjugated with various bioactive agents and targeting molecules that serve as homing devices. Poly[*N*-(2-hydroxypropyl) methacrylamide]–based systems, intended for targeted anticancer drug delivery, are well studied. Doxorubicin, for instance, may be linked to the side chain of Poly[*N*-(2-hydroxypropyl) methacrylamide] via an oligopeptide spacer (such as Gly-Phe-Leu-Gly). When the system is taken up by the target cell via endocytosis, the spacer sequence is recognized by lysosomal enzymes followed by the enzymatic hydrolysis of the linkage between the drug and the spacer. Therefore, drug is released locally with an antitumor effect, associated with a dramatic reduction of multidrug resistance [87].

Polymers as Nonviral Gene Carriers

Despite remarkable efficiency of viral carriers, nonviral gene carriers have been extensively studied over the past two decades to overcome several barriers in gene delivery. The therapeutic cargo (such as plasmid DNA) first needs to be condensed to be taken up by cells. Because the backbone of a nucleic acid is negatively charged, polymers with a series of positive charges with some degree of lipophilicity are known to condense plasmid DNA, efficiently. Poly(L-amino acids) such as poly-L-lysine and polyethylene imines are well-known examples. If the polymer–DNA complex (i.e., polyplex) needs to be directed toward a specific target, targeting molecules may be conjugated to such condensing polymers. For instance, the terplex gene carrier was developed in mid-1990s that consisted of hydrophobized poly-L-lysine, low-density lipoprotein, and plasmid DNA, forming a complex ("terplex"). The size of the complex ranged from 100 to 400 nm, which can be taken up by cultured smooth muscle cells. If the poly-L-lysine is modified with galactose via PEG spacer, the system can target the liver [88].

In the next phase, the polymer with degradable linkages is considered for reduced cellular toxicity and for enhancing cargo release, once the polyplexes are taken up by the cells. One example is a polycationic polymer that is very similar to poly-L-lysine but has a degradable ester backbone, poly[alpha-(4-aminobutyl)-L-glycolic acid] (PAGA) [89], as a less toxic nonviral gene carrier. Koh et al. [90] demonstrated that the delivery of interleukin-10 encoding plasmid by using PAGA in nonobese diabetic mice could prevent progression of autoimmune insulitis. In addition, Maheshwari and coworkers [91] showed that tumor growth was inhibited and survival rate improved in subcutaneous tumor-bearing BALB/c mice after repeated treatments with interleukin-12 gene delivery using PAGA polymer.

SUMMARY

Whether natural, synthetic, or semisynthetic, polymers have established their position in the pharmaceutical industry as an effective and functional excipient to improve and enhance the efficacy of dosage forms. They are currently being used with drugs for controlled release, protection, targeted delivery, taste masking, stabilizing dispersions, formulating transdermal patches, and extemporaneous pharmacy compounding. Many of these applications for polymers are made feasible due to desirable molecular weights, adhesion properties, and thermodynamic solubility and swellability in an aqueous medium. Furthermore, advanced polymer systems have been introduced that possess complex structure, temperature-dependent solution behavior, biocompatibility, and biodegradability. Such polymers are now being developed as injectable sustained-release platforms and implantable systems for prolonged delivery of large biomolecules such as peptides, polypeptides, and proteins, as well as potentially toxic drugs.

REVIEW QUESTIONS

1. A pharmaceutical company has been getting complaints from customers that their tablet dosage form of metformin has a bad fishy smell and horrible taste. What might the company do to formulate this product into a more patient-acceptable dosage form? What type of polymers would most likely be in this improved tablet?
2. Describe the difference between a monomer, polymer, homopolymer, copolymer, and polymer blend.
3. What properties are most likely to change when a hydrophilic polymer becomes cross-linked?
4. Water-soluble cellulose derivatives are commonly found in many pharmaceutical dosage forms. Cellulose itself is not water soluble; however, methylation of cellulose produces water-soluble methylcellulose. Can you suggest why adding a hydrophobic methyl group to cellulose improves its water solubility?

REFERENCES

1. Omidian H, Park K, Sinko P. Pharmaceutical polymers. In: Martin A, Sinko P, Singh Y, eds. *Martin's Physical Pharmacy and Pharmaceutical Sciences*, 6th ed. Baltimore, MD: Lippincott Williams & Wilkins; 2011:492–515.
2. Colorcon. Properties of solutions of Methocel. 2002. Available at: http://www.colorcon.com/literature/marketing/mr/Extended%20Release/METHOCEL/English/prop_of_solutions.pdf. Accessed May 22, 2012.
3. Salunke S, Giacoia G, Tuleu C. The STEP (safety and toxicity of excipients for paediatrics) database. Part 1-A need assessment study. *Int J Pharm*. 2012;435(2):101–111.

4. Food and Drug Administration. Guidance for Industry: Nonclinical Studies for the Safety Evaluation of Pharmaceutical Excipients. 2005. Available at: http://www.fda.gov/ohrms/dockets/98fr/2002d-0389-gdl0002.pdf. Accessed May 20, 2012.

5. Patterson DL, Yunginger JW, Dunn WF, Jones RT, Hunt LW. Anaphylaxis induced by the carboxymethylcellulose component of injectable triamcinolone acetonide suspension (Kenalog). *Ann Allerg Asthma Immunol.* 1995;74(2):163–166.

6. Bigliardi PL, Izakovic J, Weber JM, Bircher AJ. Anaphylaxis to the carbohydrate carboxymethylcellulose in parenteral corticosteroid preparations. *Dermatology.* 2003;207(1):100–103.

7. Chen H, Yuan L, Song W, Wu Z, Li D. Biocompatible polymer materials: Role of protein–surface interactions. *Prog Polym Sci.* 2008;33(11):1059–1087.

8. Mansour HM, Sohn M, Al-Ghananeem A, Deluca PP. Materials for pharmaceutical dosage forms: molecular pharmaceutics and controlled release drug delivery aspects. *Int J Mol Sci.* 2010;11(9):3298–3322.

9. Ikada Y, Tsuji H. Biodegradable polyesters for medical and ecological applications. *Macromol Rapid Commun.* 2000;21(3):117–132.

10. Mastropietro DJ, Omidian H. Prevalence and trends of cellulosics in pharmaceutical dosage forms. *Drug Dev Ind Pharm.* 2013;39(2):382–392.

11. Rowe RC, Sheskey PJ, Owen SC. *Handbook of Pharmaceutical Excipients,* 5th ed. London: Pharmaceutical Press; 2006.

12. The ConsultingRoom™. Stylage®: Product Summary. 2012; Available at: http://www.consultingroom.com/treatments/stylage. Accessed May 20, 2012.

13. Chen BW, Hiu WM, Lam SK, Cho CH, Ng MM, Luk CT. Effect of sucralfate on gastric mucosal blood flow in rats. *Gut.* 1989;30(11):1544–1551.

14. GlaxoSmithKline Consumer Healthcare L.P. Citrucel FAQ: The fiber chronicles, answers to your questions. 2012. Available at: http://www.citrucel.com/Ch5_FAQ.aspx. Accessed May 25, 2012.

15. Allergan Inc. Refresh Liquigel. 2009. Available at: http://www.refreshbrand.com/html/practitioner/home.asp. Accessed May 23, 2012.

16. Chandran S, Asghar LF, Mantha N. Design and evaluation of ethyl cellulose based matrix tablets of ibuprofen with pH modulated release kinetics. *Indian J Pharm Sci.* 2008;70(5):596–602.

17. Enayatifard R, Saeedi M, Akbari J, Tabatabaee YH. Effect of hydroxypropyl methylcellulose and ethyl cellulose content on release profile and kinetics of diltiazem HCl from matrices. *Trop J Pharm Res.* 2009;8(5):425–432.

18. Malmud LS, Charkes ND, Littlefield J, et al. The mode of action of alginic acid compound in the reduction of gastroesophageal reflux. *J Nucl Med.* 1979;20(10):1023–1028.

19. Mandel KG, Daggy BP, Brodie DA, Jacoby HI. Review article: Alginate-raft formulations in the treatment of heartburn and acid reflux. *Aliment Pharmacol Ther.* 2000;14(6):669–690.

20. GlaxoSmithKline. Gavison FAQ's. 2012. Available at: http://www.gaviscon.ca/FAQ.aspx. Accessed May 24, 2012.

21. Capsugel. Performance qualification of a new hypromellose capsule. 2010. Available at: http://capsugel.com/media/library/performance-qualification-of-a-new-hypromellose-capsule-part-i.pdf. Accessed May 26, 2012.

22. Tuleu C, Khela MK, Evans DF, Jones BE, Nagata S, Basit AW. A scintigraphic investigation of the disintegration behaviour of capsules in fasting subjects: A comparison of hypromellose capsules containing carrageenan as a gelling agent and standard gelatin capsules. *Eur J Pharm Sci.* 2007;30(3–4):251–255.

23. Thompson JE, Davidow LW. *A Practical Guide to Contemporary Pharmacy Practice,* 3rd ed. Philadelphia: Wolters Kluwer Health/Lippincott Williams & Wilkins; 2009.

24. Hiorth M, Kjøniksen A-L, Knudsen KD, Sande SA, Nyström B. Structural and dynamical properties of aqueous mixtures of pectin and chitosan. *Eur Polym J.* 2005;41(8):1718–1728.

25. Morris GA, Castile J, Smith A, Adams GG, Harding SE. The effect of different storage temperatures on the physical properties of pectin solutions and gels. *Polym Degrad Stab.* 2010;95(12):2670–2673.

26. Lyseng-Williamson KA. Fentanyl pectin nasal spray in breakthrough pain in opioid-tolerant adults with cancer. *CNS Drugs.* 2011;25(6):511–522.

27. Tonariya Y, Shimizu H, Wada Y, et al., Inventors; Kaisha, Ohta Seiyaku Kabushiki, assignee. X-ray contrast medium comprising barium and xanthan gum for examination of large intestine and small intestine. U.S. patent 5,518,711, 1996.

28. Tobyn MJ, Staniforth JN, Baichwal AR, McCall TW. Prediction of physical properties of a novel polysaccharide controlled release system .1. *Int J Pharm.* 1996;128(1–2):113–122.

29. Precision Foods Inc. AquaCareH2O: The next-generation of thickened beverages for dysphagia 2011. Available at: http://www.thickitretail.com/Products/AquaCareHsub2subO.aspx. Accessed May 27, 2012.

30. Denkbas EB, Ottenbrite RM. Perspectives on: chitosan drug delivery systems based on their geometries. *J Bioact Compatible Polym.* 2006;21(4):351–368.

31. Shukla RK, Tiwari A. Carbohydrate polymers: Applications and recent advances in delivering drugs to the colon. *Carbohydr Polym.* 2012;88(2):399–416.

32. Actavis Elizabeth LLC. Kadian full prescribing information. 2010. Available at: http://www.kadian.com/NR/rdonlyres/805E2900-ADBA-4FE4-A69E-173E4B9C151B/577/KADIAN_Prescribing_Information.pdf. Accessed May 24, 2012.

33. Balch RJ, Trescot A. Extended-release morphine sulfate in treatment of severe acute and chronic pain. *J Pain Res.* 2010;3:191–200.

34. DeMerlis CC, Schoneker DR. Review of the oral toxicity of polyvinyl alcohol (PVA). *Food Chem Toxicol.* 2003;41(3):319–326.

35. Camarco W, Ray D, Druffner A. Selecting superdisintegrants for orally disintegrating tablet formulations. *Pharm Technol.* 2006: Excipient Supplement, 30:s28–s37.

36. Muramatsu M, Kanada K, Nishida A, et al. Application of Carbopol® to controlled release preparations I. Carbopol® as a novel coating material. *Int J Pharm.* 2000;199(1):77–83.

37. *The United States Pharmacopeia and National Formulary (USP 31-NF 26).* Vol 1. Rockville, MD: United States Pharmacopeia Convention; 2007.

38. Chung TW, Lin SY, Liu DZ, Tyan YC, Yang JS. Sustained release of 5-FU from Poloxamer gels interpenetrated by crosslinking chitosan network. *Int J Pharm.* 2009;382(1–2):39–44.

39. Chaudhry NC, Saunders L. Sustained release of drugs from ion exchange resins. *J Pharm Pharmacol.* 1956;8(1):975–986.

40. Rohm and Haas Company. Duolite AP143/1093. 2006. Available at: http://www.rohmhaas.com/ionexchange/pharmaceuticals/Formulations_doc/english/143_1093.pdf. Accessed May 4, 2012.

41. Rohm and Haas. Amberlite IRP64 Pharmaceutical grade cation exchange resin. 2006. Available at: http://www.dow.com/assets/attachments/business/process_chemicals/amberlite_and_duolite_pharmaceutical_grade_resins/amberlite_irp64/tds/amberlite_irp64.pdf. Accessed April 29, 2012.

42. Riippi M, Antikainen O, Niskanen T, Yliruusi J. The effect of compression force on surface structure, crushing strength, friability and disintegration time of erythromycin acistrate tablets. *Eur J Pharm Biopharm.* 1998;46(3):339–345.

43. Jani R, Gan O, Ali Y, Rodstrom R, Hancock S. Ion-exchange resins for ophthalmic delivery. *J Ocul Pharmacol.* 1994;10(1):57–67.

44. Walker JR, Brown K, Rohatagi S, et al. Quantitative structure-property relationships modeling to predict in vitro and in vivo binding of drugs to the bile sequestrant, colesevelam (Welchol). *J Clin Pharmacol.* 2009;49(10):1185–1195.

45. Sterns RH, Rojas M, Bernstein P, Chennupati S. Ion-exchange resins for the treatment of hyperkalemia: are they safe and effective? *J Am Soc Nephrol.* 2010;21(5):733–735.

46. Porter SC. Controlled-release film coatings based on ethylcellulose. *Drug Dev Ind Pharm.* 1989;15(10):1495–1521.

47. Santus G, Baker RW. Osmotic drug delivery: a review of the patent literature. *J Control Release.* 1995;35(1):1–21.

48. Stephan RM. Intra-oral hydrogen-ion concentrations associated with dental caries activity. *J Dent Res.* 1944;23(4):257–266.

49. Chourasia MK, Jain SK. Pharmaceutical approaches to colon targeted drug delivery systems. *J Pharm Pharmac Sci.* 2003;6(1):33–66.

50. Ekpe A, Jacobsen T. Effect of various salts on the stability of lansoprazole, omeprazole, and pantoprazole as determined by high-performance liquid chromatography. *Drug Dev Ind Pharm.* 1999;25(9):1057–1065.

51. Harris WS. Fish oil supplementation: evidence for health benefits. *Cleve Clin J Med.* 2004;71(3):208–210.

52. Merck Sharp & Dohme Corp. Proscar (finasteride) highlights of prescribing information. 2012. Available at: http://www.merck.com/product/usa/pi_circulars/p/proscar/proscar_pi.pdf.

53. WebMD LLC. Asacol (mesalamine) delayed-release tablets 2012. Available at: http://www.rxlist.com/asacol-drug.htm. Accessed May 30, 2012.

54. Cortot A, Colombel J-F, Rutgeerts P, et al. Switch from systemic steroids to budesonide in steroid dependent patients with inactive Crohn's disease. *Gut.* 2001;48(2):186–190.

55. Sohi H, Sultana Y, Khar RK. Taste masking technologies in oral pharmaceuticals: recent developments and approaches. *Drug Dev Ind Pharm.* 2004;30(5):429–448.

56. Cima Labs Inc. Taste-masking expertise: Technical notes. 2012. Available at: http://www.cimalabs.com/technology/taste-masking-expertise. Accessed May 29, 2012.

57. Abbott Laboratories. Omnicef (cefdinir) full prescribing information. 2007. Available at: http://www.rxabbott.com/pdf/omnicef.pdf. Accessed May 30, 2012.

58. European Medicines Agency. Azopt product information: Scientific discussion. 2004. Available at: http://www.ema.europa.eu/docs/en_GB/document_library/EPAR_-_Scientific_Discussion/human/000267/WC500030362.pdf. Accessed May 31, 2012.

59. Kandavilli S, Nair V, Panchagnula R. Polymers in transdermal drug delivery systems. *Pharm Technol.* 2002:26(5):62–81

60. WebMD LLC. Transderm-Nitro (nitroglycerin) transdermal therapeutic system. 2012. Available at: http://www.rxlist.com/transderm-nitro-drug.htm. Accessed May 30, 2012.

61. Venkatraman S, Gale R. Skin adhesives and skin adhesion. 1. Transdermal drug delivery systems. *Biomaterials.* 1998;19(13):1119–1136.

62. 3M. 3M transdermal components. 2012. Available at: http://solutions.3m.com/wps/portal/3M/en_WW/3M-DDSD/Drug-Delivery-Systems/Transdermal-Microneedle-Directory/Componentry. Accessed May 30, 2012.

63. Sah ML, Saini TR. Formulation development and release studies of indomethacin suppositories. *Indian J Pharm Sci.* 2008;70(4):498–501.

64. Paddock Laboratories Inc. ORA-PLUS oral suspending vehicle. 2010. Available at: http://www.paddocklabs.com/html/products/pdf/Ora-Plus%20Sell%20Sheet.pdf. Accessed May 31, 2010.

65. Heller J. Use of polymers in controlled release of active agents. In: Robinson JR, Lee VH, eds. *Controlled Drug Delivery Fundamentals and Applications*, 2nd ed. New York: Marcel Dekker; 1987. pp. 180–210.

66. Winzenburg G, Schmidt C, Fuchs S, Kissel T. Biodegradable polymers and their potential use in parenteral veterinary drug delivery systems. *Adv Drug Deliv Rev.* 2004;56(10):1453–1466.

67. Eliaz RE, Kost J. Characterization of polymeric PLGA-injectable implant delivery system for the controlled release of proteins. *J Biomed Mater Res.* 2000;50:388–396.

68. van de Weert M, van Steenbergen MJ, Cleland JL, Heller J, Hennink WE, Crommelin DJ. Semisolid, self-catalyzed poly(ortho ester)s as controlled-release systems: protein release and protein stability issues. *J Pharm Sci.* 2002;91(4):1065–1074.

69. Zentner GM, Rathi R, Shih C, et al. Biodegradable block copolymers for delivery of proteins and water-insoluble drugs. *J Control Release.* 2001;72:203–215.

70. Jeong B, Bae YH, Lee DS, Kim SW. Biodegradable block copolymers as injectable drug-delivery systems. *Nature.* 1997;388:860–862.

71. Jeong B, Bae YH, Kim SW. In situ gelation of PEG-PLGA-PEG triblock copolymer aqueous solutions and degradation thereof. *J Biomed Mater Res.* 2000;50:171–177.

72. DuVall GA, Tarabar D, Seidel RH, Elstad NL, Fowers KD. Phase 2: a dose-escalation study of OncoGel (ReGel/paclitaxel), a controlled-release formulation of paclitaxel, as adjunctive local therapy to external-beam radiation in patients with inoperable esophageal cancer. *Anticancer Drugs.* 2009;20(2):89–95.

73. Vukelja SJ, Anthony SP, Arseneau JC, et al. Phase 1 study of escalating-dose OncoGel (ReGel/paclitaxel) depot injection, a controlled-release formulation of paclitaxel, for local management of superficial solid tumor lesions. *Anticancer Drugs.* 2007;18(3):283–289.

74. Jeong B, Bae YH, Kim SW. Thermosensitive gelation of PEG-PLGA-PEG triblock copolymer aqueous solutions. *Macromolecules.* 1999;32:7064–7069.

75. Jeong B, Bae YH, Kim SW. Drug release from biodegradable injectable thermosensitive hydrogel of PEG-PLGA-PEG triblock copolymers. *J Control Release.* 2000;63:155–163.

76. Lee DS, Shim MS, Kim SW, Lee H, Park I, Chang T. Novel thermoreversible gelation of biodegradable PLGA-block-PEO-block-PLGA triblock copolymers in aqueous solution. *Macromol Rapid Commun.* 2001;22:587–592.

77. Kim YJ, Choi S, Koh JJ, Lee M, Ko KS, Kim SW. Controlled release of insulin from injectable biodegradable triblock copolymer. *Pharm Res.* 2001;18:548–550.

78. Choi S, Baudys M, Kim SW. Control of blood glucose by novel GLP-1 delivery using biodegradable triblock copolymer of PLGA-PEG-PLGA in type 2 diabetic rats. *Pharm Res.* 2004;21:827–831.

79. Chen G, Hoffman AS. Graft copolymers that exhibit temperature-induced phase transitions over a wide range of pH. *Nature.* 1995;373:49–52.

80. Han CK, Bae YH. Inverse thermally reversible gelation of aqueous N-isopropylacrylamide copolymer solution. *Polymer.* 1998;39:2809–2814.

81. Vernon B, Kim SW, Bae YH. Thermosensitive copolymer gels for extracellular matrix. *J Biomed Mater Res.* 2000;51:69–79.

82. Bae YH, Okano T, Kim SW. "On-off" thermocontrol of solute transport. I. Temperature dependence of swelling of N-isopropylacrylamide networks modified with hydrophobic components in water. *Pharm Res.* 1991;8:531–537.

83. Bae YH, Okano T, Kim SW. "On-off" thermocontrol of solute transport. II. Solute release from thermosensitive hydrogels. *Pharm Res.* 1991;8:624–628.

84. Yang J, Yamato M, Shimizu T, et al. Reconstruction of functional tissues with cell sheet engineering. *Biomaterials.* 2007;28(34):5033–5043.

85. Hinds K, Koh JJ, Joss L, Liu F, Baudys M, Kim SW. Synthesis and characterization of poly(ethylene glycol)-insulin conjugates. *Bioconjugate Chem.* 2000;11:195–201.

86. Cooksley WG, Piratvisuth T, Lee SD, et al. Peginterferon alpha-2a (40 kDa): an advance in the treatment of hepatitis B e antigen-positive chronic hepatitis B. *J Viral Hepat.* 2003;10(4):298–305.

87. Kopecek J, Kopecková P. HPMA copolymers: origins, early developments, present, and future. *Adv Drug Deliv Rev.* 2010;62(2):122–149.

88. Benns JM, Kim SW. Tailoring new gene delivery designs for specific targets. *J Drug Target.* 2000;8(1):1–12.

89. Lim YB, Han SO, Kong HU, et al. Biodegradable polyester, poly[alpha-(4-aminobutyl)-L-glycolic acid], as a non-toxic gene carrier. *Pharm Res.* 2000;17(7):811–816.

90. Koh JJ, Ko KS, Lee M, Han S, Park JS, Kim SW. Degradable polymeric carrier for the delivery of IL-10 plasmid DNA to prevent autoimmune insulitis of NOD mice. *Gene Ther.* 2000;7(24):2099–2104.

91. Maheshwari A, Han S, Mahato RI, Kim SW. Biodegradable polymer-based interleukin-12 gene delivery: role of induced cytokines, tumor infiltrating cells and nitric oxide in anti-tumor activity. *Gene Ther.* 2002;9(16):1075–1084.

CHAPTER

8

MULTIFUNCTIONAL NANOCARRIERS FOR TUMOR DRUG DELIVERY AND IMAGING

GEMMA NAVARRO, SARA MOVASSAGHIAN, AND VLADIMIR P. TORCHILIN

CHAPTER OBJECTIVES

Upon completing this chapter, the reader should be able to

▸ Explain the advantages and disadvantages of nanoscaled delivery systems over the traditional formulation of anticancer drugs.

▸ List and define the main classes of nanocarriers currently used in anticancer drug delivery.

▸ Recognize the factors and physicochemical properties of the drug, protein, or imaging agent that must be considered to select the appropriate nanocarrier.

▸ Demonstrate knowledge of the general considerations for a rational design of nanocarriers that address the tumor microenvironment.

> ▸ Understand the following concepts: multifunctional nanocarrier, passive/active targeting, prolonged circulation, stimuli sensitivity, and enhanced intracellular delivery. Give examples of moieties and chemistries required to endow the carriers with such functionalities.

CHAPTER OUTLINE

INTRODUCTION

Pharmaceutical nanocarriers such as liposomes, micelles, and polymeric or lipidic nanoparticles have demonstrated enhanced *in vivo* stability and efficiency as drugs, genes, and diagnostic agents [1]. Surface engineering of nanocarriers can provide unique properties to the system, such as longevity in the blood; specific recognition of different tissues, cell types, and even cellular organelles; and real-time tracking of carrier and payload by the incorporation of contrast materials. It is evident from the literature that the technology to implement each one of these "functionalities" separately is quite well established. The benefits of nano-scaled delivery systems are clearly supported by numerous preclinical and clinical data [2, 3] and several commercialized products (Table 8-1). Therefore, researchers are moving forward trying to combine two or more of these useful properties in a single carrier in an attempt to produce more powerful multifunctional carriers.

In the particular case of cancer, the design of novel multifunctional nanocarriers needs to address some general requirements concerning anticancer drug delivery systems such as high loading capacity, low plasma protein binding affinity, and nuclear/mitochondrial specificity. At the same time, it has to consider the physiological characteristics of the tumor site (i.e., leaky vasculature, low pH) that can influence the biodistribution and release of the drug. The next generation of multifunctional nanocarriers will harmonize all these factors to simultaneously or sequentially demonstrate the following set of properties: (1) prolonged circulation in the blood; (2) ability to accumulate, specifically or nonspecifically, in the required pathological zone; (3) responsiveness to local stimuli, such as pH and/or temperature changes, resulting, for example, in accelerated

TABLE 8-1 Examples of Nanocarrier-Based Formulations Approved for Clinical Application

Nanocarrier	Drug	Route	Trade Name	Indication
Liposome	Cytarabine	Intrathecal	DepoCyt®	Malignant lymphomatous meningitis
	Daunorubicin	IV	DaunoXome®	AIDS-related Kaposi's sarcoma
	Vincristine	IV	Onco-TSC®	Aggressive non-Hodgkin's lymphoma
	Doxorubicin	IV	Myocet®	Metastatic breast cancer
PEGylated liposome	Doxorubicin	IV	Doxil®	Ovarian cancer, AIDS-related Kaposi's sarcoma, multiple myeloma
	Doxorubicin	IM	Caelyx®	Metastatic breast and ovarian cancer
Albumin-NP	Paclitaxel	IV	Abraxane®	Metastatic breast cancer
Polymeric micelles	Paclitaxel	IV	Genexol®	Metastatic breast cancer
Drug–polymer conjugates	PEG-asparaginase	IV	Oncaspar®	Acute lymphoblastic leukemia
Iron nanoparticle	Contrast agent	IV	Feridex®	MRI imaging of liver tumors
	Contrast agent	IV	Magnevist®	MRI tumor imaging

drug release; (4) effective intracellular drug delivery, including individual cell organelles; and (5) bear a contrast/reporter moiety.

In this chapter, we first review some important aspects and tips regarding the rational design of multifunctional nanocarriers for cancer diagnosis and treatment. Second, we illustrate the current status of multifunctional nanocarriers by giving some examples of multiple combinations of long circulation, targetability, and stimuli sensitivity with special attention on micelles, liposomes, and nanoparticles. At this point, it is worthwhile mentioning that we do not discuss here in depth those nanocarriers (also called multifunctional) that simultaneously contain more than one anticancer molecule. Combinations of two different cytotoxic chemicals and combinations of chemotherapy with hormone or gene therapy in a single carrier can be found elsewhere [4–8].

NANOSCALE DELIVERY SYSTEMS VERSUS CONVENTIONAL FORMULATIONS

Solubility in aqueous media is essential for anticancer drugs to enter the circulation by parenteral administration, reach disseminated tumors, and exert their therapeutic effects. Aggregation of poorly soluble drugs upon intravenous administration is associated with serious complications such as embolism and local toxicity. Because of a lack of appropriate formulations, a large percentage of new chemical entities (40%) that show anticancer activity are abandoned from further development because of their poor solubility in water [9]. The traditional formulation of poorly soluble chemotherapeutics involves decrease of the particle size, adjustment of pH, and the use of co-solvents and surfactants that are occasionally toxic [10]. For example, Cremophor EL, a surfactant used for intravenous administration of paclitaxel, is associated with neurotoxicity and acute hypersensitivity reactions. Another major problem with the classical formulation of anti-cancer drugs and diagnostic agents is the lack of targeted delivery to tumor. This is associated with undesirable drug side effects due to non-specific drug exposure of healthy tissues and low accumulation of drug in the tumor area, resulting in limited dosing schedules, limited therapeutic effects, and, eventually, development of tumor drug resistance [11]. Premature degradation and elimination, especially in protein or nucleic acid delivery, can also contribute to treatment failure. In the case of cancer diagnostic imaging, targeted and enhanced accumulation of contrast moieties must be substantial to differentiate small tumors from surrounding tissues.

The inclusion of drugs and imaging agents into a nano-scaled delivery system has emerged as an alternative to solve the problems. Nanocarriers are useful in drug delivery because they can alter the pharmacokinetics and biodistribution of their associated therapeutics. Precise changes in the composition, size, and hydrophobicity of nanocarriers leads to substantial changes in pharmacokinetics/biodistribution of the drug or the contrast agent. For example, by simply coupling L-asparaginase (indicated for acute lymphoblastic leukemia) to the hydrophilic polymer polyethylene glycol (PEG), the plasma half-life of the enzyme can be prolonged from hours (8–30) to days (12) and the dosage schedule reduced from daily administration for 4 weeks to one perfusion each for 2 weeks [12]. The use of nanocarriers is advantageous even when the pharmacokinetics of the drug–carrier duet is close to the free drug alone (i.e., rapid drug release from the carrier). Nanocarriers can avoid the excipient and/or drug aggregation-related toxicities of conventional anticancer formulations. For example, human albumin-stabilized paclitaxel nanoparticles (Abraxane®) provide several practical advantages over Cremophor EL–paclitaxel (Taxol®). Premedication for Cremophor EL hypersensitivity reactions is not required and paclitaxel can be dissolved in a smaller volume of normal saline. Thus, the infusion time is shortened from 3 hours for Taxol® to 30 minutes for Abraxane® [13, 14].

THE RIGHT CARRIER FOR THE RIGHT DRUG: OPPORTUNITIES AND CHALLENGES OF AVAILABLE NANOSYSTEMS

Pharmaceutical nanocarriers are engineered constructs, assemblies, architectures, and particulate systems with a nanometer scale size ranging from a few nanometers resembling those of native macromolecules, as in the case of drug–polymer conjugates or dendrimers, to a few hundred nanometers for liposomes or nanoparticles (**Figure 8-1**).

Among all, the most popular and well-investigated nanocarriers are polymeric nanoparticles, liposomes, and micelles. Polymeric nanoparticles are typically agglomerates of polymer chains. Examples of commonly used polymers for nanoparticles include synthetic polymers such as poly (lactide-co-glycolic acid), poly (lactic acid),

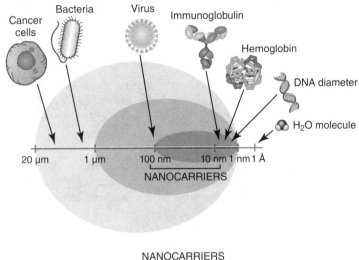

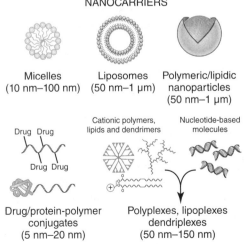

FIGURE 8-1 Classes of nanoscale delivery systems.

polycaprolactone, and polyalkylcyanoacrylates and natural polymers such as gelatin, chitosan, and hyaluronic acid. Nanoparticles can load therapeutics either by absorption onto the polymeric matrix or by surface attachment. Liposomes and micelles are spherical carriers with amphiphile-based unilamellar or multilamellar structures that separate the inner aqueous compartment from the external aqueous solvent [15, 16]. In this way, they can be loaded with a variety of water-soluble drugs (into the inner compartment) or water-insoluble drugs (into the hydrophobic compartment of the amphiphile layer). Liposomes are constructed as phospholipid vesicles, mimicking the plasma membrane of mammalian cells. They are biologically inert and cause few if any toxic or antigenic reactions. Micelles are colloidal dispersions spontaneously formed by thermodynamically favored aggregation of amphiphiles at or above the critical micellar concentration. Micelle amphiphiles are often constructed from lipid or polymeric moieties as hydrophobic blocks capping hydrophilic polymer chains. Common examples are PEG-poly (lactic acid)–based or PEG-phosphatidylethanolamine (PE)–based micelles [17, 18]. Because of their small sizes, micelles demonstrate spontaneous penetration into the tumor interstitium [15, 19]. Thus, they are attractive carriers for tumor targeting, although their stability *in vivo* can be an issue because of their dilution below the critical micellar concentration after intravenous injection. Hoang and coworkers [20] reported results of pharmacokinetics and biodistribution studies of radioactively labeled micelles and unimers administered below the critical micellar concentration up to 48 hours. Radioactivity remaining in the blood at 48 hours post-injection was significantly higher with micelles compared with unimers (4% vs 0.6% injected dose/mL). Biodistribution studies revealed significant accumulation of the micelles at the tumor site via passive targeting, but it was limited primarily to the tumor periphery.

The suitability of a specific nanocarrier or the location of the drug within the nanocarrier depends on the potency/efficacy, degradability, molecular weight, solubility, and charge of the drug. Polymer drug conjugates are the choice for potent molecules (enzymes, interleukins, and hormones [21]) because they can carry only few molecules, whereas the potency of the drug may not be an important issue for liposomes due to their high loading capacity. Liposomal doxorubicin has trapping efficiencies near 100% [22, 23]. Drug wt% of 5% to 23% was reported for doxorubicin–polymer conjugates [24]. Nanoparticles and liposomes provide good protection of very labile molecules such as plasmid DNA or oligonucleotides against enzymatic degradation upon administration. However, very-large-molecular-weight proteins or highly hydrophobic molecules may not be suitable if encapsulation compromises the maximum 100- to 200-nm size restriction required for their parenteral administration. In such cases, alternative delivery systems with small sizes such as micelles or molecular polymer conjugates can be used. In any case, nanoparticulate and liposomal systems always offer the possibility of incorporating imaging or the therapeutic molecules on the carrier surface by direct chemical attachment or by electrostatic or hydrophobic interactions between therapeutic and surface components [25–28].

When choosing a carrier platform, questions regarding elimination rate, degradability, or toxicity of the delivery system are also extremely important. Maintaining an optimal balance among stability, local drug availability, and toxicity remains challenging. Nanocarrier features that may improve blood stability may also increase the toxicity of the carrier and vice versa. The retention time of a given nanocarrier depends mostly on the hydrodynamic diameter or molecular weight. Low-molecular-weight molecules, below 40 kDa (hydrodynamic radius of 4.5 nm), can be eliminated by glomerular filtration in the kidneys. The association of small therapeutics, such as doxorubicin (579 Da), paclitaxel (853 Da), and interferon (19 kDa), with small nanocarriers, such as middle-generation dendrimers (3–28 kDa) or polymers (PEG, 30 kDa; dextran, 40 kDa), can slow the glomerular filtration of the conjugate [29–32]. One strategy to extend the half-life of the delivery system without impairing the elimination of the carrier from the body is to include biodegradable linkers between carrier and bioactive compound. Such systems have long circulation before degradation and are quickly eliminated right after degradation [33, 34]. On the other hand, larger nanoparticulate carriers that cannot be filtered by the kidneys are rapidly eliminated through the mononuclear phagocyte system (MPS) clearance. When they enter the circulation, nanoparticulate delivery systems immediately interact with plasma proteins (opsonins) and with the macrophages of the MPS in the blood, liver, and spleen [35]. Liposomes and micelles remain stable in the blood for a time depending on their composition but eventually disassemble and are phagocytized by MPS cells [36]. Once internalized into cells, a nanocarrier's intracellular fate is largely determined by its composition. Biodegradable particles are digested in lysosomes, where active degradation processes occurring under the action of the lysosomal enzymes take place, whereas non-biodegradable particles (e.g., metal colloids, ceramics) accumulate in cells for extended periods of time. Some interesting biological and regulatory considerations regarding the toxicity and safety of nanocarriers are discussed elsewhere [37, 38].

TAILORING NANOCARRIERS FOR TUMOR DELIVERY

Uptake of diagnostic and therapeutic agents differs dramatically between tumor and normal tissue. Solid tumors are characterized by a disorganized and leaky vasculature and a lack of functional lymphatic vessels. Because of their small size, "plain" nanocarriers can extravasate and accumulate in the tumor interstitium. By functionalizing their surface with synthetic polymers and adequate ligands, nanocarriers can take advantage of other peculiarities of the tumor surroundings and certain receptors that are overexpressed in cancer cells. Such approaches can enhance detection sensitivity in medical imaging, improve therapeutic effectiveness, and decrease side effects.

TUMOR MICROENVIRONMENT

The heterogeneities of the blood supply, disturbed architecture, and permeability of tumor vessels together with poor lymphatic drainage are the main reasons for the abnormal microenvironment that exists in solid tumors. Tumor vasculature does not follow the typical branching pattern of normal vessels, that is, successively smaller vessels that end in one-cell-thick capillary walls. Tumor overexpression of certain pro-angiogenic molecules, such as vascular endothelial growth factor, leads to a rapid formation of a vasculature necessary for the nutritional supply of the growing tumoral mass. In consequence, the new vasculature is chaotic, dilated, and irregularly distributed, leaving low- or non-perfused regions in the tumor. This latter fact is the main cause of the characteristic hypoxia, low pH, and necrosis of the tumor environment that acts to promote tumor resistance and aid progression [39, 40].

The structure of tumor vessels is also abnormal: The endothelial cells lining the vessels have aberrant morphology, the basement membrane is either unusually thick or absent, and the pore diameters may be several hundred nanometers or even a few micrometers depending on tumor types [41, 42]. Overall, tumor vasculature is leaky and hypermeable. In addition, proliferating tumor cells can compress blood and lymphatic vessels, especially in inner tumor regions, and cause their collapse. Therefore, the blood flow can be slow and the lymphatic drainage inefficient, promoting a high interstitial pressure in tumor tissues. This phenomenon led to coining of the term "enhanced permeability and retention effect" (EPR effect) of macromolecules in solid tumors. Macromolecules are entrapped in solid tumors and retained there at high concentrations for prolonged periods (more than 100 hours), whereas low-molecular-weight substances are not retained but returned to the circulating blood by diffusion [43, 44]. However, the benefits of nanoparticulate sizes in the accumulation by the EPR effect may be impaired by their slow diffusion through the tumoral matrix [45]. Passive targeting of nanocarriers was shown to be strongly dependent on the cut-off size of the tumor blood vessel wall that also varies among tumor types [46].

Another feature of the tumor's environment is acidosis. More than 80% of measured pH values in extratumoral blood showed pHs lower (6.5–7.2) than normal arterial blood (7.4) [47–49]. The low pH within solid tumors is the consequence of oncogene activation, loss of tumor suppressor activity, adaptation to hypoxia, and the ability of tumor cells to extrude acids such as lactic acid and carbonic acid that are generated by a shift in glucose metabolism from oxidative phosphorylation to glycolysis [50]. The existence of an acidic tumor pH has prompted the development of pH-sensitive nanocarriers that demonstrate accelerated delivery of drugs and genes to the tumor interstitium [51].

Site-specific therapy is also possible because of the presence of an increased number of overexpressed receptors on tumor cells compared with normal cells. To differentiate such cells, ligands are designed to have high affinity to their cognate receptors and have innate abilities to induce receptor-mediated endocytosis. Targeting ligands are generally presented on the exterior of the carrier. Transferrin is a very prominent target for cancer therapeutics. It is a serum, non-heme, iron-binding glycoprotein that helps transport iron to proliferating cells. Transferrin receptor is expressed on the surface of cerebral endothelial cells, hepatocytes, and highly proliferating cells such as erythroblasts and tumor cells [52]. A wide range of tumors overexpress epidermal growth factor receptor, including breast, lung, colorectal, and brain cancers. Expression on glioblastomas is 100-fold greater than on non-tumoral cells [53]. Likewise, the folate receptor is overexpressed in ovarian, lung, brain, head and neck, renal cell, and breast cancer [54].

TUNING OF NANOCARRIER'S SURFACE

To take the advantage of the peculiarities of solid tumors, it may be useful to have nanocarriers simultaneously carrying on their surface various moieties that enable the performance of multiple functions. Carriers can be transformed into stable and long-circulating ones by modifying their surface with protective polymers (e.g., PEG) to accumulate (via EPR effect) in the tumor. Tumor accumulation can be further boosted by attaching specific ligands such as antibodies, peptides, folate, transferrin, or sugar moieties. Enhanced intracellular and targeted organelle delivery of anticancer drugs and nucleic acids can be achieved by decorating the surface of nanocarriers with cell-penetrating peptides and other moieties. Some carriers can be engineered to activate and rapidly release the drug content by a change of chemical stimulus (changes in the environmental pH, pO_2 and redox balance) by the application of a rapidly oscillating magnetic field or by application of light or an external heat source. Finally, the carrier can incorporate heavy metal–based diagnostics or contrast moieties via chelating compounds, such as ethylenediaminetetraacetic acid, diethylenetriaminepentaacetic acid, or deferoxamine (**Figure 8-2**).

Combining all these moieties/functionalities in a single carrier is quite a challenge. First, the chemistries used for the attachment of molecules on the carriers are often associated with several problems regarding the control of the bioconjugate valence, orientation of the targeting moiety, and a loss of activity due to moiety–moiety or carrier–carrier cross-linking. In addition, it is not always possible to efficiently purify the final product

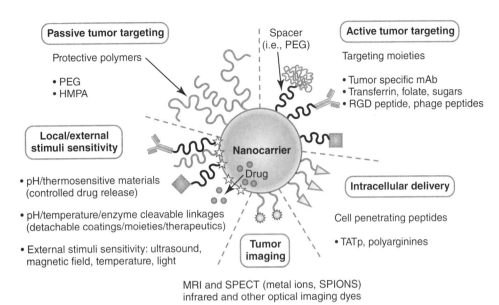

FIGURE 8-2 Multifunctional nanocarriers tailored to the tumor.

(i.e., low-conjugate valence and similar size between carrier and ligand). Obviously, the complexity of these chemistries and protocols multiplies when two or more molecules need to be incorporated in the same carrier. Second, the multifunctional approach usually involves a sequential display of the different functionalities from the application site to the intracellular destination. Multifunctional carriers should be ables to switch on (exposure) and switch off (hinder/lose) the attached functional group along the way in an orchestrated manner (**Figure 8–3**).

The combination of long circulation and targetability functionalities in a single system can serve as an example. Upon intravenous application, PEG surface modification of liposomes prolongs their blood circulation and masks targeting ligands or surface functional groups by reducing their association with plasma proteins and tissues nonspecifically. Once the tumor site is reached, however, the targeting moieties should readily interact with tumor cells. The PEG protective function is no longer needed. Moreover, it may prevent the association of the targeted carrier with the cell surface. To deal with this inconvenience, detachable protective coatings are used. A cleavable PEG-coating may provide the prolonged circulation time of liposomes and micelles and reconstitute the tumor cellular affinity for such carriers after arriving at the tumor location by detachment of the protective polymer chains at the relatively acidic pH of the tumoral mass [55, 56].

Chemical or physical conjugation of proteins, peptides, polymers, and other molecules to a carrier required to produce a multifunctional pharmaceutical nanocarrier can proceed covalently or non-covalently. The attachment can be performed covalently, via reactive groups generated on the carrier surface and by certain groups in the molecule. From a practical point of view, some of the most frequently used reactions for chemical attachment of moieties include (1) the reaction between an activated carboxyl group and amine group to yield an amide bond, (2) the reaction between maleimide groups and thiols to yield thioether bonds, (3) reactions between pyridyldithiols and thiols to yield disulfide bonds, and (4) the reaction between a succinimidyl group and amine to yield amide bonds.

Carbodiimide activation (i.e., 1-ethyl-3-(3-dimethylaminopropyl) carbodiimide hydrochloride, EDC) is one of the most popular bioconjugate reactions between carboxylated nanocarriers and aminated moieties or vice versa. Poly (lactide-co-glycolic

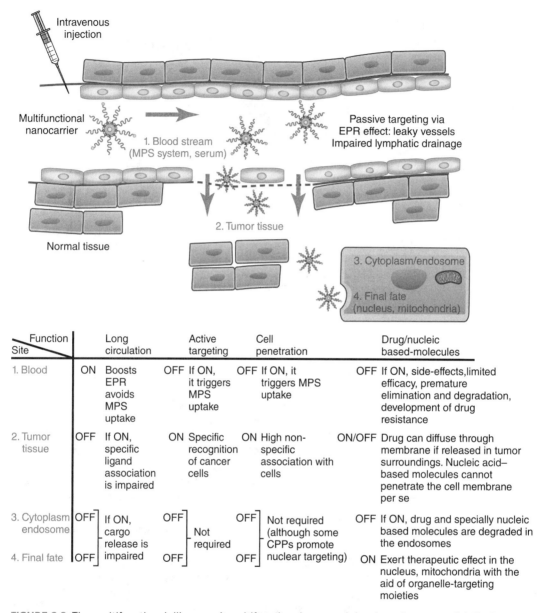

Function / Site	Long circulation		Active targeting		Cell penetration		Drug/nucleic based-molecules	
1. Blood	ON	Boosts EPR avoids MPS uptake	OFF	If ON, it triggers MPS uptake	OFF	If ON, it triggers MPS uptake	OFF	If ON, side-effects, limited efficacy, premature elimination and degradation, development of drug resistance
2. Tumor tissue	OFF	If ON, specific ligand association is impaired	ON	Specific recognition of cancer cells	ON	High non-specific association with cells	ON/OFF	Drug can diffuse through membrane if released in tumor surroundings. Nucleic acid–based molecules cannot penetrate the cell membrane per se
3. Cytoplasm endosome	OFF	If ON, cargo release is impaired	OFF	Not required	OFF	Not required (although some CPPs promote nuclear targeting)	OFF	If ON, drug and specially nucleic based molecules are degraded in the endosomes
4. Final fate	OFF		OFF		OFF		ON	Exert therapeutic effect in the nucleus, mitochondria with the aid of organelle-targeting moieties

FIGURE 8-3 The multifunctional dilemma. A multifunctional approach involves the sequential display of different functionalities along the way between the application site and the therapeutic target. Multifunctional nanocarriers should be able to switch on (exposure) and switch off (hinder/lose) the attached functional moieties in an orchestrated order that depends on their location in the body.

acid) nanoparticles were activated via EDC/NHS (N–hydroxysuccinimide) and further reacted with RGD (L–arginine, glycine and L–aspartic acid) peptide and epidermal growth factor antibody to produce efficient and targeted delivery of anticancer drugs to breast cancer [57]. Similarly, activated immunoglobulins can be attached to the exposed ethanolamine groups of PE-containing liposomes [58]. The main disadvantage of EDC activation is the instability of the intermediate reactive that is easily hydrolyzed. The excess of EDC reagent required for the complete activation of carboxylic groups may overactivate the carrier surface and lead to the precipitation of the conjugate. On the other hand, carboxylic- (aspartic acid, glutamic acid) and amine- (hystidine, lysine) containing amino acids are generally equally present in most proteins and antibodies. Activation of carboxylic acids can drive protein–protein cross-linking or a random orientation of the antibody with a subsequent decrease of the binding activity [59]. By contrast, the presence of thiol groups is either less ubiquitous in proteins or absent. In the case of non-thiol–containing proteins, the thiol group can be added via heterobifunctional cross-linkers such as *N*-succinimidyl-3(2-pyridyldithio) propionate and others [60, 61]. Reactions between thiol-containing proteins or antibodies and maleimide or pyridyldithiol modified carriers are highly effective and selective [62]. Apart from thiolation of proteins and antibodies, the formation of a carbonyl via formation of Schiff bases can be used between amino groups in the protein- (antibody) and carbohydrate-containing carriers (glycolipids) [63] or vice versa [64]. Covalent attachment reactions of antibodies and proteins are reviewed in detail elsewhere [60, 65].

Non-covalent methods used to bind polymers and ligands to a nanocarrier surface proceed via the hydrophobic absorption of certain intrinsic or specially inserted hydrophobic moieties in the ligands. Our group reported a novel approach for targeting liposomes through their fusion with purified coat proteins of a target-specific landscape phage. The "membranophilic" nature of phage coat proteins drives them to integrate into liposomes and micelles without further chemical modification [66]. In most other cases, however, ligands and polymers need to be modified to be adsorbed on the hydrophobic surface nanoparticles or incorporated into the phospholipid membrane of liposomes or hydrophobic core of micelles. Nanoparticles can be easily decorated with protective polymers (poloxamer) by hydrophobic interactions. The adsorbed polymers, however, are prone to desorb upon administration. Therefore, covalent attachment between PEG with another biodegradable polymer, such as poly(lactic acid), poly(lactide-co-glycolic acid), or polyalkylcyanoacrylates, are typically used to achieve long-term circulation and MPS avoidance of nanoparticles [67].

Different moieties can be incorporated into micelles or liposomes by incubation of hydrophobically modified proteins (monoclonal antibody 2C5), peptides (trans-activating transcriptional activator, TAT, peptide), polymers (polyethylenimine, PEG), or small molecules (ascorbate) with preformed plain liposomes or micelles via a postinsertion technique [68]. Such a protocol offers several advantages over direct chemical attachment protocols. Because no reactive groups are generated in the carrier, postinsertion protocols prevent side reactions with drug or other lipid components. In addition, this process ensures the correct orientation of ligand moieties facing out on the surface of the liposomes. Among the hydrophobic blocks, phosphatidyelthanolamine (PE) is frequently used because it can be easily derivatized into a variety of functional groups such as maleimido or pyridyldithiopropionoylamino that are very convenient for bioconjugation purposes.

Another useful tool for the design of multifunctional systems is the use of PEG chains as spacer arms between the functional moiety (ligand) and the hydrophobic anchor group. A careful selection and combination of the different commercially available PEG lengths can provide, for example, a better selective targeting of antibodies in long-circulating systems. By attaching ligands via the PEG spacer (long PEG chain) to the carrier, the ligand is extended out of the masking PEG coat (shorter PEG chain) avoiding steric hindrances for its binding to the targeted receptors [69, 70]. Similarly, different PEG-PE lengths have been used to optimize the selectivity of double-targeted doxorubicin liposomes. Monoclonal antibody (150 kDa) and folic acid (441 Da) were coupled to PEG-PE 2000 Da and PEG-PE 3350 Da, respectively, to account for the different molecular weight of the attached moieties [71]. With these possibilities in mind, several types of end-group functionalized PEG-PE were developed, including pyridyldithiopropionoylamino-PEG-PE [72], maleimido-PEG [73], and p-nitrophenylcarbonyl-PEG-PE [74].

The carboxylic group of folic acid is preferentially modified by carboiimide activation to react with amine groups of nanocarriers such as albumin [75] or chitosan [76]. Non-covalent attachment of folic acid lipoplexes for gene delivery showed greater efficacy than that of folic acid conjugated lipoplexes [77]. Sugar ligands, such as galactosamine or galactose, were attached to albumin nanoparticles via carboiimide chemistry to provide specific recognition of asialoglycoprotein receptors of liver cancer cells [78, 79]. The same functionalization of micelles improved cytotoxicity to HepG2 cells by delivering encapsulated paclitaxel intracellularly [80].

ACTIVE/PASSIVE TARGETED NANOCARRIERS: A PROLONGED CIRCULATION AND TARGETABILITY COMBINATION

Each level of biological organization presents unique barriers to the delivery of therapeutic agents such as binding to non-specific molecules in blood circulation, opsonization and increase in rate of clearance, nonspecific uptake, selectivity and permeability of biological membranes, metabolizing enzymes, and endosomal/lysosomal degradation. Considering these barriers, the focus of drug delivery systems should be on optimization of pharmacokinetics and biodistribution parameters. Practically, pharmaceutical agents are distributed within the body rather evenly, proportionally to the regional blood flow. To reach the site of action, they have to cross many biological barriers, where they can be inactivated or produce undesirable effects on normal tissues. As a result, to achieve the required therapeutic concentration within a body compartment, one has to administer the drug in large quantities. The greater part is wasted, however, in normal tissues. Additional widespread cytotoxic or immunogenic side effects are inevitable. Drug targeting helps bring a solution to these problems. The goal of designing a targeted drug delivery system is to increase accumulation of an active pharmaceutical ingredient in therapeutic target sites rather than in non-specific tissues and improve the therapeutic index.

Tumor passive targeting relies on the EPR phenomenon [44]. As mentioned above, those nanoparticles that gain interstitial access to the tumor have higher retention times than normal tissues. Clearly, an EPR-based type of targeting requires macromolecular drugs and drug delivery systems with a prolonged systemic circulation time to provide a sufficient level of accumulation at an abnormal site. Because the immune system recognizes plain nanocarriers as foreign particles and rapidly removes them from the circulation, almost all nanocarriers should be constructed to have a long-circulating property to facilitate the EPR effect. This also helps to achieve a better targeting effect for targeted (specific ligand modified) drugs and drug carriers when more time is allowed for their interaction with the target.

The most common method for prolonging the circulation of carriers is to "mask" them by modifying their surface with certain water-synthetic polymers, such as PEG [81,82]. In addition to its U.S. Food and Drug Administration approval, PEGylation provides a very attractive combination of properties as a protective polymer, including excellent solubility in water, high flexibility of the polymeric chain, and very low toxicity and immunogenicity [83]. PEG coating protects the nanocarrier and decreases the opsonization of drugs and drug carriers and their clearance by the MPS by several mechanisms, including shielding of the surface charge, increased surface hydrophobicity [84], enhanced repulsive interaction between coated nanocarriers and blood [85], and formation of a polymeric layer over the carrier surface, which is impermeable to opsonins even at low PEG concentrations [86]. Commonly used molecular weights of PEG for modification of drugs range from 1,000 to 20,000 Da.

The PEG coating approach is best developed for liposomes [16]. Long-circulating liposomes and other nanocarriers demonstrate dose-independent, non-saturable, log-linear kinetics and increased bioavailability [87]. The anticancer drug doxorubicin incorporated into long-circulating PEG-coated liposomes currently used in clinical conditions has high efficacy in EPR-based tumor therapy and strongly diminishes doxorubicin's side effects [88]. PEG-b-poly(amino acid)–based micelles loaded with cisplatin were designed for passive drug targeting into tumors and are now undergoing clinical trials [89].

Although passive targeting approaches form the basis of clinical therapy, they suffer from several limitations. Ubiquitously targeting cells within a tumor is not always feasible because some drugs cannot diffuse efficiently and the random nature of the approach makes it difficult to control the process. This lack of control may induce multiple-drug resistance [90]. One way to overcome these limitations is to program the nanocarriers so they actively bind to specific cells (active targeting) after extravasation. This binding is achieved by attachment of targeting molecules such as antibodies, sugars, or ligand–receptor binding moieties to the surface of the nanocarrier by a variety of conjugation chemistries [16].

In fact, combining the property of the specific target recognition to the carrier's ability to circulate for a prolonged period is one of the best-developed approaches for the production of more-than-one-function nanocarriers. Receptor-directed targeting of ligand-bearing drug-loaded nanocarriers results in selective binding to tumor cells and intracellular delivery of the drug. A number of targeting ligands have been tested in recent years, including antibodies against growth factor receptors, such as anti-epidermal growth factor receptor and anti-Her2 [91]; antibodies targeting the tumor cell surface [92]; and natural ligands to commonly over-expressed receptors in cancer cells, such as luteinizing hormone-releasing hormone, somatostatin, transferrin, and folate [54, 93, 94].

Among the specific ligands, antibodies provide the broadest opportunity in terms of diversity of targets and specificity of interaction. Antibody fragments containing only the variable region of the antibody are now more commonly used for active targeting of therapeutics because they retain the specificity for their target and lack the constant Fc effector region that can result in complement activation or undesirable interaction with other cells, potentially leading to premature phagocytosis of the drug delivery system [95]. An important limiting factor in the use of antibodies for therapeutic purposes has been their immunogenicity. More recently, to address this problem, antibodies that are 100% human have been developed. The final concern for the incorporation methods is to maintain the antibody specificity. Antibodies can be bound to the nanocarrier in a number of ways, some of which can block access to the binding site and consequently decrease the activity of the antibody [96]. If the immunonanoparticle attaches to vascular endothelial cells via a non-internalizing epitope, high local concentrations of the drug will be available on the outer surface of the target cell. Although this has a higher efficiency than free drug released into the circulation, only a fraction of the released drug will be delivered to the target cell. In most cases, internalization of the nanoparticle is important for effective delivery of some anticancer drugs, especially in gene delivery, gene silencing, and other biotherapeutics [97]. To achieve a better selective targeting by PEG-coated liposomes or other particulates, targeting ligands are attached to nanocarriers via the PEG spacer arm, so that ligand is extended out of the dense PEG brush [74, 98]. It was shown that PEG-immunoliposomes prepared by the conjugation of antibody fragments (Fab' or single-chain Fv) to liposome-grafted PEG chains do not increase tumor localization with respect to only PEGylated liposomes but to increased internalization and are correlated with superior antitumor activity in animal models.

A nice example of how the addition of the targeting function onto long-circulating drug-loaded nanocarriers can significantly enhance the activity of the drug was obtained when we showed that the nucleosome-specific monoclonal antibody, 2C5 mAb, capable of recognition of various tumor cells by cell-surface binding of nucleosomes improved Doxil® (doxorubicin in PEGylated liposomes) targeting to tumor and increased its cytotoxicity against various tumor cell lines [99] and against primary and metastatic tumors in mice [70, 100]. Studies had involved the coupling of transferrin or folate to PEGylated liposomes to combine longevity and targetability for improved therapeutic activity [101, 102]. PEG-polycaprolactone–based particles were surface modified with folate and, after loading with paclitaxel, increased cytotoxicity [103]. A dual-ligand long-circulating liposomal system composed of a specific ligand and a cell-penetrating peptide (CPP) was described that enhanced selectivity and cellular uptake [104].

ADDING LOCAL/EXTERNAL STIMULI SENSITIVITY TO NANOCARRIERS

Further development of the multifunctional approach involves the addition of certain stimuli-sensitive functions to long-circulating and targeted pharmaceutical nanocarriers to respond specifically to pathological triggers unique to sites of disease (e.g., temperature, pH or enzymatic catalysis, light, or magnetic fields).

PH-SENSITIVE NANOCARRIERS

Changes in pH are particularly useful for exploitation of the tumor environment and elaboration of suitable anti-cancer drug delivery systems. Apart from tumor acidosis, the low pH of endosomes can be used to maximize intracellular delivery of anticancer therapeutics. Current approaches toward the development of such systems generally involve either incorporation of "titratable" groups in the carrier platform to provoke the disruption of the endosomes or linkages that degrade under acidic conditions.

The most studied class of pH-sensitive liposomes requires fusogenic lipids in the liposome's composition, such as unsaturated 1,2-dioleoylphosphatidylethanolamine (DOPE), to render pH sensitivity to liposomes [105]. Such liposomes are capable of protonation and formation of non-bilayered structures at decreased pH and destabilizing liposomal, or both liposomal and endosomal, membranes with the subsequent drug/DNA release from liposomes or from liposomes plus endosomes [106]. Multifunctional, long-circulating, PEGylated, DOPE-containing, pH-sensitive liposomes, although having a decreased pH sensitivity, still effectively deliver their contents into the cytoplasm [107]. Serum-stable, long-circulating PEGylated, pH-sensitive liposomes were also prepared on the same liposome with a combination of a PEG and pH-sensitive terminally alkylated copolymer of N-isopropylacrylamide and methacrylic acid [108]. Combination of liposome pH sensitivity and a specific ligand for cytosolic targeting was described for transferrin-targeted liposome [109]. Promising results in terms of pH sensitivity and resistance to serum degradation were also obtained using a novel liposome formulation composed of phospahatidylcholine (PC), cholesterol hemisuccinate (CHEMS), oleyl alcohol, and Tween-80 [110]. Compared with DOPE-based pH-sensitive liposomes, the above formulation showed much better retention of its pH-sensitive properties in the presence of 10% serum. In addition, pH-responsive, membrane-destabilizing synthetic polymers have been investigated to enhance the cytoplasmic delivery of therapeutic genes or oligonucleotides.

Polyethylenimine or polyamidoamine dendrimers, known as proton sponge polymers, have the ability to strongly protonate under the acidic pH inside endosomes and to interact with endosomal membrane, inducing its destabilization and promoting the release of the condensed genetic material to the cytoplasm [111]. As an alternative to the systemic toxicity associated with cationic polymers, anionic pH-responsive polymers such as alkylamine derivatives of poly (styrene–alt–maleic anhydride) have been developed recently. These are amphiphilic polymers that contain a critical balance of acidic carboxyl groups and hydrophobic moieties. The carboxylate ions of these polymers become protonated at endosomal pH values, and the polymers undergo a change from a hydrophilic and biologically inert state to a hydrophobic and membrane-destabilizing one. Poly (styrene–alt–maleic anhydride) was incorporated in a micellar carrier to simultaneously load therapeutic small interfering RNA (siRNA) and doxorubicin for drug-resistant ovarian cancer treatment [112].

A special case of a stimulus-sensitive system is the long-circulating nanocarrier capable of losing its PEG protective coat under the influence of low pH or increased temperature. As mentioned previously, PEG chains protect the target carrier from opsonization in the blood but also may prevent the ligand from cell surface recognition and may delay the release of the DNA/drug content in the cytoplasm. A variety of liposomes [113] and polymeric micelles [114] has been described that includes components with acid-labile bonds as well as a variety of drug conjugates capable of releasing drugs such as paclitaxel [115], and doxorubicin [116–118] under acidic conditions.

The stimuli-sensitive PEG coatings are especially interesting for multifunctional approaches because they allow preparation of carriers with hidden functions. So-called SMART delivery systems based on targeted PEG-PE micelles and PEGylated liposomes that display several functionalities have been described [119]. These SMART carriers specifically recognized cells in tumors or infarcted areas by an attached antinucleosome antibody or antimyosin antibody with a long PEG spacer and nonspecifically by an attached TAT peptide (non-specific cell-penetrating peptide, TATp) via a short PEG spacer. The PEG-PE used for the preparation of the liposomes or micelles was degradable by insertion of a pH-cleavable linkage. At normal pH, TATp function was shielded by the long, degradable PEG chains. The carriers showed high specific binding via the antibody but low internalization due to TATp shielding. After pre-incubation at lower pH values (5.0–6.0), however, these SMART nanocarriers lost the PEG coating and were effectively internalized via TATp.

Another interesting approach to revealing targeted ligands in response to the weakly acidic tumor tissue was proposed by Lee and collaborators [120]. The system includes a mixture of PEG–poly (l-histidine) and ligand-functionalized poly (l-lactic acid)–PEG–poly (l-histidine)–biotin. At pH 7.4, biotin ligands are buried within the PEG shell at the interface between the hydrophilic corona and the hydrophobic core. A slight decrease in pH preferentially ionizes the histidine side chains in the poly (l-lactic acid)–PEG–poly (l-histidine)–biotin segment of the micelle, increases the hydrophilicity of the biotin-terminated poly (l-histidine) block, and allows its extension into the hydrophilic corona to display the biotin beyond the PEG shell to then markedly increase the carrier's uptake in breast adenocarcinoma cells expressing biotin receptors. Extension of this approach to a TATp moiety produced a 30-fold increase in cellular uptake at pH 7.0 and in greater doxorubicin cytotoxicity for micelles than for free doxorubicin in drug-resistant breast tumor cells [121].

Another nice example of how a stimuli-sensitive PEG coat can help to harmonize prolonged circulation times without impairing ligand binding and uptake by target cells was reported [122]. Cysteine-cleavable phospholipid–PEG was used to "mask" folate-targeted liposomes. Long, cleavable PEG–phospholipid conjugates mask folate during circulation to enable passive targeting but detach at the tumor site by external administration of cysteine. The resultant exposure of folate enables targeting to cells that over-express the folate receptor. *In vivo* studies confirmed enhanced intracellular delivery when tumor-bearing animals received targeted liposomes containing cleavable phospholipid–PEG 5000 followed by a cysteine infusion.

Temperature-Sensitive Nanocarriers

Many pathological areas demonstrate distinct hyperthermia (e.g., 42°C in human ovarian carcinoma). This can be used to design nanocarriers responsive to high temperature. In addition, tumor cells seem to be more sensitive to heat-induced damage than normal cells, and this can also be used as an adjunct to radiation or chemotherapy. This technique is called the magnetic thermal ablation technique [123]. Most clinical studies with hyperthermia have used super-paramagnetic iron oxide–containing liposomes or nanoparticles [124]. Nanocarriers provide a method for localization of the iron oxide particles. It is appealing because unlike the external probes that can heat the surrounding normal tissues, magnetic nanoparticle hyperthermia offers a way to largely ensure that only the intended target is heated [125] (see Magnetically Sensitive Nanocarriers).

For construction of smart materials showing a thermo-responsive function, temperature-responsive polymers, which change their conformation and physical properties in response to temperature change, have been extensively used in the drug delivery field. They undergo coil-to-globule transitions in water above a specific temperature, called the lower critical solution temperature. A series of poly (N–substituted acrylamide) derivatives are known to have thermal phase transitions at various temperatures, depending on their individual chemical structures. For delivery of adriamycin to a target site, thermo-responsive polymeric micelles were prepared from amphiphilic block copolymers composed of *N*-isopropylacrylamide (to provide a thermo–responsive outer shell) and styrene (a hydrophobic inner core) [126].

Temperature-sensitive liposomes frequently include dipalmitoylphosphatidylcholine (DPPC) as their key component, because liposomes usually become leaky at a gel-to-liquid crystalline phase transition. This transition for DPPC takes place at 41°C [127]. Liposomes can also be made temperature sensitive via the incorporation of certain polymers that display a lower critical solution temperature slightly above the typical physiological one [128]. Thermosensitive liposomes composed of DPPC lipid and Brij [78] demonstrate faster release of doxorubicin at 40 to 41°C (100% release in 2–3 minutes) compared with the lyso-lipid temperature-sensitive liposomes (composed of dipalmitoyl phosphatidylcholine, DPPC, myristoyl-2-stearoyl-sn-glycerol-3-phosphocholine, MSPC, and 1,2-distearoyl-sn-glycerol-3-phosphoethanolamine-N-[amino(polyethylene glycol)-2000] DSPE-PEG), a formulation that is currently in clinical trials. The new formulation showed increased drug delivery to the locally heated tumor compared with lyso-lipid temperature-sensitive liposomes and enhanced drug uptake compared with free doxorubicin. A single dose of the thermo-sensitive liposomes in combination with localized hyperthermia enhanced tumor regression and exhibited little toxicity [129]. Finally, multifunctional pH- and thermo-sensitive polymeric micelles were prepared from triblock copolymers composed of a thermo-sensitive block, a pH-sensitive block, and another hydrophobic block [130].

Redox Potential-Sensitive Nanocarriers

Redox-responsive vehicles are designed to disassemble and release drugs in the cytosol, which contains a two- to three-order of magnitude higher level of glutathione (approximately 2–10 mM) than the extracellular fluids (approximately 2–20 μM) [131]. The two distinct redox environments of intra- and extracellular spaces provide an opportunity for programmed delivery of drugs and genes. A drug or gene molecule can be entrapped or encapsulated in a nanocarrier that is held together by disulfide bonds. Once the disulfide bonds of a nanocarrier are reduced in the presence of a low reducing potential due to an excess of reduced glutathione inside the cell, the drug or gene present in the nanocarrier is released [132]. Redox-responsive liposomes have been prepared from the standard phospholipids with the addition of a small quantity of a lipid in which its head and tail are linked by the disulfide bond [133]. Redox-responsive long-circulating liposomes with a detachable PEG coat were also investigated [134]. Disulfide bonds have been used to improve intracellular delivery of plasmid DNA [135, 136] and oligonucleotides [137]. We developed redox-responsive micelles for siRNA delivery. Double-stranded siRNA was attached to PE via a disulfide bond and incorporated into PEG-PE micelles. The siRNA was well protected against degradation by nucleases and easily released from the micelles in a free and bioactive form in the presence of glutathione at typical intracellular concentrations [138].

MAGNETICALLY SENSITIVE NANOCARRIERS

Another approach to the use of drug carriers is to co-load them with magnetic nanoparticles to allow for the manipulation of a system in a magnetic field or with metallic nanoparticles, which respond to the external electromagnetic fields and control the rate of drug release by oscillation or heating of the carrier [139]. Magnetic nanoparticles were first designed for magnetic resonance imaging (MRI) via passive targeting. Currently, some superparamagnetic iron oxide nanoparticles (SPIONs) are in early clinical trials, and several formulations have been approved for medical imaging, such as Feridex®, Combidex®, or Ferumoxytol® [140]. SPIONs consist of cores made of iron oxides that can be targeted to an area of interest by external magnets. In addition to their superparamagnetic properties, SPION sizes can vary between several nanometers and several hundred nanometers in diameter [141], and they are biocompatible and biodegradable [142]. Because of these properties, magnetic drug targeting with SPIONs has received increased attention using advances in nanotechnology. To increase their stability, circulation half-life, and biocompatibility, SPIONs are coated with polymers including dextran [143], organic silane [144] or PEG, and polyethylene oxide. Targeting of magnetic polycaprolactone nanoparticles loaded with gemcitabine in a pancreatic cancer xenograft mouse model was reported using external magnets [145]. Cinteza et al. [146] also reported co-loading polymeric micelles of diacylphospholipid-PEG with the photosensitizing drug 2-[1-hexyloxyethyl]-2-devinyl pyropheophorbide and magnetic SPIONs for magnetic drug targeting *in vitro* [146].

LIGHT-SENSITIVE NANOCARRIERS

Light-responsive nanocarriers have also gained some recent attention. Design of light-sensitive systems that undergo reverse micellization/disruption by light exposure is an attractive idea that allows external control of drug release [147]. The potential biomedical utility of such carriers was first shown with PEG micelles that released their contents under infrared light exposure [148]. Later on, light-induced fusion [149] or destabilization [150] of liposomes was reported.

Photodynamic therapy is also a promising approach for the treatment of malignant tumors and macular degeneration. Photodynamic therapy involves the systemic administration of photosensitizers, followed by the local application of a laser with a specific wavelength to a diseased site [151]. Photo-irradiation generates highly reactive singlet oxygen, thereby generating light-induced cytotoxicity (photocytotoxicity). In photodynamic therapy, the development of delivery systems for photosensitizers has received much attention for improvement of the selectivity and effectiveness of photodynamic therapy as well as the prevention of side effects such as skin hypersensitivity. Polymeric micelles [152] have been studied as vehicles for photosensitizers.

A novel photo-activated targeted chemotherapy was developed by photochemical internalization (PCI) of glutathione-sensitive polymeric micelles incorporating camptothecin prepared from thiolated camptothecin and thiolated PEG-b-poly (glutamic acid). PCI allows macromolecules located in the carrier to reach the cytosol and exert their effect instead of being degraded by lysosomal hydrolases. PCI uses light with relevant wavelengths in the near infrared region that allows a therapeutic effect on lesions deeper in the targeted tissues with negligible damage to adjacent healthy tissue. In addition, after PCI the macromolecules become exposed to the extremely reductive environment of the cytosol because the concentration of glutathione in the cytosol is 100 to 1,000 times higher than that in blood. PCI can be an efficient stimulus for specific drug carrier activation. Consequently, the combination of PCI and drug carriers responsive to a reductive environment idealizes the spatial and temporal triggering of a drug's action after photo-irradiation of polymeric micelles for the delivery of chemotherapeutics and photosensitizing agents both *in vitro* and *in vivo* [153, 154].

ULTRASOUND-SENSITIVE NANOCARRIERS

Drug delivery and release from nanocarriers may also be triggered by external ultrasound. The drug release may be induced by the mechanical effects associated with ultrasound, such as transient cavitation, where liposomes containing a small quantity of air or perfluorated hydrocarbon (initially developed as an ultrasound contrast agent) can be loaded with various drugs that are released after applied ultrasound [155, 156]. Ultrasound has been used for targeted delivery to a tumor by local sonication after the injection of a micellar encapsulated drug. In addition to tumor uptake, this technique promotes the uniform distribution of micelles and drug throughout the tumor [157].

OTHER STIMULI-SENSITIVE NANOCARRIERS

Nanocarriers may also be activated by an enzyme overexpressed in a tumor by release of the drug from a nanocarrier by the cleavage of a linker of the carrier polymers. For example, a drug–polymer conjugate was created by conjugating methotrexate to dextran via a peptide linker that could be cleaved by metalloproteinase-2 and metalloproteinase-9, two important tumor-associated enzymes [158]. Interestingly, PEG linkages that cleaved in the presence of a metalloproteinase-rich environment were incorporated into long-circulating conjugates that enhanced cellular uptake and endosomal escape of systemically administered siRNA [159].

INTRACELLULAR PENETRATION AND SUBCELLULAR TARGETING OF NANOCARRIERS

The ability of multifunctional nanocarriers to specifically and non-specifically accumulate in a tumor does not guarantee successful delivery of anticancer drugs. Most anticancer drugs and macromolecules must be delivered intracellularly to exert a therapeutic effect in the cytoplasm (e.g., tubulin-targeted cisplatin, antisense oligonucelotides, siRNA), the nucleus (e.g., doxorubicin, plasmid DNA), or other organelles such as mitochondria (e.g., pro-apoptotic drugs). In general, anticancer drugs diffuse through the cell membrane by virtue of their small size and/or hydrophobicity, although evidence suggests a number of active uptake and efflux mechanisms may be responsible for the increased or reduced accumulation of drug in sensitive or resistant cancer cells, respectively [160]. By contrast, large therapeutic macromolecules and a drug with hydrophilic nature cannot cross the cellular membrane unless they are associated with a carrier for active transport.

The therapeutic significance of targeted nanocarriers carrying anticancer drugs remains difficult to predict and may vary depending on the tumor model used and on the ligand-receptor interaction [161, 162]. Even if molecules (loaded or not in nanocarriers) enter the cells by an endocytic pathway, they can become entrapped by endosomes and lysosomes where enzymatic degradation significantly decreases the availability of the therapeutic molecules, especially nucleic acid–based ones. Therefore, there is a clear necessity to impart, in addition to long circulation and targetability functions, additional mechanisms that enhance the penetration of the carriers into the cytoplasm, aid escape from endosomal entrapment, and target specific organelles.

CHARGE MODIFICATION OF NANOCARRIERS

The easiest way to improve intracellular delivery of drug-loaded nanocarriers is the addition of positive charge via incorporation of cationic polymers or lipids. Cationization of nanocarriers has been extensively used for gene delivery [163–165]. When negatively charged nucleic acid–based molecules (DNA, antisense oligonucleotides, siRNA) are mixed with cationic lipids or polymers, complexes are formed through sequence-independent electrostatic interactions between negatively charged phosphate groups of the nucleic acid and protonated (positively charged) primary amino groups on the carrier, giving rise to particles termed polyplexes, lipoplexes, or dendriplexes depending on the carriers nature (polymeric, lipidic, or dendrimeric). The overall slightly positive charge of the nanocarrier facilitates the interaction of the particle with proteoglycans responsible for the negative charge on the cell surface. Among cationic carriers, polyethylenimine, polyamidoamine, or polypropylenimine dendrimers and the lipids N-[1-(2,3-Dioleoyloxy)propyl]-N,N,N-trimethylammonium chloride (DOTAP) or N-[1-(2,3-dioleyloxy)propyl]-N,N,N-trimethylammonium chloride (DOTMA) have demonstrated enhancement of intracellular delivery *in vitro* and *in vivo* [166–168]. As discussed above (see pH–Sensitive Nanocarriers), some of these cationic carriers are considered to be proton sponges that provide an intrinsic mechanism for escape from endosomes and achievement of a high transgene expression.

INTRACELLULAR DELIVERY OF ANTICANCER DRUGS AND GENES BY CPPS

An interesting and relatively recent approach in intracellular delivery of drugs and genes is the use of certain proteins and peptides that have the unique ability to penetrate cells by a so-call transduction phenomenon. CPPs or membrane permeant peptides are known to be good vehicle moieties that improve the intracellular uptake of macromolecules such as proteins [169, 170] and nanoparticulate systems [171, 172]. They consist of short amino acid chains, fewer than 20 amino acids, made mainly of positively charged arginine and lysine that are responsible for the translocation of peptides through the plasma membrane [173]. Examples of such CPPs include transportan, VP22, Antennapedia, and synthetic polyarginines such as HIV-1 Rev or DNA-binding peptides (c-Jun, c-Fos) [174, 175].

TATp, an 11-mer peptide derived from HIV-1, is an example of an arginine-rich cell-penetrating peptide. TATp is highly cationic with six arginine and two lysine residues. This positive charge is essential for its promotion of cellular uptake. The substitution of basic (cationic) residues with neutral alanine reduced the activity of the peptide, whereas substitution of TATp's neutral residues had no effect [176, 177]. It has been hypothesized that the positive charge in TATp provides for a strong electrostatic interaction with anionic species at the extracellular surface of cell membranes, including lipid head groups, proteins like nucleolin, and proteoglycans such as heparin sulfate [178, 179]. Regarding the cell entry mechanism of CPPs, more than one mechanism has been proposed that depends on the size of the cargo attached to the CPPs [180]. Single CPPs or CPPs conjugating small molecules penetrate cells via energy independent electrostatic interactions or hydrogen bonding and translocate through the formation of micromicelles at the membrane [181] or by direct translocation through the lipid bilayer [182, 183]. CPP-mediated transport of large molecules and nanoparticles has been reported to occur via energy-dependent routes such as via caveolae, macropinocytosis [184], a clathrin-dependent pathway, and others [180]. The prevalence of one route over the others may depend on several factors such as the concentration, the net charge, the hydrophobicity, and other physicochemical parameters of the CPPs; the nature of the cargo; the cell line; and the conditions of incubation [180].

Since the discovery two decades ago of TATp transduction and its use to deliver macromolecules into cells [185–187], an impressive variety of TATp-linked nanocarriers and cargoes have been investigated both *in vitro* and *in vivo*. TATp-mediated cytoplasmic uptake of nucleic acids, drugs, polymers, nanoparticles, liposomes, and micelles into cells of all organ types and, interestingly, the brain have been reported [188, 189]. The precise mechanism of CPPs translocation through the highly discriminating blood–brain barrier, however, remains unclear [189, 190].

The cell-penetrating function can be combined with the stimuli-sensitivity function. As noted, the combination of PEGylated liposomes or micelles with TATp can enhance uptake in a pH-sensitive carrier (see SMART carriers, above). The exploitation of an acidic extracellular pH has also been described for HA-2 peptide [191] and the TAT-HA chimera [192] as well as enzymatically cleavable TAT conjugates [193].

CPPs are highly efficient *in vitro*. However, the *in vivo* use of CPPs appears to be much more complicated. CPP nanocarriers and their corresponding cargoes are dispersed almost everywhere upon injection. After intraperitoneal injection, TATp fused to β-galactosidase was found in the lung, liver, kidney, and other tissues [194]. To overcome their absence of specificity, a combination of CPP moieties and active targeting moieties has been proposed. For example, we suggested liposomes or PEG-PE micelles decorated simultaneously with TATp and nucleosome-specific antibody (2C5 mAb) [119]. Polyethylene oxide-b-polycaprolactone micelles simultaneously targeted with TATp and the integrin-specific ligand RGD demonstrated intracellular co-delivery of doxorubicin and siRNA targeted to P-glycoprotein and tumor targeting in an animal model [195].

IMAGE-GUIDED DRUG DELIVERY AND DIAGNOSTIC THERANOSTIC NANOCARRIERS

When talking about design of multifunctional nanocarriers, contrast reporter moieties are the cherry on the cake. The simultaneous delivery of therapeutic and contrast agents in a nanosized carrier, called a theranostic carrier, gives essential information to physicians such as the visualization of real-time biodistribution of an anticancer drug, the target accumulation, visualization of drug release, and information to help predict the drug response.

A great variety of contrast agents is used in imaging modalities, such as near-infrared imaging, MRI, positron emission tomography, and others. Usually, theranostic multifunctional systems are composed of a core material (platform), the therapeutic cargo, the imaging cargo, and functionalities to enhance blood circulation duration or tumor targeting. The development of nanosystems carrying different imaging agents for multimodal imaging is also an emerging field [196]. For example, a multimodal imaging system based on superparamagnetic particles (for MRI) was covalently attached with paclitaxel (an anticancer drug), rhodamine (for optical imaging), and folate (a targeting moiety) and showed targeting enhancement of apoptosis and simultaneous tracking of their intracellular pathways due to its optical and magnetic properties [197]. In another study, multimodal nanoparticles consisting of dextran-coated superparamagnetic nanoparticles (for MRI), labeled with Cy5.5 dye (for near-anfrared fluorescence imaging, NIRF), conjugated to a synthetic siRNA duplex targeting a gene of interest, and modified with myristoylated polyarginine peptides to provide membrane translocation were investigated [198]. The delivery of the probe was monitored *in vivo* by MRI and optical imaging, and efficient gene silencing was achieved in 9L rat gliosarcoma tumors.

Among theranostic carriers, liposomes and micelles are receiving greater attention. Liposomes have been widely used as gamma and MRI contrast carriers. They can easily incorporate heavy metal ions in their interior via chelation with a soluble chelator, such as diethylenetriaminepentaacetic acid, or in the liposome exterior via hydrophobic interaction of the liposome surface and hydrophobic-modified diethylenetriaminepentaacetic acid, during or after the preparation of the liposomes [199]. In addition, polychelating amphiphilic polymers have been used to improve the loading and increase the signal of the contrast agent of the carrier. Polychelating amphiphilic polymers consist of a main polymer chain with multiple side chelating groups that are able to bind many contrast agents and to be incorporated into hydrophobic nanoparticles, liposomes, or micelles [200]. Apart from metal ions (Gd, ^{99m}Tc, ^{111}In), nanoparticles [201], liposomes [202], and polymeric micelles [203] can be loaded or surface-modified with SPIONs as an alternative approach to direct conjugation of SPIONs with drugs [204, 205] and targeting moieties [203, 206]. In this regard, we recently developed and characterized PEG-PE–based micelles co-loaded with paclitaxel and SPIONs. The co-loading did not impair the properties of the drug or the SPIONs. The theranostic micelles showed good MRI contrast properties and high toxicity against cancer cells [216].

Stimuli sensitivity combined with a theranostic agent can promote controlled and locally targeted drug delivery. Multifunctional targeted pH-responsive SPION/doxorubicin loaded polymer vesicles were investigated [207]. The vesicles were formed in an aqueous solution by self-assembly of amphiphilic triblock copolymers: doxorubicin conjugated to polyglutamate via an acid-cleavable hydrazone bond and two different PEG acrylate segments (5000 and 2000 Da). Because of thermodynamic stabilization, the long PEG segments bearing folate or methoxy groups were segregated mostly on the outer hydrophilic PEG layer of the vesicle, providing active tumor targeting, whereas the short PEG segments bearing the acrylate groups were segregated primarily on the inner hydrophilic PEG layer of the vesicle, making cross-linking for improved *in vivo* stability possible. In addition, the vesicles exhibited strong pH-dependent drug release behavior. After 30 minutes, 40% of the drug was released at pH 5.3, whereas no drug release was observed at a neutral pH for up to 70 minutes. This result was highlighted as a desirable property that will minimize premature drug release in the circulation. Folate-conjugated vesicles exhibited higher cellular uptake than folate-free vesicles and led to higher cytotoxicity as well as enhanced MRI contrast, thereby making targeted cancer therapy and diagnosis possible.

FUTURE PERSPECTIVES

It is clear from the multiple examples illustrated in this chapter that the design and development of multifunctional carriers has achieved a high level of sophistication and mastery (Table 8-2). The most important issue that still needs to be addressed is the translation of these proven experimental concepts into products and clinical applications that will eventually use combined therapeutic and diagnostic nanocarriers that could dramatically improve the efficacy and accuracy of current traditional systems.

TABLE 8-2 Examples of Multifunctional Nanocarriers

Carrier	Therapeutic Agent	Functional Group 1	Functional Group 2	Functional Group 3	Reference
Liposome	Plasmid DNA	Esterase-cleavable PEG	Integrin-targeting peptides	—	208
PEI[1]	Plasmid DNA	Cleavable PEG via disulfide linkage	Tumor vasculature targeting cNGR peptide	—	136
Lipoplex	Plasmid DNA	Short ethylene glycol with ester linkage	Trifunctional peptides (DNA binding, integrin targeting, and endosomal enzymatic clevable linker)	—	209
Liposome	Plasmid DNA	PEG	Integrin targeting RGD peptide	Stearylated octaarginine (R8)	210
Liposome	siRNA	PEG	Gadolinium (MRI)	Rhodamine and Alexa Fluor (optical imaging)	211
Liposome	—	PEG	Folate	Gadolinium (MRI) Rhodamine (optical Imaging)	212
Micelle	Nile red	Acid-sensitive THP-protected HEMA (hidrophylic block)	Temperature-sensitive PNIPAM (hidrophobic block)	Disulfide bond (redox-sensitive linker)	213
Micelle	siRNA and doxorubicin	Integrin Rvβ3-specific ligand (RGD4C)	TAT peptide	Doxorubicin conjugated via hydrazone linkage	195
Nanoparticle (PLGA)	Dodetaxel	Folate	Quantum dots (-NIRF imaging)	—	214
Nanoparticle (SPION)	Paclitaxel	Folate	Rhodamine (optical imaging)	—	197
Drug–polymer conjugate	Temozolomide	PEG	Trileucine (pH-sensitive, endosomal scape)	Anti-transferrin receptor monoclonal antibody	215

PEI, polyethylenimine; cNGR, cyclic peptides containing the Asparagine-Glycine-Arginine motif; RGD (L-arginine, glycine and L-aspartic acid) peptide, THP Tetrahydropyran; HEMA, 2-hydroxyethyl methacrylate; PNIPAM, Poly(N-isopropylacrylamide; PLGA, poly(lactic-co-glycolic acid; NIRF near-infrared imaging.

SUMMARY

The use of nanocarriers for the delivery of therapeutic and diagnostic agents for cancer treatment has received significant attention in recent years. Several pharmaceutical nanocarriers have already demonstrated enhanced *in vivo* stability and efficiency, including some clinically approved liposome drug formulations and metallic imaging agents. The next generation of nanoscale delivery systems should be strategically engineered to simultaneously recognize malignant cells, visualize them by bearing contrast agents for enhanced sensitivity of medical imaging, improve drug effectiveness, and reduce side effects through selective targeting. To take advantage of the peculiarities of solid tumors, it may be useful to have nanocarriers simultaneously carrying on their surface various moieties that enable the performance of multiple functions. Carriers can be transformed into stable and long-circulating ones by modifying their surface with protective polymers (e.g., PEG) that accumulate (via the EPR effect) in the tumor. Tumor accumulation can be further boosted by attachment of specific ligands such as antibodies, peptides, folate, transferrin, or sugar moieties. Enhanced intracellular and targeted organelle delivery of anticancer drugs and nucleic acids can be achieved by decorating the surface of nanocarriers with CPPs and other moieties. Some of the carriers can be engineered to activate and rapidly release the drug content by a change of chemical stimulus (changes in the local environmental pH, Po_2, and redox balance), by the application of a rapidly oscillating magnetic field, or by application of a light or external heat source. Finally, the carrier can incorporate heavy metal–based diagnostics or contrast moieties via chelating compounds, such as ethylenediaminetetraacetic acid, diethylenetriaminepentaacetic acid, or deferoxamine.

REVIEW QUESTIONS

1. Discuss the state of the art of multifunctional nanocarriers by providing examples of multifunctional liposomes combining two, three, and four functionalities.
2. Explain why Doxil® (PEGylated liposomal doxorubicin) preferentially accumulates in tumors.
3. Discuss why it is important to provide multifunctional nanocarriers with a switch on/switch off mechanism. Give an example.
4. Propose how the treatment of other diseases can take advantage of the multifunctional approach.

REFERENCES

1. Torchilin V, ed. *Nanoparticulates as Drug Carriers*. London: Imperial College Press; 2006.
2. Fanciullino R, Ciccolini J. Liposome-encapsulated anticancer drugs: still waiting for the magic bullet? *Curr Med Chem.* 2009;16(33):4361–4371.
3. Peer D, Karp JM, Hong S, Farokhzad OC, Margalit R, Langer R. Nanocarriers as an emerging platform for cancer therapy. *Nat Nanotechnol.* 2007;2(12):751–760.
4. Dicko A, Mayer LD, Tardi PG. Use of nanoscale delivery systems to maintain synergistic drug ratios in vivo. *Expert Opin Drug Deliv.* 2010;7(12):1329–1341.
5. Magadala P, van Vlerken L, Shahiwala A, Amiji M. Multifunctional polymeric nanosystems for tumor-targeted delivery. In: Torchilin V, ed. *Multifunctional Pharmaceutical Nanocarriers*. Vol. 4. London: Springer Science+Business Media; 2008, 33–66.

6. Wang Y, Gao S, Ye WH, Yoon HS, Yang YY. Co-delivery of drugs and DNA from cationic core-shell nanoparticles self-assembled from a biodegradable copolymer. *Nat Mater.* 2006;5(10):791–796.

7. Ahmed F, Pakunlu RI, Brannan A, Bates F, Minko T, Discher DE. Biodegradable polymersomes loaded with both paclitaxel and doxorubicin permeate and shrink tumors, inducing apoptosis in proportion to accumulated drug. *J Control Release.* 2006;116(2):150–158.

8. Aryal S, Hu CM, Zhang L. Combinatorial drug conjugation enables nanoparticle dual-drug delivery. *Small.* 2010;6(13):1442–1448.

9. Stegemann S, Leveiller F, Franchi D, de Jong H, Linden H. When poor solubility becomes an issue: from early stage to proof of concept. *Eur J Pharm Sci.* 2007;31(5):249–261.

10. Soo PL, Dunne M, Liu J, Allen C. Nano-sized advanced delivery systems as parenteral formulation strategies for hydrophobic anti-cancer drugs. In: Villiers MM, Aramwit, P Kwon GS, eds. *Nanotechnology in Drug Delivery.* Vol. 10. New York: American Association of Pharmaceutical Scientists; 2009:349–383.

11. Liang XJ, Chen C, Zhao Y, Wang PC. Circumventing tumor resistance to chemotherapy by nanotechnology. *Methods Mol Biol.* 2010;596:467–488.

12. Vicent MJ, Duncan R. Polymer conjugates: nanosized medicines for treating cancer. *Trends Biotechnol.* 2006;24(1):39–47.

13. Stinchcombe TE. Nanoparticle albumin-bound paclitaxel: a novel Cremphor-EL-free formulation of paclitaxel. *Nanomedicine.* 2007;2(4):415–423.

14. Gardner ER, Dahut WL, Scripture CD, et al. Randomized crossover pharmacokinetic study of solvent-based paclitaxel and nab-paclitaxel. *Clin Cancer Res.* 2008;14(13):4200–4205.

15. Torchilin VP. Micellar nanocarriers: pharmaceutical perspectives. *Pharm Res.* 2007;24(1):1–16.

16. Torchilin VP. Recent advances with liposomes as pharmaceutical carriers. *Nat Rev Drug Discov.* 2005;4(2):145–160.

17. Discher DE, Ahmed F. Polymersomes. *Annu Rev Biomed Eng.* 2006;8:323–341.

18. Sawant RR, Torchilin VP. Polymeric micelles: polyethylene glycol-phosphatidylethanolamine (PEG-PE)-based micelles as an example. *Methods Mol Biol.* 2010;624:131–149.

19. Tang N, Du G, Wang N, Liu C, Hang H, Liang W. Improving penetration in tumors with nanoassemblies of phospholipids and doxorubicin. *J Natl Cancer Inst.* 2007;99(13):1004–1015.

20. Hoang B, Lee H, Reilly R, Allen C. Non-invasive monitoring of the fate of 111In-labeled block copolymer micelles by high resolution and high sensitivity MicroSPECT/CT imaging. *Mol Pharm.* 2009;6(2):581–589.

21. Duncan R. Polymer conjugates as anticancer nanomedicines. *Nat Rev Cancer.* 2006;6(9):688–701.

22. Johnston MJ, Edwards K, Karlsson G, Cullis PR. Influence of drug-to-lipid ratio on drug release properties and liposome integrity in liposomal doxorubicin formulations. *J Liposome Res.* 2008;18(2):145–157.

23. Mayer LD, Tai LC, Bally MB, Mitilenes GN, Ginsberg RS, Cullis PR. Characterization of liposomal systems containing doxorubicin entrapped in response to pH gradients. *Biochim Biophys Acta.* 1990;1025(2):143–151.

24. Sirova M, Mrkvan T, Etrych T, et al. Preclinical evaluation of linear HPMA-doxorubicin conjugates with pH-sensitive drug release: efficacy, safety, and immunomodulating activity in murine model. *Pharm Res.* 2010;27(1):200–208.

25. Wang J, Liu W, Tu Q, et al. Folate-decorated hybrid polymeric nanoparticles for chemically and physically combined paclitaxel loading and targeted delivery. *Biomacromolecules.* 2011;12(1):228–234.

26. Kievit FM, Wang FY, Fang C, et al. Doxorubicin loaded iron oxide nanoparticles overcome multidrug resistance in cancer in vitro. *J Control Release.* 2011;152(1):76–83.

27. Wang Z, Chui WK, Ho PC. Design of a multifunctional PLGA nanoparticulate drug delivery system: evaluation of its physicochemical properties and anticancer activity to malignant cancer cells. *Pharm Res.* 2009;26(5):1162–1171.

28. Schwendener RA, Schott H. Liposome formulations of hydrophobic drugs. *Methods Mol Biol.* 2010;605:129–138.

29. Sugahara S, Kajiki M, Kuriyama H, Kobayashi TR. Complete regression of xenografted human carcinomas by a paclitaxel-carboxymethyl dextran conjugate (AZ10992). *J Control Release.* 2007;117(1):40–50.

30. Bansal R, Post E, Proost JH, de Jager-Krikken A, Poelstra K, Prakash J. PEGylation improves pharmacokinetic profile, liver uptake and efficacy of Interferon gamma in liver fibrosis. *J Control Release.* 2011;154(3):233–240.

31. Zhang L, Zhu S, Qian L, Pei Y, Qiu Y, Jiang Y. RGD-modified PEG-PAMAM-DOX conjugates: In vitro and in vivo studies for glioma. *Eur J Pharm Biopharm.* 2011;79(2):232–240.

32. Dosio F, Arpicco S, Brusa P, Stella B, Cattel L. Poly (ethylene glycol)-human serum albumin-paclitaxel conjugates: preparation, characterization and pharmacokinetics. *J Control Release.* 2001;76(1–2):107–117.

33. Shiah JG, Dvorak M, Kopeckova P, Sun Y, Peterson CM, Kopecek J. Biodistribution and anti-tumour efficacy of long-circulating N-(2-hydroxypropyl)methacrylamide copolymer-doxorubicin conjugates in nude mice. *Eur J Cancer.* 2001;37(1):131–139.

34. Gillies ER, Dy E, Frechet JM, Szoka FC. Biological evaluation of polyester dendrimer: poly (ethylene oxide) "bow-tie" hybrids with tunable molecular weight and architecture. *Mol Pharm.* 2005;2(2):129–138.

35. Dobrovolskaia MA, Aggarwal P, Hall JB, McNeil SE. Preclinical studies to understand nanoparticle interaction with the immune system and its potential effects on nanoparticle biodistribution. *Mol Pharm.* 2008;5(4):487–495.

36. Mougin-Degraef M, Bourdeau C, Jestin E, et al. Doubly radiolabeled liposomes for pretargeted radioimmunotherapy. *Int J Pharm.* 2007;344(1–2):110–117.

37. Aillon KL, Xie Y, El-Gendy N, Berkland CJ, Forrest ML. Effects of nanomaterial physicochemical properties on in vivo toxicity. *Adv Drug Deliv Rev.* 2009;61(6):457–466.

38. Gaspar R, Duncan R. Polymeric carriers: preclinical safety and the regulatory implications for design and development of polymer therapeutics. *Adv Drug Deliv Rev.* 2009;61(13):1220–1231.

39. Hockel M, Vaupel P. Tumor hypoxia: definitions and current clinical, biologic, and molecular aspects. *J Natl Cancer Inst.* 2001;93(4):266–276.

40. Brown JM. Tumor hypoxia in cancer therapy. *Methods Enzymol.* 2007;435:297–321.

41. Jain RK. Normalization of tumor vasculature: an emerging concept in antiangiogenic therapy. *Science.* 2005;307(5706):58–62.

42. Hobbs SK, Monsky WL, Yuan F, et al. Regulation of transport pathways in tumor vessels: role of tumor type and microenvironment. *Proc Natl Acad Sci USA.* 1998;95(8):4607–4612.

43. Noguchi Y, Wu J, Duncan R, et al. Early phase tumor accumulation of macromolecules: a great difference in clearance rate between tumor and normal tissues. *Jpn J Cancer Res.* 1998;89(3):307–314.

44. Matsumura Y, Maeda H. A new concept for macromolecular therapeutics in cancer chemotherapy: mechanism of tumoritropic accumulation of proteins and the antitumor agent smancs. *Cancer Res.* 1986;46(12 Pt 1):6387–6392.

45. Jain RK, Stylianopoulos T. Delivering nanomedicine to solid tumors. *Nat Rev Clin Oncol.* 2010;7(11):653–664.

46. Yuan F, Dellian M, Fukumura D, et al. Vascular permeability in a human tumor xenograft: molecular size dependence and cutoff size. *Cancer Res.* 1995;55(17):3752–3756.

47. Engin K, Leeper DB, Cater JR, Thistlethwaite AJ, Tupchong L, McFarlane JD. Extracellular pH distribution in human tumours. *Int J Hyperthermia.* 1995;11(2):211–216.

48. Ojugo AS, McSheehy PM, McIntyre DJ, et al. Measurement of the extracellular pH of solid tumours in mice by magnetic resonance spectroscopy: a comparison of exogenous (19)F and (31)P probes. *NMR Biomed.* 1999;12(8):495–504.

49. van Sluis R, Bhujwalla ZM, Raghunand N, et al. In vivo imaging of extracellular pH using 1H MRSI. *Magn Reson Med.* 1999;41(4):743–750.

50. Chiche J, Brahimi-Horn MC, Pouyssegur J. Tumour hypoxia induces a metabolic shift causing acidosis: a common feature in cancer. *J Cell Mol Med.* 2010;14(4):771–794.

51. Lee ES, Gao Z, Bae YH. Recent progress in tumor pH targeting nanotechnology. *J Control Release.* 2008;132(3):164–170.

52. Wagner E, Curiel D, Cotten M. Derivery of drugs, proteins and genes into cells using transferrin as a ligand for receptor-mediated endocytosis. *Adv Drug Deliv Rev.* 1994;14:113–135.

53. Nicholson RI, Gee JM, Harper ME. EGFR and cancer prognosis. *Eur J Cancer.* 2001;37 (Suppl 4):S9–S15.

54. Zhao X, Li H, Lee RJ. Targeted drug delivery via folate receptors. *Expert Opin Drug Deliv.* 2008;5(3):309–319.

55. Lee ES, Na K, Bae YH. Polymeric micelle for tumor pH and folate-mediated targeting. *J Control Release.* 28 2003;91(1–2):103–113.

56. Bae Y, Nishiyama N, Kataoka K. In vivo antitumor activity of the folate-conjugated pH-sensitive polymeric micelle selectively releasing adriamycin in the intracellular acidic compartments. *Bioconjug Chem.* 2007;18(4):1131–1139.

57. Acharya S, Dilnawaz F, Sahoo SK. Targeted epidermal growth factor receptor nanoparticle bioconjugates for breast cancer therapy. *Biomaterials.* 2009;30(29):5737–5750.

58. Dunnick JK, McDougall IR, Aragon S, Goris ML, Kriss JP. Vesicle interactions with polyamino acids and antibody: in vitro and in vivo studies. *J Nucl Med.* 1975;16(6):483–487.

59. Catimel B, Nerrie M, Lee FT, et al. Kinetic analysis of the interaction between the monoclonal antibody A33 and its colonic epithelial antigen by the use of an optical biosensor. A comparison of immobilisation strategies. *J Chromatogr A.* 1997;776(1):15–30.

60. Nobs L, Buchegger F, Gurny R, Allemann E. Current methods for attaching targeting ligands to liposomes and nanoparticles. *J Pharm Sci.* 2004;93(8):1980–1992.

61. Carlsson J, Drevin H, Axen R. Protein thiolation and reversible protein-protein conjugation. N-Succinimidyl 3-(2-pyridyldithio)propionate, a new heterobifunctional reagent. *Biochem J.* 1978;173(3):723–737.

62. Algar WR, Prasuhn DE, Stewart MH, et al. The controlled display of biomolecules on nanoparticles: a challenge suited to bioorthogonal chemistry. *Bioconjug Chem.* 2011;22(5):825–858.

63. Heath TD, Macher BA, Papahadjopoulos D. Covalent attachment of immunoglobulins to liposomes via glycosphingolipids. *Biochim Biophys Acta.* 1981;640(1):66–81.

64. Kircheis R, Kichler A, Wallner G, et al. Coupling of cell-binding ligands to polyethylenimine for targeted gene delivery. *Gene Ther.* 1997;4(5):409–418.

65. Manjappa AS, Chaudhari KR, Venkataraju MP, et al. Antibody derivatization and conjugation strategies: application in preparation of stealth immunoliposome to target chemotherapeutics to tumor. *J Control Release.* 2011;150(1):2–22.

66. Jayanna PK, Torchilin VP, Petrenko VA. Liposomes targeted by fusion phage proteins. *Nanomedicine.* 2009;5(1):83–89.

67. Owens DE, 3rd, Peppas NA. Opsonization, biodistribution, and pharmacokinetics of polymeric nanoparticles. *Int J Pharm.* 2006;307(1):93–102.

68. Sawant RR, Torchilin VP. Design and synthesis of novel functional lipid-based bioconjugates for drug delivery and other applications. *Methods Mol Biol.* 2011;751:357–378.

69. Hansen CB, Kao GY, Moase EH, Zalipsky S, Allen TM. Attachment of antibodies to sterically stabilized liposomes: evaluation, comparison and optimization of coupling procedures. *Biochim Biophys Acta.* 1995;1239(2):133–144.

70. Elbayoumi TA, Torchilin VP. Tumor-specific anti-nucleosome antibody improves therapeutic efficacy of doxorubicin-loaded long-circulating liposomes against primary and metastatic tumor in mice. *Mol Pharm.* 2009;6(1):246–254.

71. Saul JM, Annapragada AV, Bellamkonda RV. A dual-ligand approach for enhancing targeting selectivity of therapeutic nanocarriers. *J Control Release.* 2006;114(3):277–287.

72. Allen TM, Brandeis E, Hansen CB, Kao GY, Zalipsky S. A new strategy for attachment of antibodies to sterically stabilized liposomes resulting in efficient targeting to cancer cells. *Biochim Biophys Acta.* 1995;1237(2):99–108.

73. Kirpotin D, Park JW, Hong K, et al. Sterically stabilized anti-HER2 immunoliposomes: design and targeting to human breast cancer cells in vitro. *Biochemistry.* 1997;36(1):66–75.

74. Torchilin VP, Levchenko TS, Lukyanov AN, et al. p-Nitrophenylcarbonyl-PEG-PE-liposomes: fast and simple attachment of specific ligands, including monoclonal antibodies, to distal ends of PEG chains via p-nitrophenylcarbonyl groups. *Biochim Biophys Acta.* 2001;1511(2):397–411.

75. Ulbrich K, Michaelis M, Rothweiler F, et al. Interaction of folate-conjugated human serum albumin (HSA) nanoparticles with tumour cells. *Int J Pharm.* 2011;406(1–2):128–134.

76. Yang SJ, Lin FH, Tsai KC, et al. Folic acid-conjugated chitosan nanoparticles enhanced protoporphyrin IX accumulation in colorectal cancer cells. *Bioconjug Chem.* 2010;21(4):679–689.

77. Duarte S, Faneca H, de Lima MC. Non-covalent association of folate to lipoplexes: a promising strategy to improve gene delivery in the presence of serum. *J Control Release.* 2011;149(3):264–272.

78. Shen Z, Wei W, Tanaka H, et al. A galactosamine-mediated drug delivery carrier for targeted liver cancer therapy. *Pharmacol Res.* 2011;64(4):410–419.

79. Gao S, Chen J, Xu X, et al. Galactosylated low molecular weight chitosan as DNA carrier for hepatocyte-targeting. *Int J Pharm.* 2003;255(1–2):57–68.

80. Wang YC, Liu XQ, Sun TM, Xiong MH, Wang J. Functionalized micelles from block copolymer of polyphosphoester and poly(epsilon-caprolactone) for receptor-mediated drug delivery. *J Control Release.* 2008;128(1):32–40.

81. Klibanov AL, Maruyama K, Torchilin VP, Huang L. Amphipathic polyethyleneglycols effectively prolong the circulation time of liposomes. *FEBS Lett.* 1990;268(1):235–237.

82. Zalipsky S. Functionalized poly (ethylene glycol) for preparation of biologically relevant conjugates. *Bioconjug Chem.* 1995;6(2):150–165.

83. Yamaoka T, Tabata Y, Ikada Y. Distribution and tissue uptake of poly (ethylene glycol) with different molecular weights after intravenous administration to mice. *J Pharm Sci.* 1994;83(4):601–606.

84. Gabizon A, Papahadjopoulos D. The role of surface charge and hydrophilic groups on liposome clearance in vivo. *Biochim Biophys Acta.* 1992;1103(1):94–100.

85. Needham D, McIntosh TJ, Lasic DD. Repulsive interactions and mechanical stability of polymer-grafted lipid membranes. *Biochim Biophys Acta*. 1992;1108(1):40–48.

86. Torchilin VP, Omelyanenko VG, Papisov MI, et al. Poly(ethylene glycol) on the liposome surface: on the mechanism of polymer-coated liposome longevity. *Biochim Biophys Acta*. 1994;1195(1):11–20.

87. Allen TM, Hansen C. Pharmacokinetics of stealth versus conventional liposomes: effect of dose. *Biochim Biophys Acta*. 1991;1068(2):133–141.

88. Gabizon A, Shmeeda H, Barenholz Y. Pharmacokinetics of pegylated liposomal Doxorubicin: review of animal and human studies. *Clin Pharmacokinet*. 2003;42(5):419–436.

89. Plummer R, Wilson RH, Calvert H, et al. A Phase I clinical study of cisplatin-incorporated polymeric micelles (NC-6004) in patients with solid tumours. *Br J Cancer*. 2011;104(4):593–598.

90. Gottesman MM, Fojo T, Bates SE. Multidrug resistance in cancer: role of ATP-dependent transporters. *Nat Rev Cancer*. 2002;2(1):48–58.

91. Baselga J, Arteaga CL. Critical update and emerging trends in epidermal growth factor receptor targeting in cancer. *J Clin Oncol*. 2005;23(11):2445–2459.

92. Torchilin V. Antibody-modified liposomes for cancer chemotherapy. *Expert Opin Drug Deliv*. 2008;5(9):1003–1025.

93. Schally AV. New approaches to the therapy of various tumors based on peptide analogues. *Horm Metab Res*. 2008;40(5):315–322.

94. Daniels TR, Delgado T, Helguera G, Penichet ML. The transferrin receptor part II: targeted delivery of therapeutic agents into cancer cells. *Clin Immunol*. 2006;121(2):159–176.

95. Chapman AP. PEGylated antibodies and antibody fragments for improved therapy: a review. *Adv Drug Deliv Rev*. 2002;54(4):531–545.

96. Lee LS, Conover C, Shi C, Whitlow M, Filpula D. Prolonged circulating lives of single-chain Fv proteins conjugated with polyethylene glycol: a comparison of conjugation chemistries and compounds. *Bioconjug Chem*. 1999;10(6):973–981.

97. Atobe K, Ishida T, Ishida E, et al. In vitro efficacy of a sterically stabilized immunoliposomes targeted to membrane type 1 matrix metalloproteinase (MT1-MMP). *Biol Pharm Bull*. 2007;30(5):972–978.

98. Blume G, Cevc G, Crommelin MD, Bakker-Woudenberg IA, Kluft C, Storm G. Specific targeting with poly(ethylene glycol)-modified liposomes: coupling of homing devices to the ends of the polymeric chains combines effective target binding with long circulation times. *Biochim Biophys Acta*. 1993;1149(1):180–184.

99. Elbayoumi TA, Torchilin VP. Enhanced cytotoxicity of monoclonal anticancer antibody 2C5-modified doxorubicin-loaded PEGylated liposomes against various tumor cell lines. *Eur J Pharm Sci*. 2007;32(3):159–168.

100. El Bayoumi TA, Torchilin VP. Tumor-targeted nanomedicines: enhanced antitumor efficacy in vivo of doxorubicin-loaded, long-circulating liposomes modified with cancer-specific monoclonal antibody. *Clin Cancer Res*. 2009;15(6):1973–1980.

101. Ishida O, Maruyama K, Tanahashi H, et al. Liposomes bearing polyethyleneglycol-coupled transferrin with intracellular targeting property to the solid tumors in vivo. *Pharm Res*. 2001;18(7):1042–1048.

102. Gabizon A, Tzemach D, Gorin J, et al. Improved therapeutic activity of folate-targeted liposomal doxorubicin in folate receptor-expressing tumor models. *Cancer Chemother Pharmacol*. 2011;66(1):43–52.

103. Park EK, Lee SB, Lee YM. Preparation and characterization of methoxy poly(ethylene glycol)/poly(epsilon-caprolactone) amphiphilic block copolymeric nanospheres for tumor-specific folate-mediated targeting of anticancer drugs. *Biomaterials*. 2005;26(9):1053–1061.

104. Takara K, Hatakeyama H, Ohga N, Hida K, Harashima H. Design of a dual-ligand system using a specific ligand and cell penetrating peptide, resulting in a synergistic effect on selectivity and cellular uptake. *Int J Pharm*. 2010;396(1–2):143–148.

105. Shalaev EY, Steponkus PL. Phase diagram of 1,2-dioleoylphosphatidylethanolamine (DOPE): water system at subzero temperatures and at low water contents. *Biochim Biophys Acta*. 1999;1419(2):229–247.

106. Fattal E, Couvreur P, Dubernet C. "Smart" delivery of antisense oligonucleotides by anionic pH-sensitive liposomes. *Adv Drug Deliv Rev*. 2004;56(7):931–946.

107. Simoes S, Moreira JN, Fonseca C, Duzgunes N, de Lima MC. On the formulation of pH-sensitive liposomes with long circulation times. *Adv Drug Deliv Rev*. 2004;56(7):947–965.

108. Roux E, Passirani C, Scheffold S, Benoit JP, Leroux JC. Serum-stable and long-circulating, PEGylated, pH-sensitive liposomes. *J Control Release*. 2004;94(2–3):447–451.

109. Kakudo T, Chaki S, Futaki S, et al. Transferrin-modified liposomes equipped with a pH-sensitive fusogenic peptide: an artificial viral-like delivery system. *Biochemistry*. 2004;43(19):5618–5628.

110. Sudimack JJ, Guo W, Tjarks W, Lee RJ. A novel pH-sensitive liposome formulation containing oleyl alcohol. *Biochim Biophys Acta*. 2002;1564(1):31–37.

111. Tros de Ilarduya C, Sun Y, Duzgunes N. Gene delivery by lipoplexes and polyplexes. *Eur J Pharm Sci.* 2010;40(3):159–170.

112. Benoit DS, Henry SM, Shubin AD, Hoffman AS, Stayton PS. pH-responsive polymeric siRNA carriers sensitize multidrug resistant ovarian cancer cells to doxorubicin via knockdown of polo-like kinase 1. *Mol Pharm.* 2010;7(2):442–455.

113. Roux E, Stomp R, Giasson S, Pezolet M, Moreau P, Leroux JC. Steric stabilization of liposomes by pH-responsive N-isopropylacrylamide copolymer. *J Pharm Sci.* 2002;91(8):1795–1802.

114. Lee ES, Shin HJ, Na K, Bae YH. Poly(L-histidine)-PEG block copolymer micelles and pH-induced destabilization. *J Control Release.* 2003;90(3):363–374.

115. Potineni A, Lynn DM, Langer R, Amiji MM. Poly (ethylene oxide)-modified poly (beta-amino ester) nanoparticles as a pH-sensitive biodegradable system for paclitaxel delivery. *J Control Release.* 2003;86(2–3):223–234.

116. Suzawa T, Nagamura S, Saito H, et al. Enhanced tumor cell selectivity of adriamycin-monoclonal antibody conjugate via a poly(ethylene glycol)-based cleavable linker. *J Control Release.* 2002;79(1–3):229–242.

117. Yoo HS, Lee EA, Park TG. Doxorubicin-conjugated biodegradable polymeric micelles having acid-cleavable linkages. *J Control Release.* 2002;82(1):17–27.

118. Lu C, Xing MM, Zhong W. Shell cross-linked and hepatocyte-targeting nanoparticles containing doxorubicin via acid-cleavable linkage. *Nanomedicine.* 2011;7(1):80–87.

119. Sawant RM, Hurley JP, Salmaso S, et al. "SMART" drug delivery systems: double-targeted pH-responsive pharmaceutical nanocarriers. *Bioconjug Chem.* 2006;17(4):943–949.

120. Lee ES, Na K, Bae YH. Super pH-sensitive multifunctional polymeric micelle. *Nano Lett.* 2005;5(2):325–329.

121. Lee ES, Gao Z, Kim D, Park K, Kwon IC, Bae YH. Super pH-sensitive multifunctional polymeric micelle for tumor pH(e) specific TAT exposure and multidrug resistance. *J Control Release.* 2008;129(3):228–236.

122. McNeeley KM, Karathanasis E, Annapragada AV, Bellamkonda RV. Masking and triggered unmasking of targeting ligands on nanocarriers to improve drug delivery to brain tumors. *Biomaterials.* 2009;30(23–24):3986–3995.

123. Hilger I, Hiergeist R, Hergt R, Winnefeld K, Schubert H, Kaiser WA. Thermal ablation of tumors using magnetic nanoparticles: an in vivo feasibility study. *Invest Radiol.* 2002;37(10):580–586.

124. Jin H, Kang KA. Application of novel metal nanoparticles as optical/thermal agents in optical mammography and hyperthermic treatment for breast cancer. *Adv Exp Med Biol.* 2007;599:45–52.

125. Ponce AM, Vujaskovic Z, Yuan F, Needham D, Dewhirst MW. Hyperthermia mediated liposomal drug delivery. *Int J Hyperthermia.* 2006;22(3):205–213.

126. Chung JE, Yokoyama M, Okano T. Inner core segment design for drug delivery control of thermo-responsive polymeric micelles. *J Control Release.* 2000;65(1–2):93–103.

127. Yatvin MB, Weinstein JN, Dennis WH, Blumenthal R. Design of liposomes for enhanced local release of drugs by hyperthermia. *Science.* 1978;202(4374):1290–1293.

128. Kono K. Thermosensitive polymer-modified liposomes. *Adv Drug Deliv Rev.* 2001;53(3):307–319.

129. Tagami T, Ernsting MJ, Li SD. Efficient tumor regression by a single and low dose treatment with a novel and enhanced formulation of thermosensitive liposomal doxorubicin. *J Control Release.* 2011;152(2):303–309.

130. Qu T, Wang A, Yuan J, Gao Q. Preparation of an amphiphilic triblock copolymer with pH- and thermo-responsiveness and self-assembled micelles applied to drug release. *J Colloid Interface Sci.* 2009;336(2):865–871.

131. Schafer FQ, Buettner GR. Redox environment of the cell as viewed through the redox state of the glutathione disulfide/glutathione couple. *Free Radic Biol Med.* 2001;30(11):1191–1212.

132. Saito G, Swanson JA, Lee KD. Drug delivery strategy utilizing conjugation via reversible disulfide linkages: role and site of cellular reducing activities. *Adv Drug Deliv Rev.* 2003;55(2):199–215.

133. West KR, Otto S. Reversible covalent chemistry in drug delivery. *Curr Drug Discov Technol.* 2005;2(3):123–160.

134. Kirpotin D, Hong K, Mullah N, Papahadjopoulos D, Zalipsky S. Liposomes with detachable polymer coating: destabilization and fusion of dioleoylphosphatidylethanolamine vesicles triggered by cleavage of surface-grafted poly(ethylene glycol). *FEBS Lett.* 1996;388(2–3):115–118.

135. Sheng R, Luo T, Zhu Y, et al. The intracellular plasmid DNA localization of cationic reducible cholesterol-disulfide lipids. *Biomaterials.* 2011;32(13):3507–3519.

136. Son S, Singha K, Kim WJ. Bioreducible BPEI-SS-PEG-cNGR polymer as a tumor targeted non-viral gene carrier. *Biomaterials.* 2010;31(24):6344–6354.

137. Mehiri M, Upert G, Tripathi S, et al. An efficient biodelivery system for antisense polyamide nucleic acid (PNA). *Oligonucleotides.* 2008;18(3):245–256.

138. Musacchio T, Vaze O, D'Souza G, Torchilin VP. Effective stabilization and delivery of siRNA: reversible siRNA-phospholipid conjugate in nanosized mixed polymeric micelles. *Bioconjug Chem.* 2010;21(8):1530–1536.

139. Sukhorukov GB, Rogach AL, Garstka M, et al. Multifunctionalized polymer microcapsules: novel tools for biological and pharmacological applications. *Small.* 2007;3(6):944–955.

140. Veiseh O, Gunn JW, Zhang M. Design and fabrication of magnetic nanoparticles for targeted drug delivery and imaging. *Adv Drug Deliv Rev.* 2010;62(3):284–304.

141. Gupta AK, Gupta M. Synthesis and surface engineering of iron oxide nanoparticles for biomedical applications. *Biomaterials.* 2005;26(18):3995–4021.

142. Weissleder R, Stark DD, Engelstad BL, et al. Superparamagnetic iron oxide: pharmacokinetics and toxicity. *AJR Am J Roentgenol.* 1989;152(1):167–173.

143. Anzai Y, Prince MR. Iron oxide-enhanced MR lymphography: the evaluation of cervical lymph node metastases in head and neck cancer. *J Magn Reson Imaging.* 1997;7(1):75–81.

144. Narayanan TN, Mary AP, Swalih PK, et al. Enhanced bio-compatibility of ferrofluids of self-assembled superparamagnetic iron oxide-silica core-shell nanoparticles. *J Nanosci Nanotechnol.* 2011;11(3):1958–1967.

145. Gang J, Park SB, Hyung W, et al. Magnetic poly epsilon-caprolactone nanoparticles containing Fe3O4 and gemcitabine enhance anti-tumor effect in pancreatic cancer xenograft mouse model. *J Drug Target.* 2007;15(6):445–453.

146. Cinteza LO, Ohulchanskyy TY, Sahoo Y, Bergey EJ, Pandey RK, Prasad PN. Diacyllipid micelle-based nanocarrier for magnetically guided delivery of drugs in photodynamic therapy. *Mol Pharm.* 2006;3(4):415–423.

147. Rapoport N. Physical stimuli-responsive polymeric micelles for anticancer drug delivery. *Progr Polym Sci.* 2007;32(8–9):962–990.

148. Goodwin AP, Mynar JL, Ma Y, Fleming GR, Frechet JM. Synthetic micelle sensitive to IR light via a two-photon process. *J Am Chem Soc.* 2005;127(28):9952–9953.

149. Kostarelos K, Emfietzoglou D, Tadros TF. Light-sensitive fusion between polymer-coated liposomes following physical anchoring of polymerisable polymers onto lipid bilayers by self-assembly. *Faraday Discuss.* 2005;128:379–388.

150. Miller CR, Clapp PJ, O'Brien DF. Visible light-induced destabilization of endocytosed liposomes. *FEBS Lett.* 2000;467(1):52–56.

151. Renno RZ, Miller JW. Photosensitizer delivery for photodynamic therapy of choroidal neovascularization. *Adv Drug Deliv Rev.* 2001;52(1):63–78.

152. Le Garrec D, Taillefer J, Van Lier JE, Lenaerts V, Leroux JC. Optimizing pH-responsive polymeric micelles for drug delivery in a cancer photodynamic therapy model. *J Drug Target.* 2002;10(5):429–437.

153. Jang WD, Nakagishi Y, Nishiyama N, et al. Polyion complex micelles for photodynamic therapy: incorporation of dendritic photosensitizer excitable at long wavelength relevant to improved tissue-penetrating property. *J Control Release.* 2006;113(1):73–79.

154. Nishiyama N, Arnida, Jang WD, Date K, Miyata K, Kataoka K. Photochemical enhancement of transgene expression by polymeric micelles incorporating plasmid DNA and dendrimer-based photosensitizer. *J Drug Target.* 2006;14(6):413–424.

155. Huang SL, MacDonald RC. Acoustically active liposomes for drug encapsulation and ultrasound-triggered release. *Biochim Biophys Acta.* 2004;1665(1–2):134–141.

156. Tartis MS, McCallan J, Lum AF, et al. Therapeutic effects of paclitaxel-containing ultrasound contrast agents. *Ultrasound Med Biol.* 2006;32(11):1771–1780.

157. Gao ZG, Fain HD, Rapoport N. Controlled and targeted tumor chemotherapy by micellar-encapsulated drug and ultrasound. *J Control Release.* 2005;102(1):203–222.

158. Gullotti E, Yeo Y. Extracellularly activated nanocarriers: a new paradigm of tumor targeted drug delivery. *Mol Pharm.* 2009;6(4):1041–1051.

159. Hatakeyama H, Akita H, Ito E, et al. Systemic delivery of siRNA to tumors using a lipid nanoparticle containing a tumor-specific cleavable PEG-lipid. *Biomaterials.* 2011;32(18):4306–4316.

160. Burger H, Loos WJ, Eechoute K, Verweij J, Mathijssen RH, Wiemer EA. Drug transporters of platinum-based anticancer agents and their clinical significance. *Drug Resist Updat.* 2011;14(1):22–34.

161. Gabizon AA, Shmeeda H, Zalipsky S. Pros and cons of the liposome platform in cancer drug targeting. *J Liposome Res.* 2006;16(3):175–183.

162. Elbayoumi TA, Torchilin VP. Liposomes for targeted delivery of antithrombotic drugs. *Expert Opin Drug Deliv.* 2008;5(11):1185–1198.

163. Li W, Szoka FC Jr. Lipid-based nanoparticles for nucleic acid delivery. *Pharm Res.* 2007;24(3): 438–449.

164. Pack DW, Hoffman AS, Pun S, Stayton PS. Design and development of polymers for gene delivery. *Nat Rev Drug Discov.* 2005;4(7):581–593.

165. Merdan T, Kopecek J, Kissel T. Prospects for cationic polymers in gene and oligonucleotide therapy against cancer. *Adv Drug Deliv Rev.* 2002;54(5):715–758.

166. Kircheis R, Wightman L, Wagner E. Design and gene delivery activity of modified polyethylen-imines. *Adv Drug Deliv Rev.* 2001;53(3):341–358.

167. Morille M, Passirani C, Dufort S, et al. Tumor transfection after systemic injection of DNA lipid nanocapsules. *Biomaterials.* 2011;32(9):2327–2333.

168. Dufes C, Uchegbu IF, Schatzlein AG. Dendrimers in gene delivery. *Adv Drug Deliv Rev.* 2005;57(15):2177–2202.

169. Lindgren M, Hallbrink M, Prochiantz A, Langel U. Cell-penetrating peptides. *Trends Pharmacol Sci.* 2000;21(3):99–103.

170. Prochiantz A. Messenger proteins: homeoproteins, TAT and others. *Curr Opin Cell Biol.* 2000;12(4):400–406.

171. Torchilin VP, Levchenko TS, Rammohan R, Volodina N, Papahadjopoulos-Sternberg B, D'Souza GG. Cell transfection in vitro and in vivo with nontoxic TAT peptide-liposome-DNA complexes. *Proc Natl Acad Sci USA.* 2003;100(4):1972–1977.

172. Sawant R, Torchilin V. Intracellular delivery of nanoparticles with CPPs. *Methods Mol Biol.* 2011;683:431–451.

173. Mahat RI, Monera OD, Smith LC, Rolland A. Peptide-based gene delivery. *Curr Opin Mol Ther.* 1999;1(2):226–243.

174. Torchilin V. Multifunctional and stimuli-sensitive pharmaceutical nanocarriers. *Eur J Pharm Biopharm.* 2009;71(3):431–444.

175. El-Sayed A, Futaki S, Harashima H. Delivery of macromolecules using arginine-rich cell-penetrating peptides: ways to overcome endosomal entrapment. *AAPS J.* 2009;11(1):13–22.

176. Wright LR, Rothbard JB, Wender PA. Guanidinium rich peptide transporters and drug delivery. *Curr Protein Pept Sci.* 2003;4(2):105–124.

177. Vivès E, Granier C, Prevot P, Lebleu B. Structure–activity relationship study of the plasma membrane translocating potential of a short peptide from HIV-1 Tat protein *Lett Peptide Sci.* 1997;4:429–436.

178. Ziegler A, Blatter XL, Seelig A, Seelig J. Protein transduction domains of HIV-1 and SIV TAT interact with charged lipid vesicles. Binding mechanism and thermodynamic analysis. *Biochemistry.* 2003;42(30):9185–9194.

179. Goncalves E, Kitas E, Seelig J. Binding of oligoarginine to membrane lipids and heparan sulfate: structural and thermodynamic characterization of a cell-penetrating peptide. *Biochemistry.* 2005;44(7):2692–2702.

180. Vives E, Schmidt J, Pelegrin A. Cell-penetrating and cell-targeting peptides in drug delivery. *Biochim Biophys Acta.* 2008;1786(2):126–138.

181. Derossi D, Calvet S, Trembleau A, Brunissen A, Chassaing G, Prochiantz A. Cell internalization of the third helix of the Antennapedia homeodomain is receptor-independent. *J Biol Chem.* 1996;271(30):18188–18193.

182. Thoren PE, Persson D, Esbjorner EK, Goksor M, Lincoln P, Norden B. Membrane binding and translocation of cell-penetrating peptides. *Biochemistry.* 2004;43(12):3471–3489.

183. Thoren PE, Persson D, Lincoln P, Norden B. Membrane destabilizing properties of cell-penetrating peptides. *Biophys Chem.* 2005;114(2–3):169–179.

184. Kaplan IM, Wadia JS, Dowdy SF. Cationic TAT peptide transduction domain enters cells by macropinocytosis. *J Control Release.* 2005;102(1):247–253.

185. Fawell S, Seery J, Daikh Y, et al. Tat-mediated delivery of heterologous proteins into cells. *Proc Natl Acad Sci USA.* 1994;91(2):664–668.

186. Mann DA, Frankel AD. Endocytosis and targeting of exogenous HIV-1 Tat protein. *EMBO J.* 1991;10(7):1733–1739.

187. Frankel AD, Pabo CO. Cellular uptake of the tat protein from human immunodeficiency virus. *Cell.* 1988;55(6):1189–1193.

188. Rao KS, Reddy MK, Horning JL, Labhasetwar V. TAT-conjugated nanoparticles for the CNS delivery of anti-HIV drugs. *Biomaterials.* 2008;29(33):4429–4438.

189. Herve F, Ghinea N, Scherrmann JM. CNS delivery via adsorptive transcytosis. *AAPS J.* 2008;10(3):455–472.

190. Simon MJ, Kang WH, Gao S, Banta S, Morrison B, 3rd. TAT is not capable of transcellular delivery across an intact endothelial monolayer in vitro. *Ann Biomed Eng.* 2011;39(1):394–401.

191. Wagner E, Plank C, Zatloukal K, Cotten M, Birnstiel ML. Influenza virus hemagglutinin HA-2 N-terminal fusogenic peptides augment gene transfer by transferrin-polylysine-DNA complexes: toward a synthetic virus-like gene-transfer vehicle. *Proc Natl Acad Sci USA.* 1992;89(17):7934–7938.

192. Wadia JS, Stan RV, Dowdy SF. Transducible TAT-HA fusogenic peptide enhances escape of TAT-fusion proteins after lipid raft macropinocytosis. *Nat Med.* 2004;10(3):310–315.

193. Vocero-Akbani AM, Heyden NV, Lissy NA, Ratner L, Dowdy SF. Killing HIV-infected cells by transduction with an HIV protease-activated caspase-3 protein. *Nat Med.* 1999;5(1):29–33.

194. Schwarze SR, Ho A, Vocero-Akbani A, Dowdy SF. In vivo protein transduction: delivery of a biologically active protein into the mouse. *Science.* 1999;285(5433):1569–1572.

195. Xiong XB, Lavasanifar A. Traceable multifunctional micellar nanocarriers for cancer-targeted co-delivery of MDR-1 siRNA and doxorubicin. *ACS Nano.* 2011;5(6):5202–5213.

196. Zheng J, Jaffaray DA, Allen C. Nanosystems for multimodality In vivo Imaging. In: Torchilin VP, ed. *Multifunctional Pharmaceutical Nanocarriers.* Vol. 4. London: Springer Science+Business; 2008:409–430.

197. Das M, Bandyopadhyay D, Mishra D, et al. "Clickable", trifunctional magnetite nanoparticles and their chemoselective biofunctionalization. *Bioconjug Chem.* 2011;22(6):1181–1193.

198. Medarova Z, Pham W, Farrar C, Petkova V, Moore A. In vivo imaging of siRNA delivery and silencing in tumors. *Nat Med.* 2007;13(3):372–377.

199. Torchilin VP. Polymeric contrast agents for medical imaging. *Curr Pharm Biotechnol.* 2000; 1(2):183–215.

200. Erdogan S, Torchilin VP. Gadolinium-loaded polychelating polymer-containing tumor-targeted liposomes. *Methods Mol Biol.* 2010;605:321–334.

201. Jain TK, Richey J, Strand M, Leslie-Pelecky DL, Flask CA, Labhasetwar V. Magnetic nanoparticles with dual functional properties: drug delivery and magnetic resonance imaging. *Biomaterials.* 2008;29(29):4012–4021.

202. Gultepe E, Reynoso FJ, Jhaveri A, et al. Monitoring of magnetic targeting to tumor vasculature through MRI and biodistribution. *Nanomedicine.* 2010;5(8):1173–1182.

203. Nasongkla N, Bey E, Ren J, et al. Multifunctional polymeric micelles as cancer targeted, MRI-ultrasensitive drug delivery systems. *Nano Lett.* 2006;6(11):2427–2430.

204. Kohler N, Sun C, Fichtenholtz A, Gunn J, Fang C, Zhang M. Methotrexate-immobilized poly(ethylene glycol) magnetic nanoparticles for MR imaging and drug delivery. *Small.* 2006;2(6):785–792.

205. Hwu JR, Lin YS, Josephrajan T, et al. Targeted paclitaxel by conjugation to iron oxide and gold nanoparticles. *J Am Chem Soc.* 2009;131(1):66–68.

206. Guthi JS, Yang SG, Huang G, et al. MRI-visible micellar nanomedicine for targeted drug delivery to lung cancer cells. *Mol Pharm.* 2010;7(1):32–40.

207. Yang X, Grailer JJ, Rowland IJ, et al. Multifunctional stable and pH-responsive polymer vesicles formed by heterofunctional triblock copolymer for targeted anticancer drug delivery and ultrasensitive MR imaging. *ACS Nano.* 2010;4(11):6805–6817.

208. Grosse SM, Tagalakis AD, Mustapa MF, et al. Tumor-specific gene transfer with receptor-mediated nanocomplexes modified by polyethylene glycol shielding and endosomally cleavable lipid and peptide linkers. *FASEB J.* 2010;24(7):2301–2313.

209. Mustapa MF, Grosse SM, Kudsiova L, et al. Stabilized integrin-targeting ternary LPD (lipopolyplex) vectors for gene delivery designed to disassemble within the target cell. *Bioconjug Chem.* 2009;20(3):518–532.

210. Kibria G, Hatakeyama H, Ohga N, Hida K, Harashima H. Dual-ligand modification of PEGylated liposomes shows better cell selectivity and efficient gene delivery. *J Control Release.* 2011;153(2):141–148.

211. Kenny GD, Kamaly N, Kalber TL, et al. Novel multifunctional nanoparticle mediates siRNA tumour delivery, visualisation and therapeutic tumour reduction in vivo. *J Control Release.* 2011;149(2):111–116.

212. Kamaly N, Kalber T, Thanou M, Bell JD, Miller AD. Folate receptor targeted bimodal liposomes for tumor magnetic resonance imaging. *Bioconjug Chem.* 2009;20(4):648–655.

213. Klaikherd A, Nagamani C, Thayumanavan S. Multi-stimuli sensitive amphiphilic block copolymer assemblies. *J Am Chem Soc.* 2009;131(13):4830–4838.

214. Pan J, Liu Y, Feng SS. Multifunctional nanoparticles of biodegradable copolymer blend for cancer diagnosis and treatment. *Nanomedicine.* 2010;5(3):347–360.

215. Patil R, Portilla-Arias J, Ding H, et al. Temozolomide delivery to tumor cells by a multifunctional nano vehicle based on poly(beta-L-malic acid). *Pharm Res.* 2010;27(11):2317–2329.

216. Upponi J, Torchilin VP. Development and characterization of micellar theranostic agent for simultaneous magnetic resonance imaging and cancer therapy. Abstract # 72. In: 38th Annual Meeting of the Controlled Released Society: 2011; Baltimore, MD.

ORAL DELIVERY

SONG GAO, YONG MA, ZHEN YANG, WEN JIANG, AND MING HU

CHAPTER OBJECTIVES

Upon completing this chapter, the reader should be able to

- ▸ Understand the rationale for oral drug delivery
- ▸ Describe the physicochemical barriers to oral delivery of drugs
- ▸ Identify the biological barriers to oral delivery of drugs
- ▸ Describe various oral dosage forms
- ▸ Discuss how various dosage forms perform in the context of bioavailability

CHAPTER OUTLINE

Introduction

Bioavailability Barriers to Orally Administered Drugs

    Physicochemical Barriers

    Biological Barriers

INTRODUCTION

Oral delivery is the preferred route of administration for most drugs, especially if the drugs are intended to manage a chronic disease such as hypertension. A number of advantages are associated with oral delivery, such as ease of use, lower cost of administration (e.g., self-administration), and better patient compliance. Common formulations for oral delivery are solid (e.g., tablet, capsule), semisolid (e.g., soft gel), or liquid (e.g., oral solution, suspension, emulsion) forms. For solid oral administration, additional advantages include longer shelf-life and a variety of delivery rates (i.e., sustained and controlled delivery). Not every drug, however, can be adminstrated orally because of the following reasons: (1) drug concentration needs to be precisely controlled in the systemic circulation (e.g., for chemotherapeutic drugs), (2) drug has unfavorable physicochemical prosperities (e.g., high molecular weight), and (3) drug absorption is limited by the hostile gastrointestinal (GI) barriers (e.g., protein drugs). In addition, although some drugs can be easily absorbed from the GI tract, first-pass elimination is extensive, which results in a short half-live and necessitates frequent dosing (more than three times per day) for desired efficacy. The need for frequent dosing is often the reason a drug may not be developed, because it may rapidly lose its market share when that drug with less-frequent dosing is developed.

To overcome some of the challenges identified, various types of modified or controlled-release formulations are developed for oral delivery. Modified or controlled-release formulations offer advantages over conventional formulations including maintenance of optimized drug concentration in plasma, increase of the duration of therapeutic effects, reduction in the frequency of administration, and/or lessening of the duration and/or severity of side effects. Modified or controlled-release formulations, however, also have distinctive challenges. For example, a controlled-release formulation usually contains higher amounts of drugs than conventional formulation, and if the formulation is damaged, the drug will be released as a bolus (i.e., dose dumping), resulting in a serious overdose problem. Nevertheless, the advantages of modified or controlled delivery often overweigh their disadvantages, and more and more drugs are now available as modified- or controlled-release dosage forms. Furthermore, as we are able to establish new relationships between pharmacokinetic and pharmacodynamics clinically, we should be able to design newer and more effective oral delivery formulation for patients.

Because oral drug delivery is the most popular route of administration, we first describe barriers to oral drug delivery and then some of the most common formulations used for oral delivery. The formulation technology, such as the production process and procedures of a certain solid dosage form (e.g., a tablet), is not the focus of this chapter. Instead, we describe different oral formulations from the bioavailability point of view by discussing the rationale and purposes of different formulations. We believe the information provided in this way will be more useful to doctor of pharmacy and graduate students and to practicing pharmacists, doctors, and nurses. Pharmaceutical researchers and other interested readers who are more specialized in oral delivery should find a review of the basic information helpful.

BIOAVAILABILITY BARRIERS TO ORALLY ADMINISTERED DRUGS

Two types of barriers keep a drug from being delivered into the systemic circulation: the physicochemical properties of the drug itself (e.g., solubility and chemical stability) and the physiological barriers of the human digestive system, including the penetration or permeability barrier, metabolism barrier, and microflora barrier [1]. Because of these factors, only a portion of drugs delivered reach their *in vivo* targets. Bioavailability, which is defined by the rate and extent of drug exposure in the systemic circulation, is the governing factor that determines how much drug could reach the site of action [1].

PHYSICOCHEMICAL BARRIERS

Physicochemical barriers are primarily the results of a drug molecule's chemical structure, which impacts its solubility, dissolution, and stability. In addition to chemical structure, the physical state of the drug molecule (solid, different crystal forms, solution, etc.) may also be part of the challenge that a drug molecule must overcome to become available for absorption. In this section, we will briefly describe the main physicochemical barriers.

Solubility

Solubility is defined as the maximum amount of a chemical substance (in solid, liquid, or gaseous state) that can be dissolved in a certain volume of a particular liquid solvent to form a homogeneous mass. Solubility is important for oral bioavailability because only dissolved substance can be absorbed across the GI epithelium. For most drugs (which are solids in the pure state), solubility is a physical property of the drug solids, which is affected by physicochemical characteristics of the drug substance (e.g., chemical structure, crystalline state), compositions of the solvent (e.g., solvent type, pH), temperature, and even the dissolution procedure [4]. Another equally important and related parameter is the dissolution rate, or the speed at which a substance is dissolved in liquid. The GI tract has established rhythm and motility, and an orally administered dose of drug normally has 4 to 6 hours to be absorbed. After this, the remaining dose is lost and nonabsorbable. Therefore, it is often desirable to get orally administered drug to dissolve rapidly but certainly within a desired period of time (e.g., 2–4 hours), especially for immediate-release oral products that release their contents in 0.5 hours or less.

Stability

Stability in the GI tract has a direct impact on drug performance *in vivo*. For most drugs (especially those developed after 1980s), stability is not a major problem because stability in the GI tract is a screening criterion for drug candidates in the early stage of preclinical development. Quite a few drugs developed before 1980s, however, and occasionally even drugs developed after the 1980s are unstable in the GI tract. Unstable compounds in the GI tract reduce amounts available for absorption, resulting in poor bioavailability and poor biological performances. In addition, degradation of drugs could change the pharmacological effects and even result in toxicity. Although stability is a chemical characteristic of drug molecules, the environment of the GI tract could accelerate the decomposition of an unstable drug. The most critical factor that influences chemical degradation of a drug is the pH value of the GI tract. Gastric fluid is very acidic, with a pH of 1 to 3. The small intestine has highly variable pH, starting at pH 5.5 in the duodenum and gradually increasing along the intestinal tract to pH 7 and 8 in the colon [5]. Drugs whose stability is sensitive to pH (e.g., certain esters) degrade at variable rates in different segments of the GI tract. Moreover, the microflora in the GI tract could also decompose certain drugs [6,7]. For example, reduction and ring fissions are the major degradation pathways enabled by microflora [8,9].

BIOLOGICAL BARRIERS

Biological barriers are mainly composed of epithelial membrane, which limit the absorption of certain xenobiotics physically, and metabolic machinery, which catalyze the formation of metabolites that are usually inactive and easy to eliminate from the body.

Permeation

Permeation is the next step in the bioavailability continuum, and only soluble drug molecules are considered available for permeation. Although nanoparticles and other small particles may also be taken up by the enterocytes, they are often processed differently from molecules present in solution. The intestinal epithelium is the first biological barrier for orally administered drugs; therefore, a better understanding of the specific cellular mechanisms involved in the permeation processes is of interest when assessing drug absorption [10].

The primary physiological function of the small intestine is to digest and absorb nutrients from the gut lumen and to sense environmental toxins, which facilitate necessary immune reactions to clear the toxins or the organisms that produce the toxins [10]. For most drugs the relevant functions of the GI tract are those that are relevant to nutrient absorption and metabolism. Orally delivered vaccines (e.g., polio vaccine), however, rely on the immune functions of the GI tract to exert their functions.

Structures and functions of intestinal epithelium membrane have been well described [11]. Briefly, the intestinal epithelium is consisted of a single layer of epithelial cells that undergo rapid and continuous renewal, with an average life span of 14 days. As the intestinal cells mature, they possess all the necessary machinery (i.e., transporters and enzymes) that play an essential part in the digestion and absorption of nutrients. In the small intestine, epithelia have significant "super" structures that protrude into the lumen, and on each of those protruded structure are thousands of finger-shaped projectiles or villi, 0.5 to 1.5 mm in length. Each of these villi has many intestinal cells that are tightly linked together by cellular junctional proteins (especially the tight junctions), and each mature enterocyte (that sit on the top one-third of the villi) has thousands of microvilli, and together they form the brush-border membrane of the small intestine. This "super" structure is especially important because it gives intestinal epithelial an enormous area for drug absorption, estimated at 100 to 200 m² (Note: A tennis court has a surface area of 100 m²). It is generally believed that absorption may occur on 90% to 95% of the villus surface, although it would be more difficult to gain access to the lower part of each villi because a thick mucous layer generally cover the villus.

Permeability measures the ability of a drug molecule to traverse a biomembrane (in this case, the intestinal epithelium) barrier. Together with drug concentration, permeability also determines the drug absorption rate across the intestinal epithelium. Absorption of a drug molecule across the intestinal epithelium is a complex process that may involve a single mechanism or multiple pathways (**Figure 9-1**). The absorption of the drug is determined by two major factors, uptake and efflux. The intestinal uptake/efflux takes place via transcellular/paracellular passive diffusion and facilitated/active transport mechanisms separately or in combination.

Passive Diffusion

Permeability is usually higher for lipophilic drugs than for hydrophilic ones when passive diffusion is the main mechanism, because most compounds are set to permeate across a lipid bilayer of the biomembrane [10]. Moreover, unionized molecules are more permeable compared with ionized ones, because charge molecules are less likely to partition into the lipid bilayer than their uncharged counterparts. The molecular size is also critical. For example, very few molecules are able to diffuse across the intestinal membrane when their molecular weight exceeds 1000 Da. For compounds to permeate via paracellular pathway, their molecular weight is usually less than 200 Da. For compounds with molecular weights between 200 and 1000 Da, Lipinski's rule of five states that in order for a drug molecule to be well absorbed via passive diffusion, the drug molecule should have no more than 5 hydrogen bond donors, no more than 10 hydrogen bond acceptors, a molecular mass of less than 500 Da, and an octanol–water partition coefficient log P not greater than 5 [12]. Although this rule is not always precise and accurate, it indicates that lipophilicity, hydrogen bond numbers, and molecular size are important factors that determine the permeability of drugs via passive diffusion.

Transporter–Mediated Uptake and Efflux

The human intestinal epithelial wall expresses several families of uptake and efflux transporters, including solute transporters such as peptide transporter 1, organic anion-transporting polypeptides, and ATP-binding cassette (ABC) transporters [13–15]. Apically located uptake transporters are important for nutrient absorption and together with relevant gut-excreted or intestinal brush-border enzymes facilitate the uptake of nutrients like glucose, amino acids, and small peptides (two to four amino acid residues). Typically, gut-excreted and brush-border enzymes digest the food stuff that are typically macromolecules (e.g., proteins, starch, and DNAs) into much smaller molecules that are amenable for uptake by these nutrients carriers. When drug molecules have structures similar to these nutrient molecules or have structures that can bind to and be transported by the nutrient carriers, they are taken up by these nutrient carriers into the cells.

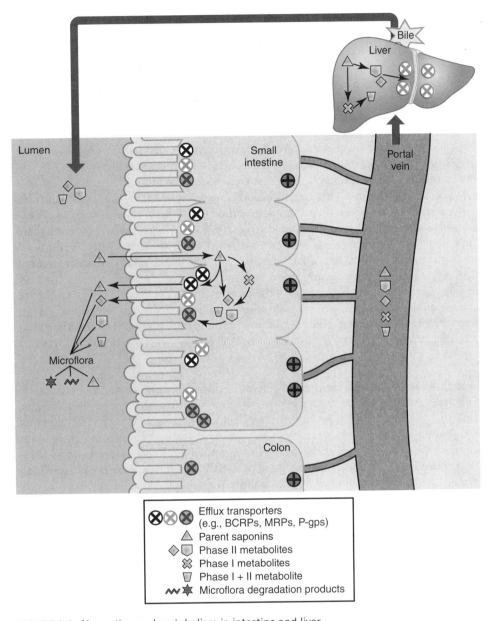

FIGURE 9-1 Absorption and metabolism in intestine and liver.

The most important nutrient carriers for orally administered drugs are peptide transporter 1, nucleoside transporters, and amino acid transporters. Other important transporters are organic anion-transporting polypeptides, bile acid transporters, mono-carboxylic acid transporters, and organic cation transporters. Among these transporters, peptide transporter 1 has the most impressive coverage, because it can transport a large number of drugs with diverse structures. Known substrates of peptide transporter 1 include, in addition to thousands of small di- and tripeptides (e.g., gly-sar), many β–lactam antibiotics (e.g., cephalexin and loracarbef), several antiviral drugs (e.g., valan-cyclovir), and a variety of peptidyl prodrugs [16]. Important organic anion-transporting polypeptide substrates include many statins (e.g., rosuvastatin and pravastatin), angiotensin-converting enzyme inhibitors (e.g., enalapril), and quite a few other drugs (e.g., fexofenadine [17].

ABC transporters with relevant drug substrates include P-glycoprotein, multidrug resistance proteins (MRPs), and breast cancer resistance protein (BCRP) [18–22]. The apically located uptake transporters facilitate drug absorption from the intestinal lumen into the enterocytes, whereas apically located efflux transporters pump drugs present within the enterocyte back into the lumen [23]. On the contrary, basolaterally located efflux transporters facilitate the transport of drug from the enterocyte to the blood, whereas basolaterally located uptake transporters could remove drug from the blood and transport it to the enterocyte. Although there are many basolaterally located efflux transporters (e.g., amino acid and sugar transporters) whose functions are similar or identical to the apically located uptake transporters of the same class (e.g., amino acid transporters), very few basolaterally located uptake transporters have been carefully characterized.

The apically located efflux transporters are well studied by scientists who deal with bioavailability issues, because these efflux transporters substantially affect the bioavailabilies of orally administrated drugs that are their substrates [24, 25]. The most pharmacologically relevant and well-studied apically located ABC transporters are P-glycoprotein (ABCB1), MRP2 (ABCC2), and breast cancer resistance protein (ABCG2). Transporters may impact bioavailability of their substrates by mediating biliary and/or direct intestinal excretion of these compounds. For more detailed description of these efflux transporters, interested readers should consult recent review articles that deal with human intestinal efflux transporters and their distribution and functions [26].

Metabolism

In addition to providing a formidable defense against indiscriminate entry of xenobiotics by preventing nonselective absorption, the intestinal epithelial membrane also catalyzes the metabolism of drugs and dietary chemicals via various metabolic enzymes. Xenobiotics that possess suitable structures are rapidly absorbed into the enterocytes, and for absorbed drugs, metabolism in the intestinal epithelial cells and/or in hepatocytes becomes a major barrier to their bioavailability. These barriers are classically termed "first-pass" metabolism, or metabolism that occurs before xenobiotics reach the systemic circulation for the first time. Drug metabolic pathways are normally divided phase I and phase II metabolic pathways. The functions of the metabolic processes is to change the structure of active drugs, making the metabolic end-products less bioactive (most of the time), more water soluble, or both, which would then facilitate their removal by organs such as liver and kidney.

Phase I Metabolism

Phase I metabolism includes oxidation (e.g., hydroxylation and dealkylation), reduction, hydrolysis, and several rare miscellaneous reactions [27]. Phase I hydrolases catalyzed enzymatic reactions are essential for the digestion of nutrients such as protein and polysaccharides, but these enzymes are usually not actively involved in metabolism of small molecular drugs (except for certain prodrugs). Hydrolytic enzymes in the GI tract, however, are a main reason why oral delivery of protein drugs remains an elusive goal.

The most important enzyme mediating phase I metabolism of drugs is called cytochrome P450 (CYP). The CYPs are a superfamily of enzymes with over 2000 individual members in almost all biological species ranging from bacteria to humans [27]. In human and other mammalian species, CYP1, CYP2, and CYP3 families are primarily associated with phase I metabolism of drugs and xenobiotics. Several databases are available to search human CYP substrates, reactions types, inducers, and inhibitors (e.g., www.gentest.com). Although most tissues and organs are well populated with CYPs, the liver is usually believed to be the most important phase I metabolic organ. Oxidation, methylation, demethylation, and reduction are some of the most common phase I reactions. Usually, introduction of a reactive functional group, such as a hydroxyl group, is the result of phase I metabolism, which makes it suitable to be eliminated through phase II metabolism or another direct route of elimination (e.g., via the kidney). Phase I reaction occurs to most hydrophobic drugs. The metabolite could be less active or more active than the parent drugs, although most metabolites are less active than the parent drug.

Phase II Metabolism

Some of the drug is a good substrate for certain intestinal and hepatic phase II enzymes. Most drugs subjected to phase II metabolism are substrates of uridine-5′-diphosphate-glucuronosyltransferases and/or sulfotransferases. A glucuronic acid or a sulfate moiety will be added to the drug, which is called phase II metabolism or conjugation. Phase II metabolism substrate often has an electrophile group (e.g., hydroxyl group) in the structure. Phase II metabolism may occur in intestinal epithelial cells, and metabolites may be transported to the liver via the portal vein (Figure 9-1). Moreover, the conjugated metabolites are often good substrates of apically located efflux transporters such as MRPs and breast cancer resistance proteins [24, 28]. Hence, significant amounts of conjugates are excreted back into the intestinal lumen. These phase II metabolites may also be good substrates of basolaterally located efflux transporters (e.g., MRP3), which facilitate their entry into the mesenteric blood. For those drugs that escape intestinal metabolism, the liver is the next organ to metabolize a large portion (if not all) of the escaped drugs via a variety of phase II mechanisms (sulfation and glucuronidation), and the drugs themselves and/or their metabolites may also be excreted via bile or be transported to sinusoidal blood and eventually enter the systemic circulation.

The excreted intact drugs from the bile or enterocytes can be reabsorbed by the intestine epithelial cells. It is commonly believed with substantial experimental data that many phase II metabolites (e.g., glucuronides and sulfates) can be hydrolyzed by microflora enzymes into aglycones, which can then be reabsorbed, thereby completing the recycling loop. A portion of the unabsorbed drugs and their metabolites could also be further metabolized by the microflora into smaller molecules, as described above. An unanticipated benefit of this extensive metabolism via conjugation and extensive excretion of the metabolites into the intestinal lumen by enterocytes and via bile and subsequent return to the aglycone is that compounds heavily metabolized via the phase II pathway could have reasonable apparent half-lives, even though they have very poor bioavailabilities. An example of this drug is raloxifene, which has a bioavailability of 5% or less but has an apparent half-life of more than 24 hours [29].

Microbial Metabolism

Other than metabolism by the intestine and liver, microflora can also metabolize the xenobiotics to limit their bioavailability. Our knowledge, however, about microbial metabolism other than those for degradation of glucuronide and sulfate as well as for certain nutrients is very limited. This is because adult human gut is estimated to contain conservatively 100 trillion microbial organisms that belong to more than 2000 species [30, 31], and we have just begun to understand this complex ecosystem [32, 33]. A complex dynamic relationship between the host and its GI tract microbiome exists shortly after birth, and this relationship remains relatively constant when adulthood is reached [34]. The benefits of GI microbiome include regulation of host epithelial development, induction of innate immunity, and stimulation of the host intestinal angiogenesis [35]. It has also been shown that the indigenous intestinal microbiome is involved in metabolism of xenobiotics, which can result in the production of metabolites that are more active or more toxic than their precursors.

RESIDENCE TIME

For oral delivery, the dosage form and drugs that are part of the dosage form usually move together with food stuff, driven by the GI motility. The residence time of solid food in the GI tract is affected by many factors, such as the volume of stomach, the type of food (high fat versus high sugar), the completeness of digestion (e.g., particle size of the food), and patient behaviors. The common recognized residence time in the stomach of liquid or semiliquid food stuff is about 15 to 30 minutes and of solid food about 120 to 240 minutes. The residence time in the small intestine is about 2 to 5 hours and in the colon about 12 to 48 hours [36–38]. Because of the differences in digestion patterns, the residence time of liquid food stuff is very different from solid food stuff in each segment of the GI tract. In addition, the present or absence of food also affects the residence time of a drug molecule in a very different manner. The residence time of orally administrated drugs in the GI tract is expected to be the same as that of food. Because most drugs are absorbed in the upper part of the intestine (duodenum, jejunum, and ileum), the total effective time for drug absorption is estimated to be from 3 to 8 hours [37, 38]. If the absorption time is slower than the residence time, drugs will move out of the absorption zone and the bioavailability will be affected. The drug residence time can be prolonged, however, by using different formulations (described below).

PATIENTS IN SPECIAL SITUATIONS (PEDIATRIC AND DISABLED)

Ordinary orally administrated drugs are in solid dosage forms such as tablets and capsules. The solid drug forms need to be swallowed by the patient during the administration. A significant percentage of patients in special situations (e.g., pediatric and disabled), however, may experience major difficulty with swallowing. For instance, stroke patients or Parkinson's disease patients have difficulty swallowing solid oral dosage forms [39, 40]. These patients have difficulty in swallowing a whole formulation or have lost the swallowing function altogether; therefore, alternative solid dosage forms or even liquid dosage forms are sometimes needed. Because of their small number, however, many of these special formulations are compounded in a pharmacy, whose quality control is usually not as rigorous as that made by manufacture under GLP procedure. These special formulations must be used with caution, because shelf-life and drug uniformity may not reach the high standard commonly associated with the dosage forms manufactured under the good manufacturing practice standards.

TABLETS

The GI tract is the most suitable site for drug absorption compared with other noninvasive dosing routes (i.e., skin, buccal, and ophthalmic administrations) [41]. The tablet is the most common solid dosage form for oral delivery, accounting for approximately 50% of all dosage forms on the market [42]. It is used for accurate dosing while maintaining good physical and chemical stability of active ingredients. More importantly, patients usually do not have acceptance issues for the tablet formulation, as evidenced by its long history of use [43].

MANUFACTURING PROCESSES AND TABLET PROPERTIES

The tablet is a compressed dosage form that consists of one or more active ingredients together with various inert excipients. The manufacturing processes of tablets are quite complex, and understanding the basic processes of tableting (e.g., compression) requires a good understanding of basic chemistry, material sciences, structural mechanics, and other related disciplines. Design of proper tableting processes and procedures requires a good understanding of active pharmaceutical ingredient form (crystalline/amorphous, free form/salt), stability in various solvents (e.g., water or alcohol), in-transit heat environment (during compression), and in-transit high pressure environment (during compression). It also requires a good understanding of a powder mixture's mechanical properties, including variables such as stress and strain and plasticity and elasticity of the materials. The modern tableting machine can produce hundreds of thousands of tablets per hour, and, therefore, the powder mixture used for feeding into the machine has to have excellent flowability so the tablets will not adhere to punch or die after the tableting processes. Because of these requirements, tableting processes are driven sometimes by engineering principles; a formulator's experience also has an impact on the dosage form design. Our focus here is on the basic processes and how these processes are necessary for the production of tablets and the direct impact on dosage form performance in humans. For a graphic overview of the tablet process, go to http://en.wikipedia.org/wiki/File:Tablet_press_animation.gif.

The major manufacturing methods for tablet manufacture include direct compression, dry granulation, and wet granulation. Direct compression is ideal for powder that can be mixed well and does not require further granulation steps before the tablet press. Nevertheless, direct compression may not be practical because of certain unfavorable characteristics of active ingredients. Granulation is usually needed to (1) prevent segregation/aggregation of certain components in the powder mixture (e.g., between active ingredients and certain excipients), (2) improve the flow ability of powder mixture, and (3) improve the compressibility of the mixture.

Dry granulation refers to the formation of a granular and free-flowing blend of uniformly sized particles/powders without the use of a liquid (binder) solution. It is suitable for active ingredients that are sensitive to moisture and/or heat that may be produced during wet granulation processes. If the powders are very fine and will not compress, addition of liquid binders to the powder mixture may be needed to ensure that active pharmaceutical ingredients are evenly distributed within the powder mixture fed to a tableting machine. Other traditional granulations, including fluid bed granulation, foam granulation, and melt extrusion granulation, are also used to make different types of tablets.

The properties of tablets are usually evaluated with respect to various physical parameters such as appearance, hardness, friability, uniformity of active ingredients, disintegration, and dissolution. Tablet mechanical strength can be measured by hardness and friability, which measures the breaking strength and resistance to abrasion and chipping. For safe handling, the limit of hardness should not be less than 4 kg/cm^2, and friability results should not be more than 2% by using a friabilator. Disintegration of different tablets has to meet different requirements based on the intended purpose of the tablet. *In vitro* dissolution tests are performed for two purposes: to assess the lot-to-lot quality variability of tablets and to guide the design of the bioequivalence study (see http://www.fda.gov/downloads/Drugs/.../Guidances/ucm070246.pdf). In general, immediate-release tablets should disintegrate within 15 minutes by using water as a medium, whereas coated tablets should disintegrate within 30 to 60 minutes at 37° ± 2°C [44]. Enteric-coated tablets should not disintegrate within 120 minutes in an acidic medium (0.1 M hydrochloric acid) without disc[1] and disintegrate within 60 minutes in mixed phosphate buffer medium (pH 6.8) with an addition of disc [45]. Finally, dispersible and

[1]A cylindrical disc made of a suitable, transparent plastic material that is commonly used in the disintegration test.

soluble tablets should disintegrate within 3 minutes using water as the medium at 24 to 26°C, and effervescent tablets should disintegrate within 5 minutes [46].

EXCIPIENTS

Many types of excipients are used in the powder mixture fed to the tablet machine to produce high-quality tablets. Excipients are not supposed to alter (neither diminish nor enhance) the activities of the active ingredient. In other words, excipients should be inert. Several major types of excipients are briefly described below.

Diluents and Fillers

These are the inert substances used to increase bulk of the compressible dosage forms (or tablets) when the mass of active ingredient alone cannot provide a practical shape and size. Widely used fillers are lactose, dextrin, microcrystalline cellulose, pregelatinized starch, powdered sucrose, kaolin, mannitol, sodium chloride, and calcium phosphate [47].

Binders and Adhesives

These materials are used to enhance adhesion of particles, which enable preparation of granules and maintenance of the integrity of the final tablets. Binders and adhesives work together to stabilize the granules and tablets during and after the manufacturing processes. Examples of binders and adhesives include natural gums, cellulose derivatives, gelatin, synthetic polymers, glucose, polyvinyl pyrrolidone, hydroxypropyl methylcellulose, pregelatinized starch, and sodium alginate [48]. Too much binder and adhesive, however, can cause the tablet to fail in the disintegration and dissolution process, so other agents (e.g., disintegrants) are added to counter the action of these agents for optimal (drug) release rates *in vivo*.

Disintegrants

These are agents that facilitate the disintegration of the tablet to smaller particles in the fluid of the stomach and/or GI tract. Disintegration is important for the dissolution of drugs contained in a dosage form, which is the necessary first step before absorption. In general, disintegrants are able to expand in the presence of water in the GI tract, and it is the expansion of the disintegrants that facilitates the rupture (i.e., disintegration) of the tablets. Typical disintegrants include starches, pregelatinized starch, sodium starch glycolate, sodium carboxymethylcellulose, microcrystalline cellulose, polyvinyl pyrrolidone, and crospovidone [49]. Although disintegrants are chemically and/or physically similar to certain binders, adhesives, and even diluents, they are often added to the powder mixture after the granulation process has been completed.

Lubricants

Lubricants are manufacturing aids that are necessary for modern tableting machines because these machines produce tablets at a very high speed and demand that the powder mixture flows evenly without segregation. In general, lubricants have three major types: (1) lubricants, which improve the ejection of tablets from the die wall and smooth the production of tablets by reducing friction between sliding surface; (2) glidants, which reduce the friction between particles and improve the flow properties of granules or powder and decrease the variation of tablet weight; and (3) antiadherents, which prevent sticking problems to certain machine surfaces (e.g., tablet punches). These excipients include metallic stearates, stearic acid, colloidal silicas, and talc. Like binders, too much lubricant could impede disintegration and/or dissolution of the tablets, which in turn affects a tablet's performance *in vivo*.

Flavoring/Coloring Agents and Sweeteners

These excipients are not necessary for the manufacturing of tablets, but certain oral formulations, such as chewable, buccal, and sublingual tablets and lozenges, require flavoring agents to improve palatability. Some bitter-tasting drugs also have added sweetening agents to cover unfavorable tastes. Coloring agents are used to disguise the off-colored drugs or improve tablet identification and appearance. Coloring agent is generally limited to 0.05% of the total tablet weight for safety considerations.

TYPES OF TABLETS

Tablets can be divided into different categories based on delivery mechanisms and/or release profiles. Except for immediate-release tablets for quick action, tablets are also formulated as controlled-release dosage forms to achieve targeted delivery and/or sustained release. Most controlled-release tablets fall in the category of matrix, reservoir, or multilayer systems [50]. The major types of tablets are presented below.

Compressed Tablets or Uncoated Tablets

These are the standard uncoated tablets that are made by direct compression or granulation after mixing of active ingredients and excipients. There are single or multiple layers, and each layer of the multiple-layered tablets can provide different drug-release profiles. The details are below.

Coated Tablets

The uncoated core tablet could be coated with one or more layers of additional excipient substances, often for a defined purpose. Depending on the purpose, the coating can be further divided. Tablets coated for sustained or controlled delivery are discussed below.

The first type is sugar-coated tablets, and the purpose is to mask the unpleasant taste, smell, color, or a combination thereof. The coating is achieved using a sugar solution with other additives as appropriate. This coating is used less in modern pharmaceutical manufacturing because sugar coating could reduce the shelf-life of the final product.

The second is (thin) film-coated tablets, which is quite common because the thin film is commonly used to enhance appearance of the tablets and to improve its other physical attributes (e.g., integrity and photosensitivity). This method of coating can also mask the unpleasant taste, smell, color, or a combination thereof, but additives additional to the polymer are needed. Thin-film coating in combination with other ingredients could also protect the active ingredient from moisture and/or oxidation.

The third is enteric-coated tablets, and the purpose is to functionally change the release site where the tablet is disintegrated from the stomach to the intestine. Enteric-coated tablets are covered by gastric-resistant coating polymers, which cause the tablets to release their active ingredients in the intestinal fluid instead of the gastric fluid. Enteric-coated tablets are commonly used to protect unstable drugs in the acidic environment of stomach and enable high absorption in the small intestine. This coating may also be used to prevent the release of certain active ingredients that are either harmful or irritating to the stomach (e.g., aspirin).

Multilayered Tablets

A multilayered tablet usually consists of a hydrophilic matrix core containing the active ingredient and impermeable or semipermeable polymeric coatings that function as the barrier layers to adjust the hydration or swelling rate of the core [50]. Some incompatible active ingredients can be loaded in different layers, and formulators can insert an inert layer in between to prevent possible interactions (Figure 9–2). They can provide different release profiles to achieve desirable therapeutic effects [51]. For example, fast release for immediate bioavailability and controlled released for a whole day can be achieved in a single tablet without multiple doses. It also provides good patient compliance because a single tablet containing multiple medications is more convenient than separate tablets and more useful in patients with, for example, Alzheimer's disease.

Disintegrating Tablets

Orally disintegrating tablets can disintegrate within approximately 30 seconds in the oral cavity without the need for chewing or drinking liquids. This dosage form was initially designed for pediatric and geriatric patients who may experience compliance problems with conventional tablets because of impaired swallowing and for patients whose adherence to the compliance may be difficult (e.g., for psychiatric disorders). In addition to having compliance advantages, orally disintegrating tablet also share the advantages of conventional tablet dosage forms, like better stability as a solid dosage form, easier production process, and a pleasant taste. Maxalt MLT® and Zofran ODT® are two examples of orally disintegrating tablets. Most orally disintegrating tablets are considered to be bioequivalent with regular tablets, but certain orally disintegrating tablet products could achieve fast onset or higher exposure due to significant absorption in the oral cavity (e.g., Staxyn®).

Chewable Tablets

Chewable tablets disintegrate rapidly when chewed. They usually contain flavoring agents to improve taste and are especially useful for pediatric and geriatric patients. Mannitol is an ideal excipient for the preparation of chewable tablets containing moisture-sensitive drugs and can also mask the taste of active components with objectionable tastes and/or smells. Antacids are typically formulated as chewable tablets. The drug molecules released from chewable tablets are absorbed in the oral cavity (through the buccal membrane), which could bypass first-pass metabolism in intestine and liver. The bioavailability of chewable tablets is expected to be higher than intestinal absorption formulation, if the drugs are subjected to extensive first-pass metabolism.

Dispersible Tablets

There are two types of dispersible tablets: an immediate-release tablet, which instantaneously disintegrates in the mouth when it comes in contact with saliva, and an uncoated

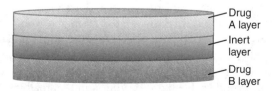

FIGURE 9-2 Several incompatible or different release rates require drugs to be separated by an inert layer in a single multilayered tablet.

or film-coated tablet, which produces a uniformly dispersed liquid before administration. Both have a short disintegrating time, usually less than 1 minute. To achieve this rapid disintegration, tablets must be highly porous and able to rapidly absorb water and saliva by incorporating hydrophilic excipients for a rapid disintegration. They are convenient formulations for pediatric patients and also useful formulations for nonstable drugs. The main disadvantage of this formulation is the lack of high mechanical resistance because of rapid deaggregation of the matrices and lower doses of active drugs [52, 53].

Effervescent Tablets

Effervescent tablets are intended to be dissolved in the mouth or dispersed in water before administration. These are uncoated tablets containing acidic and base substances that react rapidly in water to release carbon dioxide. They provide fast onset of action and are easy for patients who cannot swallow tablets. Effervescent tablets are also useful for drugs that are not stable in water, and they can be dissolved in water right before administration (**Figure 9-3**). It is extensively applied to many drugs, nutrients, and supplements due to better dissolution behaviors.

Lozenges and Sublingual/Buccal Tablets

These tablets are dissolved in the mouth, and active ingredients have immediate local or systemic effect by direct absorption through mucosa to avoid first-pass metabolism. Because of relatively high permeability and rich vascular supply at the oral site, these formulations can also be categorized into intraoral delivery. Faster onset and higher absorption rate constant are two critical advantages, in addition to bypassing first-pass metabolism. This type of tablets is usually applied to drugs that need fast onset, such as migraine, cardiac disorder, analgesia, and insomnia. Nitroglycerine sublingual tablets are well-known examples of this tablet type.

Sustained- and Controlled-Release Tablets

It is sometimes desirable to have drugs released slowly over a prolonged period of time to decrease the difference between peak and valley drug concentrations for reduced side effects and/or enhanced efficacy, to decrease the frequency of drug administration (e.g., from three to two times a day), and to protect the patent length, a practice also called "life cycle" management [54, 55].

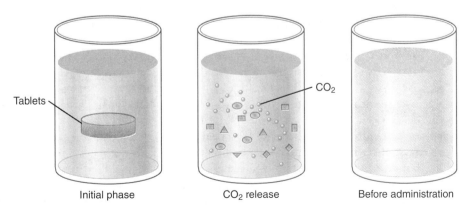

FIGURE 9-3 Effervescent tablets contain acidic and base substances that react rapidly in water to release carbon dioxide and break down quickly to form uniform solution before administration.

Erosion Type Controlled-Release Tablets

The drug release mechanism for the erosion type is usually dissolution controlled [55]. In other words, drug release depends on dissolution of drugs from the dosage form. This dissolution process is sometimes controlled by the slow release of drugs, whereas in other instances it is controlled by the slow erosion of the excipients that surrounds the active drug solids [55]. Many if not most sustained-release formulations are of the erosion type because of the low cost of production versus membrane-controlled or osmotic pump tablets. The main advantage is associated with the relative ease with which this type of device is designed and manufactured. The major disadvantage is the lack of precise control over the rate of drug release. In addition, zero-order release cannot be achieved (i.e., cost release over time), as is desired in many controlled-release formulations.

Membrane Controlled-Release Tablets

The drug release mechanism for membrane-controlled devices is usually diffusion [55]. In this type of device, the rate of drug release is controlled by a membrane, usually made from a biocompatible polymer. Rate of release depends on the thickness and composition of the membrane, saturated drug concentration inside the membrane, and diffusivity of the drug molecules across the membrane. The main advantage is that the release rate could be constant over time, at a rate that can be predicted based on *in vitro* experiments. The main disadvantage is that the cost of manufacturing is high, so there must be a justification for this type of device. In addition, because vast majority of this type of device is not designed to release 100% of its contents during passage *in vivo* (to maintain constant concentration inside the device), any dosage form failure results in serious dose dumping. Dose dumping is a general risk for controlled/sustained delivery dosage forms [55] but is more acute for membrane-controlled drug delivery devices. This is because all drugs are likely to be released at once if the dosage form is somehow compromised.

Osmotic Pump Tablets

The drug release mechanism for this type of device is osmotic pressure difference across the dosage form. Osmotic pump tablets achieve controlled drug delivery by controlling the rate at which water is able to cross a semipermeable membrane coating the tablet. Unlike other types of controlled-release devices, the rate of delivery is not controlled by the physicochemical characteristics of the drug solids or molecules. Rather, it is controlled by the rate of water diffusion across the semipermeable membrane and the size of the orifice from which the drug contents (usually a paste) is expelled from the dosage form. The core of this type of device is usually made of two layers containing the active and osmotic agents. It uses osmosis to release drugs at a constant rate. The advantage of osmotic pump tablets is a reduced risk of adverse reaction by slowly releasing drugs at a zero-order delivery rate to achieve sustained release. It also has a high degree of *in vitro–in vivo* correlation. Because the release rate is controlled by the permeation of water, its *in vivo* drug release behaviors can be accurately predicted based on its *in vitro* drug release behavior. Elementary osmotic pump tablets work well for water-soluble drugs, but with improved technology, many poorly water-soluble drugs can also be made into osmotic pump tablets. Nifedipine osmotic pump (Procardia XL® and Adalat®) and glipizide osmotic pump (Glucotrol®) are good examples of osmotic pump tablets (**Figure 9-4**) [56, 57]. A major disadvantage of the osmotic pump tablet is the high cost of manufacturing and capital investment (for a laser drill that is used to make the orifice), which could limit its application to many drugs due to economical consideration.

Gastroretentive Tablets

The purpose of gastroretentive tablets is to increase the drug absorption within the "absorption window" by retaining the tablet in the gastric fluid for a prolonged period of time, thus extending its residence time in the relevant segment of the GI tract that contains the absorption window. The gastroretentive approaches include swelling devices that result in increased size of the dosage form after administration (expandable systems, biodegradable hydrogels), floating systems that delay the gastric emptying after administration (bioadhesive, superporous, low-density, and high-density systems), and other devices that apply basic physicochemical characteristics (e.g., magnetic systems; **Figure 9–5**) [58]. The gastroretentive tablets are particularly appealing for drugs that are locally active or absorbed only in the stomach and/or upper part of the GI tract

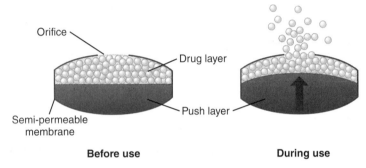

FIGURE 9-4 An osmotic pump-driven tablet consists of core tablet coated with a semipermeable membrane with orifices and push layer with osmotic agents. It uses osmosis to release drugs at a constant rate.

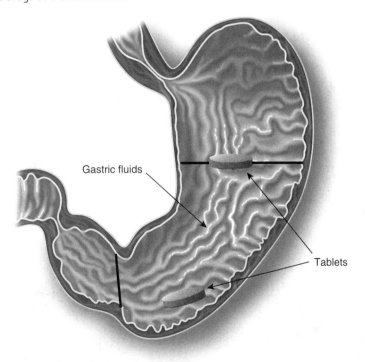

FIGURE 9-5 Tablets may float in gastric fluid (low density) or be retained in the bottom of stomach (high density).

(e.g., drugs absorbed primarily in the duodenum). For certain drugs that are unstable in intestinal environments or exhibit low solubility at high pH values or those that can disrupt the normal colonic microflora, the strategy of using gastroretentive floating tablets can potentially alleviate or avoid these adverse effects [59, 60].

Summary

Various tablet formulations are designed to address different demands from delivery requirements to patient needs. In addition to conventional tablet technology, the use of nanoparticles, solid dispersions, and other pharmacokinetic/permeation enhancers are applied more frequently to tablet formulations with technology advancement. Compared with conventional tablets, sustained- and/or controlled-release tablets were designed to achieve sustained or targeted delivery or improve convenience and compliance. Ultimately, the pharmacokinetic profile of an orally administered drug in a conventional/enabled or controlled-release tablet will determine if the tablet has achieved its desirable pharmacokinetic and pharmacodynamics effects. These are the goals that researchers and medical professionals care about most because they directly affect how our patients respond to these drugs in a proper dosage form.

CAPSULES

The word "capsule" in English is originally derived from a Latin word *capsula*, which means a small container. In pharmacy terms, capsules are referred to as small enveloping shells that contain a dose of bioactive substances. Capsules for drug formulation were invented several hundred years ago, and now they account for a considerable proportion of all prescriptions dispensed every year, even though they are not nearly as popular as tablets [61].

A wide range of drugs are formulated as capsules. In general, capsules can be divided into two main classes: hard-shell capsules and soft-shell capsules (**Figure 9-6**) [62]. Solids, semisolids, or liquids can be encapsulated into the shells by various techniques during the manufacture of capsules. Solid drugs are usually sized as powders, minipellets, or minitablets and then enclosed into hard-shell capsules. In contrast, soft-shell capsules contain liquids or semisolids and are often used for those ingredients that are oil-like or are dissolved or suspended in oil [63]. The liquid contents within the soft-shell capsules should not dissolve the shells.

For both hard- and soft-shell capsules, the manufacturing materials of the shells are mainly gelatin, a natural substance derived from animal skin and bones [64]. Gelatin is selected because its major component is animal protein, which is nontoxic for humans. Gelatin can be rapidly dissolved in the fluid of the GI tract after oral administration.

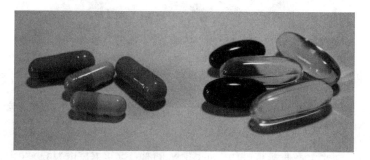

FIGURE 9-6 Hard-shell capsules (left) and soft-shell capsules (right).

More recently, other materials, for example, plant-derived or synthesized polysaccharides, are also used to produce shells [65].

Formulation of drugs in capsules has many advantages. The shells could provide a protection from drugs with unpleasant flavor or tastes, especially those that are irritating to the oral mucosa [66]. The contents in the capsules are usually not as compact as pills or tablets, making fast dissolution of the drugs possible. Moreover, the loading dose in each capsule can be matriculated according to the actual situation or practical requirements. Capsules may also be used in additional routes of drug administration (e.g., rectal or vaginal). Moreover, it is simpler to formulate the powder/granules present in the capsules than those used for tablets. However, their disadvantages or limitations are also evident. A highlighted problem is safety, because capsules can be easily tampered with. Because of the properties of shells, storage of capsules at low humidity is required, and efforts are also needed to prevent microbial growth. The total cost of manufacturing is also higher for most capsules than for regular tablets.

Although capsules have been a primary dosage form in pharmacies for a long time, the design and manufacture of capsules are still being optimized for an improved effect on drug delivery. New types of capsules are also being invented for specific purposes. Some of them are designed to have superior functions (see below).

CAPSULE SHELL MATERIALS

Gelling Agents

Both hard- and soft-shell capsules are usually made of gelling agents. Naturally occurring gelling agents are proteins or polysaccharides. Gelatin, a protein derived from the collagen of animal skin or bone, is a primary substance used in the manufacture of shells. These capsules are referred to as gelatin capsules. Besides gelatin, certain polymers, usually polysaccharides, are also developed as alternative materials for the manufacture of capsules. Capsules made of plant polysaccharides or their derivatives are sometimes called vegetable capsules [67].

Gelatin Capsules

Gelatin capsules are classified into two types, based on the different methods used to pretreat raw materials before extraction. Type A gelatins are often produced by treating raw materials such as pig skin with acid solutions, whereas type B gelatins are often produced by treating raw materials such as bovine bones with alkali solutions [68]. The sources of raw materials and the processes of manufacturing significantly impact the properties of gelatin produced. Thus, when selecting a suitable gelatin type for the capsule formulation, the compatibility between the gelatin wall and the contents (especially the active ingredient) should be considered, especially for soft gelatin capsules.

Dried gelatin films are colorless, flavorless, and brittle. At room temperature it is in solid state. Gelatin will melt upon moderate heat and turn into a solid again when cooled down. A highly viscous solution can be formed when gelatin is dissolved in water, and when cooled down the solution turns into a semisolid gel. The phase change is reversible and often occurs within a few degrees above room temperature. These properties make gelatin an ideal gelling agent to serve as additives in foods, pharmaceuticals, and cosmetics [69]. Gelatin is selected as the primary component of the capsule shells because it has several advantages. The decent aqueous solubility at body temperature makes it readily dissolved in biological fluids. As animal proteins, gelatin is easily digested in the GI tract, and it is a safe material to be used in humans. Because of its good gelling ability, gelatin is easy to process into thin films with various shapes, which is used to form the capsule shells. The thin films made of gelatin and other ingredients are usually strong enough to bear the mechanic tension of stretching and bending during the encapsulating and packaging processes [70].

The thin films of gelatin used as capsule shells still contain 10% to 15% water. If the moisture is lost completely, the shells become extremely brittle and cannot bear any tension. Thus, a main disadvantage of gelatin capsules is their vulnerability to environmental humidity [71]. If stored improperly, gelatin capsules may either lose or absorb water in air and lose their integrity or function. For the same reason, drugs that are hygroscopic or labile in moisture are not suitable to be filled in gelatin capsules. Meanwhile, because of religious and cultural customs or dietary habits, certain consumer populations require capsules made of materials other than animal proteins. In addition, in stressful environments such as high temperature and humidity, gelatin cross-linking may occur [72]. This phenomenon may help to explain the adverse effects of prolonged storage on capsule disintegration and drug dissolution. These and other significant limitations of gelatin have led to the search for alterative materials.

Vegetable Capsules

In the last two decades certain polymers have been developed as substitutes for gelatin in the manufacturing of the gelatin capsules. Most of them are polysaccharides, like carrageenan, pullulan, and chitosan. Modified starch and cellulose from plants may also be used as substitutes for gelatin. Capsules made of these materials are referred to as plant or vegetable capsules. Among them, the most commonly used is hypromellose, which is a short name for hydroxypropyl methylcellulose.

Hypromellose is a semisynthetic polymer derived from cellulose. The hydroxyl groups in each unit of cellulose are methylated or hydroxypropylated in the synthesis of hypromellose, bringing new thermal properties to the product. At low temperature, hypromellose dissolves in water and gets hydrated, forming a viscous liquid. When the temperature increases, hypromellose gradually loses hydrating water and the liquid becomes less viscous. When the liquid is heated to above a critical temperature, interactions between polymers result in the congealing of the system [73]. In production, a gelling aid, usually carrageenan, gellan gum, or pectin, is often added to the solution of hypromellose to help congealing, as well as a gelation promoter like potassium chloride [67].

The main advantage of hypromellose capsules is that they contain much less water than gelatin capsules. Thus, they are a better choice for hygroscopic drugs than gelatin capsules. Hypromellose capsules are still strong enough to bear certain mechanic tension even when they are totally anhydrous. It was shown that after 1 year of storage under conditions as stressful as 40°C and 60% relative humidity, the dissolution profiles of hypromellose capsules filled with model drugs did not change. In the same test, however, the dissolution profiles of gelatin capsules were significantly prolonged due to gelatin cross-linking [74].

Hypromellose capsules are also different from gelatin capsules with respect to dissolution behaviors [75]. When products from different companies are compared, dissolution profiles of regular gelatin capsules are not as diverse as those of hypromellose capsules. This is because different types and contents of gelling aids may result in distinctively different dissolution profiles of hypromellose capsules. In addition, pH and ionic strength of the medium also influence the dissolution of hypromellose capsules. For example, at pH lower or equal to 5.8, a rapid dissolution of hypromellose capsules containing carrageenan occurs between 10 and 55°C. If, however, pH is increased to 6.8, the dissolution time of the same capsules is prolonged and becomes more variable [76]. For hypromellose capsules that are free of gelling aids, their dissolution profiles are independent of pH and ionic strength and exhibit lag times, which are not observed in the dissolution of gelatin capsules [75]. For hypromellose capsules prepared with gellan gum and potassium chloride, the dissolution is hindered under acidic conditions and in the presence of K^+.

Other Ingredients

Besides the gelling agents, several other ingredients are also included in the shell of capsules. These ingredients are minor but are still important in determining the properties of the capsule shells. For example, the difference between hard-shell capsules and softgels in texture is due to the different ratio of plasticizers to gelatin in the gelling solutions from which they are made. The plasticizers are a class of agents often used to increase the plasticity (flexibility) of polymeric materials. Polyols such as glycerin and sorbitol are often used as plasticizers for gelatin. The shells of softgels contain more plasticizers than those of hard-shell capsules; thus, they are softer and more flexible. Plasticizers may also alter other physiochemical properties of capsules, ranging from the appearance to the dissolution behavior. Thus, types and amounts of plasticizers in capsule manufacture should be carefully determined. Potential interactions between filling contents (active and excipients) and plasticizers should also be considered during the dosage-form design process.

Approved dyes and pigments are usually included as colorants, which include titanium dioxide, iron oxide, aluminum lake, and vegetable colors. These colorants may be applied individually or in combination. Titanium oxide is the most commonly used opaquing agent in the shells, shielding the contents from lights. Preservatives are sometimes included in the capsules to prevent bacterial growth during storage. If the capsules give off an unpleasant odor, flavoring agents may also be added to mask the odor. In chewable softgels, sugars like sucrose may be included to provide the sweetness. In addition, information about product codes and drug strengths may be printed on the shells using pharmaceutical-grade inks, usually after the capsules are filled.

TYPES OF CAPSULES

Hard-Shell Capsules

A hard-shell capsule is usually made of two pieces, a telescoping cap and a body. The length of the cap is usually slightly shorter than that of the body. When the cap is pressed on the body, the two pieces fit firmly and form a closed space inside for the drug load. Indentations are usually found around the seam of the cap and body, providing an interlock between the two half-shells to prevent accidental decapping.

Typically, solids like powders, minipellets, and minitablets are filled into the hard-shell capsules. These solids usually include uniformly mixed bioactive ingredients and excipients. The superficial areas of the solids in hard-shell capsules are much bigger than those of pills or tablets, resulting in higher dissolution rates in the GI fluid. Thus, quick absorption may be observed after the rupture of the shell. Occasionally, liquids are also filled into hard-shell capsules. These liquids are often nonaqueous solutions or suspension of active gradients and excipients. In cases where liquids are easier to handle, some solids are liquefied during the filling process and then turn solid again at room temperature. In manufacturing, filled hard-shell capsules are sometimes further sealed by wrapping the seam with an additional layer of gelatin or fusing the two pieces with volatile solvents, especially when the contents in the capsules are mobile at room temperature [77].

Soft-Shell Capsules

Soft-shell capsules are also known as softgels. Contents in softgels are often surrounded by a continuous and closed soft shell, and thus sometimes softgels are also called one-piece capsules. The shells of softgels are often thicker than those of hard-shell capsules.

Softgels are available in mainly three different shapes: oblong, oval, and round. Besides these, softgels with some other shapes can be designed for specific requirements. For each shape, more than 10 different sizes are available, ranging from very tiny ones to those with a volume over 5 mL.

Different from the hard-shell capsules, softgels are usually filled with liquids or semisolids, not solids. Softgels are effective in oral delivery of liquids, providing an alternative dosage form to solutions and other liquid preparations. For certain poorly soluble drugs, the softgel is a good choice because drugs can be dissolved or suspended in liquids, which may help the active ingredients disperse in the GI fluid. For solid drugs with problematic powder flow and/or compressibility, which make them unsuitable for tablets, these drugs can be filled in the softgels with certain liquid vehicles to achieve dosage uniformity. The liquid vehicles in softgels can be water-immiscible liquids such as vegetable oils, esters, and ethers or water-miscible liquids such as polyethylene glycols and polysorbates [78].

Specific Capsules and New Innovations

Although capsules have traditionally served as a primary dosage form for oral drug delivery, a variety of innovations is continuing in the development of new capsules with desired properties and specific functions. These innovations may either improve certain properties of the capsule shells or lead to totally new capsule systems. Most commonly, capsules can be used to change drug-release profiles along the GI tract.

Controlled-Release Capsules

To avoid potential drug inactivation or mucosal irritation in the stomach, a delayed release of drug from capsules is sometimes required. The rupture of capsules should be ensured to occur after they pass the stomach. One strategy is to build the shells with acid-resistant materials. More commonly, the capsules or the encapsulated drug particles are coated with certain pH-sensitive polymers. The capsules with a thin layer of polymers outside the shells are referred to as enteric-coated capsules. The most used polymers include cellulose acetate phthalate, polyvinyl acetate phthalate, hydroxypropyl methylcellulose acetate succinate, and polymethacrylates, which are all available as commercial pharmaceutical excipients [79]. The polymers remain unionized and insoluble in the gastric fluid, and when the pH increases in the intestine, the dissolved polymer layers allow the contact between the capsule shells and the intestinal fluid, thereby releasing the drugs within the capsules.

Controlled-release capsules are also used in the targeted delivery of drugs to certain locations along the GI tract, especially the colon. In colon-directed drug delivery, the most important issue is how to trigger drug release selectively in the colon. Various release mechanisms can be used to achieve this goal. For example, intestinal pressure-controlled colon delivery capsules rupture and release the drug after they enter the colon, due to the increased luminal pressure [80]. Controlled-release capsules relying on the biodegradation actions of the colonic microflora are usually considered to be the most site selective. A capsule system named CODES™ uses shells made of certain polysaccharides, which are only degraded by bacteria in the colon [81]. In another system, conventional capsules are coated with the two specific polysaccharides, pectin and galactomannan, that impede capsule rupture and drug release until they reach the colon (**Figure 9-7**) [82].

Chewable Softgels

Conventionally, orally administered capsules are usually swallowed as a whole with water. Recently, chewable softgels have been developed as an innovative dosage form

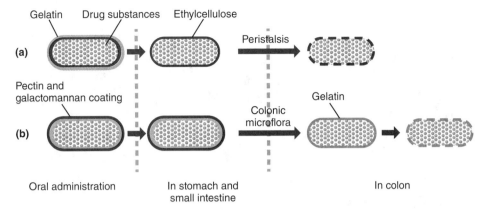

FIGURE 9-7 Two controlled-release capsule systems designed for colon targeted drug delivery. (a) Pressure-controlled colon delivery capsules (Data from R. Pahwa, N. Saini, V. Kumar, and K. Kohli. Chitosan-based gastroretentive floating drug delivery technology: an updated review. *Expert Opin Drug Deliv.* 9:525–539 (2012); 61. M. Helliwell and D. Taylor. Solid oral dosage forms. *Professional Nurse* (London, England). 8:313–317 (1993); and R. Schrieber and H. Gareis. *From Collagen to Gelatine. Gelatine Handbook.* Wiley-VCH Verlag GmbH & Co. KGaA2007, pp. 45–117.) (b) Pectin- and galactomannan-coated capsules. (Data from Yang L, Chu JS, Fix JA. Colon-specific drug delivery: new approaches and *in vitro/in vivo* evaluation. *Int J Pharm.* 2002;235:1–15.)

with promising market prospects. The shells of chewable softgels are made of gelatin with glycerin as the plasticizer, providing the suitable hardness and texture for chewing. These softgels are usually filled with oil or emulsions, containing the bioactive ingredients. Flavors and sweeteners are usually supplemented in the shell and/or content to improve the taste and offer a pleasant mouth feel.

Chewable softgels may be more convenient than conventional capsules because water is not necessary when they are taken. They are particularly suitable for administrating analgesics and nutrients, like vitamins, minerals, and fish oil. Consumers can also enjoy the natural flavors of nutrients when they are supplied as chewable softgels. More importantly, chewable softgels may provide more compliance in populations who have difficulty or physiological discomfort in swallowing whole capsules, especially children. Today, various brands of docosahexaenoic acid (DHA) chewable softgels for children are already on the market [83]. Just like chewable tablets, chewable softgels may also be endowed with additional functions such as oral hygiene products.

Pulsatile Capsules

The maximum efficacy of certain drugs used during therapy can only be obtained by achieving peak plasma drug concentrations at certain optimal time points. A typical "pulsatile" release consists of a predetermined lag time without any release and then a rapid and complete release at a particular time point. To treat certain diseases with peak symptoms at night or to control body functions influenced by circadian rhythm, a pulsatile drug–release pattern is more advantageous than a continuous–release pattern [84]. Several kinds of pulsatile capsules have been proposed for time- or site-controlled release in oral drug administration. Different from the controlled-release capsules mentioned above, these pulsatile capsules are often innovative in the design of the total capsule system, not limited to the shells. Pulsincap, a representative of pulsatile capsules, consists of an insoluble gelatin body coated with ethyl cellulose and a soluble gelatin cap [85]. The drug is sealed in the capsule body with hydrogel polymer as a plug. After the cap is

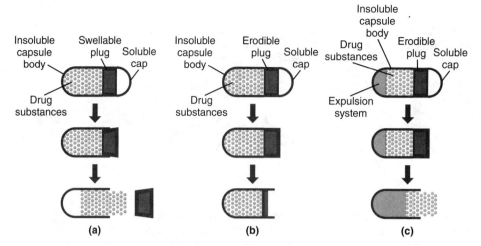

FIGURE 9-8 Pulsatile capsules. (a) Pulsatile capsules with swellable plugs. (b) Pulsatile capsules with erodible plugs. (c) Pulsatile capsules with expulsion systems.(Data from R. Pahwa, N. Saini, V. Kumar, and K. Kohli. Chitosan-based gastroretentive floating drug delivery technology: an updated review. *Expert Opin Drug Deliv.* 9:525–539 (2012); 61. M. Helliwell and D. Taylor. Solid oral dosage forms. *Professional Nurse* (London, England). 8:313–317 (1993); and R. Schrieber and H. Gareis. *From Collagen to Gelatine. Gelatine Handbook.* Wiley-VCH Verlag GmbH & Co. KGaA2007, pp. 45–117.)

dissolved, the hydrogel plug absorbs water and swells in GI fluids. During this process the hydrogel is pulled out of the capsule body gradually, and thus the drug is exposed and released eventually. The swelling rate of the hydrogel plug can be modulated to preset optimal releasing times for different drugs. Besides swellable plugs, erodible and bacterial-degradable materials may also be exploited to build the controlling barrier for release [85, 86]. By organizing components in pulsatile capsules carefully, it is also possible to achieve multiple pulses of drug release in one capsule (Figure 9-8) [87].

TRANSMUCOSAL DRUG DELIVERY SYSTEMS

Oral thin film, patch, and medicated chewing gum belong to oral transmucosal drug delivery systems, which deliver the drug through the oral mucosa. It has been explored intensively during the last decade to overcome the disadvantages of oral drug delivery via the GI tract. Because the oral mucosa is highly vascularized, drugs are transported across the oral mucosa membranes and could then have direct access to the systemic circulation via capillaries and venous drainage, which could bypass the first-pass effect from hepatic and intestinal metabolism. Saliva provides a water-rich environment in the oral cavity, facilitating the release of drugs from the formulation. The rate of blood flow through the oral mucosa is substantial and is generally not considered to be the rate-limiting factor in the absorption of drugs via this route [5]. The bioavailability of oral thin film, patch, and gum is higher than other formulations that are delivered through GI tract, if the drugs are extensively metabolized due to the first-pass effects. These formulations are designed to deliver the drug for rapid release, pulsatile release, or sustained/controlled release for an extended period of time.

The major challenge of the oral transmucosal drug delivery system is the drug residence time. In this delivery system, a drug is supposed to be absorbed in the oral cavity, which does not store food and other substances like the GI tract does. Solids in the oral cavity go to the throat, esophagus, and then the stomach, accomplished by the swallowing function. Liquid is washed into the GI tract, accompanied by swallowing of the saliva. Saliva excretion is 0.5 to 2.0 L daily; however, the volume of saliva constantly available in the oral cavity is about 1.0 mL [5]. The swallowing of saliva is extremely frequent. Therefore, the drug residence time in the oral cavity is limited.

Another challenge is the relatively small surface area of the oral cavity, which means only small quantities of drug can be delivered via the oral route. Because of this, most drugs delivered via buccal route are intended for topical application and local ailments. Highly potent drugs are desirable for optimal effects.

ORAL THIN FILM/PATCH

Oral thin film/patch is a formulation prepared using hydrophilic polymers that rapidly dissolve on the tongue or buccal cavity. The formulation is usually a postage stamp–sized rectangle with drugs in the material that dissolve in seconds when placed on the tongue. The drug is then delivered to the systemic circulation via the absorption in the mouth. The clear advantage is that drugs absorbed via the oral cavity bypass first-pass metabolism (phase I and/or phase II) in the intestine and liver. Therefore, bioavailability is improved by using oral thin films/patch delivery. Additional advantages include quick release, enhanced safety, high precision during dose administration compared with liquid forms, and high level of patient compliance.

Because the oral thin film/patch releases the drug instantly, this dosage form can be formulated to treat diseases such as local pain, allergies, sleep disturbances, anxiety, and gastric problems, which require a fast onset of action. Moreover, because of the convenience, oral thin films are also preferred by patients suffering from dysphasia, motion sickness, repeated emesis, and mental disorders because they are unable to swallow large amounts of water. The advantages of convenient dosing and portability of oral thin films have also led to a wide applicability of this dosage form in pediatric and geriatric patients.

The first commercial launch of oral thin films, Triaminic and Theraflu Thin Strips, for systemic drug delivery occurred in 2004 [88]. This formulation is still in the beginning stages and has a bright future because it fulfils most patient needs except for the limitation of low delivery quantities. In the U.S. market, the over-the-counter films of pain management and motion sickness are commercialized. More importantly, prescription oral thin films have now been approved in the United States, European Union, and Japan, the three major regions of drug usages and development [89]. These approved drugs have the potential to dominate other oral dosage forms of the same drug. The value of the overall oral thin film market may grow significantly.

MEDICATED CHEWING GUM

Medicated chewing gum is defined by the European Pharmacopoeia as single-dose preparations with a base consisting mainly of gum that is intended to be chewed but not to be swallowed, providing a slow steady release of the medicine contained within the dosage form [90]. A medicated chewing gum usually contains water-insoluble gum base and water-soluble ingredients such as sweeteners, colors, flavoring agents, and medications. It can be used for the treatment of local (oral cavity) diseases or treatment of systemic diseases by absorption via oral cavity and/or GI tract.

The advantages of medicated chewing gum include faster onset of action for local treatment, rapid drug release, ease of administration, fewer side effects, higher local bioavailability, less first-pass impact, better patient compliance, and more acceptance by children. Some major disadvantages, however, limit the use of this formulation. For example, many drugs have objectionable taste and smell that cannot be efficiently masked, rendering them unavailable for this dosage form. In addition, chewing and swallowing habits are highly variable between individuals; therefore, the drug release and absorption in the oral cavity tend to be more variable. For systemic treatment, the drug is partially absorbed in the oral cavity and partially in the GI tract, because unabsorbed drugs will be swallowed and available for absorption in the intestine. As a result, bioavailability depends on the habit of chewing and swallowing.

The first commercial chewing gum, state of Maine pure spruce gum, was introduced into the U.S. market in 1848, and the first medicated chewing gum product, Aspergum®, containing acetylsalicylic acid for headache was launched in 1928 [90]. The successful launch of nicotine chewing gum in the 1980s further enticed pharmaceutical companies to develop this formulation. Medicated chewing gum is an alternative to traditional dosage forms for drugs intended for the treatment of oral cavity diseases such as toothache, periodontal disease, oral bacterial and fungal infections, aphthous, and dental stomatitis. Medicated chewing gum can also be used to treat motion sickness, nausea, pain, allergy, infection, and even hypertension [90].

ORAL LIQUIDS (SOLUTION/SUSPENSION)

Oral solutions contain one or more active ingredients dissolved in a suitable vehicle, whereas oral suspensions contain one or more active ingredients suspended in a suitable vehicle with sufficient quantities of suspending agents. The former is a solution and the latter is a relative uniform suspension with designed thermodynamic stability to prevent caking and aggregation. In oral liquid formulations, drug solids are dissolved or suspended in the vehicle, which means a drug can be absorbed faster than those in regular solid formulations (e.g., tablets). This is especially true when the drug is hydrophobic with poor water solubility. Drug absorption still occurs in the GI tract for oral liquid, however, and epithelial permeability is still the main barrier. In addition, if the drug is a substrate of metabolism enzymes, first-pass effect in the intestine and liver cannot be avoided. Clinical trials showed no significantly bioavailability differences between oral liquid and tablet formulations [91]. However, oral liquids are broadly used in patients in special situations (e.g., pediatric, disabled, geriatric) due to the need for flexible dosing and the danger of airway obstruction that interfere with swallowing [91]. The major challenge associated with oral liquid dosage forms are the shorter shelf-life (compared with tablets or capsules), inability to mask unpleasant taste and/or smells, and instability of the drug molecules in the aqueous environment. Many drugs are much more stable in the solid state than in the liquid (especially aqueous) state [91].

Oral liquid formulations include vehicles (may contain syrup or flavoring agents to enhance taste), suspending agents (for suspension), color additives, and preservatives. If the drug is not completely soluble in water, a suspending agent is required to prepare an oral suspension, because suspended solid particles are normally unstable thermodynamically and require suspending agents to stabilize them. Carboxymethylcellulose and methylcellulose are the most common suspending agents used to enhance dose uniformity and physical stability, because they increase the viscosity of the liquid [91]. Syrup is often used to adjust the taste and to keep the osmotic pressure high, which suppresses microbial growth. The pH value of the liquid and suspension is usually about 4 to 5. Unlike solid formulations, oral liquids and suspensions contain plenty of water, which means bacteria could grow easily (hence the need for preservative) and the chemical stability of the drug could be questionable (hence the shorter shelf-life). For suspension,

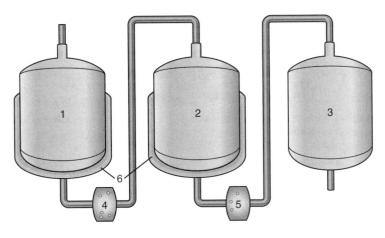

1. Sugar melting vessel   4. Online sugar filter
2. Syrup vessel   5. Online syrup filter
3. Storage vessel   6. Heating jacket

FIGURE 9-9 A schematic diagram of automatic oral liquid process equipment.

physical stability of the suspension is also a very critical issue and needs to be considered and evaluated. The storage condition is also more critical than solid formulations because hydrolysis, light, high temperature, and oxygen could accelerate the degradation of the drug in liquid or suspension. A schematic diagram of automatic oral liquid process equipment is shown in **Figure 9-9**.

Cetirizine hydrochloride is an oral liquid antihistamine drug used to temporarily relieve symptoms due to hay fever or other upper respiratory allergies. The formulation is made by mixing cetirizine hydrochloride (5 mg/5 mL) with other inactive ingredients, including calcium acetate, grape flavor, glacial acetic acid, glycerin, methylparaben, propylene glycol, propylparaben, and purified water [71].

MICROEMULSIONS

Microemulsion is an isotropic, thermodynamically stable transparent (or translucent) systems of oil, water, and surfactant frequently in combination with a cosurfactant with particles of droplet sizes usually in the range of 20 to 200 nm [93]. A microemulsion system usually has very low oil–water interfacial tension. Because the particles or droplet size is less than 25% of the wavelength of visible light, microemulsions are transparent. The system is usually formed readily and spontaneously, without high-energy input. According to the structure, there are three types of microemulsions: oil-in-water, water-in-oil, and biocontinuous systems. In all three types of microemulsions the interface is stabilized by an appropriate combination of surfactants (and/or cosurfactants) to enhance the thermodynamic stability.

Advantages of microemulsion over other formulations are obvious. Microemulsion systems increase water solubility of insoluble drugs. As a result, the absorption of poorly water-soluble drugs is increased, which could lead to the enhanced oral bioavailability. This system is suitable for hydrophobic drugs with poor solubility. Advantages other than the enhanced absorption are numerous and not limited to the following: (1) it is a liquid formulation and can be used by patients with special conditions (e.g., disabled, pediatric), (2) it decreases the variability in absorption rates because dissolution is not necessary, (3) it provides protection from hydrolysis and oxidation when drugs are in the oil phase of microemulsion, and (4) it could help in masking tastes and smells [93]. On the other hand, the disadvantages of microemulsion limit its usage in drug development. The system uses large amounts of concentrated surfactants with/without cosurfactants to stabilize the droplets or particles. The surfactant and cosurfactant must be nontoxic for pharmaceutical usage, which has been proven to be elusive for the most part. The most visible commercial product is a cyclosporine A microemulsion formulation called Neoral [94]. In addition, the stability of the microemulsion system is influenced by environmental parameters such as pH and temperature, which could change during delivery to patients.

The original term of "microemulsion" was used in 1959 to describe a multiphase system consisting of water, oil, surfactant, and alcohol, which forms a transparent solution [95]. The first attempt at using microemulsion as a potential drug delivery vehicle was reported in 1974 [96]. This is a novel drug delivery system whose full potential is yet to be realized. Many innovations are expected to come in the field of microemulsion technology.

SUMMARY

This chapter describes various factors that impact the bioavailability of drugs delivered via the oral route. We describe and summarize the properties of major oral formulations, including tablets, capsules, oral thin film/patch, medicated chewing gum, oral liquid, and microemulsion. We focused our efforts on outlining factors that are considered when designing each type of dosage forms and how these factors could impact the *in vivo* performance in humans.

Tablets remain the most common solid dosage form for oral delivery due to ease of use, long shelf-lives, and excellent patient compliance. Multiple types of controlled-release tablets are available to overcome different delivery challenges, including rapid release tablets, coated/uncoated tablets, multilayered tablets, orally disintegrating tablets, chewable tablets, dispersible tablets, effervescent tablets, lozenges and sublingual/buccal tablets, controlled- and/or sustained-release tablets, osmotic pump tablets, gastroretentive tablets, and drug combination tablets.

Capsule is the second most used formulation for oral drug delivery. The major advantage of capsules is that the shell can be used to deliver drugs with unpleasant flavor or tastes, especially those that are irritating to the oral mucosa. Moreover, the contents in capsules are usually not as compressed as pills or tablets, making a quick dissolution of the drugs possible. Furthermore, a capsule's contents could be easily dispersed for patients who cannot swallow it whole. For oral liquid formulations, the drug is dissolved or suspended in the vehicle and can be absorbed faster than those in solid formulations, especially when the drug is hydrophobic with poor water solubility. Another advantage of oral liquid is that the liquid is suitable for patients with special situations when swallowing is impaired due to age or diseased conditions. The advantage of microemulsion is that increments of water solubility for insoluble drugs result in enhanced oral bioavailability.

Oral thin film, patch, and medicated chewing gum belong to the oral transmucosal drug delivery system. The biggest advantage of these formulations is that drug molecules transported across the oral mucosa membranes have direct access to the systemic circulation via capillaries and venous drainage, which could bypass first-pass effects. Although advantages are obvious for controlled-release formulations, limitations still exist. In drug development, whether or not to use innovative formulation depends on multiple factors such as the physicochemical property of the drug, the conditions of the targeted patient population, and cost.

REVIEW QUESTIONS

1. What are the advantage and disadvantage of oral delivery as compared to other routes of drug delivery?
2. What are the barriers that can limit the bioavailability of a drug used in oral administration?
3. How many types of drug metabolism pathways are available in liver and intestine, and what are major types of the enzymes responsible for these metabolisms?
4. What are the major manufacturing methods for tablet manufacture and tablet properties?
5. What are the advantages and disadvantages of using capsules as compared to other oral dosage forms?
6. How is drug release triggered in the colon when using capsules for colon-targeted drug delivery?

REFERENCES

1. Hurst S, Loi CM, Brodfuehrer J, El-Kattan A. Impact of physiological, physicochemical and bio pharmaceutical factors in absorption and metabolism mechanisms on the drug oral bioavailability of rats and humans. *Expert Opin Drug Metab Toxicol.* 2007;3:469–489.
2. Keberle H. Physico-chemical factors of drugs affecting absorption, distribution, and excretion. *Acta Pharmacol Toxicol.* 1971;29(Suppl 3):30–47.
3. Avdeef A. Physicochemical profiling (solubility, permeability and charge state). *Curr Top Med Chem.* 2001;1:277–351.
4. Edward LD, Kerns H. *Drug-like Properties: Concepts, Structure Design and Methods for ADME to Toxicity Optimization.* New York: Elsevier; 2008.
5. Patel VF, Liu F, Brown MB. Advances in oral transmucosal drug delivery. *J Control Release.* 2011;153:106–116.
6. Blaut M, Clavel T. Metabolic diversity of the intestinal microbiota: implications for health and disease. *J Nutr.* 2007;137:751S–755S.
7. van Nuenen MH, Venema K, van der Woude JC, Kuipers EJ. The metabolic activity of fecal microbiota from healthy individuals and patients with inflammatory bowel disease. *Dig Dis Sci.* 2004;49:485–491.
8. Booth AN, Deeds F, Jones FT, Murray CW. The metabolic fate of rutin and quercetin in the animal body. *J Biol Chem.* 1956;223:251–257.
9. Braune A, Gutschow M, Engst W, Blaut M. Degradation of quercetin and luteolin by *Eubacterium ramulus. Appl Environ Microbiol.* 2001;67:5558–5567.
10. Gaoand S, Hu M. Bioavailability challenges associated with development of anti-cancer phenolics. *Mini Rev Med Chem.* 2010;10:550–567.
11. Morteau O, ed. *Oral Tolerance: The Response of the Intestinal Mucosa to Dietary Antigens.* New York, NY: Kluwer Academic/Plenum; 2004.
12. Lipinski CA, Lombardo F, Dominy BW, Feeney PJ. Experimental and computational approaches to estimate solubility and permeability in drug discovery and development settings. *Adv Drug Deliv Rev.* 2001;46:3–26.
13. Leibach FH, Ganapathy V. Peptide transporters in the intestine and the kidney. *Annu Rev Nutr.* 1996;16:99–119.
14. Tamai I. Oral drug delivery utilizing intestinal OATP transporters. *Adv Drug Deliv Rev.* 2012;64:508–514.
15. Englund G, Rorsman F, Ronnblom A, et al. Regional levels of drug transporters along the human intestinal tract: co-expression of ABC and SLC transporters and comparison with Caco-2 cells. *Eur J Pharm Sci.* 2006;29:269–277.
16. Smith DE, Clemencon B, Hediger MA. Proton-coupled oligopeptide transporter family SLC15: physiological, pharmacological and pathological implications. *Mol Aspects Med.* 2013;34:323–336.
17. Kalliokoski A, Niemi M. Impact of OATP transporters on pharmacokinetics. *Br J Pharmacol.* 2009;158:693–705.

18. Choi YH, Yu AM. ABC transporters in multidrug resistance and pharmacokinetics, and strategies for drug development. *Curr Pharm Des.* 2014;20(5):793–807.

19. Marquez B, Van Bambeke F. ABC multidrug transporters: target for modulation of drug pharmacokinetics and drug-drug interactions. *Curr Drug Targets.* 2011;12:600–620.

20. Sharom FJ. ABC multidrug transporters: structure, function and role in chemoresistance. *Pharmacogenomics.* 2008;9:105–127.

21. Glavinas H, Krajcsi P, Cserepes J, Sarkadi B. The role of ABC transporters in drug resistance, metabolism and toxicity. *Curr Drug Deliv.* 2004;1:27–42.

22. Jiang W, Hu M. Mutual interactions between flavonoids and enzymatic and transporter elements responsible for flavonoid disposition via phase II metabolic pathways. *RSC Adv.* 2012;2:7948–7963.

23. Yang Z. The roles of membrane transporters on the oral drug absorption. *J Mol Pharm Org Proc Res.* 2013;1:e102. doi:10.4172/jmpopr.1000e102 doi: 10.4172/jmpopr.1000e102.

24. Yang Z, Zhu W, Gao S, et al. Breast cancer resistance protein (ABCG2) determines distribution of genistein phase II metabolites: reevaluation of the roles of ABCG2 in the disposition of genistein. *Drug Metab Dispos.* 2012;40:1883–1893.

25. Yang Z, Gao S, Wang J, et al. Enhancement of oral bioavailability of 20(S)-ginsenoside Rh2 through improved understanding of its absorption and efflux mechanisms. *Drug Metab Dispos.* 2011;39:1866–1872.

26. Alvarez AI, Real R, Perez M, Mendoza G, Prieto JG, Merino G. Modulation of the activity of ABC transporters (P-glycoprotein, MRP2, BCRP) by flavonoids and drug response. *J Pharm Sci.* 2010;99:598–617.

27. Lewis DF. Human cytochromes P450 associated with the phase 1 metabolism of drugs and other xenobiotics: a compilation of substrates and inhibitors of the CYP1, CYP2 and CYP3 families. *Curr Med Chem.* 2003;10:1955–1972.

28. McGhie TK, Walton MC. The bioavailability and absorption of anthocyanins: towards a better understanding. *Mol Nutr Food Res.* 2007;51:702–713.

29. Kosaka K, Sakai N, Endo Y, et al. Impact of intestinal glucuronidation on the pharmacokinetics of raloxifene. *Drug Metab Dispos.* 2011;39:1495–1502.

30. Savage DC. Microbial ecology of the gastrointestinal tract. *Annu Rev Microbiol.* 1977;31:107–133.

31. Berg RD. The indigenous gastrointestinal microflora. *Trends Microbiol.* 1996;4:430–435.

32. Kumari A, Catanzaro R, Marotta F. Clinical importance of lactic acid bacteria: a short review. *Acta Biomed.* 2011;82:177–180.

33. Festi D, Schiumerini R, Birtolo C, et al. Gut microbiota and its pathophysiology in disease paradigms. *Dig Dis.* 2011;29:518–524.

34. Salminen S, Benno Y, de Vos W. Intestinal colonisation, microbiota and future probiotics? *Asia Pac J Clin Nutr.* 2006;15:558–562.

35. Hooper LV, Gordon JI. Commensal host-bacterial relationships in the gut. *Science.* 2001;292:1115–1118.

36. Patel VF, Liu F, Brown MB. Advances in oral transmucosal drug delivery. *J Control Release.* 2011;153:106–116.

37. Adebisi A, Conway BR. Gastroretentive microparticles for drug delivery applications. *J Microencapsul.* 2011;28:689–708.

38. Sathish D, Kumar YS, Rao YM. Floating drug delivery systems for prolonging gastric residence time: a review. *Curr Drug Deliv.* 2011;8(5):494–510.

39. Salat-Foix D, Suchowersky O. The management of gastrointestinal symptoms in Parkinson's disease. *Expert Rev Neurother.* 2012;12:239–248.

40. Cecconi E, Di Piero V. Dysphagia—pathophysiology, diagnosis and treatment. *Front Neurol Neurosci.* 2012;30:86–89.

41. Yang Z, Teng Y, Wang H, Hou H. Enhancement of skin permeation of bufalin by limonene via reservoir type transdermal patch: formulation design and biopharmaceutical evaluation. *Int J Pharm.* 2013;447(1–2):231–40.

42. Deyand P, Maiti S. Orodispersible tablets: A new trend in drug delivery. *J Nat Sci Biol Med.* 2010;1:2–5.

43. Mrsny RJ. Oral drug delivery research in Europe. *J Control Release.* 2012;161:247–253.

44. Gupta A, Hunt RL, Shah RB, Sayeed VA, Khan MA. Disintegration of highly soluble immediate release tablets: a surrogate for dissolution. *AAPS PharmSciTech.* 2009;10:495–499.

45. Cora LA, Romeiro FG, Americo MF, et al. Gastrointestinal transit and disintegration of enteric coated magnetic tablets assessed by ac biosusceptometry. *Eur J Pharm Sci.* 2006;27:1–8.

46. Parkash V, et al. Fast disintegrating tablets: Opportunity in drug delivery system. *J Adv Pharm Technol Res.* 2011;2:223–235.

47. Gabrielsson J, Sjostrom M, Lindberg NO, Pihl AC, Lundstedt T. Multivariate methods in the development of a new tablet formulation: excipient mixtures and principal properties. *Drug Dev Ind Pharm*. 2006;32:7–20.
48. Saha S, Shahiwala AF. Multifunctional coprocessed excipients for improved tabletting performance. *Expert Opin Drug Deliv*. 2009;6:197–208.
49. Mehta S, De Beer T, Remon JP, Vervaet C. Effect of disintegrants on the properties of multiparticulate tablets comprising starch pellets and excipient granules. *Int J Pharm*. 2012;422:310–317.
50. Efentakisand M, Peponaki C. Formulation study and evaluation of matrix and three-layer tablet sustained drug delivery systems based on Carbopols with isosorbite mononitrate. *AAPS PharmSciTech*. 2008;9:917–923.
51. Patel VM, Prajapati BG, Patel MM. Formulation, evaluation, and comparison of bilayered and multilayered mucoadhesive buccal devices of propranolol hydrochloride. *AAPS PharmSciTech*. 2007;8:22.
52. Schiermeier S, Schmidt PC. Fast dispersible ibuprofen tablets. *Eur J Pharm Sci*. 2002;15:295–305.
53. Fini A, Bergamante V, Ceschel GC, Ronchi C, de Moraes CA. Fast dispersible/slow releasing ibuprofen tablets. *Eur J Pharm Biopharm*. 2008;69:335–341.
54. Robinson JR. *Sustained and Controlled Release Drug Delivery Systems*. Marcel Dekker; 1978.
55. Wen H, Park K. *Oral Controlled Release Formulation Design and Drug Delivery: Theory to Practice*. Hoboken, NJ: John Wiley & Sons; 2011.
56. Zhang ZH, Dong HY, Peng B, et al. Design of an expert system for the development and formulation of push-pull osmotic pump tablets containing poorly water-soluble drugs. *Int J Pharm*. 2011;410:41–47.
57. Okimoto K, Tokunaga Y, Ibuki R, et al. Applicability of (SBE)7m-beta-CD in controlled-porosity osmotic pump tablets (OPTs). *Int J Pharm*. 2004;286:81–88.
58. Arza RA, Gonugunta CS, Veerareddy PR. Formulation and evaluation of swellable and floating gastroretentive ciprofloxacin hydrochloride tablets. *AAPS PharmSciTech*. 2009;10:220–226.
59. Pahwa R, Saini N, Kumar V, Kohli K. Chitosan-based gastroretentive floating drug delivery technology: an updated review. *Expert Opin Drug Deliv*. 2012;9:525–539.
60. Talukder R, Fassihi R. Gastroretentive delivery systems: a mini review. *Drug Dev Ind Pharm*. 2004;30:1019–1028.
61. Helliwell M, Taylor D. Solid oral dosage forms. *Profess Nurse*. 1993;8:313–317.
62. Singh SK, Naini V. Dosage forms: non-parenterals. In: Swarbrick J (ed). *Encyclopedia of Pharmaceutical Technology*, 3rd ed. Boca Raton, FL: CRC Press. 2006:988–1000.
63. Bergstrom DH, Tindal S, Dang W. Capsules, soft. In: Swarbrick J (ed). *Encyclopedia of Pharmaceutical Technology*, 3rd ed. Boca Raton, FL: CRC Press. 2006:419–430.
64. Schrieberand R, Gareis H. *From Collagen to Gelatine. Gelatine Handbook*. Berlin, Germany: Wiley-VCH Verlag GmbH & Co.; 2007:45–117.
65. Jones BE. Capsules, hard. In: Swarbrick J (ed). *Encyclopedia of Pharmaceutical Technology*, 3rd ed. Boca Raton, FL: CRC Press. 2006:406–418.
66. Morris H. Administering drugs to patients with swallowing difficulties. *Nursing Times*. 2005;101:28–30.
67. Al-Tabakha MM. HPMC capsules: current status and future prospects. *J Pharm Pharmac Sci*. 2010;13:428–442.
68. Francis FJ. *Wiley Encyclopedia of Food Science and Technology*, 2nd ed. Vols. 1–4. Hoboken, NJ: John Wiley & Sons; 1999.
69. Schrieber R, Gareis H. *Introduction. Gelatine Handbook*. Wiley-VCH Verlag GmbH & Co.; 2007:1–44.
70. Tsou AH, Hord JS, Smith GD, Schrader RW. Strength analysis of polymeric films. *Polymer*. 1992;33:2970–2974.
71. Dupont AL. Study of the degradation of gelatin in paper upon aging using aqueous size-exclusion chromatography. *J Chromatogr A*. 2002;950:113–124.
72. Digenis GA, Gold TB, Shah VP. Cross-linking of gelatin capsules and its relevance to their in vitro-in vivo performance. *J Pharm Sci*. 1994;83:915–921.
73. Li CL, Martini LG, Ford JL, Roberts M. The use of hypromellose in oral drug delivery. *J Pharm Pharmacol*. 2005;57:533–546.
74. Nagata S. Advantages to HPMC capsules: a new generation's drug delivery technology. *Drug Devel Deliv*. 2002;2:34–39.
75. Sherry Ku M, Li W, Dulin W, et al. Performance qualification of a new hypromellose capsule: Part I. Comparative evaluation of physical, mechanical and processability quality attributes of Vcaps Plus®, Quali-V® and gelatin capsules. *Int J Pharm*. 2010;386:30–41.
76. Ku MS, Lu Q, Li W, Chen Y. Performance qualification of a new hypromellose capsule: Part II. Disintegration and dissolution comparison between two types of hypromellose capsules. *Int J Pharm*. 2011;416:16–24.

77. Stegemann S. Hard gelatin capsules today—and tomorrow. *Capsugel Library* 1999;1–23.
78. Jimerson RF, Scherer RP. Soft gelatin capsule update. *Drug Dev Indust Pharm.* 1986;12:1133–1144.
79. Felton LA, McGinity JW. Enteric film coating of soft gelatin capsules. *Drug Deliv Technol.* 2003;3(6).
80. Muraoka M, Hu Z, Shimokawa T, et al. Evaluation of intestinal pressure-controlled colon delivery capsule containing caffeine as a model drug in human volunteers. *J Control Release.* 1998;52:119–129.
81. Katsuma M, Watanabe S, Takemura S, et al. Scintigraphic evaluation of a novel colon-targeted delivery system (CODES™) in healthy volunteers. *J Pharm Sci.* 2004;93:1287–1299.
82. Yang L, Chu JS, Fix JA. Colon-specific drug delivery: new approaches and in vitro/*in vivo* evaluation. *Int J Pharm.* 2002;235:1–15.
83. Haug IJ, Sagmo LB, Zeiss D, et al. Bioavailability of EPA and DHA delivered by gelled emulsions and soft gel capsules. *Eur J Lipid Sci Technol.* 2011;113:137–145.
84. Maroni A, Zema L, Cerea M, Sangalli ME. Oral pulsatile drug delivery systems. *Expert Opin Drug Deliv.* 2005;2:855–871.
85. Ross AC, Macrae RJ, Walther M, Stevens HNE. Chronopharmaceutical drug delivery from a pulsatile capsule device based on programmable erosion. *J Pharm Pharmacol.* 2000;52:903–909.
86. Krögel I, Bodmeier R. Pulsatile drug release from an insoluble capsule body controlled by an erodible plug. *Pharm Res.* 1998;15:474–481.
87. Li B, Zhu J, Zheng C, Gong W. A novel system for three-pulse drug release based on "tablets in capsule" device. *Int J Pharm.* 2008;352:159–164.
88. Novartis launches first systemic OTC in film strip format. *In* pharmatechnologist.com, Breaking News on Global Pharmaceutical Technology & Manufacturing, 2004. http://www.in-pharmatechnologist.com/Ingredients/Novartis-launches-first-systemic-OTC-in-film-strip-format. Accessed April 4, 2014.
89. Nehal Siddiqui GG, Sharma PK. A short review on a novel approach in oral fast dissolving drug delivery system and their patents. *Adv Biol Res.* 2011;5:291–303.
90. Chaudhary SA, Shahiwala AF. Medicated chewing gum—a potential drug delivery system. *Expert Opin Drug Deliv.* 2010;7:871–885.
91. Lam MS. Extemporaneous compounding of oral liquid dosage formulations and alternative drug delivery methods for anticancer drugs. *Pharmacotherapy.* 2011;31:164–192.
92. Zorin S, Kuylenstierna F, Thulin H. In vitro test of nicotine's permeability through human skin. Risk evaluation and safety aspects. *Ann Occup Hyg.* 1999;43:405–413.
93. Talegaonkar S, Azeem A, Ahmad FJ, Khar RK, Pathan SA, Khan ZI. Microemulsions: a novel approach to enhanced drug delivery. *Recent Pat Drug Deliv Formul.* 2008;2:238–257.
94. Johnston A, Belitsky P, Frei U, et al. Potential clinical implications of substitution of generic cyclosporine formulations for cyclosporine microemulsion (Neoral) in transplant recipients. *Eur J Clin Pharmacol.* 2004;60:389–395.
95. Schulman SW. Mechanism of formation and structure of microemulsions by electron microscopy. *J Phys Chem.* 1959;63:1677–1680.
96. Attwood L, Elworthy PH. Study of solubilized micellar solutions. I. Phase studies and particle size analysis of solutions with nonionic surfactants. *J Colloid Interface Sci.* 1974;46:249–256.

CHAPTER 10

Ocular Drug Delivery

Aswani Dutt Vadlapudi, Kishore Cholkar, Supriya Reddy Dasari, and Ashim K. Mitra

CHAPTER OBJECTIVES

Upon completing this chapter, the reader should be able to

- Describe the anatomy and physiology of the eye.
- Understand the importance of various routes of drug administration to the eye.
- Describe various barriers to ocular drug delivery and constraints with conventional ocular therapy.
- Determine the ideal physicochemical properties for ocular drug candidates.
- Acquire sound knowledge of various approaches to increase ocular drug absorption.
- Understand the utility, recent progress, and specific development issues relating to dendrimers, cyclodextrins, nanoparticles, liposomes, nanomicelles, microneedles, implants, *in situ* gelling systems, and contact lens in ocular drug delivery.
- Explore key advances in the application of nanotechnology for gene delivery to the eye.

CHAPTER OUTLINE

INTRODUCTION

Drug delivery to the eye has been one of the most challenging tasks to pharmaceutical scientists. The unique anatomy and physiology of the eye renders it a highly protected organ, and the unique structure restricts drug entry at the target site of action. Drug delivery to the eye can be generally classified into anterior and posterior segments. Conventional delivery systems, including eye drops, suspensions, and ointments, cannot be considered optimal; however, more than 90% of the marketed ophthalmic formulations indicated for the treatment of debilitating vision-threatening ophthalmic disorders are in the form of eye drops. These formulations primarily target diseases of the front of the eye (anterior segment). Most topically instilled drugs do not offer adequate bioavailability due to the wash off of the drugs from the eye by various mechanisms (lacrimation, tear dilution, and tear turnover). In addition, the human cornea composed of epithelium, substantia propria, and endothelium hinders drug entry; consequently, less than 5% of administered drug enters the eye.

Alternative approaches are continuously sought to facilitate significant drug absorption into the eye. Currently, the treatment of disorders of the back of the eye (posterior segment) still remains a formidable task for the ocular pharmacologists and physicians. The tight junctions of blood–retinal barrier (BRB) limit the entry of systemically administered drugs into the retina. High vitreal drug concentrations are required for the treatment of posterior segment diseases. This can be accomplished only with local administration (intravitreal [IVT] injections/implants and periocular injections). Periocular injections are associated with fairly high patient compliance relative to IVT injections. Nevertheless, structural variations of each layer of ocular tissue can pose a significant barrier upon drug administration by any route (i.e., topical, systemic, and periocular). To date, remarkable changes have been observed in the field of ophthalmic drug delivery.

This chapter offers great insight into anatomical and physiological features of the eye and various routes of ocular drug administration. Furthermore, this chapter emphasizes the role of various ocular transporters, prodrug strategies, colloidal dosage forms, implants, contact lens, *in situ* gelling systems, and other recent developments in drug delivery strategies, including gene therapy.

ANATOMY OF THE EYE

The eye is an isolated, highly complex, and specialized organ for photoreception. A complex anatomy and physiology renders it a highly protected organ [1]. Generally, the eye can be divided into two segments: anterior and posterior. The anterior segment of the eye is composed of cornea, conjunctiva, iris, ciliary body, aqueous humor, and lens, whereas the posterior segment includes sclera, choroid, retina, and vitreous body (**Figure 10-1**). The front part of the eye is bound by a transparent cornea and a minute part of the sclera. The cornea and sclera join together through the limbus. Cornea is devoid of blood vessels and receives nourishment and oxygen supply from the aqueous humor and tear film, whereas the corneal periphery receives nourishment from the limbal capillaries. The human cornea measures approximately 12 mm in diameter and 520 μm in thickness. It is composed of six layers: the epithelium, Bowman's membrane, stroma, Dua's layer, Descemet's membrane, and endothelium (**Figure 10-2**) [2]:

- Epithelium: The corneal epithelium is a stratified, squamous, nonkeratinized layer approximately 50 μm in thickness. It serves as an outer protective barrier comprising five to six cell layers, including two to three layers of flattened superficial cells, wing cells, and a single layer of columnar basal cells separated by a 10- to 20-nm intercellular space. Desmosome-attached cells can communicate by gap junctions through which small molecules permeate. The superficial epithelial cell layers are sealed by tight junctions called zonulae occludens that prevent the permeation of compounds with low lipophilicity across the cornea. Thus, the corneal epithelium is a rate-limiting barrier and hinders the permeation of hydrophilic drugs and macromolecules.
- Bowman's membrane: This acellular thin basement layer is made up of collagen fibrils. It is not considered as a rate-limiting barrier.

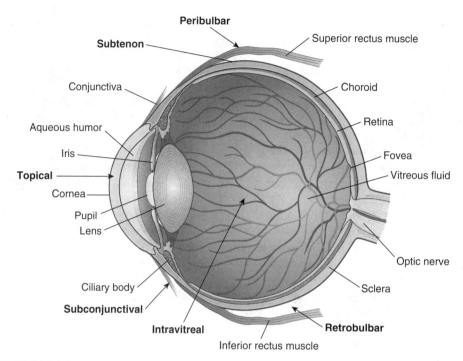

FIGURE 10-1 Anatomy of the eye and various routes of ocular drug administration.

- Stroma: Constituting about 90% of the cornea, this layer is abundant in hydrated collagen. Because of its hydrophilic nature, the stroma offers minimal or low resistance to diffusion of highly hydrophilic drugs.
- Dua's layer: It is a newly identified, well-defined, acellular, strong layer in the pre-Descemet's cornea. Its functional role is yet to be determined [3].
- Descemet's membrane: It is a thin homogeneous layer sandwiched between the stroma and the endothelium.
- Endothelium: It is a single-layered squamous epithelium posterior to the corneal surface. The stroma and Descemet's membrane cover the inner endothelial cells, which contain macula adherens. The endothelial cells do not act as a barrier to permeant molecules due to lack of tight junctions.

Conjunctiva is a vascularized mucous membrane lining the inner surface of eyelids and the anterior surface of sclera up to the limbus. It facilitates lubrication in the eye by generating mucus and helps with tear film adhesion. It offers less resistance to drug permeation relative to cornea. Iris, the most anterior portion of the uveal tract, is the pigmented portion of the eye consisting of pigmented epithelial cells and circular muscles (constrictor iridial sphincter muscles). The opening in the middle of the iris is called the pupil. The iris sphincter and dilator muscles aid in tuning the pupil size, which regulates the entry of light into the eye. The ciliary body, a ring-shaped muscle attached to the iris, is produced by ciliary muscles and the ciliary processes. The aqueous humor, a fluid present in the anterior segment, is secreted by the ciliary processes into the posterior segment at the rate of 2 to 2.5 μL/min. It supplies most nutrition and oxygen to avascular tissues (lens and cornea). It flows continuously from the posterior to the anterior through the pupil and leaves the eye via trabecular meshwork and Schlemm's canal. Such continuous flow maintains the intraocular pressure (IOP). The lens is a crystalline and flexible structure enclosed in a capsule. It is suspended from the ciliary muscles by

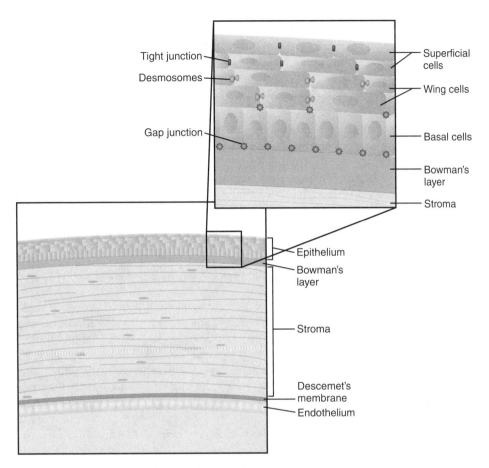

FIGURE 10-2 Cornea and its cellular organizations depicting various barriers to drug transport. The outer superficial epithelial cells possess tight junctions and exhibit the tightest monolayer. The wing and basal cells exhibit gap junctions. The stroma, Dua's layer, and Descemet's membrane covers the inner endothelial cells, display macula adherens, and are more permeable.

very thin fibers called the zonules. It is very important for vision and offers protection to the retina from ultraviolet radiation in conjunction with ciliary muscles.

The posterior segment comprises the retina, vitreous humor, choroid, sclera, and the optic nerve. The retina is a multilayered sensory, light-sensitive tissue that lines the back of the eye. It consists of a neural layer, pigment epithelium, and millions of photoreceptors (rods and cones) that capture and subsequently convert light rays into electrical impulses. Such impulses are transferred by the optic nerve to brain where images are formed. The vitreous humor is a jelly-like substance between the retina and lens. This hydrogel matrix consists of hyaluronic acid, proteoglycans, and collagen fibrils. Separated from the anterior segment by hyaloid membrane, the vitreous is joined to the retina via ligaments. Choroid is a highly vascularized tissue located between the retina and sclera. Its major function is to provide nourishment to the photoreceptor cells in the retina. Sclera is the whitish outermost layer, surrounding the globe, and is called the "white of the eye." It is composed of collagen bundles, mucopolysaccharides, and elastic fibers. This tissue acts as a principal shield to protect the intraocular contents. The scleral tissue is about 10 times more permeable than the cornea and at least half as permeable as the conjunctiva. Hence, permeants can diffuse and enter the posterior segment through the transscleral route.

ROUTES OF OCULAR DRUG ADMINISTRATION

Ophthalmic diseases are primarily treated conventionally by medications administered via either the topical or systemic route. Topical application remains the most preferred route due to ease of administration, low cost, and patient compliance. It is generally useful in the treatment of anterior segment disorders [4]. Drug delivery to the posterior segment still is a major challenge to pharmaceutical scientists. Anatomical and physiological barriers obstruct drug entry into posterior ocular tissues such as retina and choroid. After topical instillation, a large fraction (about 90%) of the applied dose is lost due to nasolacrimal drainage, tear dilution, and tear turnover, leading to poor ocular bioavailability. Less than 5% of the administered dose reaches the aqueous humor after topical administration [5]. Frequent dosing is required, which ultimately results in patient discomfort and inconvenience. Two major absorption routes have been proposed for drugs instilled via topical route: corneal route (cornea–aqueous humor–intraocular tissues) and noncorneal route (conjunctiva–sclera–choroid/retinal pigment epithelium [RPE]). The preferred mode of absorption depends on the physicochemical properties of the permeant [6, 7].

Conventional topical formulations require frequent large doses to produce therapeutic amounts in the back of the eye. Therefore, oral delivery alone [8–10] or in combination with topical delivery [11] has also been investigated because the oral route is considered as noninvasive and high in patient compliance, especially for chronic retinal disorders. High doses are required to achieve significant amounts in the retina. Such high doses, however, lead to systemic adverse effects, and safety and toxicity become a major concern. Oral administration is not predominant and may be highly beneficial only if the drug possesses high oral bioavailability. Nevertheless, molecules in systemic circulation should be able to cross the blood–aqueous barrier (BAB) and BRB after oral administration.

Systemic administration is often preferred for the treatment of posterior segment disorders. A major disadvantage with this route, however, is that it only allows 1% to 5% of administered drug into the vitreous chamber. After systemic administration, the availability of drug is restricted by the BAB and BRB, which are the major barriers for anterior segment and posterior segment ocular drug delivery, respectively. The BAB consists of two distinct cell layers: the endothelium of the iris/ciliary blood vessels and the nonpigmented ciliary epithelium. Both layers prevent drug entry into the intraocular tissues, including aqueous humor, because of the presence of tight junctions [12]. In a similar manner, BRB prevents drug entry from blood into the posterior segment. BRB is composed of two types: retinal capillary endothelial cells (inner BRB) and RPE cells (outer BRB) (Figure 10-3). RPE is a monolayer of highly specialized cells sandwiched between neural retina and the choroid. It selectively transports molecules between photoreceptors and choriocapillaris [13]. Tight junctions of RPE, however, also restrict intercellular drug transport.

Drug entry into the posterior ocular tissues is mainly governed by the BRB. It is selectively permeable to highly hydrophobic drug molecules. To maintain high drug concentrations, frequent dosing is necessary, which often leads to systemic adverse effects [14]. Drawbacks such as lack of adequate ocular bioavailability and failure to deliver therapeutic drug concentration to the retina led ophthalmic scientists to explore alternative administration routes.

Over the past decade, IVT injections have drawn significant attention to scientists, researchers, and physicians. This method involves injection of the drug solution directly into the vitreous via the pars plana using a 30-G needle. This route provides higher drug concentrations in the vitreous and retina. Unlike other routes, the drug can be directly

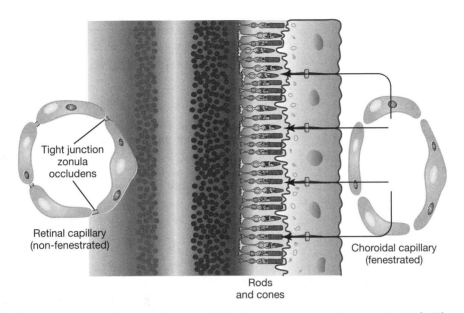

Tight junction zonula occludens

Retinal capillary (non-fenestrated)

Choroidal capillary (fenestrated)

Rods and cones

FIGURE 10-3 Retinal cellular architecture: RPE cells, and retinal capillary endothelial (RCE) cells represent the outer and inner retinal barriers, respectively. RPE and RCE represent major drug transport barriers. The outer layer of RPE possesses tight junctions (zonula occludens). Inner RCE expresses tight junctions and are usually nonfenestrated as opposed to choroidal capillary endothelial cells.

injected into the vitreous cavity; however, drug distribution is not uniform. Although small molecules can rapidly diffuse throughout the vitreous fluid, the distribution of macromolecules is restricted or limited. After IVT administration, drug elimination depends on the molecular weight of the compound as well as the pathophysiological condition [15]. For example, macromolecules, which are linear and globular–shaped compounds (especially protein and peptide drugs) with molecular weights between 40 and 70 kDa, tend to cause longer retention in the vitreous humor [16]. The half-life of the drug in the vitreous fluid is also a major determinant of therapeutic efficacy. Elimination of a drug after IVT administration may occur via the anterior or posterior route. The anterior route of elimination involves drug diffusion to the aqueous from the vitreous humor via zonular spaces followed by elimination through aqueous turnover and uveal blood flow. On the other hand, the posterior route of elimination involves drug transport across the BRB, which necessitates optimal passive permeability or active transport. Consequently, drug molecules with higher molecular weight and hydrophilicity tend to be retained in the vitreous humor for longer periods due to longer half-lives of the compounds [13]. Although IVT administration is advantageous in achieving larger drug concentrations in the retina, frequent administration is often associated with complications such as endophthalmitis, retinal detachment, and IVT hemorrhages, leading to poor patient outcome [17].

Periocular administration has also been considered as an efficient route for drug delivery to the posterior segment. Periocular refers to the periphery of the eye or the region surrounding the eye. This route includes peribulbar, posterior juxtascleral, retrobulbar, subtenon, and subconjunctival routes (Figure 10-1). Drugs administered by the periocular route can reach the posterior segment of the eye by three different pathways: transscleral pathway, systemic circulation through the choroid, and anterior pathway through the tear film, cornea, aqueous humor, and vitreous humor [18].

Subconjunctival injection involves the introduction of an active ingredient beneath the conjunctiva. Conjunctival epithelium serves as a rate-limiting barrier for the permeability of water-soluble compounds. As a result, the transscleral pathway bypasses the cornea–conjunctiva barrier. Various dynamic, static, and metabolic barriers, however, impede drug entry to the back of the eye. Several publications reported rapid drug elimination via these pathways after subconjunctival administration [19–21]. Therefore, most of the administered dose drains into the systemic circulation, leading to poor ocular bioavailability. However, molecules that escape conjunctival vasculature may pass through sclera and choroid and ultimately reach the neural retina and photoreceptor cells. Sclera offers less resistance to drug transport and is more permeable than the cornea [22]. Unlike corneal and conjunctival tissues, scleral permeability is independent of lipophilicity/hydrophobicity but is dependent on the molecular radius [13, 23]. On the other hand, high choroidal blood flow can reduce substantial fractions of the dose reaching the neural retina. Moreover, BRB also hinders drug availability to the photoreceptor cells. Although the periocular route is considered suitable for sustained-release drug delivery systems, several anterior segment complications, such as increased IOP, cataract, hyphema, strabismus, and corneal decompensation, have been observed [24, 25].

Subtenon injection usually involves injection into the tenon's capsule located around the upper portion of the eye and into the belly of the superior rectus muscle. The tenon's capsule is a fibrous membrane that covers the globe from the corneal margin to the optic nerve. A blunt-tipped cannula needle is generally inserted into the tenon's capsule after a surgical incision into the subtenon's space. This technique is widely used during anesthesia for ocular surgery because the cannula approach reduces sharp-needle complications [22].

Retrobulbar injections usually involve the injection in the conical compartment within the rectus muscles and intramuscular septa. These injections provide higher local drug concentrations with negligible influence on IOP. The peribulbar route involves the injection in the extracellular spaces of the rectus muscles and their intramuscular septa. Although drug administration through the peribulbar route is safer, it is less effective than the retrobulbar route. Posterior juxtascleral injection using a blunt-tipped curved cannula delivers the drug directly onto the outer surface of sclera. This route may allow sustained delivery to the macula. Retrobulbar injections are considered the most efficient among all periocular routes but are associated with serious complications, such as retrobulbar hemorrhage, globe perforation, and respiratory arrest.

ROLE OF EFFLUX AND INFLUX TRANSPORTERS IN THE EYE

One conventional approach to enhance ocular bioavailability is to modify the parent drug chemically to achieve desired solubility and lipophilicity with minimal toxicity. A more coherent approach, however, would be a transporter-targeted ligand modification of the drug. Transporter-targeted delivery has turned out to be a powerful strategy to deliver drugs to target ocular tissues because of the ability of the transporter to translocate the cargo inside the cell as well as into intracellular organelles at a higher rate. Transporters are membrane-associated proteins that are actively involved in the translocation of nutrients across cellular membranes. Of particular interest in ocular drug delivery are efflux and influx transporters [6, 26, 27]. Efflux transporters belong to the ATP binding cassette superfamily, whereas influx transporters belong to the solute carrier (SLC) superfamily of proteins. Efflux transporters carry molecules out of cell membrane and cytoplasm, thereby resulting in low bioavailability. Major efflux proteins identified on various ocular tissues include P-glycoprotein, multidrug resistance protein (MRP), and breast cancer resistance protein. P-glycoprotein extrudes lipophilic compounds from both normal and malignant cells and is involved in the emergence of drug resistance. Functional and molecular aspects of P-glycoprotein have been characterized on various ocular cell lines and tissues, such as the cornea [28–30], conjunctiva [31, 32], and RPE [33–35]. MRP also works in a similar manner but effluxes organic anions and conjugated compounds. Three of nine isoforms of the MRP family have been identified on ocular tissues. MRP1 is primarily expressed on rabbit conjunctival epithelial cells [36] and RPE [37], whereas MRP2 and MRP5 have been identified on corneal epithelium [38, 39]. The molecular presence of breast cancer resistance protein was also reported on the corneal epithelium [40]. Breast cancer resistance protein-mediated transport occurs in conjunction with nonpolar substrates in the lipid bilayer and can function as a drug flippase, transferring drugs from the inner to the outer portion of the membrane. Expression levels and patterns of these transporter proteins in cells may differ based on its origin and culture conditions.

On the other hand, influx transporters are involved in transporting xenobiotics and essential nutrients, such as amino acids, vitamins, glucose, lactate, and nucleobases, into cells. Influx transporters are often targets for prodrug delivery because these derivatives can improve absorption of poorly diffusing parent drugs. The prodrug is not a good substrate for efflux transporters. In addition, physicochemical properties of the active (i.e., solubility and stability) can be enhanced. Influx transporters usually targeted for ophthalmic drug delivery are amino acid, vitamins, and peptide transporters. These proteins facilitate physiological roles of transporting various amino acids, vitamins, and nutrients into ocular tissues. Amino acid transporters belonging to the SLC1, SLC6, and SLC7 gene families were detected in ocular tissues, mainly on corneal epithelium and RPE cells. Five high-affinity glutamate transporters (EAAT1–EAAT5) and two neutral amino acid transporters (ASCT1 and ASCT2) compose the SLC1 family. ASCT1 (SLC1A4) was detected on rabbit cornea and in rabbit primary corneal epithelial cells [41], whereas ASCT2 was expressed in retinal Müller cells [42]. Alanine and serine translocated by ASCT1 and 2, respectively. $B^{(0, +)}$, a neutral and cationic amino acid transporter with broad substrate specificity, has been identified on cornea [43] and conjunctiva [44]. This system is associated with arginine transport across cornea and conjunctiva. Also, a sodium-independent large neutral amino acid transporter, LAT1, has been detected on human and rabbit corneas [45], whereas expression of LAT2 was confirmed on ARPE-19 and hTERT-RPE cells [46, 47]. These carriers translocate phenylalanine into ocular tissues.

Gene products from the SLC gene families, such as sodium-dependent multivitamin transporter (SMVT), derived from *SLC5A6* gene, are responsible for translocation and absorption of vitamins such as biotin, pantothenate, and lipoate. SMVT specifically carries biotin as directed by the Na^+ gradient [48, 49]. Functional and molecular aspects of biotin uptake via SMVT have been delineated on cornea and retina of both human-derived [50] and rabbit-derived cells [51, 52]. SMVT has been explored by designing targeted lipid based drug conjugates that can significantly enhance absorption of a parent drug [48]. Peptide transporters have been extensively studied for ocular drug delivery. Oligopeptide transporter has been identified on rabbit cornea [53]. Both PEPT1 and PEPT2 have been detected on the newly introduced clonetics human corneal epithelium (cHCE) cell line and on human cornea [54, 55]. A proton-coupled dipeptide transport system on conjunctival epithelial cells can mediate the uptake of dipeptide L-carnosine [56]. Furthermore, peptide transporter expression was also studied in retinal Müller cells [57] and neural retina [58].

In addition to amino acid, vitamin, and peptide transporters, several others, including organic cation/anion [55, 59], monocarboxylate [60], folate [61], ascorbate [62], and nucleoside transporters [63], have been characterized on various ocular tissues. Overall, influx and efflux transporters play vital roles in the absorption of vital nutrients and drugs. These proteins also deal with the elimination of waste and harmful xenobiotics.

PRODRUG STRATEGIES FOR INCREASING OCULAR DRUG ABSORPTION

Prodrugs are bioreversible derivatives of drug molecules that are enzymatically or chemically transformed *in vivo* to release the active parent drug, which can then elicit the desired pharmacodynamic response [6, 64]. Prodrugs have been primarily designed to improve physicochemical, biopharmaceutical, and pharmacokinetic properties of pharmacologically active ophthalmic drugs. In particular, most prodrugs are designed to increase solubility, improve drug shelf life, or stability both chemically and metabolically so these conjugates can reach their physiological target, minimize the side effects, and aid in formulation [65]. In addition to facilitating improved therapeutic efficacy, prodrug strategy can cause evasion of efflux pumps. Lipophilic prodrugs of acyclovir (ACV) and ganciclovir (GCV) caused enhancement of drug transport across corneal epithelium [66–68]. Apparent permeability of the valerate ester prodrug of GCV across cornea is about six times higher than the parent drug GCV [67]. Pilocarpine and some natural prostaglandins also demonstrated enhanced corneal and scleral permeation after lipophilic prodrug derivatization [69, 70].

Malik et al. [71] investigated transscleral retinal delivery of celecoxib, an anti-inflammatory and anti–vascular endothelial growth factor (VEGF) agent, which is poorly water soluble and, moreover, binds readily to melanin pigment in choroid-RPE. These researchers developed three hydrophilic amide prodrugs of celecoxib: celecoxib succinamidic acid (CSA), celecoxib maleamidic acid (CMA), and celecoxib acetamide (CAA). These prodrugs have been developed to improve solubility of celecoxib, reduce pigment binding, and enhance retinal delivery. Aqueous solubilities of CSA, CMA, and CAA were 300-, 182-, and 76-fold higher than celecoxib, respectively. *In vitro* transport studies across isolated bovine sclera and sclera-choroid-RPE demonstrated eight-fold higher transport for CSA than celecoxib. The rank order for cumulative percent transport across bovine sclera was CSA > CMA > CAA ~ celecoxib and across bovine sclera-choroid-RPE was CSA > CMA ~ CAA ~ celecoxib (**Figure 10-4**). *In vivo* delivery in pigmented brown Norway rats showed concentrations of total celecoxib (free + prodrug) were significantly higher in the CSA group compared with the celecoxib group for all posterior eye tissues except choroid-RPE and periocular tissues [71].

A crystalline lipid prodrug, octadecyloxyethyl-cyclic-cidofovir, was developed for the treatment of cytomegalovirus retinitis. Intraocular pharmacokinetics of octadecyloxyethyl-cyclic-cidofovir after IVT injection was evaluated in rabbits. IVT injection of ^{14}C-octadecyloxyethyl-cyclic-cidofovir displayed biphasic drug elimination. The initial phase lasted from the time of injection to day 21, whereas the second phase was observed from day 21 to day 63. Noncompartment analysis demonstrated a half-life of 5.5 days for the first phase and a terminal half-life of 25 days. The maximum concentration (C_{max}) values were calculated as 130.43 ± 24.42 µg/mL, 45.22 ± 10.98 µg/mL, and 16.10 ± 1.66 µg/mL in the vitreous, retina, and choroid, respectively. This prodrug generated more drug exposure to the retina than the vitreous [72].

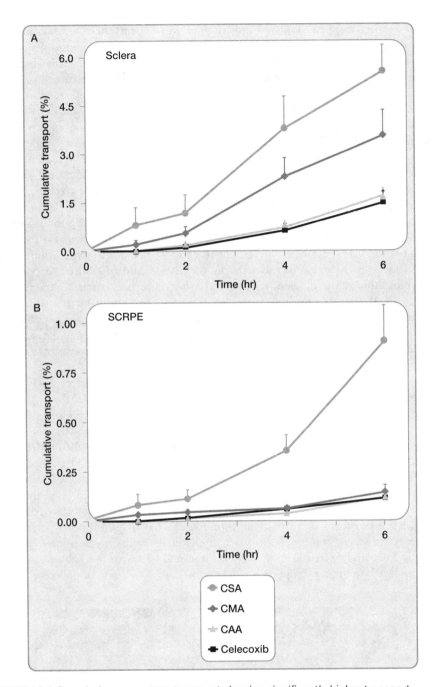

FIGURE 10-4 Cumulative percentage transport showing significantly higher transport for celecoxib succinamidic acid (CSA) than celecoxib across bovine sclera and sclera-choroid-RPE. Cumulative percentage transport of celecoxib and its amide prodrugs across bovine (a) sclera and (b) sclera-choroid-RPE. (Reproduced from Malik P, Kadam RS, Cheruvu NP, Kompella UB. Hydrophilic prodrug approach for reduced pigment binding and enhanced transscleral retinal delivery of celecoxib. *Mol Pharm.* Mar 5, 2012;9[3]:605–614. © American Chemical Society.)

Membrane transporter targeted prodrug design has been the most exciting of all current drug delivery strategies. Prodrugs targeted toward nutrient transporters and receptors expressed on various epithelial cells are designed to enhance the absorption of poorly permeating drug molecules. Influx transporters recognize such prodrugs as substrates and transported the entire cargo across the epithelial membrane. Most studies have been directed toward peptide transporters to improve ocular bioavailability of ACV or GCV after oral, systemic, or topical administrations [73–76]. Mitra and coworkers developed a series of stereoisomeric valine-valine based dipeptide ester prodrugs of ACV. Prodrugs including LLACV, LDACV, DLACV, and DDACV were designed to facilitate enhanced residence time of intact prodrug in the systemic circulation, thus enabling targeting transporters on blood–ocular barriers after oral or systemic administration. Hydrolytic enzymes such as peptidases and esterases responsible for bioreversion of dipeptide prodrugs are stereospecific and show high affinity for L-isomers. Therefore, D–isomers were incorporated into the dipeptide moieties at a particular position to modulate the rate of conversion of the prodrugs. Such incorporation enabled prodrugs to be more stable in the systemic circulation and to facilitate recognition and translocation by the nutrient transporters at blood–ocular barriers. Among these prodrugs, LLACV and LDACV hydrolyzed in Caco-2 cell homogenate and LDACV was relatively more stable of the two compounds (Table 10-1). Incorporation of two D-Valine moieties into a dipeptide moiety, however, enhanced the enzymatic stability but abolished the affinity of these prodrugs (DDACV and DLACV) toward the peptide transporter [77].

Several dipeptide ester prodrugs of GCV (L-valine-L-valine, L-tyrosine-L-valine, and L-glycine-L-valine) were synthesized and evaluated for their vitreal pharmacokinetics in anesthetized rabbit model by an ocular microdialysis technique. These prodrugs appeared to permeate deeper into the retina after IVT administration relative to GCV [78]. Subsequently, vitreal pharmacokinetics of various GCV prodrugs was also studied in a conscious animal model. A comparison of vitreous pharmacokinetic parameters of valine-valine-GCV and regenerated valine-GCV and GCV after IVT administration of valine-valine-GCV in conscious and anesthetized rabbit models is summarized in Table 10-2 [79]. The data suggest lowering the exposure of drug and prodrug levels in conscious animals, although vitreal half-lives did not change.

A novel prodrug strategy that imparts lipophilicity and site specificity has been designed. This study utsed a lipid raft with one end conjugated to the parent drug (ACV) molecule to impart lipophilicity and the other end to a targeting moiety (biotin)

TABLE 10-1 Stability in Caco-2 homogenate—first-order degradation rate constants and half lives of all prodrugs

Drug	$K \times 10^3$ (h^{-1})	t_{v2} (h)
LLACV	92.23 ± 4.79	7.52 ± 0.40
LDACV	13.33 ± 1.96	52.80 ± 8.42
DLACV	*	*
DDACV	*	*
D-VAl-ACV	29.86 ± 4.71	23.56 ± 3.42

*No degradation during the time of study. Each value is represented as mean ± S.D. (n − 3).

Reproduced from Talluri RS, Samanta SK, Gaudana R, Mitra AK. Synthesis, metabolism and cellular permeability of enzymatically stable dipeptide prodrugs of acyclovir. *International Journal of Pharmaceutics*. Sep. 1, 2008; 361(1–2):118–124, with permission from Elsevier.

TABLE 10-2 Conscious animal vitreous pharmacokinetic parameters of Valine-Valine-Ganciclovir and regenerated Valine-Ganciclovir and Ganciclovir after intravitreal administration of Valine-Valine-Ganciclovir

Parameters	Val-Val-GCV		P Value (<0.05>)
	Conscious animal	Anesthetized animal	
AUC (mg · min · mL^{-1})	6. 3 ± 0.3	29.4 ± 3.2	*
λ_z (× 10^{-3}/min)	17.4 ± 6.9	10.1 ± 2.2	NS
$t_{1/2}$ (min)	44.8 ± 19.2	68.6 ± 12.3	NS
V_{ss} (mL)	1.9 ± 0.2	1.3 ±0.3	*
Cl (µL/min)	35.3 ± 1.8	8.9 ± 1.8	*
MRT$_{last}$ (min)	50.5 ± 6.4	138.4 ± 25.6	*
C_{last} (µg/mL)	0.8 ± 0.2	7.2 ± 1.1	*
T_{last} (min)	293.3 ± 11.5	600	*
Regenerated Val-GCV from Val-Val-GCV			
AUC (mg · min · mL^{-1})	1.5 ± 0.6	2.2 ± 0.5	NS
C_{max} (µg/mL)	3.6 ± 1.9	3.9 ± 1.6	NS
T_{max} (min)	120 ± 105.8	460 ± 105	*
MRT$_{last}$ (min)	304.5 ± 15.3	333 ± 28	NS
Regenerated GCV from Val-Val-GCV			
AUC (mg · min · mL^{-1})	2.7 ± 1.0	3.5 ± 1.2	NS
C_{max} (µg/mL)	12.5 ± 7.2	6.3 ± 1.6	NS
T_{max} (min)	140 ± 69.3	420 ± 96	*
MRT$_{last}$ (min)	231.8 ± 64.6	349 ± 48	*

*Represents significant difference at $P < 0.05$.

Abbreviations: AUC, area under curve; C_{last}, last measured plasma concentration; GCV, ganciclovir; MRT, mean residence time; NS, not significant; Val, valine; V_{ss}, volume of distribution at steady state.
Reproduced from Janoria KG, Boddu SH, Natesan S, Mitra AK. Vitreal pharmacokinetics of peptide-transporter-targeted prodrugs of ganciclovir in conscious animals. *J Ocul Pharmacol Th.*: the official journal of the Association for Ocular Pharmocology and Therapeutics. Jun 2010;26(3):265-271.

that can be recognized by a specific transporter/receptor (SMVT). Lipophilic prodrugs readily diffused across the cell membrane by facilitated diffusion, whereas transporter/receptor targeted prodrugs translocated compounds across the cell membrane via active transport by transporter recognition. Marginal improvement in cellular uptake was evident from both approaches. However, this novel approach combines both lipid and transporter/receptor targeted delivery to generate a synergistic effect. Compared with ACV, the uptake of targeted lipid prodrugs (biotin–ricinoleicacid–acyclovir [B–R–ACV] and biotin–12hydroxystearicacid–acyclovir [B–12HS–ACV]) increased by 13.6 and 13.1 times, respectively, whereas the uptake of B–ACV, R–ACV, and 12HS–ACV was higher by only 4.6, 1.8, and 2.0 times, respectively, in HCEC cells (**Figure 10-5**) [80]. The targeted lipid prodrugs B–R–ACV and B–12HS–ACV exhibited much higher cellular accumulation than B–ACV, R–ACV, and 12HS–ACV. Both the targeted lipid prodrugs

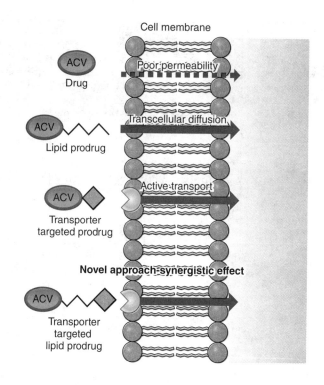

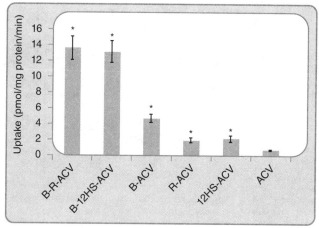

FIGURE 10-5 Novel targeted lipid prodrug strategy showing advantage of this strategy over lipophilic prodrug derivatization and transporter targeted prodrug approaches. Cellular accumulation of B-R-ACV, B-12HS-ACV, B-ACV, R-ACV, 12HS-ACV, and ACV on HCEC cells. (With kind permission from Springer Science+Business Media: Vadlapudi AD, Vadlapatla RK, Earla R, et al. Novel biotinylated lipid prodrugs of acyclovir for the treatment of herpetic keratitis [HK]: Transporter recognition, tissue stability and antiviral activity. *Pharmaceutical research,* May 9 2013.)

B-R-ACV and B-12HS-ACV demonstrated higher affinity toward SMVT than B-ACV. These promising results suggest that the lipid raft may facilitate enhanced interaction of prodrugs with membrane transporters/receptors probably assisting docking of the targeted ligand into the binding domain of transporter/receptor protein. The net effect observed is rapid translocation of the cargo across the cell membrane. This novel prodrug design may also allow for enhanced plasma membrane uptake of hydrophilic therapeutic agents such as genes, silent interfering RNA, nucleosides, nucleotides, oligonucleotides or antisense oligonucleotides, peptides, and proteins [48].

COLLOIDAL DOSAGE FORMS FOR ENHANCING OCULAR DRUG ABSORPTION

DENDRIMERS

Dendrimers may be defined as artificial macromolecular core shell-like structures consisting of three architectural components: a central core; an interior shell made of repeating branch of monomeric units; and peripheral functional groups. In general, dendrimer/dendrons are synthesized from branched monomer units in a stepwise manner following two approaches: convergent and divergent methods (**Figure 10-6, A** and **B**). Examples of dendrimers that find application in drug delivery include poly(amidoamine) (PAMAM) and polypropylenimine. Becasue these macromolecules are artificially synthesized, it is possible to precisely control their molecular size, shape, dimension, density, polarity, flexibility, and solubility with appropriate selection of building units and surface functional groups. Dendrimers with terminal primary amine functional groups are named as "full generation" (G2, G3, G4, etc.), whereas those with carboxylate or ester terminal functional groups are named as "half generation" (G2.5, G3.5, G4.5, etc.) dendrimers, where "G" stands for generation. As the number of branches in dendrimers increase, it leads to the development of higher generation dendrimers. Low generation dendrimers possess empty core and open conformations, which helps to encapsulate hydrophobic drug molecules [81]. In addition, the presence of high surface density functional groups ($-NH_2$, $-COOH$, $-OH$) such as in PAMAM, allows improved solubility for many drugs and also permits surface conjugation of targeting ligands and/or drugs (**Figure 10-7**)

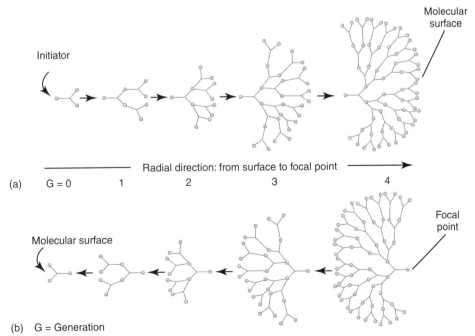

FIGURE 10-6 Synthesis of dendrimers: (a) divergent method and (b) convergent method.

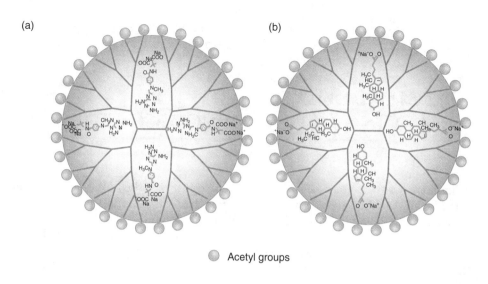

Acetyl groups

FIGURE 10-7 (i) Proposed inclusion structures of acetylated G4 polypropylenimine dendrimer/drug complexes: (a) methotrexate sodium; (b) sodium deoxycholate. (ii) Synthesis of triphenylphosphonium (ligand) conjugated, fluorescently labeled, acetylated G(5)-PAMAM dendrimer. (Part a reproduced from Wang F, Cai X, Su Y, et al. Reducing cytotoxicity while improving anti-cancer drug loading capacity of polypropylenimine dendrimers by surface acetylation. *Acta Biomater.* Dec. 2012;8[12]:4304–4313, with permission from Elsevier. Part b reproduced from Biswas S, Dodwadkar NS, Piroyan A, Torchilin VP. Surface conjugation of triphenylphosphonium to target poly[amidoamine] dendrimers to mitochondria. *Biomaterials.* Jun 2012;33[18]:4773–4782, with permission from Elsevier.)

[82–85]. Different shapes may be observed depending on the dendrimer generation. The PAMAM dendrimers of low generation (G0 to G3) with an ethylenediamine core have ellipsoidal shape, whereas high generations (G4 to G10) with well-defined core display roughly spherical shapes [86]. Encapsulation of active agents into dendrimers is drawing a lot of attention in drug delivery. Mode of interactions with dendrimers may be subdivided into three types: simple encapsulation, electrostatic interactions, and covalent conjugation.

Dendrimers may be suitable as vehicles for ocular drug delivery. These dendritic polymers can accommodate hydrophobic agents in their cavity and provide sustained release. Vandamme and Brobeck [87] studied a series of PAMAM dendrimers for controlled ocular delivery of pilocarpine nitrate and tropicamide. PAMAM dendrimers with primary amino (G2, G4), hydroxyl (G2, G4), and carboxylate (G1.5, G3.5) terminal group were studied. Miotic and mydriatic effects have been evaluated in New Zealand albino rabbits. The duration of mitoic/mydriatic response was defined as the time interval between topical administration of drug treatment and the time at which the pupil

TABLE 10-3 Notation of the ocular lesions (conjunctiva, iris and cornea), determination of the maximum ocular irritating index, 1-hour post-instillation and evaluation of the mean residence time post-instillation of different solutions on the cornea

Formulation	Notation of Ocular Lesion			Ocular Irritating Index	Mean Residence Time (min) ± SE
	Conjunctiva	Iris	Cornea		
DG2 (2.0%)	2.7	0	0	2.7	100 ± 60.5
DG2.5 (0.25%)	—	—	—	—	300 ± 34.5
DG2.5 (0.5%)	—	—	—	—	260 ± 17.5
DG2.5 (2.0%)	3.3	0	0	3.3	260 ± 0.0
DG4 (2.0%)	4.7	0	0	4.7	203 ± 83.5
DG4.5 (2.0%)	1.3	0	0	1.3	220 ± 69.0
DG2(OH) (2.0%)	0.7	0	0	0.7	300 ± 0.0
DG4(OH) (2.0%)	0	0	0	0	300 ± 0.0
Carbopol® 980 NF (0.2%)	7.3	1.7	0	9	270 ± 30.0
HPMC (0.2%)	4.7	1.7	0	6.3	26 ± 11.0
Phosphate buffer, pH 7.4	4.7	0	0	4.7	21 ± 5.0

Dendrimers and linear polymers are in different pH solutions as described in the text. DG, dendrimer generation; HPMC, hydroxypropylmethylcellulose; carbopol 980 NF, linear poly(acrylic) acid.

Reproduced from Vandamme TF, Brobeck L. Poly(amidoamine) dendrimers as ophthalmic vehicles for ocular delivery of pilocarpine nitrate and tropicamide. *J Control Release.* Jan 20 2005;102(1):23–38, with permission from Elsevier.

diameter returned to its normal pretreatment value. *In vivo* studies have been conducted with topical instillation of various generation dendrimer solutions. All formulations tested were weakly irritant with minor lesions to anterior ocular tissues (up to a concentration of 2.0% w/v). The dendrimer formulations improved fluorescein ocular mean residence time relative to phosphate buffer (Table 10–3) [87].

Low polymer concentrations (dendrimer G2.5) demonstrated better ocular compatibility than high concentrations (2.0% w/v). Mitoic and mydriatic activities are improved and prolonged with dendrimers G4 amino and hydroxyl terminal groups (2.0% w/v). Pharmacokinetic parameters for miotic/mydriatic activities with topical dosing demonstrated statistically significant improvement in bioavailability for both drugs. Dendrimer G4 with amino and hydroxyl group terminals encapsulating pilocarpine nitrate and tropicamide exhibited higher area under the curve (AUC) of 213.5 ± 7.8 and 559.5 ± 4.3 min mm $\pm$ SE, respectively, compared with phosphate buffer (134.5 ± 3.8 min mm $\pm$ SE). The nature of surface functional groups on the dendrimers helps to improve bioadhesion properties. Therefore, higher drug bioavailability is due to bioadhesive property of dendrimers and subsequent slow release of encapsulated drug from the core.

Dendrimers not only sustain drug release but also translocate drug molecules across ocular tissues. To demonstrate the application of dendrimers in enhancing drug permeation, Yao et al. [88] conducted studies across excised cornea with dendrimer: drug physical mixture and complex. Cationic dendrimers of generations (G3, G4, and G5) with amino terminal and half generation (G3.5 and G4.5) with carboxylate terminal functional group have been studied. A mixture was prepared with peurarin and dendrimer in phosphate-buffered saline, whereas a complex was prepared by solvent evaporation with methanol. Peurarin has low aqueous solubility of 4 mg/mL. The solubility of peurarin is dependent on dendrimer concentration. The dendrimer complex sustained peurarin release (*in vitro*) and reduced burst release by ~25%. Higher generation dendrimer caused ~85% of peurarin released in less than 2 hours [89]. Corneal permeability of dendrimer is dependent on molecular weight, size, and method of formulation preparation. Molecular weight and size of dendrimer have shown inverse relationships with peurarin permeability across the cornea (i.e., G3 > G4 > G5) with cationic dendrimers. Apparent permeability of peurarin is reduced approximately 50% from 3.07 ± 0.07 to 1.68 ± 0.02 cm.h^{-1} $\times$ 10^{-2}, respectively, for G3 and G5 PAMAM dendrimers. The physical mixture generated two times higher peurarin permeability (Papp) relative to complex. The reason for the higher permeability of peurarin with a dendrimer physical mixture is that PAMAM dendrimer incorporates into the corneal lipid epithelial bilayer, thereby loosening epithelial tight junctions. Peurarin released from PAMAM dendrimer core then permeates across the cornea through narrow epithelial intercellular spaces through the paracellular pathway. Aqueous humor pharmacokinetic studies with cationic dendrimer physical mixtures (G3, G4, and G5) have been conducted in rabbits following a microdialysis technique [90]. The dendrimer physical mixture G4 demonstrated higher AUC, C_{max}, and maximum time of 107.32 ± 23.83 μg mL^{-1}min^{-1}, 1.11 ± 0.31 μg mL^{-1}, and 90 minutes, respectively, relative to G3 and G5. Increasing dendrimer size and molecular weight improved corneal bioavailability but lowered bioavailability with the G5 physical mixture. It can be attributed to the G5 physical mixture causing ocular irritation, which can lead to higher blinking and drug drainage from the ocular surface.

Cationic dendrimers composed of poly-L-lysine (PLL), polyamidoamine, and polyethyleneimine (PEI) can encapsulate plasmid DNA, gene, or short hairpin RNA and deliver the cargo to RPE and retinal ganglionic cells [91]. Marano et al. [91] designed and synthesized a lipid-lysine dendrimer to encapsulate an anti-VEGF agent, ODN-1, and deliver the complex into retinal cell nuclei. *In vivo* studies were conducted in a neovascularized rat model with IVT injection of the complex. The composition was well tolerated, and a significant suppression of VEGF expression was achieved. The complex was retained in retinal tissues for more than 2 months.

Drug delivery and *in vivo* performance of dendrimers can be further improved with surface modification. Several dendritic conjugates such as PEGylated, guanidinylated, and glucosamine conjugated dendrimers have been studied for ocular drug delivery [92, 93]. Cationic dendrimers such as PAMAM carry a high density of positive surface charge, due to the amino functional group. The surface density is dependent on the generation (i.e., G5 has greater density than G3). The positive surface of PAMAM expresses higher affinity or electrostatic interaction with negatively charged components of bacteria cell membrane, such as lipopolysaccharide or lipoteichoic acid. Binding of dendrimer to the bacterial surface does not induce antimicrobial effect. Dendrimers induce their antibacterial effect probably by disrupting the bacterial cell membrane. Dendrimer penetration and diffusion across the bacterial cell membrane into the cytoplasm may also be required to induce antibacterial effect. To facilitate this process, a net balance between the positive charge, size, and hydrophobicity is required. It is known that G5 has higher amino group density than G3 but suffers from larger size, which prevents its permeation across the bacterial cell wall. Therefore, G3 appears to induce more significant antimicrobial effect than G5. This dendrimer is toxic to normal corneal cells. To reduce toxicity, Lopez et al. [93] synthesized polyethylene glycol (PEG) conjugated dendrimers (G3 and G5). Different PEG chain lengths with varying degrees of PEG surface density have been synthesized and evaluated for antibacterial activity and cytotoxicity. Surface PEGylation demonstrated reduction in antibacterial activity due to smaller number of free $-NH_2$ groups and partial shielding by PEG. An enhancement in antibacterial effect with longer PEG chain lengths has been revealed. Reasons can be attributed to cationic character of dendrimer and dual lipophilic/hydrophilic character of PEG chains. This study confirmed that surface PEGylated dendrimers serve three purposes: reduced toxicity induced to corneal cells, development of a new antimicrobial polymer, and optimization of PEG chain length and density leading to maximal antimicrobial effect.

CYCLODEXTRINS

Cyclodextrins (CDs) are biodegradable, biocompatible cyclic oligosaccharides available as α, β, and γ depending on the number of sugar units 6, 7, and 8, respectively (Table 10 4). Derivatives of CDs with cyclic ring structures appear to improve delivery properties (Figure 10-8). A comparison between the naturally available CDs and their derivatives show that β-CD is most commonly and widely used. The ring size of CD enlarges with the number of sugar units (Table 10-4). These cyclic sugars consist of an outer hydrophilic corona of hydroxyl groups and an inner hydrophobic core (Figure 10-8) [94]. CDs have a wide range of applications in pharmaceutical

TABLE 10-4 Cyclodextrins and their properties				
Cyclodextrin	Glucopyranose Units	Mol. Wt. (Da)	Central Cavity Diameter (ext./int., Å)	Aqueous Solubility (at 25°C, g/100 mL)
A	6	972	5.3/4.7	14.5
B	7	1135	6.5/6.0	1.85
Γ	8	1297	8.3/7.5	23.2

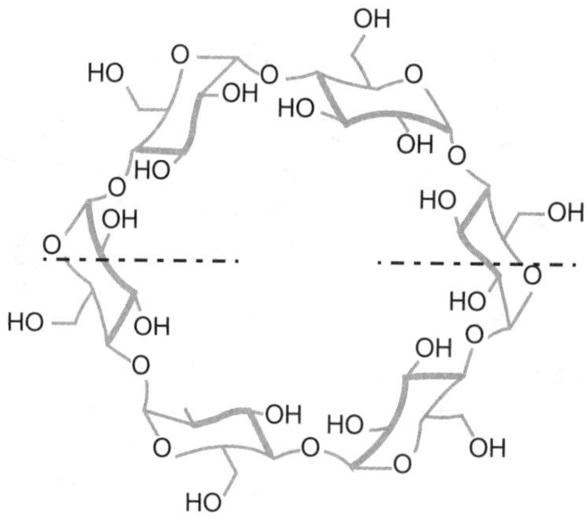

FIGURE 10-8 Structure for cyclodextrins (interior hydrophobic and corona hydrophilic).

compositions and are commonly used as solubilizers and stabilizers. CDs can also lower local drug-induced irritation, sustain drug release, and improve *in vivo* performance [95, 96]. CDs improve aqueous solubility of hydrophobic drugs by complexation. These substances are not capable of modifying the permeability of the biological barrier relative to surfactants. One example of a CD that was modified to improve aqueous solubility is hydroxypropyl (HP)-β-CD. Modification of β-CD with the HP group not only improved its aqueous solubility but also demonstrated high ocular tolerability in rabbits up to 12.5% with ophthalmic preparations [97]. This new CD derivative demonstrated improved solubility for various other drug candidates, such as but not limited to carbonic anhydrase inhibitors (acetazolamide, ethoxyzolamide), steroids (hydrocortisone, dexamethasone acetate), and nonsteroidal anti-inflammatory drugs (diclofenac sodium). Also, HP-β-CD has been found to improve stability of drugs such as tropicamide, GCV, and mycophenolate mofetil [98–105].

Fungal infections affecting the eye to date have no specific ocular formulation available. Drugs are administered systemically to treat ocular fungal infections, but local administration with topical drops is preferred. Ketoconazole, an imidazole derivative, possesses fungistatic activity against various pathogens. Its delivery, however, is limited due to poor aqueous solubility. Zhang et al. studied ocular (aqueous humor) pharmacokinetics of topically administered ketoconazole solution containing HP-β-CD in New Zealand albino rabbits [106a]. Ocular ketoconazole aqueous drops were prepared by dissolving with HP-β-CD and compared with 1.5% ketoconazole suspension. Both ketoconazole aqueous solution and suspension were instilled topically to the eye. Both formulations were well tolerated with no irritation. Ketoconazole containing HP-β-CD showed significantly higher corneal permeability relative to suspension. Aqueous humor pharmacokinetics showed a significantly higher ketoconazole level at 10 to 120 minutes relative to suspension. The ketoconazole AUC versus time profile for aqueous humor and cornea was found to be ~8.42 and ~12.85 times higher than suspension. The highest concentration (C_{max}) detected in aqueous humor and cornea was 0.44 ± 0.46 and 2.67 ± 2.9 µg/mL at 30 and 20 minutes, respectively, after a topical single dose. The addition of CD to ketoconazole significantly increased drug levels (above minimum inhibitory concentrations) in aqueous humor and cornea than suspension. Local drug administration may avoid systemic ketoconazole complications and result in therapeutic drug concentrations at the target site (ocular tissues).

NANOPARTICLES

Nanoparticles are colloidal dispersions with a size range between 10 and 1000 nm. Depending on the method of preparation, nanospheres or nanocapsules can be obtained. Nanospheres differ from nanocapsules in that they are matrix form, in which particle entire mass is solid. Nanocapsules are reservoir form, in which a solid material shell encircles a liquid or semisolid core at room temperature (15–25°C). The central core is composed of either oil or aqueous solvent. These colloidal systems have been used as drug carriers in ocular drug delivery. In general, nanoparticles offer several advantages, including increased longevity and stability of the carrier system and encapsulated drug, improved drug bioavailability, possibility to obtain a cell targeted release, and ability to overcome ocular physiological barriers. Also, a sustained or controlled release, restricted drug biodistribution, reduced drug clearance, low ocular irritation, and retarded drug metabolism can be achieved. Nanoparticle surface coated with a protective polymer can further alter all the earlier mentioned parameters [106]. Another strategy to sustain the drug release is embedding the nanoparticles in biodegradable and biocompatible thermosensitive gels [107]. Thermosensitive gel-based strategy is used for local drug delivery. More details are provided below in *In Situ* Gelling Systems.

Nanoparticles composed of lipids, proteins, and natural or synthetic polymeric systems have been studied for ocular drug delivery. Most widely used polymeric systems include but are not limited to albumin, hyaluronic acid (HA), sodium alginate, chitosan, poly(lactide-co-glycolic acid) (PLGA), poly(lactic acid) (PLA), polycaprolactone (PCL), PEG, and poly(glycolic acid) (PGA). Ocular administration of drug-loaded nanoparticles into the cul-de-sac/precorneal pocket or vitreous humor causes rapid elimination, mostly similar to aqueous solutions. To overcome such rapid elimination and improve residence time, nanoparticles are surface coated with PEG, chitosan, and/or HA or embedded in thermosensitive gels. Surface modification enhances mucoadhesive property for nanoparticles, sustains drug release, and imparts higher residence time in the eye. Suspending nanoparticles in thermosensitive or hydrogel systems reduces the rate of nanoparticle elimination, retains the particles for longer time in the precorneal pocket, improves bioavailability, and produces better therapeutic effect. To improve ocular bioavailability and retention time of dexamethasone, Gan et al. [108] prepared self-assembled liquid crystalline nanoparticles (cubosomes) following the emulsification method with monoolein and poloxamer 407 polymers. Precorneal clearance parameters for nanoparticles have been evaluated with noninvasive fluorescence imaging in rabbits. Nanoparticles labeled with ethyl rhodamine B (Rh B) have been used for studies using carbopol and Rh B solutions served as controls. A 3.5- and 2.5-fold increase in

TABLE 10-5 Precorneal ethyl Rh B clearance parameters in rabbits, after topical drop administration

Sample	AUC 0→ 180 minutes (% min)	k (min⁻¹)	A90 (%)
Rh B solution	2196.7 ± 920.1	0.031 ± 0.008	10.4 ± 5.7
Rh B carbopol gel	3104 ± 1267.9	0.026 ± 0.015	14.2 ± 5.7
Rh B cubosome F1	7715.8 ± 1050.9*,†	0.013 ± 0.002*,†	37.8 ± 2.8*,†

k, clearance rate constant; A90, activity remaining at region of interest at 90 minutes postdosing.

*$P < 0.05$, statistically significantly difference from Rh B solution.

†$P < 0.05$, statistically significantly difference from Rh B carbopol gel.

Reproduced from Gan L, Han S, Shen J, et al. Self-assembled liquid crystalline nanoparticles as a novel ophthalmic delivery system for dexamethasone: Improving preocular retention and ocular bioavailability. *International Journal of Pharmaceutics.* Aug 30 2010;396(1-2):179–187, with permission from Elsevier.

AUC was observed with nanoparticles relative to Rh B solution and Rh B carbopol gel (Table 10-5) [108]. No significant difference for clearance rate between Rh B carbopol gel and aqueous solution was observed. This indicates that nanoparticles improve ocular residence time and bioavailability of drug into ocular tissues.

To further improve precorneal residence time, nanoparticles are surface coated with chitosan. Chitosan coating imparts a positive charge to nanoparticles and hence they bind to the negatively charged corneal surface. This improves precorneal residence and decreases clearance. For instance, natamycin-lecithin nanoparticles with chitosan coating exhibited higher ocular bioavailability in rabbit relative to marketed suspension. After topical dosing, AUC (0–∞) increased by 1.47-fold and clearance was reduced by 7.4-fold, where marketed suspension served as control [109]. Musumeci et al. [110] studied melatonin-loaded PLGA nanoparticles for an IOP-lowering effect in rabbits. Melatonin nanoparticles surface coated with PEG demonstrated a significant IOP-lowering effect relative to blank PLGA nanoparticles and aqueous solution (Figure 10–9). Reduced zeta potential of nanoparticles fabricated from PLGA–PEG relative to PLGA allows better and longer interaction between nanoparticles and ocular surface. This results in effective and higher hypotensive effect for prolonged period. Other parameters for nanoparticle ocular drug delivery include size and surface property. Particle size–based studies were conducted for posterior ocular tissue drug delivery following the transscleral route. In vivo studies were conducted after periocular administration of fluorescent polystyrene nanoparticles with 20 nm, 200 nm, and 2 μm in Sprague-Dawley rats. Twenty-nanometer particles were rapidly cleared from periocular tissues and circulatory systems (conjunctival, episcleral, or other periocular circulatory systems), suggesting that small sized particles could not be retained at the retinal tissue. On the other hand, 200- and 2000-nm particles were retained at the depot site for at least 2 months [111, 112]. Hence, particle size plays an important role in drug delivery from periocular tissues to retina. An optimal particle size is necessary for their ability to overcome the ocular barriers and deliver the cargo to retinal tissues.

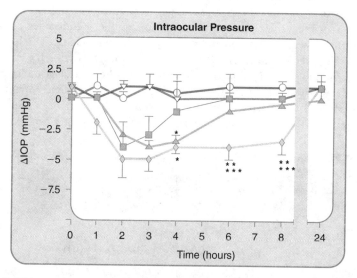

FIGURE 10-9 IOP in normotensive rabbit after topical instillation of melatonin (MEL) aqueous solution (■) or nanoparticles (NPs): RG (PLGA NPs) (O), RGP (PLGA-PEG NPs) (▽), RG-MEL1 (MEL loaded PLGA NPs) (▲), or RGP-MEL1 (MEL loaded PLGA-PEG NPs) (◆). *$P < 0.01$, **$P < 0.001$ vs. melatonin; ***$P < 0.001$ vs. RGP-MEL1. (Reproduced from Musumeci T, Bucolo C, Carbone C, Pignatello R, Drago F, Puglisi G. Polymeric nanoparticles augment the ocular hypotensive effect of melatonin in rabbits. *International Journal of Pharmaceutics*. Jan 20,2013;440(2):135-140, with permission from Elsevier.)

Another method to improve ocular bioavailability is overcoming ocular barriers and delivering high drug levels to retinal tissues is with an IVT injection. After IVT dosing, nanoparticles migrate through the retinal layers and tend to accumulate in RPE cells. The PLA nanoparticles, <350 nm, accumulated in rat RPE and were detected up to 4 months after a single IVT injection. IVT administration of nanoparticles shows great potential for achieving steady and continuous delivery to the back of the eye tissues. Zhang et al. [113] demonstrated better pharmacokinetics and tolerance for dexamethasone-loaded PLGA nanoparticles in rabbits after IVT injection. Dexamethasone levels were maintained at a steady state in vitreous humor for more than 30 days, with a mean concentration of 3.85 mg/L. On the contrary, only trace amounts of dexamethasone were detected at day 7 with IVT dexamethasone solution. Dexamethasone nanoparticles sustained drug release, thereby reducing the dosing frequency. Surface charge of nanoparticles also plays an important role in ocular drug delivery. Kim et al. [114] demonstrated that anionic surface charged human serum albumin (HSA) nanoparticles penetrated the whole rat retina and formed a depot inside RPE relative to cationic counterparts, after IVT administration. Also, movement of IVT nanoparticles depends on retinal injury. In the injured retina, HSA nanoparticles reached the choroid through the disruption site of RPE and Bruch's membrane. Therefore, the anionic surface charge on nanoparticles imparts greater permeability across ocular tissues such as the choroid region to provide effective treatment for choroidal neovascularization. Similarly, Koo et al. [115] demonstrated a correlation between nanoparticle surface property and their distribution in vitreous body and retina after IVT injection. Heterogeneous PEI/glycol chitosan (GC), HSA/GC, and HSA/HA nanoparticles have been studied. The zeta potential for nanoparticles were 20.7 ± 3.2, −1.9 ± 4.1, and −23.3 ± 4.4 for PEI/GC, HSA/GC, and HSA/HA nanoparticles, respectively. Nanoparticles were IVT injected in Long Evans rats and vitreous/retinal distribution was evaluated. **Figure 10-10** shows that PEI/GC nanoparticles easily permeated the vitreal barrier and reached the inner limiting membrane [115]. PEI/GC and HSA/GC nanoparticles, however, could not readily be

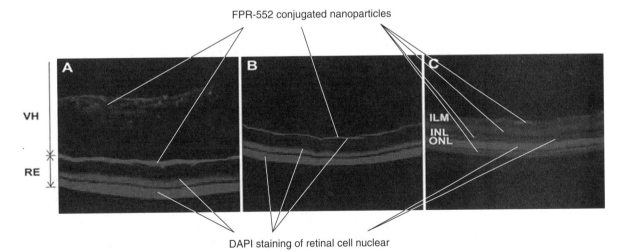

FIGURE 10-10 Vitreal and retinal distribution of intravitreally administered (A) PEI/GC heterogeneous nanoparticles, (B) HSA/GC heterogeneous nanoparticles, and (C) HSA/HA heterogeneous nanoparticles 6 hours postinjection. VH, RE, ILM, INL, and ONL represent the vitreous, retina, inner limiting membrane, inner nuclear layer, and outer nuclear layer, respectively. All images were captured at ×10 magnification. (Reproduced from Koo H, Moon H, Han H, et al. The movement of self-assembled amphiphilic polymeric nanoparticles in the vitreous and retina after intravitreal injection. *Biomaterials.* Apr 2012;33[12]:3485-3493, with permission from Elsevier.)

transported to deeper retinal layers and form aggregates in vitreous. It is hypothesized that inhibition of the interaction between HSA and the Müller cells in retina by GC limits nanoparticle translocation. Negatively charged HSA/HA nanoparticles penetrated the entire retinal structures and reached the outer retinal layers (i.e., photoreceptors and RPE). Enhanced permeation may be attributed to interactions between anionic membrane groups and Müller cells [115].

LIPOSOMES

Liposomes are vesicles/carrier systems composed of one or more phospholipid bilayers enclosing a central aqueous compartment. Liposomal carrier systems offer unique advantages in ocular drug delivery by encapsulating both hydrophobic and hydrophilic drugs. The vesicles also exhibit excellent biocompatibility due to their phospholipid bilayer, which is similar to the cell membrane. In general, size ranges between 0.08 and 10 μm. Liposomes are classified as small unilamellar vesicles (10–100 nm), large unilamellar vesicles (100–300 nm), and multilamellar vesicles (contains more than one bilayer) [116]. Attempts have been made to deliver drugs to anterior and posterior ocular tissues with liposomes as drug delivery vehicles. Despite their advantages, liposomes suffer from certain drawbacks such as low stability (both physical and chemical), sterilization, encapsulation efficiency, and intracellular lysosomal degradation.

Anterior ocular drug delivery suffers from a limitation, that is, loss of a topically applied dose in tears. Natarajan et al. [117] developed a latanoprost-loaded liposomal formulation and demonstrated long-term IOP lowering in rabbits. A single subconjunctival administration of latanoprost liposomal formulation produced somewhat similar and comparative IOP lowering with daily topical dosing up to 50 days. Further precorneal residence time of liposomes is improved by positively charged lipids forming cationic liposomes. The cationic liposomes exhibit better performance as ocular delivery systems than negatively charged and/or neutral liposomes. Positively charged cationic liposomes show higher binding with the negatively charged corneal surface. Examples of cationic lipids include didodecyldimethylammonium bromide, stearylamine, and N-(1-(2,3-dioleoyloxy)propyl)-N,N,N-trimethylammonium chloride.

Diebold et al. [118] prepared a liposome–chitosan nanoparticle complex for ocular delivery. *In vivo* studies in rabbits demonstrated higher uptake in conjunctiva relative to cornea. Law et al. prepared ACV-loaded cationic and anionic liposomes with stearylamine and dicetylphosphate as cationic and anionic charge-inducing agents, respectively [119]. *In vivo* studies in rabbits demonstrated higher corneal ACV concentrations with cationic liposome relative to anionic and free ACV solution. Concentrations of ACV in cornea were 253.3 ± 72.0 ng/g, 1093.3 ± 279.7 ng/g, and 571.7 ± 105.3 ng/g from ACV solution, ACV loaded cationic, and anionic liposomes, respectively. Also, the extent of ACV transport through the cornea was higher with cationic liposomes. The higher binding of cationic liposomes with negatively charged corneal surface through electrostatic interactions demonstrated increased residence time and improved ACV absorption [119]. Cheng et al. [120] prepared self-assembling liposomes of lipid prodrug of GCV, 1-O-hexadecylpropanediol-3-phospho-GCV. *In vivo* studies were conducted in rabbits with IVT administration of GCV, blank liposomes, and prodrugs in liposome. IVT injection of 1-O-hexadecylpropanediol-3-phospho-GCV showed 0.2 mM vitreal concentration in the rabbit retinitis model. In another study, Shen and Tu [121] prepared GCV liposomes. *In vivo* studies were conducted in rabbits with topical dosing. No significant difference in precorneal clearance was observed with liposomal formulation and GCV solution. AUC with liposomal formulation was enhanced 1.7-fold over GCV solution. Ocular tissue concentrations were 2 to 10 times higher in the sclera, cornea, iris, lens, and vitreous humor relative to GCV solution. This study indicates that liposomal formulations improve delivery across ocular tissues. Coenzyme Q10-loaded liposomes surface coated with mucoadhesive trimethyl chitosan were studied [122]. *In vivo* topical dosing studies in rabbits demonstrated a 4.8-fold increase in precorneal residence time.

Liposomes as carrier systems have been investigated for posterior ocular tissue delivery. These carrier systems have been developed to improve drug half-life, lower vitreous humor clearance, and provide protection from degradation of enzymatically labile drugs like peptides and oligonucleotides. Also, encapsulation of these molecules in liposomes sustains drug release. Gupta et al. [123] demonstrated improved fluconazole vitreal half-life from 3.08 to 23.40 hours with liposomal encapsulation. Also, the terminal vitreal elimination constant for fluconazole-loaded liposome was seven times less than drug solution. Another study by Zhang et al. [124] demonstrated better efficacy of tacrolimus (FK 506) liposomal formulation in the treatment of autoimmune uveoretinitis with IVT administration to Lewis rats. Tacrolimus concentrations were maintained over ~14 days, and the regimen suppressed experimental autoimmune uveitis. Sasaki et al. [125] developed liposomal topical drops surface modified with PLL for back of the eye delivery. Varying molecular weights and concentrations of PLL were added to surface coat liposomes. The authors identified PLL molecular weights of 15 to 30 kDa, and concentrations of 0.005% were optimal for liposomal coating. Liposomal formulation encapsulating coumarin-6 demonstrated better fluorescence intensity in the inner plexiform retinal layer (**Figure 10-11**). Enhanced intensity lasted for 30 to 90 minutes relative to uncoated liposomes. PLL-coated liposomes delivered payload to the retina during

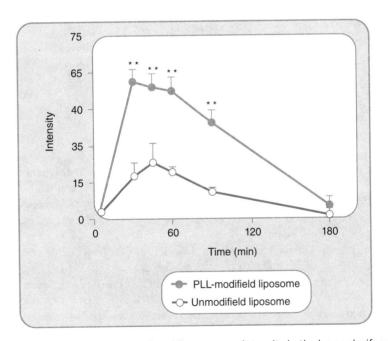

FIGURE 10-11 Time course of accumulated fluorescence intensity in the inner plexiform layer after administration of eye-drop preparations of 0.005% poly-L-lysine (PLL) 15000-modified liposomes (egg phosphatidylcholine [EPC]:dicetyl phosphate [DCP]:cholesterol = 8:0.5:1). Data are shown as mean ± SEM. Comparisons were made with the unmodified liposome preparation; **$P < 0.01$. (Reproduced from Sasaki H, Karasawa K, Hironaka K, Tahara K, Tozuka Y, Takeuchi H. Retinal drug delivery using eyedrop preparations of poly-l-lysine-modified liposomes. *Eur J Pharm Biopharm*. Vol 83. Issue 3. April 2013 pp. 364–369, with permission from Elsevier.)

the first 60 minutes and were subsequently cleared within 3 hours after topical dosing. Fluorescence quenching was attributed to diffusion of liposomes from topical drops into the circulatory system. Further, PLL-coated liposomes delivered higher coumarin-6 (higher fluorescence intensity) relative to uncoated liposomes, indicating better *in vivo* performance with surface-modified PLL (Figure 10-11) [125]. Surface modification did not influence liposomal clearance. These results suggest that liposomal formulations may be suitable as potential ocular drug delivery systems.

NANOMICELLES

Nanomicelles are colloidal structures formed from self-assembly of amphiphilic monomers/molecules with sizes from 5 to 200 nm. Monomers tend to initiate self-aggregation (i.e., micelle formation at certain concentration in solvent system). The concentration at which self-assembly of monomers is initiated is defined as the critical micellar concentration. Nanomicelles offer unique advantages such as simplicity, ease of manufacturing, and reproducibility at small and bulk scale. Monomers allow surface conjugation of targeting moiety or specific ligand allowing for targeted drug delivery. But nanomicelles suffer from a few limitations. Drug-loaded nanomicellar formulations encounter rapid tear dilution upon their topical administration. Premature drug release and lack of sustained/controlled release limit their applications. Another major disadvantage of micelles is their inability to entrap hydrophilic small molecule drugs and macromolecules. The advantages include ease of sterilization by simple filtration process, an aqueous formulation of fairly insoluble compounds. Nanomicelles can be either prepared from surfactants (ionic, nonionic, zwitterionic) or block copolymers.

Amphiphilic monomers carrying a charge (anion or cation) on their head groups are referred to as ionic surfactants. Examples include sodium dodecyl sulfate and dodecyltrimethylammonium bromide as anionic and cationic surfactants, respectively [126]. On the contrary, monomers that carry no charge on the head group are referred to as nonionic surfactant such as n-dodecyl tetra (ethylene oxide) ($C_{12}E_4$). Amphiphilic monomers that carry both positive and negative charges on the head group are referred to as zwitterionic surfactants (e.g., dioctanoyl phosphatidyl choline). Block copolymers have been synthesized to form new amphiphilic polymer monomeric units with U.S. Food and Drug Administration–approved polymers. These polymer blocks are arranged in different ways, such as diblock (A-B type), triblock (A-B-A type), and grafted/branched type copolymers, in which A and B represents any of the polymers like, but not limited to, PEG, PLL, polyethylene oxide, poly(D,L-lactic acid), polypropylene oxide, PCL, PGA, and poly(amino acids), such as poly(aspartic acid), poly(glutamic acid), poly(L-lysine), and poly(histidine).

Nanomicelles as carrier systems have drawn attention from ocular drug delivery scientists because of their ability to translocate drugs across ocular tissues and significantly improve bioavailability. Nanomicelles have been evaluated for elevating anterior ocular drug bioavailability. A twofold increase in ocular bioavailability was achieved for ketorolac when loaded in block copolymeric nanomicelles [127]. These nanomicelles are composed of copolymers of nisopropylacrylamide, vinyl pyrrolidone, and acrylic acid cross-linked with N,N'-methylene-bis-acrylamide. Topical administration showed no corneal damage, and the suspension was well tolerated. PEG and/or carbon chain (C16) conjugated polyhydroxyethyl-aspartamide system has been used to encapsulate and prepare dexamethasone nanomicelle for ocular delivery. Higher dexamethasone permeability was achieved with polyhydroxyethyl-aspartamide-C16 and polyhydroxyethyl-aspartamide-PEG-C16 micelles across primary cultured rabbit conjunctival and corneal epithelial cells relative to solutions and suspensions. *In vivo* ocular bioavailability in rabbits demonstrated higher dexamethasone bioavailability from micelles, relative to its aqueous suspension [128]. Similarly, methoxy poly(ethylene glycol)-hexylsubstituted poly(lactides) micellar formulations of cyclosporine A demonstrated excellent *in vitro* and *in vivo* ocular biocompatibility, transparency, and stability. Pilocarpine-loaded triblock copolymer pluronic F127 (poly[oxyethylene]/poly[oxypropylene]/poly[oxyethylene]) demonstrated improved pharmacokinetic parameters (duration of miotic response and area under the miosis time curve) relative to standard pilocarpine solutions [129]. Further, to improve precorneal residence time, mucoadhesive polymers like chitosan have been used in micellar formulation. Dexamethasone-loaded polyoxyethylated non-ionic surfactant pluronic F127 (F127) and chitosan demonstrated significant enhancement in ocular bioavailability (i.e., 2.4-fold relative to dexamethasone suspension) [130]. A novel photodynamic therapy with dendrimer porphyrin-loaded polyion complex micelles has been evaluated for selective accumulation in pathological corneal neovascularization. Nanomicelles demonstrated an enhanced permeability and retention effect with selective accumulation in corneal neovascularization with no detectable level in normal limbal vessels [131].

Nanomicellar constructs have been used for posterior segment drug delivery. Fluorescein isothiocyanate–poly-lysine (FITC-P[Lys]) loaded PEG-block-poly-α,β-aspartic acid micelles were used to deliver the cargo to posterior ocular tissues (choroid). *In vivo* studies were conducted in rats postinduction of choroidal neovascularization (CNV) with a diode laser photocoagulator. Rats intravenously administered with free FITC-P(Lys) died within 1 hour, suggesting high toxicity, but no death occurred in animals administered FITC-P(Lys)–polyion complex micelles. Polyion complex micelles were retained up to 7 days and showed a C_{max} at 4 hours. Micellar constructs demonstrated selective accumulation at the pathological neovascular site, due to an enhanced permeability and retention effect [132]. Mitra and colleagues [133, 134] made significant strides to deliver drugs to posterior ocular tissues with mixed nanomicellar formulations. Voclosporin-loaded mixed nanomicelles demonstrated better ocular tolerability than Restasis® in New Zealand White rabbits. Single- and multidrop instillation of voclosporin micelles in rabbits demonstrated C_{max} at 48 and 76 hours, respectively [135]. Further, dexamethasone (0.1%) and rapamycin (0.2%) mixed nanomicellar formulations demonstrated therapeutic drug concentrations in retina–choroid with single-drop instillation [136]. Therefore, small size and hydrophilic corona probably assist nanomicelles to cross ocular barriers and deliver drugs to posterior ocular tissues. A topical aqueous optically clear mixed nanomicellar formulation composed of vitamin E, D-α-tocopheryl polyethylene glycol succinate (TPGS), and octoxynol-40 loaded with 0.1% B-12HS-ACV was successfully developed for the treatment of herpetic keratitis. B-12HS-ACV–loaded nanomicelles are relatively small in size, spherical, homogenous, and devoid of aggregates. The formulations were perfectly transparent and comparable with water. Moreover, ocular biocompatibility studies indicated that mixed nanomicelles were non-toxic and noninflammatory to corneal epithelial cells [137]. Similarly, diclofenac-loaded methoxypoly(ethylene glycol)-PCL micelles were investigated for ocular delivery [138] and demonstrated no irritancy in rabbit eyes. *In vitro* corneal penetration studies across rabbit cornea demonstrated a 17-fold increase in permeability with nanomicelles relative to diclofenac phosphate-buffered saline solution. *In vivo* pharmacokinetic profile of the micelles demonstrated that diclofenac-loaded methoxypoly(ethylene glycol)-PCL micelles generated a twofold increase in AUC (0–24 hours) than diclofenac phosphate-buffered saline solution eye drops. Therefore, nanomicelles have significant potential in improving various ocular pathologies.

MICRONEEDLES

Microneedles have been used to administer drugs into ocular tissues. This administration technique has been developed to deliver drugs to the back of the eye tissues in a minimally invasive manner. Microneedle-based drug administration may reduce the risk and complications associated with IVT injections, such as retinal detachment, hemorrhage, cataract, endophthalmitis, and pseudo-endophthalmitis. It can circumvent BRB and provides an efficient treatment strategy for age-related macular degeneration (AMD), diabetic retinopathy (DR), and posterior uveitis. Microneedles are custom designed to penetrate into the sclera or suprachoroidal space (SCS), the region between sclera and choroid, so damage to deeper ocular tissues may be avoided, and deposit drug solution there. Drug solution or carrier system depot in this region may facilitate drug diffusion into deeper ocular tissues (i.e., choroid and neural retina). Various compounds have been delivered to back of the eye tissues with surface-coated microneedles in cadaver eyes and rabbits [139]. Studies have been initiated to examine sclera as a static barrier to microneedles and intrascleral dissolution of microneedle from surface-coated sulforhodamine. After microneedle scleral penetration, surface-coated drug rapidly accumulated in the microneedle penetration region, forming sulforhodamine depot. Similarly, microneedles have been used for anterior segment ocular delivery. *In vivo* studies with pilocarpine surface-coated microneedles in rabbits demonstrated rapid drug dissolution and depot formation. Such depot can sustain pilocarpine release from the cornea, thereby improving bioavailability and resulting in rapid and extensive pupil constriction [139].

Moreover, to sustain drug release, microparticles and nanoparticles are used. Microneedles have also been used as a mode of drug administration to infuse and deposit drug solutions, microparticles, and nanoparticles into sclera [140]. Carrier systems if placed near the back of the eye tissues (i.e., in SCS) can deliver high drug concentrations to the retina–choroid. Patel et al. [141] attempted to deliver drug solution, nanoparticles, and microparticles in the SCS of rabbit, pig, and cadaver eyes with microneedles and suggested that the procedure is safe, minimally invasive, and forms drug/drug carrier depot at the administration site. Evidence of drug reaching the inner retinal tissues from SCS, however, has not been firmly established [142]. *In vivo* pharmacokinetics of SCS deposited solution/suspension demonstrated longer half-lives for soluble molecules, macromolecules, nanoparticles, and microparticulates. The exact mechanism or pathway, however, for drug solution or micro/nanoparticles clearance from SCS has not been delineated, and further studies are needed. Microneedle-based administration may allow minimally invasive drug delivery to back of the eye tissues (i.e., neural retina, choroid, Bruch's membrane).

IMPLANTS

Implants are drug-eluting devices specially designed for local sustained drug release over long periods. These devices circumvent multiple ocular punctures with needles (IVT injections) and associated complications [143, 144]. Devices are surgically implanted into the vitreous humor by incision at the pars plana and drug placement near the retina. Implants are preferred over IVT injections because of sustained and local drug release for prolonged periods, reduced side effects, and ability to circumvent the BRB [143]. Two types of ocular implants are biodegradable and nonbiodegradable.

Nonbiodegradable Implants

Nonbiodegradable drug-eluting implants are prepared by using polymers like polyvinyl alcohol (PVA), ethylene vinyl acetate, and polysulfone capillary fiber [144]. Implants from such polymers offer prolonged, controlled drug release with near zero-order kinetics [145]. Examples of nonbiodegradable, U.S. Food and Drug Administration–approved, and commercially available implants include Vitrasert® and Retisert®. Other implants under clinical trials include I-vation, Renexus, NT-503, pSivida, brimonidine, and ODTx intraocular implants.

Vitrasert® is a controlled GCV-releasing intraocular implant for the treatment of cytomegalovirus retinitis. The implant/device is composed of PVA or ethylene vinyl acetate polymer containing GCV (4.5 mg) that provides drug release over 5 to 8 months [145,146]. Moreover, intraocular implants like Vitrasert® may circumvent GCV-induced systemic toxicity. Retisert® is a controlled fluocinolone acetonide–releasing implant for the treatment of chronic uveitis. The device is composed of fluocinolone acetonide encapsulated in a silicone-laminated PVA platform sustaining fluocinolone acetonide release up to 3 years. This implant was shown to effectively control inflammation, reduce uveitis recurrences, and improve visual acuity. The major side effects associated with intraocular implants include cataract formation [145–147].

I-vation (Surmodics Inc.) is a titanium helical coil surface coated with triamcinolone acetonide, poly(methyl methacrylate), and ethylene vinyl acetate for sustained triamcinolone acetonide release over a period of 2 years. The implant has completed phase I clinical trials in patients with diabetic macular edema (DME). Patients were divided into two groups, a slow-releasing group and a fast-releasing group. The slow-releasing group patients demonstrated improvement in visual acuity (greater than 0 Early Treatment Diabetic Retinopathy Study [ETDRS] letter gain from baseline) of 68% relative to the fast-releasing group of 72%. About 28.6% of patients in the fast-releasing group gained more than 15 letters. The mean macular thickness decreased in the slow-releasing group and fast-releasing group by 201 μm and 108 μm, respectively.

Renexus (formerly NT-501) is an IVT implant composed of a sealed semipermeable hollow-fiber membrane capsule covered by six strands of polyethylene terephthalate yarn loaded with genetically modified RPE cells. This implant was developed for the treatment of retinitis pigmentosa and geographical atrophy associated with AMD. RPE cells secrete recombinant human ciliary neurotrophic factor. The implant protects the contents of the device from immune response, human ciliary neurotrophic factor, and other cell metabolites in vitreous humor and also regulates nutrient exchange. Phase I results showed that Renexus was well tolerated for 6 months in patients with late-stage retinitis pigmentosa [148]. Visual acuity was stabilized and was accompanied by corresponding structural changes that were dose dependent ($p < 0.001$). The geographic atrophy (GA) area growth rate was minimized in treated eyes compared with contralateral eyes at 12 and 18 months. Also, Renexus was found to prevent secondary cone degeneration in patients with retinitis pigmentosa [149]. Phase II studies are underway for Usher syndrome (type 2 or 3) and a phase I study for macular telangiectasia.

NT-503 is currently in the development stage. It encapsulates VEGF receptor Fc-fusion protein (VEGFR-Fc)-releasing cells. VEGFR-Fc has been found to be ~20-fold more efficient in neutralizing VEGF relative to ranibizumab. *In vivo* vitreous

NT-503 implantation in rabbits demonstrated VEGFR-FC continuous release up to 12 months. Currently, this implant is under phase I clinical trial for neovascular AMD outside the United States [150]. Drug-loaded multiple reservoir systems/implants are biocompatible and nonresorbable and release optimized injectable doses triggered by laser activation. The composition of the drug reservoir implants is not known. Such reservoirs are capable of loading both small and large molecules. These agents are released via a standard, noninvasive laser activation procedure. The multiple-reservoir system allows ophthalmologists to control drug delivery by activating specific reservoirs. The inactivated reservoirs, however, remain intact for future activation and drug release. Reports indicate that the device demonstrated promising *in vivo* results for release of both small molecules and proteins.

Long-term drug release has been achieved with single nonbiodegradable implant systems. The use of implants is limited, however, because these devices have to be surgically implanted and periodically removed after drug depletion. This procedure makes the treatment expensive and noncompliant. In some cases, the drug-depleted devices are left in the vitreous and a new drug-loaded implant is introduced. Adverse events such as endophthalmitis, pseudo-endophthalmitis, vitreous haze and hemorrhage, cataract development, and retinal detachment limit their applications.

BIODEGRADABLE IMPLANTS

Biocompatible and biodegradable implants are gaining more attention currently. These biodegradable implants are not required to be surgically removed, which signifies a distinctive advantage over nonbiodegradable implants. PLA, PGA, PLGA, and PCL are the most commonly used polymers selected for fabrication of implants [144]. Examples include Surodex™ and Ozurdex®, which are now commercially available. These implants offer sustained dexamethasone release for the treatment of intraocular inflammation and macular edema [145].

Surodex™ is composed of dexamethasone enclosed in PLGA and hydroxypropyl methylcellulose implant. The implant is inserted into the anterior chamber to control postoperative inflammation in cataract patients. This implant demonstrated sustained dexamethasone release over 7 to 10 days with improved anti-inflammatory effect comparable with that of topical steroid administration [145]. Ozurdex® is another dexamethasone ocular implant indicated for the treatment of macular edema. This implant is composed of dexamethasone-enclosed PLGA polymer matrix. The implant prolonged the release of dexamethasone for up to 6 months. Randomized clinical trials have demonstrated its efficacy to stop vision loss and improve visual acuity in eyes with macular edema associated with branch retinal vein occlusion or central retinal vein occlusion. Moreover, clinical trials for treatment of diabetic retinopathy and Irvine-Gass syndrome suggested that the implant is a promising treatment option [145].

Brimonidine IVT implant is a biodegradable, rod-shaped, drug-eluting device for the treatment of retinitis pigmentosa and atrophic AMD. Currently, the implant is in phase II/III clinical trials. Brimonidine is an β_2-adrenergic agonist that can release various neurotrophins including brain-derived neurotrophic factor (BDNF), human ciliary neurotrophic factor [151], and fibroblast growth factor-basic (b-FGF) [152]. These neurotrophins provide protection to photoreceptor cells and/or RPE from apoptosis. The implant is composed of brimonidine tartrate in PLGA for sustained release. Recently, ocular inserts composed of brimonidine tartrate, 7% PVP K-90, 1.5% low-molecular-weight sodium alginate with or without ethyl cellulose coat were shown to sustain *in vitro* release of brimonidine. *In vivo* therapeutic efficacy, regarding IOP-lowering effect, showed superior and sustained effect compared with brimonidine solution in rabbits. Moreover, due to mucoadhesive property and sustained effect, one-side-coated ocular inserts have shown higher IOP-lowering effect relative to noncoated or dual-side-coated counterparts [153]. Thethadur is a biocompatible, biodegradable, honeycomb-like nanostructured porous silicon (biosilicon) device under development. The implant also offers sustained drug release and can carry a variety of drugs (i.e., small molecules, peptides, proteins, and other biologics).

CONTACT LENS

Contact lenses are thin, curve-shaped plastic discs designed to be placed over the cornea [154]. After placing over the cornea, contact lenses adhere to the surface of the eye because of interfacial tension. Both the cornea and contact lens are separated from each other by a thin tear fluid layer called postlens tear film. In general, contact lenses are prepared with polymers such as silicone hydrogel (composed of *N,N-N,N*-dimethylacrylamide, 3-methacryloxypropyltris[trimethylsiloxy]silane, bis-alpha,omega-[methacryloxypropyl] poly dimethylsiloxane, 1-vinyl-2-pyrrolidone, and ethylene glycol dimethacrylate) and poly (hydroxyethyl methacrylate) (p-HEMA) [155, 156].

Contact lenses loaded with drug and/or drug-loaded nanocarriers have been developed for ocular delivery [157, 158]. Several active drugs such as timolol, dexamethasone, dexamethasone 21 acetate, beta-blockers, antihistamines, and antimicrobials have been loaded for anterior delivery [156]. Drug-laden contact lenses exhibit longer precorneal residence time. In the postlens tear film it causes high corneal drug flux with minimal drug flow into nasolacrimal duct. Generally, contact lenses are loaded by soaking the lenses in drug solutions. Such drug-loaded contact lenses demonstrate slow drug release, minimal drug loss due to precorneal clearance, improved corneal bioavailability, and higher efficiency in delivery relative to conventional topical drops. As an example, dexamethasone loaded in p-HEMA contact lenses demonstrated higher ocular bioavailability relative to conventional topical eye drops [159].

Contact lenses surface coated with surfactants have been developed to improve drug loading and achieve sustained release. Optimizing the interactions between contact lens polymer matrices with hydrophobic tails of ionic surfactants helps to adsorb surfactant molecules on the polymer. A tight packing creates high surface charge on the contact lens. Ionic compounds adsorb on the charged surfactant-coated contact lens surfaces with high affinity. Such interactions cause reduced transport rates, leading to extended release. Anionic drug dexamethasone 21-disodium phosphate binds to p-HEMA contact lenses through cationic surfactant (cetalkonium chloride). Drug molecules adsorbed on the surfactant-covered polymer demonstrated slow diffusion along the surface with diffusivity at a lower rate than free drug. The surfactant loading accelerated duration of release from about 2 to 50 hours within 1 day using Acuvue® contact lenses [155]. These drug-loaded contact lenses have advantages over conventional topical drops but suffer from limitations such as inadequate drug loading and short-term drug release (few hours). To further improve drug loading and extend drug release, colloidal drug delivery systems such as liposomes and nanoparticles are laden into contact lenses and molecularly imprinted contact lenses have been developed.

For the preparation of particle-laden contact lenses, initially the therapeutic agent is entrapped in colloids such as liposomes, nanoparticles, or microemulsions. Furthermore, these loaded carrier systems are dispersed in the contact lens material. For example, particle-laden contact lenses have been prepared by dispersing lidocaine entrapped in microemulsions and/or liposomes followed by incorporation in p-HEMA hydrogels. Particle-loaded contact lenses demonstrated extended lidocaine release over 8 days [160, 161]. After use, contact lenses are required to be stored in drug-saturated solutions to avoid drug loss during storage. Stimuli responsive or "smart" particles that release drug only upon contact with the ocular surface may overcome such a problem.

Molecular imprinted contact lenses have demonstrated improved drug loading and drug release. Soft contact lenses fabricated by the molecular imprinting method demonstrated ~1.6 times higher timolol loading than contact lenses prepared by a conventional method. Also, molecular imprinted contact lenses demonstrated sustained timolol release that produced higher ocular tear fluid bioavailability for ketotifen fumarate relative to drug-soaked contact lens and commercially available topical drops [162]. The ketotifen fumarate molecular imprinted contact lenses demonstrated improved ocular relative bioavailability (about threefold higher) than nonimprinted lenses. The AUC for ketotifen fumarate in imprinted lens, nonimprinted lens, and eye drops were 4365 ± 1070 μg h/mL, 493 ± 180 μg h/mL, and 46.6 ± 24.5 μg h/mL, respectively [163]. Thus, molecular imprinted contact lenses have been demonstrated to possess more effectiveness over conventionally prepared drug-loaded lens and topical eye drops.

IN SITU GELLING SYSTEMS

In situ gelling systems or hydrogels refer to polymeric aqueous solutions that undergo a sol to gel transition in response to environmental or physiological stimuli. In general, thermosensitive gels are prepared with biocompatible and biodegradable polymers. Gel formation can be initiated by temperature variation, pH change, and ionic balance and/ or with ultraviolet irradiation. For ocular drug delivery, thermosensitive gels (i.e., solutions that respond to temperature changes and transform into gels) have been developed [164]. Polymers used for the development of thermosensitive gels include poloxamers and multiblock copolymers made from PCL, PEG, PLA, PGA, poly(N-isopropylacrylamide), and chitosan. These polymeric systems form temperature-dependent micellar aggregation followed by gelation at higher temperatures due to aggregation or packing [165]. Drug-loaded thermosensitive polymeric solution once in contact with the ocular surface transforms to an *in situ* gel depot. Because of the unique transition from sol-to-gel phase at physiological temperature, these gelling systems cause improvement in ocular drug bioavailability.

Effects of hydrophilic and hydrophobic polymeric additives on sol–gel transition and release profile of timolol maleate from PEG-PCL-PEG–based thermosensitive hydrogels have been studied [166]. PCL (hydrophobic additive) and PVA (hydrophilic additive) lower critical gel concentrations of the PEG-PCL-PEG triblock polymer. The effect of PCL on sol–gel transition is more pronounced than PVA (**Figure 10-12**) [167]. The effect of PVA on the release profile was more pronounced and the cumulative percentage timolol maleate release was improved from $86.4 \pm 0.8\%$ to $73.7 \pm 1.8\%$ over 316 hours. Thermosensitive gels appear to be noncytotoxic in rabbit primary corneal epithelial culture cells with/without additives, indicating PEG-PCL-PEG hydrogel matrix to be a viable drug delivery system.

Dexamethasone acetate–loaded thermosensitive gel comprising the triblock polymer PLGA-PEG-PLGA has been developed as an ocular delivery system [165]. *In vivo*

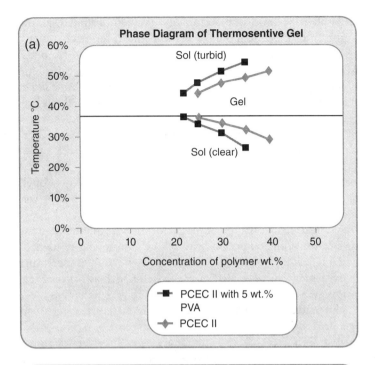

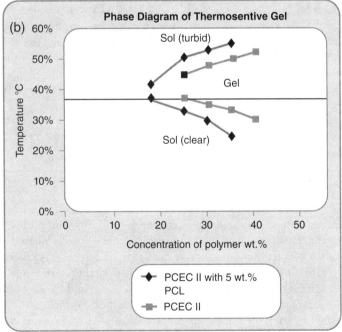

FIGURE 10-12 Sol–gel transition phase diagram. (a) PEG_{750}–PCL_{3750}–PEG_{750} (PCEC II) triblock copolymer aqueous solutions alone and with 5 wt.% PVA. (b). PCEC II triblock copolymer aqueous solutions alone and with 5 wt.% PCL. (Reproduced with kind permission from Springer Science+Business Media: Mishra GP, Tamboli V, Mitra AK. Effect of hydrophobic and hydrophilic additives on sol-gel transition and release behavior of timolol maleate from polycaprolactone-based hydrogel. *Colloid and polymer science.* Sep 2011;289[14]:1553–1562.)

studies with topical drop administration to rabbit eye demonstrated significantly higher C_{max} (125.2 µg/mL) for dexamethasone acetate in the anterior chamber with PLGA-PEG-PLGA solution relative to dexamethasone acetate solution (17.6 ± 2.18 ng/mL). Moreover, AUC was higher with PLGA-PEG-PLGA over topical solution. C_{max} and AUC were higher by ~7- and 7.98-fold from PLGA-PEG-PLGA *in situ* gel than solution. The triblock polymer comprising PLGA and PEG (ReGel™) has been studied for delivery of macromolecules such as ovalbumin [168]. *In vivo* studies with subconjunctival administration in rat eye demonstrated sustained drug release. Ovalbumin concentrations were maintained at measurable levels in the back of the eye tissues (sclera, choroid, and retina) over 14 days.

Other polymeric systems comprising cross-linked poly(*N*–isopropylacrylamide)-PEG diacrylate hydrogels have been synthesized for sustaining bovine serum albumin and immunoglobulin G release [169]. *In vitro* studies demonstrated 3-week sustained bovine serum albumin release from gel. Therefore, thermosensitive gels offer significant advantages in providing sustained drug release, improving residence time on the cornea, minimizing dosing frequency, lowering side effects, and increasing ocular bioavailability. Furthermore, drug-loaded carrier systems such as nanoparticles suspended in thermosensitive gels can be used [170]. Steroids such as dexamethasone-, hydrocortisone acetate–, and prednisolone acetate–loaded PLGA nanoparticles suspended in thermosensitive gel demonstrated zero-order drug release kinetics. The burst release from nanoparticles was minimized. *Ex vivo* studies across rabbit sclera demonstrated longer sustained drug release relative to drug-loaded nanoparticles. For targeted drug delivery, thermosensitive gels composed of PLGA-PEG-PLGA were studied. Doxorubicin-loaded micelles (PLGA-PEG-folate [FOL]) were suspended in thermosensitive gel that sustained doxorubicin release for a period of 2 weeks. *In vitro* uptake studies across Y-79 cells demonstrated about four times higher uptake than PLGA-PEG micelles [171]. These studies indicate that thermosensitive polymers form gels at physiological temperatures sustain drug release and aid in targeted delivery to both anterior and posterior ocular tissues.

GENE DELIVERY

Gene delivery to targeted cells involves safe and effective delivery of a specific, efficacious, and safe genome. The delivered genome is expected to elicit robust expression, coupled with high efficiency, high persistent levels, and long duration of expression. Two types of gene transfer vectors, viral and nonviral, have been evaluated in preclinical and clinical settings. Viral gene transfer vectors include adenovirus, adeno-associated virus (AAV), retrovirus, lentivirus (LV), alphavirus, herpes virus, and baculovirus vectors [172–174]. Of these viral vectors, adenovirus, AAV, and LV are commonly used for ocular gene transfer. These viral vectors have specific molecular sites on the capsid coat that causes it to track specific cell types of a target organ known as tropism [175]. Nonviral gene transfer vectors include plasmids, cationic lipids, and polymers. These nonviral vectors form a complex with DNA and then condense to form particles in nanometer range (<25 nm) so the complex can pass to the cell nucleus. Gene transfer vectors have specific advantages and limitations. Viral vectors are more efficient in translocating into target ocular cells. These viral vectors, however, are limited in application due to heightened concern for long-term safety and immunogenicity problems, which have not yet been overcome. Nonviral vectors do not usually elicit such safety and immunogenicity concerns. Clinical trials have revealed nonviral vectors to be considered safer than viral vectors but much less efficient in transduction relative to viral vectors [176].

ADENOVIRUS VECTORS

Adenovirus-based gene therapy can be directed to the back of the eye tissue (retina) and anterior segment tissues. Adenoviruses are nonenveloped double-stranded DNA viruses with several serotypes [177]. These viruses are obtained by partial deletion of the viral genome. Adenoviruses can accommodate 36 kb of exogenous sequences and do not integrate in the target cell. Because of the transient nature of the transgene expression in adenovirus vector, immune-mediated elimination is identified. Therefore, the desired long-lasting therapeutic gene expression required for ocular diseases is absent. Adenovirus vectors expressing the herpes virus thymidine kinase have been demonstrated to phosphorylate the GCV into the triphosphate form. This cytotoxic product of the herpes simplex thymidine kinase reaction is transported to adjacent cells through gap junctions, inhibits DNA replicates, and destroys transduced cells [178].

AAV VECTORS

Recombinant AAV (rAAV) is a small, nonpathogenic, single-stranded DNA virus that exists in over 100 distinct variants. Ocular gene transfer with AAV has received much attention recently. The rAAV vectors demonstrated several advantages, such as long-term transgene expression in the eye and lack of pathogenicity [179]. More than eight different AAV serotypes are known. These vectors have specialized tracking mechanisms to target cells that have demonstrated robust, persistent gene expression and profiles of differing kinetic expressions. The versatility, efficacy, low immunogenicity, and nonpathogenicity render rAAV vectors highly efficient for ocular gene transfer. These vectors have only one limitation: their gene-carrying capacity is restricted to 4.7 kb [180]. rAAV vectors have been used to mediate efficient transduction by deletion of coding sequences and insertion of expression cassettes between the inserted terminal repeats. Tissue specificity and expression kinetics of rAAV vectors highly depend on the vector serotype and anatomical compartment of delivery within the globe. rAAV vectors have been used for efficient transduction across RPE, photoreceptor cells, and retinal ganglionic cells [181]. In *in vivo* studies in large animal models, rAAV vectors demonstrated stable expression in the retina that was maintained over several years [180, 182, 183].

LV VECTORS

The LVs are integrating, complex, single-strand, positive sense, enveloped RNA retroviruses. These vectors possess the necessary cellular and molecular components required for stable transduction of dividing and postmitotic cells. The vectors are widely used in ocular gene delivery because of their ability to transduce nondividing cells and generate and maintain long-term transgene expression [184]. Advantages of LVs include absence of immunological complications after intraocular delivery and relatively large transgene carrying capacity (8–10 kb) compared with rAAVs, which permits multicistronic codelivery of several therapeutic genes. Such LVs have certain limitations, such as, the potential generation of replication competent lentiviruses during LV production, *in vivo* recombination with lentiviral polynucleotide sequences, and insertional addition of proviral DNA in or close to active genes, which may elicit tumor initiation or promotion [185].

In vivo studies in rodents with intracameral administration of vesicular stomatitis virus glycoprotein (VSV-G) pseudo-typed HIV-1 and equine infectious anemia virus demonstrated efficient transduction in corneal endothelium and trabecular meshwork [186–189]. Other studies with different species established that VSV-G- pseudo-typed feline immunodeficiency virus vector specifically target the trabecular meshwork [190–192]. Rabies-G pseudo-typed equine infectious anemia virus vector can transduce neuronal cells within the anterior ocular tissues with low efficiency [187]. IVT delivery of VSV-G pseudo-typed HIV-1, equine infectious anemia virus, VSV-G pseudo-typed feline immunodeficiency virus, and rabies–G pseudo-typed equine infectious anemia virus vector failed to produce efficient intraocular expression in the corneal endothelium. On the contrary, few studies suggest widespread intraocular transduction after IVT delivery of these vectors [193–195]. Subretinal delivery of LVs have been found to demonstrate efficient and stable transduction of rodents and nonhuman primate RPE cells [172].

NONVIRAL VECTORS

Nonviral vectors have been and continue to be of interest due to their safe, effective, and promising strategy for ocular gene transfer. Vectors such as compacted DNA nanoparticles may mediate gene therapy safely with sustained expression over several months [196]. These systems appear to be promising in the treatment of genetic ocular diseases. Han et al. demonstrated that DNA (CK30PEG) nanoparticles can be retained in the eye after subretinal injection. On the other hand, AAV injection exhibited vector DNA and green fluorescent protein (GFP) expression in the visual pathway of the brain. It appears that nonviral nanocarriers are a potential successful alternative to viral gene therapy [197].

Similarly, cationic core-shell liponanoparticles demonstrated higher uptake in human conjunctival cells than plasmid-laden chitosan nanoparticles and lipid-coated chitosan nanoparticles [198]. *In vivo* studies conducted in rabbits revealed that cationic core-shell liponanoparticles demonstrated ~2.5-fold rise in enhanced green fluorescent protein (EGFP) expression, indicating an alternative to viral vectors. Nanomicellar constructs prepared from polyethylene oxide-polypropylene oxide-polyethylene oxide were evaluated as a carrier for plasmid DNA with the *lacZ* gene [199]. These nanomicellar constructs demonstrated efficient and stable transfer of functional gene via topical drops in mice and rabbits, indicating the potential of block copolymers for DNA transfer. Kurosaki et al. [200] evaluated ocular gene expression using anionic ternary/plasmid DNA-PEI complex [200]. A coating of plasmid DNA-PEI complex with ternary complexes such as γ-polyglutamic acid and chondroitin sulfate demonstrated no cytotoxicity and aggregation. *In vivo* intravenous administration of ternary complex to rabbits showed high gene expression in the retina, indicating the complex to be a suitable carrier for effective and safe ocular gene therapy.

SUMMARY

Effective management of ophthalmic diseases is a challenging task for pharmaceutical scientists because of the complex nature of various diseases and the presence of ocular barriers. Challenges in ocular drug delivery have been partially met by the identification of transporters on ocular tissues and chemical modification of drug substances to target such transporters. Transporter specificity helps in targeting specific tissues, thereby lowering side effects and improving bioavailability. Ideally, therapeutically effective drug levels should be maintained for prolonged periods of time after a single application.

Invasive modes of drug delivery cannot be considered safe, effective, and patient compliant. Drug delivery via the periocular route could overcome many of these limitations and also offer sustained drug levels in various ocular pathologies affecting both the anterior and posterior segments. Targeted lipid prodrug strategy can be a promising approach for many drug molecules with poor absorption across ocular barriers. Colloidal drug delivery systems could significantly improve the state of current therapy and may emerge as an alternative after periocular administration.

Advances in nanotechnology and noninvasive drug and gene delivery techniques will remain in the forefront of designing and developing novel ocular drug delivery systems. More emphasis needs to be given to noninvasive sustained drug delivery for both anterior and posterior segment eye disorders. Further, continuous innovation in gene therapy appears to be a very exciting area for a gamut of ocular diseases. Nevertheless, a clear understanding of the complexities associated with normal and diseased conditions, physiological barriers, and pharmacokinetics would significantly hasten further drug development in this field.

ACKNOWLEDGMENT

This work was supported by National Institutes of Health grants R01 EY09171 and R01 EY10659.

REVIEW QUESTIONS

1. List the various layers of the cornea.
2. Describe the advantages and disadvantages of topical ocular drug administration.
3. What are cyclodextrins?
4. Define nanomicelles and their advantages and disadvantages.
5. What are ocular implants? Describe briefly implants used in ocular drug delivery.
6. What is gene delivery? List the vectors commonly used in gene delivery.

REFERENCES

1. Vadlapudi AD, Patel A, Cholkar K, Mitra A. Recent patents on emerging therapeutics for the treatment of glaucoma, age related macular degeneration and uveitis. *Rec Pat Biomed Eng.* 2012;5(1):83–101.
2. Barar J, Asadi M, Mortazavi-Tabatabaei SA, Omidi Y. Ocular drug delivery; impact of in vitro cell culture models. *J Ophthalm Vis Res.* 2009;4(4):238–252.
3. Dua HS, Faraj LA, Said DG, Gray T, Lowe J. Human corneal anatomy redefined: a novel pre-Descemet's layer (Dua's layer). *Ophthalmology.* 2013;120(9):1778–1785.
4. Lee VH, Robinson JR. Topical ocular drug delivery: recent developments and future challenges. *J Ocul Pharmacol.* 1986;2(1):67–108.
5. Hughes PM, Olejnik O, Chang-Lin JE, Wilson CG. Topical and systemic drug delivery to the posterior segments. *Adv Drug Deliv Rev.* 2005;57(14):2010–2032.
6. Gaudana R, Jwala J, Boddu SH, Mitra AK. Recent perspectives in ocular drug delivery. *Pharm Res.* 2009;26(5):1197–1216.

7. Ahmed I, Patton TF. Importance of the noncorneal absorption route in topical ophthalmic drug delivery. *Invest Ophthalmol Vis Sci*. 1985;26(4):584–587.

8. Santulli RJ, Kinney WA, Ghosh S, et al. Studies with an orally bioavailable alpha V integrin antagonist in animal models of ocular vasculopathy: retinal neovascularization in mice and retinal vascular permeability in diabetic rats. *J Pharmacol Exp Ther*. 2008;324(3):894–901.

9. Shirasaki Y, Miyashita H, Yamaguchi M. Exploration of orally available calpain inhibitors. Part 3. Dipeptidyl alpha-ketoamide derivatives containing pyridine moiety. *Bioorg Med Chem*. 2006; 14(16):5691–5698.

10. Kampougeris G, Antoniadou A, Kavouklis E, Chryssouli Z, Giamarellou H. Penetration of moxifloxacin into the human aqueous humour after oral administration. *Br J Ophthalmol*. 2005;89(5):628–631.

11. Sakamoto H, Sakamoto M, Hata Y, Kubota T, Ishibashi T. Aqueous and vitreous penetration of levofloxacin after topical and/or oral administration. *Eur J Ophthalmol*. 2007;17(3):372–376.

12. Pitkanen L, Ranta VP, Moilanen H, Urtti A. Permeability of retinal pigment epithelium: effects of permeant molecular weight and lipophilicity. *Invest Ophthalmol Vis Sci*. 2005;46(2):641–646.

13. Urtti A. Challenges and obstacles of ocular pharmacokinetics and drug delivery. *Adv Drug Deliv Rev*. 2006;58(11):1131–1135.

14. Duvvuri S, Majumdar S, Mitra AK. Drug delivery to the retina: challenges and opportunities. *Expert Opin Biol Ther*. 2003;3(1):45–56.

15. Mitra AK AB, Duvvuri S. Drug delivery to the eye. In: J Fischbarg, ed. *The Biology of the Eye*. New York: Academic Press; 2006:307–351.

16. Marmor MF, Negi A, Maurice DM. Kinetics of macromolecules injected into the subretinal space. *Exp Eye Res*. 1985;40(5):687–696.

17. Ausayakhun S, Yuvaves P, Ngamtiphakom S, Prasitsilp J. Treatment of cytomegalovirus retinitis in AIDS patients with intravitreal ganciclovir. *J Med Assoc Thai*. 2005;88(Suppl 9):S15–S20.

18. Ghate D, Edelhauser HF. Ocular drug delivery. *Expert Opin Drug Deliv*. 2006;3(2):275–287.

19. Hosseini K, Matsushima D, Johnson J, et al. Pharmacokinetic study of dexamethasone disodium phosphate using intravitreal, subconjunctival, and intravenous delivery routes in rabbits. *J Ocul Pharmacol Ther*. 2008;24(3):301–308.

20. Kim SH, Csaky KG, Wang NS, Lutz RJ. Drug elimination kinetics following subconjunctival injection using dynamic contrast-enhanced magnetic resonance imaging. *Pharm Res*. 2008;25(3):512–520.

21. Weijtens O, Feron EJ, Schoemaker RC, et al. High concentration of dexamethasone in aqueous and vitreous after subconjunctival injection. *Am J Ophthalmol*. 1999;128(2):192–197.

22. Raghava S, Hammond M, Kompella UB. Periocular routes for retinal drug delivery. *Expert Opin Drug Deliv*. 2004;1(1):99–114.

23. Prausnitz MR, Noonan JS. Permeability of cornea, sclera, and conjunctiva: a literature analysis for drug delivery to the eye. *J Pharm Sci*. 1998;87(12):1479–1488.

24. Chew EY, Glassman AR, Beck RW, et al. Ocular side effects associated with peribulbar injections of triamcinolone acetonide for diabetic macular edema. *Retina*. 2011;31(2):284–289.

25. Castellarin A, Pieramici DJ. Anterior segment complications following periocular and intraocular injections. *Ophthalmol Clin North Am*. 2004;17(4):583–590, vii.

26. Mannermaa E, Vellonen KS, Urtti A. Drug transport in corneal epithelium and blood-retina barrier: emerging role of transporters in ocular pharmacokinetics. *Adv Drug Deliv Rev*. 2006; 58(11):1136–1163.

27. Dey S, Anand BS, Patel J, Mitra AK. Transporters/receptors in the anterior chamber: pathways to explore ocular drug delivery strategies. *Expert Opin Biol Ther*. 2003;3(1):23–44.

28. Dey S, Gunda S, Mitra AK. Pharmacokinetics of erythromycin in rabbit corneas after single-dose infusion: role of P-glycoprotein as a barrier to in vivo ocular drug absorption. *J Pharmacol Exp Ther*. 2004;311(1):246–255.

29. Dey S, Patel J, Anand BS, et al. Molecular evidence and functional expression of P-glycoprotein (MDR1) in human and rabbit cornea and corneal epithelial cell lines. *Invest Ophthalmol Vis Sci*. 2003;44(7):2909–2918.

30. Kawazu K, Yamada K, Nakamura M, Ota A. Characterization of cyclosporin A transport in cultured rabbit corneal epithelial cells: P-glycoprotein transport activity and binding to cyclophilin. *Invest Ophthalmol Vis Sci*. 1999;40(8):1738–1744.

31. Yang JJ, Kim KJ, Lee VH. Role of P-glycoprotein in restricting propranolol transport in cultured rabbit conjunctival epithelial cell layers. *Pharm Res*. 2000;17(5):533–538.

32. Saha P, Yang JJ, Lee VH. Existence of a p-glycoprotein drug efflux pump in cultured rabbit conjunctival epithelial cells. *Invest Ophthalmol Vis Sci*. 1998;39(7):1221–1226.

33. Constable PA, Lawrenson JG, Dolman DE, Arden GB, Abbott NJ. P-Glycoprotein expression in human retinal pigment epithelium cell lines. *Exp Eye Res*. 2006;83(1):24–30.

34. Duvvuri S, Gandhi MD, Mitra AK. Effect of P-glycoprotein on the ocular disposition of a model substrate, quinidine. *Curr Eye Res*. 2003;27(6):345–353.

35. Kennedy BG, Mangini NJ. P-glycoprotein expression in human retinal pigment epithelium. *Mol Vis*. 2002;8:422–430.

36. Yang JJ, Ann DK, Kannan R, Lee VH. Multidrug resistance protein 1 (MRP1) in rabbit conjunctival epithelial cells: its effect on drug efflux and its regulation by adenoviral infection. *Pharm Res*. 2007;24(8):1490–1500.

37. Aukunuru JV, Sunkara G, Bandi N, Thoreson WB, Kompella UB. Expression of multidrug resistance-associated protein (MRP) in human retinal pigment epithelial cells and its interaction with BAPSG, a novel aldose reductase inhibitor. *Pharm Res*. 2001;18(5):565–572.

38. Karla PK, Quinn TL, Herndon BL, Thomas P, Pal D, Mitra A. Expression of multidrug resistance associated protein 5 (MRP5) on cornea and its role in drug efflux. *J Ocul Pharmacol Ther*. 2009;25(2):121–132.

39. Karla PK, Pal D, Quinn T, Mitra AK. Molecular evidence and functional expression of a novel drug efflux pump (ABCC2) in human corneal epithelium and rabbit cornea and its role in ocular drug efflux. *Int J Pharm*. 2007;336(1):12–21.

40. Karla PK, Earla R, Boddu SH, Johnston TP, Pal D, Mitra A. Molecular expression and functional evidence of a drug efflux pump (BCRP) in human corneal epithelial cells. *Curr Eye Res*. 2009;34(1):1–9.

41. Katragadda S, Talluri RS, Pal D, Mitra AK. Identification and characterization of a Na+-dependent neutral amino acid transporter, ASCT1, in rabbit corneal epithelial cell culture and rabbit cornea. *Curr Eye Res*. 2005;30(11):989–1002.

42. Dun Y, Mysona B, Itagaki S, Martin-Studdard A, Ganapathy V, Smith SB. Functional and molecular analysis of D-serine transport in retinal Müller cells. *Exp Eye Res*. 2007;84(1):191–199.

43. Jain-Vakkalagadda B, Pal D, Gunda S, Nashed Y, Ganapathy V, Mitra AK. Identification of a Na+-dependent cationic and neutral amino acid transporter, B(0,+), in human and rabbit cornea. *Mol Pharm*. 2004;1(5):338–346.

44. Hosoya K, Horibe Y, Kim KJ, Lee VH. Na(+)-dependent L-arginine transport in the pigmented rabbit conjunctiva. *Exp Eye Res*. 1997;65(4):547–553.

45. Jain-Vakkalagadda B, Dey S, Pal D, Mitra AK. Identification and functional characterization of a Na+-independent large neutral amino acid transporter, LAT1, in human and rabbit cornea. *Invest Ophthalmol Vis Sci*. 2003;44(7):2919–2927.

46. Gandhi MD, Pal D, Mitra AK. Identification and functional characterization of a Na(+)-independent large neutral amino acid transporter (LAT2) on ARPE-19 cells. *Int J Pharm*. 2004;275(1-2):189–200.

47. Nakauchi T, Ando A, Ueda-Yamada M, et al. Prevention of ornithine cytotoxicity by nonpolar side chain amino acids in retinal pigment epithelial cells. *Invest Ophthalmol Vis Sci*. 2003;44(11):5023–5028.

48. Vadlapudi AD, Vadlapatla RK, Kwatra D, et al. Targeted lipid based drug conjugates: a novel strategy for drug delivery. *Int J Pharm*. 2012;434(1–2):315–324.

49. Vadlapudi AD, Vadlapatla RK, Mitra AK. Sodium dependent multivitamin transporter (SMVT): a potential target for drug delivery. *Curr Drug Targets*. 2012;13(7):994–1003.

50. Vadlapudi AD, Vadlapatla RK, Pal D, Mitra AK. Functional and molecular aspects of biotin uptake via SMVT in human corneal epithelial (HCEC) and retinal pigment epithelial (D407) cells. *AAPS J*. 2012;14(4):832–842.

51. Janoria KG, Boddu SH, Wang Z, et al. Vitreal pharmacokinetics of biotinylated ganciclovir: role of sodium-dependent multivitamin transporter expressed on retina. *J Ocul Pharmacol Ther*. 2009;25(1):39–49.

52. Janoria KG, Hariharan S, Paturi D, Pal D, Mitra AK. Biotin uptake by rabbit corneal epithelial cells: role of sodium-dependent multivitamin transporter (SMVT). *Curr Eye Res*. 2006;31(10):797–809.

53. Anand BS, Mitra AK. Mechanism of corneal permeation of L-valyl ester of acyclovir: targeting the oligopeptide transporter on the rabbit cornea. *Pharm Res*. 2002;19(8):1194–1202.

54. Xiang CD, Batugo M, Gale DC, et al. Characterization of human corneal epithelial cell model as a surrogate for corneal permeability assessment: metabolism and transport. *Drug Metab Dispos*. 2009;37(5):992–998.

55. Zhang T, Xiang CD, Gale D, Carreiro S, Wu EY, Zhang EY. Drug transporter and cytochrome P450 mRNA expression in human ocular barriers: implications for ocular drug disposition. *Drug Metab Dispos*. 2008;36(7):1300–1307.

56. Basu SK, Haworth IS, Bolger MB, Lee VH. Proton-driven dipeptide uptake in primary cultured rabbit conjunctival epithelial cells. *Invest Ophthalmol Vis Sci*. 1998;39(12):2365–2373.

57. Berger UV, Hediger MA. Distribution of peptide transporter PEPT2 mRNA in the rat nervous system. *Anat Embryol (Berl)*. 1999;199(5):439–449.

58. Macha S, Mitra AK. Ocular pharmacokinetics of cephalosporins using microdialysis. *J Ocul Pharmacol Ther.* 2001;17(5):485–498.

59. Garrett Q, Xu S, Simmons PA, Vehige J, Flanagan JL, Willcox MD. Expression and localization of carnitine/organic cation transporter OCTN1 and OCTN2 in ocular epithelium. *Invest Ophthalmol Vis Sci.* 2008;49(11):4844–4849.

60. Majumdar S, Gunda S, Pal D, Mitra AK. Functional activity of a monocarboxylate transporter, MCT1, in the human retinal pigmented epithelium cell line, ARPE-19. *Mol Pharm.* 2005;2(2):109–117.

61. Jwala J, Boddu SH, Paturi DK, et al. Functional characterization of folate transport proteins in Staten's Seruminstitut rabbit corneal epithelial cell line. *Curr Eye Res.* 2011;36(5):404–416.

62. Talluri RS, Katragadda S, Pal D, Mitra AK. Mechanism of L-ascorbic acid uptake by rabbit corneal epithelial cells: evidence for the involvement of sodium-dependent vitamin C transporter 2. *Curr Eye Res.* 2006;31(6):481–489.

63. Majumdar S, Gunda S, Mitra A. Functional expression of a sodium dependent nucleoside transporter on rabbit cornea: Role in corneal permeation of acyclovir and idoxuridine. *Curr Eye Res.* 2003;26(3–4):175–183.

64. Rautio J, Kumpulainen H, Heimbach T, et al. Prodrugs: design and clinical applications. *Nat Rev Drug Discov.* 2008;7(3):255–270.

65. Anand BS, Dey S, Mitra AK. Current prodrug strategies via membrane transporters/receptors. *Expert Opin Biol Ther.* 2002;2(6):607–620.

66. Macha S, Duvvuri S, Mitra AK. Ocular disposition of novel lipophilic diester prodrugs of ganciclovir following intravitreal administration using microdialysis. *Curr Eye Res.* 2004;28(2):77–84.

67. Tirucherai GS, Dias C, Mitra AK. Corneal permeation of ganciclovir: mechanism of ganciclovir permeation enhancement by acyl ester prodrug design. *J Ocul Pharmacol Ther.* 2002;18(6):535–548.

68. Hughes PM, Mitra AK. Effect of acylation on the ocular disposition of acyclovir. II. Corneal permeability and anti-HSV 1 activity of 2'-esters in rabbit epithelial keratitis. *J Ocul Pharmacol.* 1993;9(4):299–309.

69. Madhu C, Rix P, Nguyen T, Chien DS, Woodward DF, Tang-Liu DD. Penetration of natural prostaglandins and their ester prodrugs and analogs across human ocular tissues in vitro. *J Ocul Pharmacol Ther.* 1998;14(5):389–399.

70. Suhonen P, Jarvinen T, Rytkonen P, Peura P, Urtti A. Improved corneal pilocarpine permeability with O,O'-(1,4-xylylene) bispilocarpic acid ester double prodrugs. *Pharm Res.* 1991;8(12):1539–1542.

71. Malik P, Kadam RS, Cheruvu NP, Kompella UB. Hydrophilic prodrug approach for reduced pigment binding and enhanced transscleral retinal delivery of celecoxib. *Mol Pharm.* 2012;9(3): 605–614.

72. Cheng L, Beadle JR, Tammewar A, Hostetler KY, Hoh C, Freeman WR. Intraocular pharmacokinetics of a crystalline lipid prodrug, octadecyloxyethyl-cyclic-cidofovir, for cytomegalovirus retinitis. *J Ocul Pharmacol Ther.* 2011;27(2):157–162.

73. Jwala J, Boddu SH, Shah S, Sirimulla S, Pal D, Mitra AK. Ocular sustained release nanoparticles containing stereoisomeric dipeptide prodrugs of acyclovir. *J Ocul Pharmacol Ther.* 2011; 27(2):163–172.

74. Kansara V, Hao Y, Mitra AK. Dipeptide monoester ganciclovir prodrugs for transscleral drug delivery: targeting the oligopeptide transporter on rabbit retina. *J Ocul Pharmacol Ther.* 2007;23(4):321–334.

75. Anand BS, Patel J, Mitra AK. Interactions of the dipeptide ester prodrugs of acyclovir with the intestinal oligopeptide transporter: competitive inhibition of glycylsarcosine transport in human intestinal cell line-Caco-2. *J Pharmacol Exp Ther.* 2003;304(2):781–791.

76. Collins PS, Han W, Williams LR, Rich N, Lee JF, Villavicencio JL. Maffucci's syndrome (hemangiomatosis osteolytica): a report of four cases. *J Vasc Surg.* 1992;16(3):364–371.

77. Talluri RS, Samanta SK, Gaudana R, Mitra AK. Synthesis, metabolism and cellular permeability of enzymatically stable dipeptide prodrugs of acyclovir. *Int J Pharm.* 2008;361(1–2):118–124.

78. Majumdar S, Kansara V, Mitra AK. Vitreal pharmacokinetics of dipeptide monoester prodrugs of ganciclovir. *J Ocul Pharmacol Ther.* 2006;22(4):231–241.

79. Janoria KG, Boddu SH, Natesan S, Mitra AK. Vitreal pharmacokinetics of peptide-transporter-targeted prodrugs of ganciclovir in conscious animals. *J Ocul Pharmacol Ther.* 2010;26(3):265–271.

80. Vadlapudi AD, Vadlapatla RK, Earla R, et al. Novel biotinylated lipid prodrugs of acyclovir for the treatment of herpetic keratitis (HK): transporter recognition, tissue stability and antiviral activity. *Pharm Res.* 2013;30(8)2063–2076.

81. Jansen JF, de Brabander-van den Berg EM, Meijer EW. Encapsulation of guest molecules into a dendritic box. *Science.* 1994;266(5188):1226–1229.

82. Yiyun C, Tongwen X. Dendrimers as potential drug carriers. Part I. Solubilization of non-steroidal anti-inflammatory drugs in the presence of polyamidoamine dendrimers. *Eur J Med Chem.* 2005;40(11):1188–1192.

83. Yang H, Morris JJ, Lopina ST. Polyethylene glycol-polyamidoamine dendritic micelle as solubility enhancer and the effect of the length of polyethylene glycol arms on the solubility of pyrene in water. *J Colloid Interface Sci.* 2004;273(1):148–154.

84. Wang F, Cai X, Su Y, et al. Reducing cytotoxicity while improving anti-cancer drug loading capacity of polypropylenimine dendrimers by surface acetylation. *Acta Biomater.* 2012;8(12):4304–4313.

85. Biswas S, Dodwadkar NS, Piroyan A, Torchilin VP. Surface conjugation of triphenylphosphonium to target poly(amidoamine) dendrimers to mitochondria. *Biomaterials.* 2012;33(18):4773–4782.

86. Tomalia DA. Birth of a new macromolecular architecture: dendrimers as quantized building blocks for nanoscale synthetic polymer chemistry. *Progr Polym Sci.* 2005;30(3–4):294–324.

87. Vandamme TF, Brobeck L. Poly(amidoamine) dendrimers as ophthalmic vehicles for ocular delivery of pilocarpine nitrate and tropicamide. *J Control Release.* 2005;102(1):23–38.

88. Yao WJ, Sun KX, Liu Y, et al. Effect of poly(amidoamine) dendrimers on corneal penetration of puerarin. *Biol Pharm Bull.* 2010;33(8):1371–1377.

89. Yao W, Sun K, Mu H, et al. Preparation and characterization of puerarin-dendrimer complexes as an ocular drug delivery system. *Drug Dev Ind Pharm.* 2010;36(9):1027–1035.

90. Yao C, Wang W, Zhou X, et al. Effects of poly(amidoamine) dendrimers on ocular absorption of puerarin using microdialysis. *J Ocul Pharmacol Ther.* 2011;27(6):565–569.

91. Marano RJ, Wimmer N, Kearns PS, et al. Inhibition of in vitro VEGF expression and choroidal neovascularization by synthetic dendrimer peptide mediated delivery of a sense oligonucleotide. *Exp Eye Res.* 2004;79(4):525–535.

92. Durairaj C, Kadam RS, Chandler JW, Hutcherson SL, Kompella UB. Nanosized dendritic polyguanidilyated translocators for enhanced solubility, permeability, and delivery of gatifloxacin. *Invest Ophthalmol Vis Sci.* 2010;51(11):5804–5816.

93. Lopez AI, Reins RY, McDermott AM, Trautner BW, Cai C. Antibacterial activity and cytotoxicity of PEGylated poly(amidoamine) dendrimers. *Mol Biosyst.* 2009;5(10):1148–1156.

94. Del Valle EMM. Cyclodextrins and their uses: a review. *Proc Biochem.* 2004;39(9):1033–1046.

95. Kurkov SV, Loftsson T. Cyclodextrins. *Int J Pharm.* 2013;453(1)167–180.

96. Loftsson T, Duchene D. Cyclodextrins and their pharmaceutical applications. *Int J Pharm.* 2007;329(1-2):1–11.

97. Jansen T, Xhonneux B, Mesens J, Borgers M. Beta-cyclodextrins as vehicles in eye-drop formulations: an evaluation of their effects on rabbit corneal epithelium. *Lens Eye Toxic Res.* 1990;7(3–4):459–468.

98. Tirucherai GS, Mitra AK. Effect of hydroxypropyl beta cyclodextrin complexation on aqueous solubility, stability, and corneal permeation of acyl ester prodrugs of ganciclovir. *AAPS Pharm Sci Tech.* 2003;4(3):E45.

99. Bertelmann E, Knapp S, Rieck P, Keipert S, Hartmann C, Pleyer U. [Transcorneal-paracorneal penetration route for topical application of drugs to the eyt. Mycophenolate mofetil as a model substance]. *Ophthalmologe.* 2003;100(9):696–701.

100. Maestrelli F, Mura P, Casini A, Mincione F, Scozzafava A, Supuran CT. Cyclodextrin complexes of sulfonamide carbonic anhydrase inhibitors as long-lasting topically acting antiglaucoma agents. *J Pharm Sci.* 2002;91(10):2211–2219.

101. Cappello B, Carmignani C, Iervolino M, Immacolata La Rotonda M, Fabrizio Saettone M. Solubilization of tropicamide by hydroxypropyl-beta-cyclodextrin and water-soluble polymers: in vitro/in vivo studies. *Int J Pharm.* 2001;213(1–2):75-81.

102. Bary AR, Tucker IG, Davies NM. Considerations in the use of hydroxypropyl-beta-cyclodextrin in the formulation of aqueous ophthalmic solutions of hydrocortisone. *Eur J Pharm Biopharm.* 2000;50(2):237–244.

103. Reer O, Bock TK, Müller BW. In vitro corneal permeability of diclofenac sodium in formulations containing cyclodextrins compared to the commercial product voltaren ophtha. *J Pharm Sci.* Sep 1994;83(9):1345–1349.

104. Loftsson T, Frithriksdottir H, Stefansson E, Thorisdottir S, Guthmundsson O, Sigthorsson T. Topically effective ocular hypotensive acetazolamide and ethoxyzolamide formulations in rabbits. *J Pharm Pharmacol.* 1994;46(6):503–504.

105. Usayapant A, Karara AH, Narurkar MM. Effect of 2-hydroxypropyl-beta-cyclodextrin on the ocular absorption of dexamethasone and dexamethasone acetate. *Pharm Res.* 1991;8(12):1495–1499.

106. Juillerat-Jeanneret L. The targeted delivery of cancer drugs across the blood-brain barrier: chemical modifications of drugs or drug-nanoparticles? *Drug Discov Today.* 2008;13(23-24):1099–1106.

106a. Zhang J, Wang L, Gao C, Zhang L, Xia H. Ocular pharmacokinetics of topically-applied ketoconazole solution containing hydroxypropyl beta-cyclodextrin to rabbits. *J Ocul Pharmacol Ther.* 2008 Oct;24(5):501–506.

107. Date AA, Shibata A, Goede M, et al. Development and evaluation of a thermosensitive vaginal gel containing raltegravir+efavirenz loaded nanoparticles for HIV prophylaxis. *Antiviral Res.* 2012;96(3):430–436.

108. Gan L, Han S, Shen J, et al. Self-assembled liquid crystalline nanoparticles as a novel ophthalmic delivery system for dexamethasone: improving preocular retention and ocular bioavailability. *Int J Pharm.* 2010;396(1–2):179–187.

109. Bhatta RS, Chandasana H, Chhonker YS, et al. Mucoadhesive nanoparticles for prolonged ocular delivery of natamycin: In vitro and pharmacokinetics studies. *Int J Pharm.* 2012;432(1–2):105–112.

110. Musumeci T, Bucolo C, Carbone C, Pignatello R, Drago F, Puglisi G. Polymeric nanoparticles augment the ocular hypotensive effect of melatonin in rabbits. *Int J Pharm.* 2013;440(2):135–140.

111. Amrite AC, Edelhauser HF, Singh SR, Kompella UB. Effect of circulation on the disposition and ocular tissue distribution of 20 nm nanoparticles after periocular administration. *Mol Vis.* 2008; 14:150–160.

112. Amrite AC, Kompella UB. Size-dependent disposition of nanoparticles and microparticles following subconjunctival administration. *J Pharm Pharmacol.* 2005;57(12):1555–1563.

113. Zhang L, Li Y, Zhang C, Wang Y, Song C. Pharmacokinetics and tolerance study of intravitreal injection of dexamethasone-loaded nanoparticles in rabbits. *Int J Nanomed.* 2009;4:175–183.

114. Kim H, Robinson SB, Csaky KG. Investigating the movement of intravitreal human serum albumin nanoparticles in the vitreous and retina. *Pharm Res.* 2009;26(2):329–337.

115. Koo H, Moon H, Han H, et al. The movement of self-assembled amphiphilic polymeric nanoparticles in the vitreous and retina after intravitreal injection. *Biomaterials.* 2012;33(12):3485–3493.

116. Kaur IP, Garg A, Singla AK, Aggarwal D. Vesicular systems in ocular drug delivery: an overview. *Int J Pharm.* 2004;269(1):1–14.

117. Natarajan JV, Chattopadhyay S, Ang M, et al. Sustained release of an anti-glaucoma drug: demonstration of efficacy of a liposomal formulation in the rabbit eye. *PLoS One.* 2011;6(9):e24513.

118. Diebold Y, Jarrin M, Saez V, et al. Ocular drug delivery by liposome-chitosan nanoparticle complexes (LCS-NP). *Biomaterials.* 2007;28(8):1553–1564.

119. Law SL, Huang KJ, Chiang CH. Acyclovir-containing liposomes for potential ocular delivery. Corneal penetration and absorption. *J Control Release.* 2000;63(1–2):135–140.

120. Cheng L, Hostetler KY, Chaidhawangul S, et al. Intravitreal toxicology and duration of efficacy of a novel antiviral lipid prodrug of ganciclovir in liposome formulation. *Invest Ophthalmol Vis Sci.* 2000;41(6):1523–1532.

121. Shen Y, Tu J. Preparation and ocular pharmacokinetics of ganciclovir liposomes. *AAPS J.* 2007;9(3):E371–E377.

122. Zhang J, Wang S. Topical use of coenzyme Q10-loaded liposomes coated with trimethyl chitosan: tolerance, precorneal retention and anti-cataract effect. *Int J Pharm.* 2009;372(1–2):66–75.

123. Gupta SK, Velpandian T, Dhingra N, Jaiswal J. Intravitreal pharmacokinetics of plain and liposome-entrapped fluconazole in rabbit eyes. *J Ocul Pharmacol Ther.* 2000;16(6):511–518.

124. Zhang R, He R, Qian J, Guo J, Xue K, Yuan YF. Treatment of experimental autoimmune uveoretinitis with intravitreal injection of tacrolimus (FK506) encapsulated in liposomes. *Invest Ophthalmol Vis Sci.* 2010;51(7):3575–3582.

125. Sasaki H, Karasawa K, Hironaka K, Tahara K, Tozuka Y, Takeuchi H. Retinal drug delivery using eyedrop preparations of poly-l-lysine-modified liposomes. *Eur J Pharm Biopharm.* 2013; 83(3):364–369.

126. Sammalkorpi M, Karttunen M, Haataja M. Ionic surfactant aggregates in saline solutions: sodium dodecyl sulfate (SDS) in the presence of excess sodium chloride (NaCl) or calcium chloride (CaCl2). *J Phys Chem B.* 2009;113(17):5863–5870.

127. Gupta AK, Madan S, Majumdar DK, Maitra A. Ketorolac entrapped in polymeric micelles: preparation, characterisation and ocular anti-inflammatory studies. *Int J Pharm.* 2000;209(1–2):1–14.

128. Civiale C, Licciardi M, Cavallaro G, Giammona G, Mazzone MG. Polyhydroxyethylaspartamide-based micelles for ocular drug delivery. *Int J Pharm.* 2009;378(1–2):177–186.

129. Pepic I, Jalsenjak N, Jalsenjak I. Micellar solutions of triblock copolymer surfactants with pilocarpine. *Int J Pharm.* 2004;272(1–2):57–64.

130. Pepic I, Hafner A, Lovric J, Pirkic B, Filipovic-Grcic J. A nonionic surfactant/chitosan micelle system in an innovative eye drop formulation. *J Pharm Sci.* 2010;99(10):4317–4325.

131. Usui T, Sugisaki K, Amano S, Jang WD, Nishiyama N, Kataoka K. New drug delivery for corneal neovascularization using polyion complex micelles. *Cornea.* 2005;24(8 Suppl):S39–S42.

132. Kataoka K, Harada A, Nagasaki Y. Block copolymer micelles for drug delivery: design, characterization and biological significance. *Adv Drug Deliv Rev.* 2001;47(1):113–131.

133. Velagaleti PRAE, Khan IJ, Gilger BC, Mitra AK. Topical delivery of hydrophobic drugs using a novel mixed nanomicellar technology to treat diseases of the anterior and posterior segments of the eye. *Drug Deliv Technol.* 2010;10(4):42–47.

134. Vadlapudi AD, Mitra AK. Nanomicelles: an emerging platform for drug delivery to the eye. *Ther Deliv.* 2013;4(1):1–3.

135. Cholkar K, Patel A, Vadlapudi AD, Mitra A. Novel nanomicellar formulation approaches for anterior and posterior segment ocular drug delivery. *Rec Pat Nanomed.* 2012;2(2):82–95.

136. Cholkar K, Patel SP, Vadlapudi AD, Mitra AK. Novel strategies for anterior segment ocular drug delivery. *J Ocul Pharmacol Ther.* 2013;29(2):106–123.

137. Vadlapudi AD, Cholkar K, Vadlapatla RK, Mitra AK. Aqueous nanomicellar formulation for topical delivery of biotinylated lipid prodrug of acyclovir: formulation development and ocular biocompatibility. *J Ocul Pharmacol Ther.* 2014;30(1):49–58.

138. Li X, Zhang Z, Li J, Sun S, Weng Y, Chen H. Diclofenac/biodegradable polymer micelles for ocular applications. *Nanoscale.* 2012;4(15):4667–4673.

139. Jiang J, Gill HS, Ghate D, et al. Coated microneedles for drug delivery to the eye. *Invest Ophthalmol Vis Sci.* 2007;48(9):4038–4043.

140. Jiang J, Moore JS, Edelhauser HF, Prausnitz MR. Intrascleral drug delivery to the eye using hollow microneedles. *Pharm Res.* 2009;26(2):395–403.

141. Patel SR, Lin AS, Edelhauser HF, Prausnitz MR. Suprachoroidal drug delivery to the back of the eye using hollow microneedles. *Pharm Res.* 2011;28(1):166–176.

142. Patel SR, Berezovsky DE, McCarey BE, Zarnitsyn V, Edelhauser HF, Prausnitz MR. Targeted administration into the suprachoroidal space using a microneedle for drug delivery to the posterior segment of the eye. *Invest Ophthalmol Vis Sci.* 2012;53(8):4433–4441.

143. Del Amo EM, Urtti A. Current and future ophthalmic drug delivery systems. A shift to the posterior segment. *Drug Discov Today.* 2008;13(3-4):135–143.

144. Bourges JL, Bloquel C, Thomas A, et al. Intraocular implants for extended drug delivery: therapeutic applications. *Adv Drug Deliv Rev.* 2006;58(11):1182–1202.

145. Lee SS, Hughes P, Ross AD, Robinson MR. Biodegradable implants for sustained drug release in the eye. *Pharm Res.* 2010;27(10):2043–2053.

146. Choonara YE, Pillay V, Danckwerts MP, Carmichael TR, du Toit LC. A review of implantable intravitreal drug delivery technologies for the treatment of posterior segment eye diseases. *J Pharm Sci.* 2010;99(5):2219–2239.

147. Jaffe GJ, McCallum RM, Branchaud B, Skalak C, Butuner Z, Ashton P. Long-term follow-up results of a pilot trial of a fluocinolone acetonide implant to treat posterior uveitis. *Ophthalmology.* 2005;112(7):1192–1198.

148. Sieving PA, Caruso RC, Tao W, et al. Ciliary neurotrophic factor (CNTF) for human retinal degeneration: phase I trial of CNTF delivered by encapsulated cell intraocular implants. *Proc Natl Acad Sci USA.* 2006;103(10):3896–3901.

149. Talcott KE, Ratnam K, Sundquist SM, et al. Longitudinal study of cone photoreceptors during retinal degeneration and in response to ciliary neurotrophic factor treatment. *Invest Ophthalmol Vis Sci.* 2011;52(5):2219–2226.

150. Noriyuki K, Fujii S. Ocular drug delivery systems for the posterior segment: A review. *Retina Today.* 2012;May/June:54–59.

151. Lonngren U, Napankangas U, Lafuente M, et al. The growth factor response in ischemic rat retina and superior colliculus after brimonidine pre-treatment. *Brain Res Bull.* 2006;71(1-3):208–218.

152. Kim HS, Chang YI, Kim JH, Park CK. Alteration of retinal intrinsic survival signal and effect of alpha2-adrenergic receptor agonist in the retina of the chronic ocular hypertension rat. *Vis Neurosci.* 2007;24(2):127–139.

153. Aburahma MH, Mahmoud AA. Biodegradable ocular inserts for sustained delivery of brimonidine tartarate: preparation and in vitro/in vivo evaluation. *AAPS PharmSciTech.* 2011;12(4):1335–1347.

154. Gupta H, Aqil M. Contact lenses in ocular therapeutics. *Drug Discov Today.* 2012;17(9-10):522–527.

155. Bengani LC, Chauhan A. Extended delivery of an anionic drug by contact lens loaded with a cationic surfactant. *Biomaterials.* 2013;34(11):2814–2821.

156. Kim J, Conway A, Chauhan A. Extended delivery of ophthalmic drugs by silicone hydrogel contact lenses. *Biomaterials.* 2008;29(14):2259–2269.

157. Soluri A, Hui A, Jones L. Delivery of ketotifen fumarate by commercial contact lens materials. *Optom Vis Sci.* 2012;89(8):1140–1149.

158. Gulsen D, Chauhan A. Ophthalmic drug delivery through contact lenses. *Invest Ophthalmol Vis Sci.* 2004;45(7):2342–2347.

159. Kim J, Chauhan A. Dexamethasone transport and ocular delivery from poly(hydroxyethyl methacrylate) gels. *Int J Pharm.* 2008;353(1-2):205–222.

160. Gulsen D, Li CC, Chauhan A. Dispersion of DMPC liposomes in contact lenses for ophthalmic drug delivery. *Curr Eye Res.* 2005;30(12):1071–1080.

161. Gulsen D, Chauhan A. Dispersion of microemulsion drops in HEMA hydrogel: a potential ophthalmic drug delivery vehicle. *Int J Pharm.* 2005;292(1–2):95–117.

162. Hiratani H, Fujiwara A, Tamiya Y, Mizutani Y, Alvarez-Lorenzo C. Ocular release of timolol from molecularly imprinted soft contact lenses. *Biomaterials.* 2005;26(11):1293–1298.

163. Tieppo A, White CJ, Paine AC, Voyles ML, McBride MK, Byrne ME. Sustained in vivo release from imprinted therapeutic contact lenses. *J Control Release.* 2012;157(3):391–397.

164. Shaunak S, Thomas S, Gianasi E, et al. Polyvalent dendrimer glucosamine conjugates prevent scar tissue formation. *Nat Biotechnol.* 2004;22(8):977–984.

165. Rajoria G, Gupta A. *In situ* gelling system: a novel approach for ocular drug delivery. *AJPTR.* 2012;2(4):24–53.

166. Mishra GP, Tamboli V, Mitra AK. Effect of hydrophobic and hydrophilic additives on sol-gel transition and release behavior of timolol maleate from polycaprolactone-based hydrogel. *Colloid Polym Sci.* 2011;289(14):1553–1562.

167. Mishra GP, Tamboli V, Mitra AK. Effect of hydrophobic and hydrophilic additives on sol-gel transition and release behavior of timolol maleate from polycaprolactone-based hydrogel. *Colloid Polym Sci.* 2011;289(14):1553–1562.

168. Gao Y, Sun Y, Ren F, Gao S. PLGA-PEG-PLGA hydrogel for ocular drug delivery of dexamethasone acetate. *Drug Dev Ind Pharm.* 2010;36(10):1131–1138.

169. Rieke ER, Amaral J, Becerra SP, Lutz RJ. Sustained subconjunctival protein delivery using a thermosetting gel delivery system. *J Ocul Pharmacol Ther.* 2010;26(1):55–64.

170. Boddu SH, Jwala J, Vaishya R, et al. Novel nanoparticulate gel formulations of steroids for the treatment of macular edema. *J Ocul Pharmacol Ther.* 2010;26(1):37–48.

171. Boddu SH, Jwala J, Chowdhury MR, Mitra AK. In vitro evaluation of a targeted and sustained release system for retinoblastoma cells using doxorubicin as a model drug. *J Ocul Pharmacol Ther.* 2010;26(5):459–468.

172. Balaggan KS, Ali RR. Ocular gene delivery using lentiviral vectors. *Gene Ther.* 2012;19(2):145–153.

173. van Adel BA, Kostic C, Deglon N, Ball AK, Arsenijevic Y. Delivery of ciliary neurotrophic factor via lentiviral-mediated transfer protects axotomized retinal ganglion cells for an extended period of time. *Hum Gene Ther.* 2003;14(2):103–115.

174. Walther W, Stein U. Viral vectors for gene transfer: a review of their use in the treatment of human diseases. *Drugs.* 2000;60(2):249–271.

175. Choi VW, McCarty DM, Samulski RJ. AAV hybrid serotypes: improved vectors for gene delivery. *Curr Gene Ther.* 2005;5(3):299–310.

176. Uddin SN. Cationic lipids used in non-viral gene delivery systems. *Biotechnol Mol Biol Rev.* 2007;2(3):58–67.

177. Harrison SC. Virology. Looking inside adenovirus. *Science.* 2010;329(5995):1026–1027.

178. Chevez-Barrios P, Chintagumpala M, Mieler W, et al. Response of retinoblastoma with vitreous tumor seeding to adenovirus-mediated delivery of thymidine kinase followed by ganciclovir. *J Clin Oncol.* 2005;23(31):7927–7935.

179. Martin KR, Klein RL, Quigley HA. Gene delivery to the eye using adeno-associated viral vectors. *Methods.* 2002;28(2):267–275.

180. Lotery AJ, Yang GS, Mullins RF, et al. Adeno-associated virus type 5: transduction efficiency and cell-type specificity in the primate retina. *Hum Gene Ther.* 2003;14(17):1663–1671.

181. Rolling F. Recombinant AAV-mediated gene transfer to the retina: gene therapy perspectives. *Gene Ther.* 2004;11(Suppl 1):S26–S32.

182. Bainbridge JW, Mistry A, Schlichtenbrede FC, et al. Stable rAAV-mediated transduction of rod and cone photoreceptors in the canine retina. *Gene Ther.* 2003;10(16):1336–1344.

183. Weber M, Rabinowitz J, Provost N, et al. Recombinant adeno-associated virus serotype 4 mediates unique and exclusive long-term transduction of retinal pigmented epithelium in rat, dog, and nonhuman primate after subretinal delivery. *Mol Ther.* 2003;7(6):774–781.

184. Bainbridge JW, Tan MH, Ali RR. Gene therapy progress and prospects: the eye. *Gene Ther.* 2006;13(16):1191–1197.

185. Maury W. Regulation of equine infectious anemia virus expression. *J Biomed Sci.* 1998;5(1):11–23.

186. Trittibach P, Barker SE, Broderick CA, et al. Lentiviral-vector-mediated expression of murine IL-1 receptor antagonist or IL-10 reduces the severity of endotoxin-induced uveitis. *Gene Ther.* 2008;15(22):1478–1488.

187. Balaggan KS, Binley K, Esapa M, et al. Stable and efficient intraocular gene transfer using pseudotyped EIAV lentiviral vectors. *J Gene Med.* 2006;8(3):275–285.

188. Challa P, Luna C, Liton PB, et al. Lentiviral mediated gene delivery to the anterior chamber of rodent eyes. *Mol Vis*. 2005;11:425–430.

189. Bainbridge JW, Stephens C, Parsley K, et al. In vivo gene transfer to the mouse eye using an HIV-based lentiviral vector; efficient long-term transduction of corneal endothelium and retinal pigment epithelium. *Gene Ther*. 2001;8(21):1665–1668.

190. Barraza RA, Rasmussen CA, Loewen N, et al. Prolonged transgene expression with lentiviral vectors in the aqueous humor outflow pathway of nonhuman primates. *Hum Gene Ther*. 2009;20(3):191–200.

191. Loewen N, Fautsch MP, Teo WL, Bahler CK, Johnson DH, Poeschla EM. Long-term, targeted genetic modification of the aqueous humor outflow tract coupled with noninvasive imaging of gene expression in vivo. *Invest Ophthalmol Vis Sci*. 2004;45(9):3091–3098.

192. Loewen N, Bahler C, Teo WL, et al. Preservation of aqueous outflow facility after second-generation FIV vector-mediated expression of marker genes in anterior segments of human eyes. *Invest Ophthalmol Vis Sci*. 2002;43(12):3686–3690.

193. Bemelmans AP, Kostic C, Crippa SV, et al. Lentiviral gene transfer of RPE65 rescues survival and function of cones in a mouse model of Leber congenital amaurosis. *PLoS Med*. 2006;3(10):e347.

194. Derksen TA, Sauter SL, Davidson BL. Feline immunodeficiency virus vectors. Gene transfer to mouse retina following intravitreal injection. *J Gene Med*. 2002;4(5):463–469.

195. Cheng L, Chaidhawangul S, Wong-Staal F, et al. Human immunodeficiency virus type 2 (HIV-2) vector-mediated in vivo gene transfer into adult rabbit retina. *Curr Eye Res*. 2002;24(3):196–201.

196. Cai X, Conley S, Naash M. Nanoparticle applications in ocular gene therapy. *Vision Res*. 2008;48(3):319–324.

197. Han Z, Conley SM, Makkia R, Guo J, Cooper MJ, Naash MI. Comparative analysis of DNA nanoparticles and AAVs for ocular gene delivery. *PLoS One*. 2012;7(12):e52189.

198. Jiang M, Gan L, Zhu C, Dong Y, Liu J, Gan Y. Cationic core-shell liponanoparticles for ocular gene delivery. *Biomaterials*. 2012;33(30):7621–7630.

199. Liaw J, Chang SF, Hsiao FC. In vivo gene delivery into ocular tissues by eye drops of poly(ethylene oxide)-poly(propylene oxide)-poly(ethylene oxide) (PEO-PPO-PEO) polymeric micelles. *Gene Ther*. 2001;8(13):999–1004.

200. Kurosaki T, Uematsu M, Shimoda K, et al. Ocular gene delivery systems using ternary complexes of plasmid DNA, polyethylenimine, and anionic polymers. *Biol Pharm Bull*. 2013;36(1):96–101.

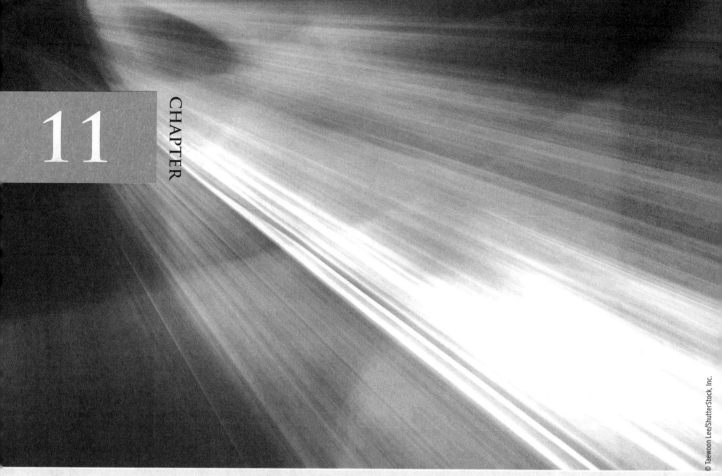

Transmucosal Drug Delivery

Navdeep Kaur, Amit Kokate, Xiaoling Li, and Bhaskara Jasti

CHAPTER OBJECTIVES

Upon completing this chapter, the reader should be able to

▶ Describe the transmucosal route and its advantages over traditional methods of drug delivery.

▶ Explain the structure of oral mucosa, the permeability barrier, and the permeation routes of absorption.

▶ Describe the methods of assessing oral mucosal absorption.

▶ List various drug delivery systems and techniques used to optimize the delivery across oral mucosa and commercialized formulations currently available in the market.

CHAPTER OUTLINE

INTRODUCTION

Transmucosal drug delivery came into existence as an alternative to traditional methods (peroral and parenteral) of drug delivery to overcome their drawbacks such as hepatic first-pass metabolism, degradation in the acidic environment of stomach, and inconvenience due to invasive nature. The various transmucosal routes available for drug delivery are oral, nasal, vaginal, rectal, and ocular. Among these, oral mucosa has an advantage over all other transmucosal routes. It is superior to nasal mucosa because it is more robust and less responsive to allergenic and irritant materials unlike nasal mucosa, which may undergo irreversible damage as a result of long-term administration of drugs. Also, rectal and vaginal routes are not preferred by patients, and the vaginal route is limited to female gender. The ocular route is mainly intended for local/topical delivery of drugs versus systemic administration [1].

The history of oral mucosal drug delivery dates back to the 1800s when Dr. Paulson observed encouraging clinical effects of certain drugs when administered in the oral cavity [2]. In 1879, Murell demonstrated the clinical effectiveness of nitroglycerin when administered sublingually [3]. Since then, a number of products have been developed for administration via oral mucosa and lot of research has been performed to understand the mechanism of transport across the oral cavity.

Drugs can be delivered through different regions in the oral cavity and can be divided as sublingual delivery, which involves administration of drug in the area beneath the tongue; buccal delivery, which entails administration of drug via buccal mucosa or lining of the cheek; and palatal, gingival, and periodontal delivery, which involves administration via soft palate, gingival membrane, and around a tooth, respectively. Of these routes of administration, delivery across buccal and sublingual mucosa has been most useful because these are nonkeratinized and highly permeable regions with the available area of 50.2 cm^2 and 26.5 cm^2, respectively [4].

This chapter reviews oral mucosal drug delivery with details regarding the structure of oral mucosa, permeation routes, methods of assessing oral mucosal absorption, and the various drug delivery systems and techniques used to optimize the delivery across oral mucosa.

ANATOMY AND STRUCTURE OF THE ORAL CAVITY/MUCOSA

Anatomically, the oral cavity can be divided into the vestibule and oral cavity proper. The vestibule is defined as the space between the teeth and inner mucosal lining of lips and cheeks (gingival and buccal), whereas the oral cavity proper is mainly composed of tongue, bounded by hard and soft palate and mucous membrane from the underside of the tongue/floor of the mouth [5]. The lining/covering of the oral cavity, called oral mucosa, is composed of multiple layers of tightly packed cells known as stratified squamous epithelium and a loose fibrous connective tissue separated from each other by means of a basement membrane. The main purpose of the epithelium is to protect the underlying tissues and organs against mechanical and chemical damage, whereas the connective tissue provides the mechanical support and nutrients for the epithelium.

Oral mucosa can be differentiated into three different types based on their function in the oral cavity: masticatory, lining, and specialized mucosa (**Figure 11-1**). These regions in the oral cavity show different adaptations of the epithelium and connective tissue. Masticatory mucosa represented by gingiva and hard palate is composed of keratinized epithelium tightly attached to underlying connective tissue, whereas lining mucosa (cheeks, floor of the mouth, soft palate, and lips) is composed of nonkeratinized stratified squamous epithelium connected to loose, elastic connective tissue. Specialized mucosa includes dorsum of the tongue and consists of keratinized as well as nonkeratinized epithelium. Lining mucosa, masticatory mucosa, and specialized mucosa represent 60%, 25%, and 15% of the total area of oral cavity, respectively [6, 7]. Oral mucosa has a total surface area of ~100 cm [2, 8].

Epithelial thickness varies in different regions of the oral cavity: hard palate, 100 to 120 μm; buccal mucosa, 500 to 600 μm; lip mucosa, 500 to 600 μm; and floor of the mouth, 100 to 200 μm [9]. The epithelium continually undergoes differentiation with cells produced in the basal region and moving toward the epithelial surface as they increase in size, become flattened, mature, and accumulate lipids and cytoplasmic protein filaments. In keratinized epithelium, cytoplasmic protein filaments representing cytokeratins differentiate and synthesize a number of specific proteins such as profillagrin and involucrin for the thickening of cell envelope, whereas in nonkeratinized epithelium these changes are less evident. The process of continuous differentiation results in a constant epithelial population as cells are shed from the surface. The amount of time it takes to renew the entire thickness of epithelium is called turnover time, found to be around 13 days for buccal mucosa, 20 days for the floor of the mouth, and 24 days for the hard palate, which is slower than that of the gastrointestinal epithelium but faster than that of skin epidermis (27 days) [7].

As shown in **Figure 11-2**, the epithelium is separated from the connective tissue by means of an irregular, continuous basement membrane called basal lamina, a noncellular

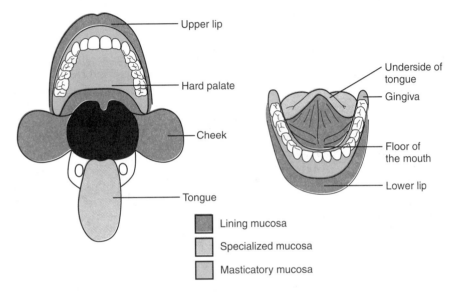

FIGURE 11-1 Regions of the oral cavity.

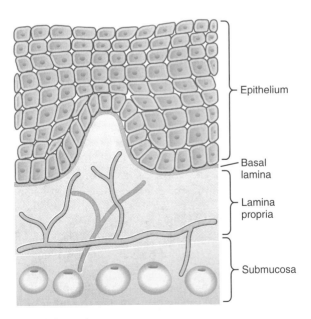

FIGURE 11-2 Structure of the oral mucosa.

TABLE 11-1 Difference between buccal and sublingual mucosae		
Parameter	**Buccal**	**Sublingual**
Epithelial thickness	500–600 μm (40–50 cell layers)	100–200 μm (8–12 cell layers)
Area	50.2 cm²	26.5 cm²
Median turnover time	13 days	20 days
Blood supply	Maxillary artery	Sublingual artery

structure with a thickness of around 1 to 2 μm. The connective tissue can be divided into lamina propria, containing collagen fibrils, blood vessels, nerves, and smooth muscles, and submucosa, which is composed of thick connective tissue containing few salivary glands [10, 11].

Branches of the external carotid artery supply blood to the oral cavity. The major branch, the maxillary artery, supplies blood to cheek, hard palate, and gingiva, whereas the facial artery and sublingual artery provide blood to lips, soft palate and tongue, and floor of the mouth, respectively (**Table 11-1**) [9].

BIOCHEMICAL COMPOSITION AND PERMEABILITY BARRIER

In keratinized regions of the oral mucosa, the permeability barrier is composed of flattened, keratin-filled cells embedded in a lipid matrix, whereas in nonkeratinized regions the barrier is located in approximately the outer one-third of the epithelium. The composition and organization of intercellular material, chiefly lipid and glycolipid content extruded from membrane coating granules, are responsible for barrier functions in the epithelium. Membrane coating granules are small, spherical, or oval cytoplasmic granules having a diameter of 100 to 300 nm [12]. Membranes of membrane coating granules fuse with that of the cells in the upper third quarter of the epithelium and release their contents in the intercellular spaces.

In nonkeratinized regions, abundance of polar lipids (i.e., phospholipids, glycosylceramides, and cholesterol esters) are present. These polar lipids are localized in the intercellular spaces and are responsible for increased fluidity and higher permeation of hydrophilic compounds. On the other hand, the keratinized regions are rich in cholesterol, fatty acids, and complex series of six types of ceramides. The ceramides and fatty acids consist of straight and saturated fatty acids that are responsible for highly structured and less permeable regions. Also, the lamellar arrangement of membrane coating granules contributes to the rigidity. Polar lipids like phospholipids and glycosylceramides are converted to ceramides and fatty acids by hydrolytic enzymes such as phospholipase and glycosidases to a great extent in keratinized epithelia. The quantity of these enzymes is fairly less in nonkeratinized regions and thus results in retained polar lipids in the epithelium. Law et al. [13] found that lipid content of buccal mucosa was greater than that of sublingual mucosa (**Table 11-2**) [14].

TABLE 11-2 Biochemical composition of buccal and sublingual mucosae

	Buccal Mucosa	Sublingual Mucosa
Sphingomyelin	16.3 ± 7.3	6.0 ± 1.0
Phosphatidylcholine	17.5 ± 7.9	9.8 ± 2.5
Phosphatidylserine	11.3 ± 4.8	6.5 ± 0.9
Phosphatidylinositol	6.0 ± 2.4	3.2 ± 0.7
Phosphatidylethanolamines	16.6 ± 7.1	9.3 ± 2.2
Cholesterol sulfate	6.1 ± 2.0	2.3 ± 1.1
Glycosylceramides	15.9 ± 7.2	4.5 ± 0.8
Ceramide 2	0.8 ± 0.3	0.2 ± 0.2
Cholesterol	20.4 ± 4.0	16.8 ± 4.1
Fatty acids	10.8 ± 2.2	4.8 ± 1.5
Triglycerides	4.7 ± 2.1	7.0 ± 1.5
Cholesterol esters	4.1 ± 3.2	9.0 ± 4.9

Values are means ± standard deviation.

SALIVA AND MUCUS

Saliva is produced by a number of salivary glands present in the oral cavity, such as parotid (under and in front of the ear), submandibular/submaxillary (beneath the floor of the mouth), sublingual (anterior to submaxillary gland, beneath the floor of the mouth), and minor salivary glands present in lips, buccal, and linings of mouth and throat. The main function of salivary secretions is to provide protection to the soft tissues in the oral cavity, maintain a moist surface, and provide lubrication [9]. The film of saliva coating the mucosa of oral cavity has a thickness of 70 to 100 µm [4]. Saliva is primarily made up of water (99%) and a complex fluid containing proteins, glycoproteins, and electrolytes. Saliva also contains enzymes such as α-amylase, lysozyme, lingual lipase, phosphatase, and esterases [11]. It has a pH of 6.5 to 7.5 and a flow rate of 0.2 to 0.4 mL/min under a resting state, which increases to 2.0 to 5.0 mL/min when stimulated [6]. The composition and flow rate of saliva varies with time of the day, degree and type of stimulation, between individuals, in disease states, and with drug therapy. The average volume of saliva produced is 750 mL/day, with 60%, 30%, 5%, and 5% to 7% contributed by submandibular, parotid, sublingual, and minor glands, respectively [15].

Mucous glycoproteins or mucins produced by minor salivary glands and sublingual glands are responsible for providing lubrication in the oral cavity, which assists in the functions of swallowing of food and talking [15]. The mucous secretions are composed mainly of water (99% by weight), macromolecular glycosylated proteins, and inorganic salts. The glycosylated proteins comprises of a protein core containing oligosaccharide chains attached to it and have a molecular mass ranging from 1 to 10 million Da [11]. Two types of mucins have been identified, secretory or soluble mucins and membrane-bound or cell-associated mucins. Secretory or soluble mucins are produced by specialized epithelial cells and possess viscoelastic and lubricating properties due to their ability to form intermolecular disulfide bonds, for example, high-molecular-weight mucin glycoprotein 1 and low-molecular-weight mucin glycoprotein 2. Membrane-bound or cell-associated mucins possess the ability to bind to membranes by means of a hydrophobic stretch of amino acids and lack the disulfide bond [16].

Mucins form a dense structure at the pH of the oral cavity, which gives it the ability to bind to the epithelial cell surface. Also, because of sugar content, mucins have considerable water-holding capacity. These qualities result in lubrication of the oral cavity and also provide a means of attaching bioadhesive dosage forms in the oral cavity for drug delivery. Few studies have reported that saliva and mucin serve as a barrier to drug delivery; however, the role of mucin as a permeability barrier is not clear. Moreover, its contribution as a barrier may be negligible relative to that posed by epithelium [15]. The oral cavity is not suitable for delivery of drugs containing ester functional groups and ester prodrugs because of the presence of esterases in the saliva and also for molecules having molecular weights greater than 30 kDa because the mucin network acts as a sieve and slows its movement. Also, an increase in salivary flow rate due to chewing gum may result in drug release and overall decrease in concentration in the oral cavity [16].

TRANSPORT ROUTES ACROSS ORAL MUCOSA

The oral mucosa possesses two major permeability barriers or routes of drug transport, transcellular and paracellular. Intercellular spaces constitute the paracellular route, which is predominantly hydrophilic and poses a barrier for lipophilic compounds. The transcellular route is the passage across the cell membrane, which is lipophilic in nature and thus restricts the permeation of hydrophilic drugs [17]. The volume of the membrane coating granules in the intracellular spaces and extrusion of lipid contents in the intercellular space determine the resistance across transcellular and paracellular routes, respectively [18].

Flux (J_P) of drugs transporting or diffusing via the paracellular route can be expressed as follows:

$$J_P = \frac{D_P \varepsilon}{h_P} C_D$$

where D_P is the diffusion coefficient in the intercellular spaces, h_P is the path length of the paracellular route, ε is the area fraction of the paracellular route, and C_D is the concentration of drug in the donor.

Goswami et al. [19] performed a study using a homologous series of polyethylene glycols as hydrophilic probes to estimate the theoretical pore size of porcine oral mucosa (buccal and sublingual). In this study the relationship between molecular weight and permeability across buccal and sublingual mucosa was explored as well as the theoretical parameters of aqueous pathway such as radius of the pore and ratio of the area fraction of the aqueous pathway to the barrier length of the membrane determined.

Two methods (i.e., Stoke's Einstein radius and radius of gyration) were used to calculate the radius of polyethylene glycols. The experimental permeability data of polyethylene glycols across porcine oral mucosa were used to calculate the values of radius of the pore (r_P) and area fraction of the aqueous path pathway to the barrier length of the membrane (ε/L) using least-squares fit with Scientist™ version 2 (Micromath, MO).

$$P_i = D_i \frac{\varepsilon}{L}\left[1-\left(\frac{r_i}{r_p}\right)^2\right]\left[1-2.104\left(\frac{r_i}{r_p}\right)+2.09\left(\frac{r_i}{r_p}\right)^3-0.95\left(\frac{r_i}{r_p}\right)^5\right]$$

where P_i, D_i, r_i, ε, and L are the permeability coefficient of the permeant through the membrane, diffusion coefficient of the permeant in water, radius of the permeant, area fraction of the aqueous pathway, and barrier length, respectively.

The results demonstrated smaller pore size in buccal mucosa (22 Å) but higher ε/L (1.42), representing pore occupancy over the length in a membrane as compared with sublingual mucosa (53 Å, 1.24, respectively). The permeability of polyethylene glycols decreased with increase in molecular weight, across sublingual mucosa from 5.31×10^{-6} cm/s to 2.72×10^{-6} cm/s and for buccal mucosa from 2.97×10^{-6} cm/s to 1.28×10^{-6} cm/s as molecular weight was increased threefold (282 to 942 Da) and twofold (282 to 546 Da), respectively [19].

Steady-state flux (J_T) across transcellular route can be represented as follows:

$$J_T = \frac{K_P D_T (1-\varepsilon)}{h_T} C_D$$

where K_p is the partition coefficient between lipophilic (cell membrane) and hydrophilic regions (intercellular space), D_T is the diffusion coefficient in the lipophilic phase, and h_T is the path length of the transcellular route. The choice of route for transport across oral mucosa depends on the physicochemical properties of the drugs and the preferred route is the one presenting least resistance [20].

METHODS OF ASSESSING ORAL MUCOSAL ABSORPTION

In vitro methods were developed with the intention of understanding the mechanism of drug absorption/transport across the oral mucosa and to get an approximation of expected *in vivo* absorption rate. Experimental methodology used in *in vitro* experiments is relatively simple because it involves clamping of a freshly dissected/excised oral mucosa from a test animal between two diffusion cells containing drug solution and the receiving media simulating systemic circulation, respectively. Repetitive samples of the receiving media are collected at predetermined time intervals to determine the amount of drug permeated across excised tissue. These studies also allow for understanding the effects of various factors such as pH, permeation enhancers, and temperatures on the permeation of drug candidates across the oral mucosa [21]. These studies have several advantages such as they are quick and easy to perform using excised tissue and experimental variables can be easily controlled, unlike in *in vivo* studies. The drawback of *in vitro* studies is that the tissue is introduced in an artificial environment and does not truly represent absorption in a complex *in vivo* system, which has constant salivary flow and systemic clearance.

Cell cultures derived from buccal region have been suggested as an *in vitro* model to study the absorption characteristics and metabolism. Cultured buccal epithelium obtained by isolating and growing hamster pouch buccal epithelium was shown to possess biochemical, morphological, and permeability characteristics similar to that of excised hamster pouch epithelium as well as of human, rabbit, and other species [22].

TR146, a cell line derived from the squamous cell carcinoma of buccal mucosa, is the most successful cell culture used for permeability studies [23]. EpiOral™ is a commercially available buccal tissue model developed by MatTek Corporation that consists of normal, human-derived epithelial cells grown into a multilayered tissue differentiated into organized basal layer and multiple noncornified layers. This model resembles the human buccal mucosa histologically and in biochemical composition [24]. The various advantages of *in vitro* studies using cell cultures are ease of handling, ability to study transport under controlled conditions, and easy manipulation of various factors influencing transport. A few points, however, need to be considered while using cell culture systems for transport studies, such as passage number, cell heterogeneity, differentiation potential, cell viability, primary culture, or a stable cell line and their phenotypic stability [10].

Despite the various advantages offered by *in vitro* studies, the inability to extrapolate absorption in an *in vivo* system makes *in vivo* studies indispensable. A simple, noninvasive test, where swirling of a buffered drug solution of known concentration and volume in the oral cavity for a given amount of time followed by expulsion and washing of the oral cavity has been used for years. The drug content was analyzed in the expelled drug solution to determine the rate and extent of drug disappearance from the oral cavity [25]. The limitations of this method include inability to localize the drug solution within a specified area of the oral cavity, salivary dilution of the drug, accidental swallowing, time consuming, and uncertainty of amount of intact drug that actually reaches systemic circulation [26, 27]. Various modifications of the method were proposed by scientists to account for the drug dilution by salivary secretion during the test and the accidental swallowing of drug solution [28]. To shorten the time needed to determine drug absorption kinetics, Tucker proposed a modification to the original method that involved multiple sampling of the drug solution being swirled in the oral cavity [29]. Before even Beckett and Triggs came up with the buccal absorption test to determine the absorption characteristics of a drug candidate across the oral mucosa, numerous scientists in the mid-1900s conducted *in vivo* experiments in human volunteers and animal models to determine the absorption of drugs based on their clinical effects [30].

To overcome the limitation of the buccal absorption test (i.e., inability to localize the drug solution in a specified region of the oral cavity) scientists devised absorption cells to perform *in vivo* studies. Kaaber used a small disc made of filter paper to determine the uptake and loss of water across the oral mucosa [31]. Other scientists such as Anders et al, used a disc made of Polytef® and filter paper, respectively, to study the absorption of drugs from the oral cavity [32]. Absorption cells were also used in the animal models to study *in vivo* absorption of drug candidates across the oral mucosa. Siegel used the rubber O-ring as the absorption cell. The O-ring was fixed onto a rat's tongue with a cyanoacrylate adhesive and the drug solution (10 μL) was introduced inside the ring. Plasma samples and samples of the test solution from the O-ring were used to determine the *in vivo* absorption profile of the drug candidate. Ritschel et al., Kurosaki et al., Kellaway, and Zhang et al. proposed or developed absorption cells of modified design and capable of holding sufficient volume of drug solution to study *in vivo* absorption characteristics [27, 33, 34].

Perfusion cells were proposed as further modification of absorption cells that provide protection of the drug solution from salivary secretions and continuous movement of drug solution across mucosal surface, which is not available in absorption cells. The study involves circulating drug solution through the device attached to the oral mucosa and collecting a fraction of the perfusion solution at different time points to evaluate the absorption characteristic. Blood samples can also be withdrawn simultaneously to obtain pharmacokinetic data. A number of studies were conducted using perfusion cells in animal models to determine the absorption characteristics of drug candidates and to evaluate the variation in the permeability of different regions of the oral mucosa [35–38].

Numerous laboratory animals such as rats, hamsters, and guinea pigs were used as *in vivo* animal models for the determination of absorption across oral mucosa, but because of their keratinized epithelium they were not considered useful in extrapolating the results to humans. Rabbit is the only rodent possessing nonkeratinized epithelium resembling that of humans and was found to be a good experimental model for extrapolating results to humans in the study of sublingual absorption of drug candidates by Dali et al. [38]. However, buccal mucosa of rabbit was found to be unsuitable for studies because of a sudden transition from nonkeratinized to keratinized regions at the margins. Various large animals such as monkeys, dogs, and pigs were used in a number of studies because of their similarity in terms of structure and composition to human oral mucosa. However, high costs of purchasing and maintaining as well as difficulties in handling make these models unsuitable [7].

In silico or a computational approach is increasingly becoming popular for predicting permeabilities across a barrier and *in vivo* absorption using molecular properties. The advantages of computational methods are saving resources because of reduced time and money involved in conducting laborious *in vivo* and *in vitro* studies and identification of drug candidates that may pose absorption problems later in the drug development. The computational approach is based on quantitative structure-property relationship that attempts to establish a quantitative relationship between molecular descriptors and the property of interest. It is important to consider a few points for obtaining a significant correlation between chemical structure and descriptors with good predictive ability, such as the data used should be free from bias and large standard errors and should not be obtained from a small sample size. It is also essential to use appropriate descriptors that describe the property of interest. In addition, the model obtained should ideally have a low standard error and a restricted number of physicochemical descriptors [39].

A number of computational models have been proposed in the area of oral and transdermal delivery to predict *in vivo* or *in vitro* permeability by establishing a correlation with the molecular descriptors of drug candidates [41, 42]. Very few attempts have been made, however, to predict the permeability or *in vivo* absorption across oral mucosa. One such model was proposed by Kokate et al. [42] for prediction of *in vitro* buccal permeability of drugs using various molecular descriptors based on structure and physicochemical properties of drug candidates. Fifteen structurally diverse molecules were chosen to build the predictive model, and it was shown that molecular volume, number of hydrogen bond donors, log $D_{6.8}$, and number of rotatable bonds were the principal descriptors describing the *in vitro* permeability coefficient:

$$\text{Log } K_p = -3.13 - 0.0128 \text{ molecular volume} - 0.617 \text{ hydrogen bond donors} + 0.263 \text{ number of rotatable bonds} + 0.654 \log D_{6.8}$$

The predictive capability of the model was assessed using an external data set, and it was found to be better than the transdermal predictive model, the Potts-Guy model, often used for prediction of *in vitro* transmucosal permeability because of lack of specific models for oral mucosa [42].

Goswami [43] developed an *in silico* model for prediction of drug permeability across the sublingual mucosa. Fourteen drugs covering a wide range of physicochemical and molecular properties were used to develop the multiple linear regression model with log P_e (permeability coefficient) as the response variable and descriptors as the predictive variable. The results demonstrated that hydrogen bond donors and log $D_{6.8}$ are the most important descriptors governing sublingual permeability:

$$\text{Log } P_e = -5.08 - 0.24 \text{ hydrogen bond donors} + 0.53 \log D$$

The difference between the significant descriptors in the buccal and sublingual *in silico* model suggests that this discrepancy could be due to the difference in the barrier properties of the two mucosae. Molecular volume and number of rotatable bonds describing the size and flexibility of a permeant were found to be insignificant for sublingual permeability, suggesting that bigger molecules may traverse the sublingual mucosa with ease as compared with buccal mucosa.

As discussed above, a number of methods have been devised to study permeability of oral mucosa. No correlation has been established, however, between the methods such as *in vitro–in vivo* correlation, which is well established for oral drug delivery.

INTRAORAL TRANSMUCOSAL DRUG DELIVERY

Intraoral transmucosal drug delivery refers to delivery of drug candidates across the mucosa of the oral cavity. The various advantages of intraoral transmucosal drug delivery are rapid absorption in the systemic circulation because of rich blood supply of the oral mucosa, avoidance of hepatic first-pass metabolism and degradation in the acidic environment of gastrointestinal tract, convenience/ease of administration, and robust/faster turnover time.

The major challenge associated with intraoral delivery is the short residence time of the drug delivery system in the oral cavity because of the continuous clearance of the drug into the gastrointestinal tract by salivary secretions. Thus, one of the main goals of intraoral delivery system designing is to prolong the retention time in the oral cavity. The various strategies used to achieve the longer retention time include usage of bioadhesive polymers, gums, lozenges, dry powder, and so on. Other points to consider while designing an oral mucosal drug delivery system are convenience/acceptability to the patient (i.e., it should not handicap drinking, eating, and sleeping).

DRUG DELIVERY SYSTEMS

Numerous drug delivery platforms have been designed to improve the delivery of drugs across the oral mucosa. A list of commercially available intraoral drug delivery systems is summarized in **Table 11-3**.

SOLID DOSAGE FORMS

The various solid dosage forms such as tablets, lozenges, and troches are intended to be placed in contact with the oral mucosa. Based on the excipients used, dosage forms adhere or disintegrate on coming in contact with the oral mucosa and salivary secretions. Solid dosage forms dissolve in saliva, and the drug gets absorbed from the mucosa of the entire oral cavity and top third of the esophageal mucosa [44]. Solid dosage forms can be classified into quick dissolving and slow dissolving based on their rate of dissolution/disintegration.

Quick-Dissolving Dosage Forms

These dosage forms disintegrate or undergo dissolution within a few seconds to a minute on coming in contact with saliva in the oral cavity, thereby releasing the drug. The ability to administer the dosage form without water, ease of swallowing, and quick onset of action are some of the advantages of quick-dissolving dosage forms. The fragility and friability of these dosage forms is a limitation that requires single-unit blister packs.

TABLE 11-3 Intraoral drug delivery systems

Dosage Form	Commercial Name	Drug	Technology	Indication	Company
Solid	Maxalt-MLT®	Rizatriptan benzoate	ODT	Migraine	Merck
	Zyprexa® Zydis®	Olanzapine	ODT	Schizophrenia	Eli Lilly
	Risperdal® M-Tablet®	Risperidone	ODT	Schizophrenia	Janssen
	Claritin® RediTabs®	Loratadine	ODT	Antihistamine	Schering/Merck
	Clarinex® Reditabs®	Desloratadine	ODT	Antihistamine	Schering/Merck
	Zomig®-ZMT	Zolmitriptan	ODT	Migraine	AstraZeneca
	FazaClo®	Clozapine	ODT	Schizophrenia	Jazz Pharmaceuticals
	Tempra® quicklets	Acetaminophen	QDT		
	Remeron® SolTab®	Mirtazapine	QDT	Depression	Organon
	Alavert®	Loratadine	QDT	Antihistamine	Pfizer
	Benadryl® Fastmelt®	Diphenhydramine citrate	QDT	Allergy	McNeil-PPC
	Zelapar®	Selegiline HCl	QDT	Parkinson's disease	Valeant Pharmaceuticals International Inc.
	Nicorette	Nicotine	Lozenge	Smoking cessation	GlaxoSmithKline
	Actiq	Fentanyl	Lozenge	Cancer pain	Cephalon
	Uprima	Apomorphine	Sublingual tablet	Erectile dysfunction	TAP Pharmaceutical Products Inc.
	Fentora	Fentanyl	Buccal tablet (OraVescent® technology)	Cancer pain	Cephalon
Semisolid	Emdogain® gel	Hydrophobic enamel	Gel	Periodontal disease	Straumann
	Biotene® oral balance gel	Protein-enzyme system	Gel	Dry mouth relief	GlaxoSmithKline
	Gelclair®	Bioadherent barrier-forming agents	Gel	Oral mucositis	Helsinn
	Aphthasol®	Amlexanox	Paste	Canker sores	Discus Dental Inc.
	Orabase® Oralone®	Triamcinolone acetonide	Paste	Mouth sores	Colgate

(cont.)

TABLE 11-3 Intraoral drug delivery systems (cont.)

Dosage Form	Commercial Name	Drug	Technology	Indication	Company
Sprays	Nitrolingual Pumpspray	Nitroglycerin	Lingual spray	Angina	Arbor Pharmaceuticals Inc.
	Oral-lyn™	Insulin	Oral spray	Diabetes	Generex Biotechnology
	Glytrin Spray®	Glyceryl trinitrate	Lingual spray	Angina	Sanofi-Aventis
	Benactiv®	Flurbiprofen	Throat spray	Oropharyngeal pain	Reckitt Benckiser
	Subsys®	Fentanyl	Sublingual spray	Breakthrough cancer pain	Insys Therapeutics, Inc.
Wafer/films	Onsolis™	Fentanyl	Buccal soluble film	Cancer pain	Meda Pharmaceuticals Inc.
	Suboxone®	Buprenorphine and naloxone	Sublingual film	Opioid dependence	Reckitt Benckiser

ODT, orally disintegrating tablet; QDT, quick dispersing tablet.

Flashdose®, OraSolv®, duraSolv®, OraVescent®, Flashtbab®, Ziplets®, Oraquick™, Wowtab®, and Rapitrol™ are a few examples of the technologies used to achieve quick dissolution/dispersion in the oral cavity.

Slow-Dissolving Dosage Forms

As the name suggests, these products dissolve slower in the oral cavity compared with quick-dissolving dosage forms (i.e., within 1 to 10 minutes). Examples include chewable tablets, sublingual tablets, lollipops, and mucoadhesive tablets.

Tablets can also be formulated into monolithic systems, containing a mixture of drug with a bioadhesive/sustained-release polymer and multilayered matrices, comprising two or more layers of polymer with or without the active pharmaceutical ingredient. Further release of the drug from the tablets can be controlled by coating the surface of tablets with an impermeable polymer to achieve a unidirectional or bidirectional release [45]. Despite being popular, there are certain limitations to the solid dosage forms, such as short residence time, accidental swallowing, and patient acceptability (mouth feel, taste, irritation). Numerous drugs have been incorporated into oral mucosal solid dosage forms and are available commercially, such as Nicorette® (nicotine lozenge), Fentora™ (fentanyl buccal tablet), Actiq® (fentanyl lozenge), and Striant® (testosterone extended-release buccal tablet) [46].

PATCHES

Intraoral mucoadhesive patches can be designed to deliver drugs locally in the oral cavity and/or systemically. Intraoral mucoadhesive patches contain a bioadhesive agent such as polyacrylic polmers, povidone, or cellulose derivatives (sodium carboxymethyl cellulose) that retain the formulation onto the oral mucosa (buccal, palatal, or gingival mucosa) and are intended for sustained or prolonged release of drug. Patches can be classified as follows: (1) monolithic matrix, type I, patches with a dissolvable matrix that slowly and completely dissolves in the oral cavity, releasing drug multidirectionally, mainly intended for local action; (2) multilayer matrix, type II, patches with a nondissolvable backing that releases the drug unidirectionally into the systemic circulation across oral mucosa, protecting it from saliva; and (3) multilayer matrix, type III, patches with a dissolvable backing designed for systemic drug delivery thta slowly dissolves completely, releasing drug unidirectionally into the oral mucosa [1, 46]. Patches have advantages over solid dosage forms in that they are flexible and are localized over a specified region, thus resulting in less inter- and intrasubject variability [41]. Limitations of patches are that the drug can only be delivered to a small area of the mucosa, thus limiting the dose that can be delivered, and patches with nondissolvable backing need to be removed from the oral cavity once the drug has been released.

AEROSOLS AND SPRAYS

Intraoral aerosol drug delivery systems are based on the similar technology as that of aerosols used for pulmonary drug delivery and are intended to deliver drugs effectively across the oral mucosa into the systemic circulation. The spray produces fine droplets of optimum size to be absorbed from the buccal mucosa but too big to be absorbed across lungs. Generex Biotechnology™ has devised an aerosol-based buccal drug delivery technology called RapidMist™. The technology consists of a proprietary formulation made up of a mixture of drug candidate, absorption enhancers, and excipients and a device to deliver the medication accurately, reliably, and safely. Using this technology, Generex Biotechnology™ has developed an intraoral (buccal) spray called Oral-lyn™ for delivering insulin across the buccal mucosa [47]. Novadel Pharma Inc. has a proprietary technology called NovaMist™ for delivering pharmaceutically active agents via spray across the oral mucosa. NitroMist™ (nitroglycerin), ZolpiMist™ (zolpidem), Zensania™ (ondansetron), Duromist™ (sildenafil), NVD-201 (sumatriptan), and NVD-301 (midazolam) are few of the products using Novadel's NovaMist™ technology [48]. The advantages of aerosol formulation are that a uniform unit dosage can be administered by means of the pump spray, thus improving the safety profile of certain drugs by lowering the dose, and the ability to administer the drug without water [46].

SEMISOLID DOSAGE FORMS

Semisolid dosage forms include medicated gels and pastes for systemic and topical delivery of drugs. Gels are made of bioadhesive polymers that provide controlled release of the drug while adhering to muocsa for long periods of time. One major disadvantage of gels is the difficulty in measuring the exact dose of drug to be administered/applied at a particular site. Miconazole oral gel is marketed as Daktarin for the treatment of oropharyngeal candidiasis [49]. Oraqix® is a local anesthetic gel containing lidocaine and prilocaine composed of a thermosetting system that when applied into the periodontal pockets thickens at body temperature into an elastic gel, thereby remaining at the site for the time required to produce anesthesia [50].

Pastes are a relatively new mode of delivering drugs via the oral cavity for local or systemic action. Clobetasol propionate is used topically in the form of lipophilic ointment in a hydrophilic base and more recently encapsulated in the lipid microspheres for the treatment of oral lichen planus [51]. Amlexanox oral paste marketed as Aphthasol® is used for healing of aphthous ulcers or canker sores [52]. An oral paste containing prednisolone acetate, rifamycin, along with parachlorophenol and iodoform was tested for improved healing after dental extractions in HIV-positive patients [53]. An oral paste containing mucoadhesive microspheres was used for controlled release of triclosan [54]. Hydrogels are the flexible formulations composed of swellable hydrophilic matrices that swell on coming in contact with saliva in the oral cavity and release the drug through the spaces in the network of hydrogels [55].

CHEWING GUMS

Medicated chewing gums have been used since 1928, when Aspergum®, a chewing gum containing acetylsalicylic acid, was introduced. In 1970, another medicated chewing gum, Nicorette®, containing nicotine for the treatment of smoking cessation, was launched in the market. A number of medicated chewing gums are available in the market: Nicotinell® containing nicotine [56], Fluogum® containing fluoride, Stay Alert® containing caffeine, Surpass® containing calcium carbonate (discontinued), Travel Gum® containing dimenhydrinate (antiemetic, available in Austria and Czech Republic), and Vitaflo CHX® containing chlorhexidine [46, 57].

Gum base is the basic component in all chewing gums apart from other excipients such as sweetening agents, flavoring agents, aromatics, and an active pharmaceutical ingredient. The gum base is mainly composed of elastomers, which provide elasticity and cohesion; emulsifiers and fats used to soften the mixture of elastomers; and fillers to provide suitable texture for the gum base [58].

Chewing gums as drug delivery systems have advantage of releasing drugs over a longer period of time, patient compliance because it is convenient to use, and controlled drug release by changing the rate and vigor of chewing [44]. It can be used to deliver drugs locally or systemically. A major limitation associated with this delivery system, however, is that a part of the drug reaches the gastrointestinal tract due to involuntary swallowing of excess saliva produced as a result of mastication.

WAFERS

Wafers are thin porous wafer-like tablets or strips formulated by lyophilization of polymer containing active pharmaceutical ingredient. The formulation instantaneously disintegrates when placed in the oral cavity, releasing the drug subsequently [46].

FILMS AND STRIPS

Films are thin flexible strips composed of a drug dissolved/dispersed/distributed in a water-dissolving polymer, which hydrates, adheres, and quickly dissolves within few seconds when placed in the oral cavity. The films are monolithic matrices that release the drug multidirectionally, and drug release from these matrices can be controlled by varying the rate of dissolution. The films are prepared by wet film or hot melt coating, which involves casting the formulation onto a moving web where it gets dried or cooled, resulting in a thin flexible film [46].

LIPOSOMES

Liposomes are artificial vesicles composed of phospholipids with the drug entrapped in their core or attached to the membrane. Depending on the composition and nature of lipids, liposomes can be designed to be acid sensitive, acid resistant, heat sensitive, plasma stable, or stealth.

Liposomes have been explored to deliver drugs across the oral mucosa. For example, liposomes were investigated for the delivery of antigens across the oral mucosa as a vaccine delivery system [59]. Also, liposomes were shown to effectively transport benzyl nicotinate across the oral mucosa, and dexamethasone sodium phosphate–loaded multilamellar vesicle liposomes were used in treating oral ulcers [60, 61]. Another liposomal formulation, called transferosomes, a highly deformable lipid vesicle, was used to deliver insulin across the buccal mucosa [62]. Franz-Montan et al. [60] showed liposome-encapsulated ropivacaine produced longer soft tissue anesthesia and reduced pain during needle insertion when administered across the oral mucosa as compared with other anesthetics used in the study. An advantage of using liposomal preparations for oral mucosal delivery is that it results in enhanced penetration through the permeability barrier [63]. Triamcinolone acetonide palmitate encapsulated in large multilamellar vesicles was used to treat oral ulcers by localizing the action of drug and thereby reducing the systemic drug absorption [64].

Polymersomes are membrane-enclosed spherical vesicular structures composed of macromolecular aggregates of amphiphilic block copolymers. The amphiphilic molecules contain a hydrophilic and hydrophobic region and self-assemble to yield an entropically stable structure on coming in contact with water. Polymersomes made up of two block copolymers, (2-(methacryloyloxy)ethyl phosphorylcholine)-poly(2-(diisopropylamino)ethyl methacrylate) and poly(ethylene oxide)-poly(2-(diisopropylamino)ethyl methacrylate), were investigated for their intra- and transepithelial permeation potential across tissue-engineered human oral mucosa. Polymersomes have the advantage over traditional liposomes in being more stable, less leaky, and capable of encapsulating hydrophilic as well as hydrophobic molecules. The study by Hearnden et al. [65] shows that polymersomes may have the potential of delivering drugs across oral mucosa.

MICROPARTICLES AND NANOPARTICLES

Holpuch et al. [66] explored the possibility of using nanoparticles for delivering a poorly water-soluble drug locally in the oral cavity. In this proof of concept study, internalization of two types of nanoparticles, solid lipid nanoparticles and polystyrene nanoparticles, was assessed using monolayer cultured human oral squamous cell carcinoma and normal human oral muocsa explants. The results demonstrated that oral squamous cell carcinoma cells internalized solid lipid nanoparticles and the nanoparticles penetrated the epithelium and basement membrane into the connective tissue, thus showing the potential of nanoparticles for systemic drug delivery across oral mucosa in addition to local delivery.

Microspheres made of poloxamer 407 containing atenolol were assessed for their delivery potential across buccal mucosa. The results demonstrated that the microsphere resulted in higher bioavailability at lower dosage as compared with oral marketed product [67].

SUMMARY

Bypassing first-pass metabolism, degradation in the gastrointestinal tract, and improved patient compliance are a few of the numerous advantages offered by transmucosal drug delivery. Of various means of delivering drugs transmucosally, the buccal and sublingual routes are particularly beneficial because of their added advantages. A number of drugs have been used for delivery across the oral mucosal route, and numerous drug delivery systems using different technologies are available commercially. The oral mucosal route has a lot of potential, and with the advent of new technologies such as nanotechnology it will further improve its utility for clinical use.

REVIEW QUESTIONS

1. Describe various methods of assessing transmucosal absorption.
2. List the permeability barrier in oral mucosa and its biochemical composition.
3. Describe the various routes of permeation across the oral mucosa.
4. List the various drug delivery systems and technologies used for intraoral drug delivery.

REFERENCES

1. Hearnden V, Sankar V, Hull K, et al. New developments and opportunities in oral mucosal drug delivery for local and systemic disease. *Adv Drug Deliv Rev.* 2012;64(1):16–28.
2. Paulson W. Sublingual medication. *Practitioner.* 1916;97:389.
3. Murrell W. Nitroglycerin as a remedy for angina pectoris. *Lancet.* 1879;1(80):113.
4. Collins LM, Dawes C. The surface area of the adult human mouth and thickness of the salivary film covering the teeth and oral mucosa. *J Dent Res.* 1987;66(8):1300–1302.
5. Gray H. *Anatomy of the Human Body*, 20th ed. Philadelphia: Lea & Febiger; 1918.
6. Nanci A. *Ten Cate's Oral Histology: Development, Structure, and Function*, 7th ed. Philadelphia: Elsevier Health Sciences; 2008.
7. Squier CA, Wertz PW. *Structure and Function of the Oral Mucosa and Implications for Drug Delivery.* Vol. 74. New York: Marcel Dekker; 1996.
8. Rossi S, Sandri G, Caramella CM. Buccal drug delivery: a challenge already won? *Drug Discov Today Technol.* 2005;2(1):59–65.
9. James C. McElnay CMH. *Drug Delivery: Buccal Route*, 3rd ed. Philadelphia: Taylor & Francis; 2006.
10. Li B, Robinson JR. *Preclinical Assessment of Oral Mucosal Drug Delivery Systems.* Vol. 145. Philadelphia: Taylor & Francis; 2005.
11. Sudhakar Y, Kuotsu K, Bandyopadhyay AK. Buccal bioadhesive drug delivery—a promising option for orally less efficient drugs. *J Control Release.* 2006;114(1):15–40.
12. Harris D, Robinson JR. Drug delivery via the mucous membranes of the oral cavity. *J Pharm Sci.* 1992;81(1):1–10.
13. Law S, Wertz PW, Swartzendruber DC, Squier CA. Regional variation in content, composition and organization of porcine epithelial barrier lipids revealed by thin-layer chromatography and transmission electron microscopy. *Arch Oral Biol.* 1995;40(12):1085–1091.
14. Kurosaki Y, Kimura T. Regional variation in oral mucosal drug permeability. *Crit Rev Ther Drug Carrier Syst.* 2000;17(5):467–508.
15. Rathbone MJ, Drummond BK, Tucker IG. The oral cavity as a site for systemic drug delivery. *Adv Drug Deliv Rev.* 1994;13(1–2):1–22.
16. Schenkels LCPM, Gurururaja TL, Levine MJ. *Salivary Mucins: Their Role in Oral Mucosal Barrier Function and Drug Delivery.* Vol. 74. New York: Marcel Dekker; 1996.
17. Zhang H, Robinson JR. *Routes of Drug Transport Across Oral Mucosa.* Vol. 74. New York: Marcel Dekker; 1996.
18. Shojaei AH, Berner B, Xiaoling L. Transbuccal delivery of acyclovir. I. In vitro determination of routes of buccal transport. *Pharm Res.* 1998;15(8):1182–1188.
19. Goswami T, Jasti BR, Li X. Estimation of the theoretical pore sizes of the porcine oral mucosa for permeation of hydrophilic permeants. *Arch Oral Biol.* 2009;54(6):577–582.
20. Gandhi RB, Robinson JR. Oral cavity as a site for bioadhesive drug delivery. *Adv Drug Deliv Rev.* 1994;13(1–2):43–74.
21. Zhang H, Robinson JR. *In Vitro Methods for Measuring Permeability of the Oral Mucosa.* Vol. 74. New York: Marcel Dekker; 1996.
22. Tavakoli-Saberi MR, Audus KL. Cultured buccal epithelium: an in vitro model derived from the hamster pouch for studying drug transport and metabolism. *Pharm Res.* 1989;6(2):160–166.
23. Nielsen HM, Rassing MR. Nicotine permeability across the buccal TR146 cell culture model and porcine buccal mucosa in vitro: effect of pH and concentration. *Eur J Pharm Sci.* 2002;16(3):151–157.
24. Epioral™. Available at: http://www.mattek.com/pages/products/epioral. Accessed February 2012.
25. Beckett ABR, Triggs EJ. Kinetics of buccal absorption of amphetamines. *J Pharm Pharmacol* 1968;20:92–7.

26. Shojaei AH, Chang RK, Guo X, Burnside BA, Couch RA. Systemic Drug delivery via the buccal mucosal route. *Pharm Technol.* 2001;June:70–81.

27. Rathbone MJ, Purves R, A. GF, Ho PC. *In Vivo Techniques for Studying the Oral Mucosal Absorption Characteristics of Drugs in Animals and Humans.* Vol. 74. New York: Marcel Dekker; 1996.

28. Dearden JC, Tomlinson E. A new buccal absorption model. *J Pharm Pharmacol.* 1971;23:68S–72S.

29. Tucker IG. A method to study the kinetics of oral mucosal drug absorption from solutions. J Pharm Pharmacol 1988;40:679–83.

30. Walton RP, Lacey CF. Absorption of drugs through the oral mucosa. *J Pharmacol Exp Therap.* 1935;54(1):61–76.

31. Kaaber S. The permeability and barrier functions of the oral mucosa with respect to water and electrolytes. Studies of the transport of water, sodium and potassium through the human mucosal surface in vivo. Acta Odontol Scand Suppl 1974;32:3–47.

32. Anders R, Merkle HP, Schurr W, Ziegler R. Buccal absorption of protirelin: an effective way to stimulate thyrotropin and prolactin. J Pharm Sci 1983;72:1481–3.

33. Rathbone MJ. Human buccal absorption. I. A method for estimating the transfer kinetics of drugs across the human buccal membrane. *Int J Pharm.* 1991;69(2):103–108.

34. Kurosaki Y, Takatori T, Nishimura H, Nakayama T, Kimura T. Regional variation in oral mucosal drug absorption: permeability and degree of keratinization in hamster oral cavity. *Pharm Res.* 1991;8(10):1297–1301.

35. Veillard MM, Longer MA, Martens TW, Robinson JR. Preliminary studies of oral mucosal delivery of peptide drugs. *J Control Release.* 1987;6(1):123–131.

36. Yamahara H, Suzuki T, Mizobe M, Noda K, Samejima M. In situ perfusion system for oral mucosal absorption in dogs. *J Pharm Sci.* 1990;79(11):963–967.

37. Weaver ML, Tanzer JM, Kramer PA. Salivary flow induction by buccal permucosal pilocarpine in anesthetized beagle dogs. *J Dent Res.* 1992;71(11):1762–1767.

38. Dali MM, Moench PA, Mathias NR, Stetsko PI, Heran CL, Smith RL. A rabbit model for sublingual drug delivery: comparison with human pharmacokinetic studies of propranolol, verapamil and captopril. *J Pharm Sci.* 2006;95(1):37–44.

39. Malkia A, Murtomaki L, Urtti A, Kontturi K. Drug permeation in biomembranes: in vitro and in silico prediction and influence of physicochemical properties. *Eur J Pharm Sci.* 2004;23(1):13–47.

40. Linnankoski J, Makela JM, Ranta VP, Urtti A, Yliperttula M. Computational prediction of oral drug absorption based on absorption rate constants in humans. *J Med Chem.* 2006;49(12):3674–3681.

41. Winiwarter S, Bonham NM, Ax F, Hallberg A, Lennernas H, Karlen A. Correlation of human jejunal permeability (in vivo) of drugs with experimentally and theoretically derived parameters. A multivariate data analysis approach. *J Med Chem.* 1998;41(25):4939–4949.

42. Kokate A, Li X, Williams PJ, Singh P, Jasti BR. In silico prediction of drug permeability across buccal mucosa. *Pharm Res.* 2009;26(5):1130–1139.

43. Goswami T. *Sublingual Drug Delivery: In Vitro Characterization of Barrier Properties and Prediction of Permeability.* Stockton, CA: University of the Pacific; 2008.

44. Zhang H, Zhang J, Streisand JB. Oral mucosal drug delivery: clinical pharmacokinetics and therapeutic applications. *Clin Pharmacokinet.* 2002;41(9):661–680.

45. Rathbone MJ, Ponchel G, Ghazali FA. *Systemic Oral Mucosal Drug Delivery and Delivery Systems.* Vol. 74. New York: Marcel Dekker; 1996.

46. Pfister WR, Ghosh TK. *Intraoral Delivery Systems: An Overview, Current Status and Future Trends.* Vol. 145. Philadelphia: Taylor & Francis Group; 2005.

47. Oral-lyn™. Available at: http://www.generex.com/index.php. Accessed February 23, 2012.

48. http://yahoo.brand.edgar-online.com/EFX_dll/EDGARpro.dll?FetchFilingHtmlSection1?Section ID=6141758-6028-23555&SessionID=JatKHvigik-axA7. Accessed April 2014.

49. Bensadoun RJ, Daoud J, El Gueddari B, et al. Comparison of the efficacy and safety of miconazole 50-mg mucoadhesive buccal tablets with miconazole 500-mg gel in the treatment of oropharyngeal candidiasis: a prospective, randomized, single-blind, multicenter, comparative, phase III trial in patients treated with radiotherapy for head and neck cancer. *Cancer.* 2008;112(1):204–211.

50. Friskopp J, Huledal G. Plasma levels of lidocaine and prilocaine after application of Oraqix, a new intrapocket anesthetic, in patients with advanced periodontitis. *J Clin Periodontol.* 2001;28(5):425–429.

51. Campisi G, Giandalia G, De Caro V, Di Liberto C, Arico P, Giannola LI. A new delivery system of clobetasol-17-propionate (lipid-loaded microspheres 0.025%) compared with a conventional formulation (lipophilic ointment in a hydrophilic phase 0.025%) in topical treatment of atrophic/erosive oral lichen planus. A phase IV, randomized, observer-blinded, parallel group clinical trial. *Br J Dermatol.* 2004;150(5):984–990.

52. Khandwala A, Van Inwegen RG, Alfano MC. 5% Amlexanox oral paste, a new treatment for recurrent minor aphthous ulcers. I. Clinical demonstration of acceleration of healing and resolution of pain. *Oral Surg Oral Med Oral Pathol Oral Radiol Endod.* 1997;83(2):222–230.

53. Ortega KL, Rezende NP, Araujo NS, Magalhaes MH. Effect of a topical antimicrobial paste on healing after extraction of molars in HIV positive patients: randomised controlled clinical trial. *Br J Oral Maxillofac Surg.* 2007;45(1):27–29.

54. Kockisch S, Rees GD, Tsibouklis J, Smart JD. Mucoadhesive, triclosan-loaded polymer microspheres for application to the oral cavity: preparation and controlled release characteristics. *Eur J Pharm Biopharm.* 2005;59(1):207–216.

55. Hoogstraate JAJ, Wertz PW. Drug delivery via the buccal mucosa. *Pharm Sci Technol Today.* 1998;1(7):309–316.

56. Nicotinell. Available at: http://nicotinell.co.uk/index.shtml. Accessed February 2012.

57. Hao J, Heng PW. Buccal delivery systems. *Drug Dev Ind Pharm.* 2003;29(8):821–832.

58. Rassing MR, Specialized oral mucosal drug delivery systems: Chewing gums. In: Rathbone, M.J. (Ed.), Oral Mucosal Drug Delivery, Marcel Dekker, New York, 1996; 319–57.

59. Zhou F, Neutra MR. Antigen delivery to mucosa-associated lymphoid tissues using liposomes as a carrier. *Biosci Rep.* 2002;22(2):355–369.

60. Erjavec V, Pavlica Z, Sentjurc M, Petelin M. *In vivo* study of liposomes as drug carriers to oral mucosa using EPR oximetry. *Int J Pharm.* 2006;307(1):1–8.

61. Farshi FS, Ozer AY, Ercan MT, Hincal AA. In-vivo studies in the treatment of oral ulcers with liposomal dexamethasone sodium phosphate. *J Microencapsul.* 1996;13(5):537–544.

62. Yang TZ, Wang XT, Yan XY, Zhang Q. Phospholipid deformable vesicles for buccal delivery of insulin. *Chem Pharm Bull.* 2002;50(6):749–753.

63. Franz-Montan M, Silva AL, Cogo K, et al. Liposome-encapsulated ropivacaine for topical anesthesia of human oral mucosa. *Anesth Analg.* 2007;104(6):1528–1531, table of contents.

64. Harsanyi BB, Hilchie JC, Mezei M. Liposomes as drug carriers for oral ulcers. *J Dent Res.* 1986;65(9):1133–1141.

65. Hearnden V, Lomas H, Macneil S, et al. Diffusion studies of nanometer polymersomes across tissue engineered human oral mucosa. *Pharm Res.* 2009;26(7):1718–1728.

66. Holpuch AS, Hummel GJ, Tong M, et al. Nanoparticles for local drug delivery to the oral mucosa: proof of principle studies. *Pharm Res.* 2010;27(7):1224–1236.

67. Monti D, Burgalassi S, Rossato MS, et al. Poloxamer 407 microspheres for orotransmucosal drug delivery. Part II. In vitro/in vivo evaluation. *Int J Pharm.* 2010;400(1–2):32–36.

TRANSDERMAL DRUG DELIVERY

MEERA GUJJAR, ANUSHREE KISHOR HERWADKAR, AND AJAY K. BANGA

CHAPTER OBJECTIVES

Upon completing this chapter, the reader should be able to

▸ Describe the anatomical and physiological factors that control drug transport across skin.

▸ Determine the ideal physicochemical properties for transdermal drug candidates.

▸ Describe the various types of transdermal patches available on the market.

▸ Describe the active transdermal technologies available to enhance percutaneous absorption.

▸ Provide advantages and disadvantages of transdermal delivery over other routes of administration.

▸ Provide counseling to patients about the proper use and precautions necessary during the application of a transdermal drug delivery system.

283

CHAPTER OUTLINE

INTRODUCTION

Topical delivery implies delivery of drugs into skin layers. This route of administration is beneficial for treatment of localized skin conditions such as eczema or atopic dermatitis. On the other hand, transdermal delivery implies delivery of drugs through the skin into the systemic circulation. This route of administration has proved to be beneficial in several cases as an alternative to oral and other routes of delivery. Major advantages associated with transdermal delivery include bypassing first-pass metabolism and providing continuous and controlled drug delivery [1]. Transdermal administration can effectively deliver low-molecular-weight, moderately lipophilic, and potent drug molecules. Several molecules, such as nicotine, scopolamine, testosterone, nitroglycerin, fentanyl, estradiol, capsaicin, selegiline, and oxybutynin, have been formulated and marketed as transdermal patches. Active enhancement techniques such as microporation, iontophoresis, electroporation, and sonophoresis are also being investigated to increase the scope of transdermal delivery [2]. The use of these technologies can assist delivery of hydrophilic molecules as well as macromolecules such as peptides and proteins [3]. In this chapter we discuss fundamentals of passive transdermal delivery and active techniques used to enhance transdermal delivery.

SKIN STRUCTURE

Skin is the largest organ of the human body, with a surface area of 2 m^2. It serves as a barrier, protecting the inner organs of the body from the environment. The structure of skin is primarily divided into two layers: epidermis and dermis (Figure 12–1).

The epidermis is the outermost layer of the skin and hence is the layer exposed to the environment. This avascular layer can be further divided into nonviable and viable epidermis. The epidermis is separated from the underlying dermis by a basement membrane. The epidermis is composed of several layers of epithelial cells. The layer above the basement membrane is called the stratum germinativum or stratum basale. Cells of the stratum germinativum differentiate to form strata known as stratum spinosum, stratum granulosum, stratum lucidum, and stratum corneum. The layers stratum germinativum, stratum spinosum, stratum granulosum, and stratum lucidum together form the viable epidermis. The stratum corneum is composed of flat, dead, keratinized cells and forms the nonviable epidermis [4].

The epithelial cells of the epidermis are known as keratinocytes and are embedded in a lipid matrix. The keratinocytes undergo continuous differentiation as they move from the stratum basale toward the stratum corneum. As the cells move toward the surface of skin, they lack oxygen and nourishment present in the basal layers. By the time they reach the surface, they are transformed into flattened, dead keratinized cells known as corneocytes. The differentiation from keratinocytes of stratum basale to corneocytes of stratum corneum takes approximately 28 days, which includes 14 days residence of the corneocytes in the stratum corneum. This is followed by a process called desquamation where one cell layer of the stratum corneum is sloughed off per day. The stratum corneum is composed of 15 to 25 layers of corneocytes stacked over each

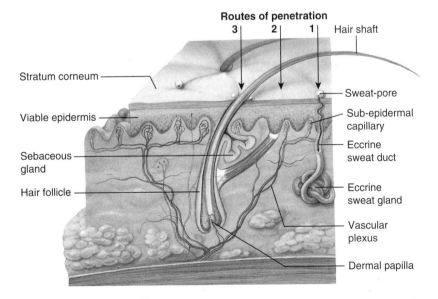

FIGURE 12-1 Anatomy of the skin.

other [5]. The corneocytes are hexagonal in shape and very closely packed. The space in between these cells is filled with a lipid matrix composed of cholesterol, ceramides, and free fatty acids. The closely packed "brick and mortar" structure of the stratum corneum makes this layer a rate-limiting barrier for transdermal transport (permeation) of molecules. Apart from keratinocytes, the epidermis contains melanocytes, which produce the pigment melanin. Additionally, Merkel cells and Langerhans cells, which form a part of the immune system, are also present in the epidermis [2].

The dermis, the thickest layer of skin, is composed of collagen and elastic fibers interspersed in proteoglycan ground substance. The dermis is predominantly hydrophilic in nature. This composition of the dermis layer is responsible for providing plasticity to skin. Skin appendages such as sweat glands, sebaceous glands, and hair follicles originate in the dermis. The appendages cover ~0.1% of the skin area but are important for transdermal delivery because they provide shunt pathways for permeation of molecules by bypassing the stratum corneum [6]. The appendageal pathway of permeation is also important for active iontophoretic transdermal delivery because charged molecules prefer to travel by the shortest (shunt) pathway [7]. In addition to appendages, the dermis is also supplied with nerves, blood vessels, lymphatic vessels, fibroblasts, and mast cells. The layer of subcutaneous fat underlying the dermis is usually several millimeters thick and serves as mechanical support to the skin and insulation for the body.

The thickness of skin varies at different anatomical sites on the body of an individual and also varies from person to person. Typically, the total thickness of the skin ranges from 2 to 5 mm, and the thickness of stratum corneum is usually 10 to 15 μm. Epidermal thickness varies from 0.06 mm on eyelids to 0.8 mm on palms and soles [4].

ADVANTAGES OF TRANSDERMAL DELIVERY

Transdermal drug delivery offers several advantages over conventional routes of administration such as oral or parenteral delivery. Transdermal delivery helps to bypass first-pass metabolism [8] and gastrointestinal degradation of drugs [9] and can potentially improve their bioavailability. It is also beneficial for drugs that cause gastrointestinal irritation, such as several nonsteroidal anti-inflammatory drugs. Delivery of drugs through the skin is noninvasive and painless and can serve as a potential alternative to parenteral delivery. Skin offers a large surface area for drug delivery that is readily accessible. This allows initiation and termination of delivery as required. This route is suitable for continuous administration of drugs and hence is particularly beneficial for drugs with short half-lives. Sustained drug delivery is also possible [1]. In addition, drug delivery can be modulated according to patient needs using active enhancement techniques, such as iontophoresis.

FACTORS INFLUENCING TRANSDERMAL DRUG DELIVERY

PHYSICOCHEMICAL FACTORS

Molecular Size

The molecular size of a compound is an important parameter determining the extent of its transdermal permeation. Molecular volume is ideally the most appropriate measure for estimating permeability of a compound. Molecular volumes are difficult to measure, however, and conventionally molecular weight has been used as a criterion to select potential compounds for transdermal delivery. Compounds having a molecular weight <500 Da are ideal for transdermal delivery [10]. Typically, drugs used as transdermal formulations have molecular weights ranging from 100 to 500 Da. It is important to note, however, that in this molecular weight range, other factors, such as partition coefficient or solubility, may have more influence in determining permeability of a molecule [4].

Partition Coefficient

To permeate across skin, a drug has to partition into the stratum corneum from the vehicle in which it is dissolved or suspended and also partition out of the stratum corneum into the underlying hydrophilic layers of skin to reach the blood circulation. Therefore, the partition coefficient forms an important factor influencing transdermal delivery [1]. This parameter is typically measured as a log P/log K octanol–water partition coefficient and is the logarithm of a ratio of concentration of a unionized solute in the oil phase (typically octanol) to its concentration in water:

$$\log P = \log\left(\frac{\text{solute in octanol}}{\text{unionized solute in water}}\right)$$

Higher log P values indicate higher lipophilicity of the molecule. Compounds having log P values ranging between 1 and 3 are ideal candidates for transdermal permeation [11]. The partition coefficient and lipophilicity of a compound also determine its predominant pathway of permeation through the skin. Compounds with higher log P values usually permeate through lipid-rich regions between keratinocytes [4].

Ionization

Generally, unionized molecules are better candidates for transdermal permeation compared with ionized molecules. Charged molecules, however, may sometimes penetrate through appendageal shunt pathways. The choice of vehicles used and pH of the formulation can influence the extent of drug ionization. Formulation parameters can be optimized for each drug molecule to control ionization.

FORMULATION FACTORS

Concentration and Dose

An increase in the concentration of a drug in a formulation increases transdermal flux. Concentration gradient across skin is the driving force for passive transdermal delivery; hence, a higher concentration of drug in the donor formulation results in higher transdermal delivery. An increase in drug concentration also improves thermodynamic activity of the drug in the formulation, thereby increasing flux. It is important to note that when comparing transdermal formulations, the permeant should have the same thermodynamic activity in different vehicles. This can be achieved by ensuring the same level of saturation (i.e., drug equivalent to 90% saturation solubility) in different formulations. In this case, the drug concentration in each vehicle may vary, but the thermodynamic activity is the same.

Drug delivery through skin can be carried out using finite or infinite dosing. Finite dosing implies that the drug would be expected to deplete from the formulation/skin surface during the period of permeation. Several marketed topical preparations such as creams or gels contain finite doses of drugs. Infinite dosing, on the other hand, implies a negligible change in concentration or thermodynamic activity of the drug in the formulation during the course of permeation. Infinite dosing may be used to obtain steady-state fluxes in transdermal delivery, and most marketed transdermal patches are designed this way.

pH

The degree of ionization of ionizable compounds can be controlled by pH of the vehicle in which they are dissolved. The pH of the vehicle can be adjusted to obtain an ionization state that can maximize the transdermal flux of the compound. In general, unionized compounds have higher skin permeability as compared with ionized molecules. To determine the degree of ionization of a compound at a certain pH, the Henderson-Hasselbalch equation for weak acids and weak bases may be used. For a weak acid,

$$pH = pKa - \log([HA]/[A^-])$$

where [HA] and [A⁻] are the concentrations of unionized and ionized species, respectively, at that particular pH. For a weak base,

$$pH = pKa - \log([BH^+]/[B])$$

where [BH⁺] and [B] are the concentrations of ionized and unionized species, respectively, at that particular pH.

Buffers may be used to control the degree of ionization. The use of a buffer two to three pH units below the pKa of a weak acid ensures negligible ionization. Similarly, the use of buffer two to three pH units above the pKa of a weak base ensures negligible ionization.

PHYSIOLOGICAL FACTORS

Physiological factors such as body site, race, age, pathological conditions, and skin hydration can also play a role in determining flux of molecules through skin. Different body sites have varying skin thickness, and some parts of the body can be more permeable than others [4]. The most commonly used sites for transdermal delivery are the stomach and abdomen (trunk), arms, and the region behind the ears (postauricular). A pharmacokinetic absorption study carried out on Ortho Evra® contraceptive patch evaluated absorption of norelgestromin and ethinyl estradiol from the abdomen, buttock, outer upper arm, and upper torso. Results from this study indicated that all four body sites delivered therapeutically equivalent amounts of drugs.

Aging of the skin causes a loss in its moisture content. Blood flow to the dermal tissue also decreases with aging. This may cause reduction in permeability of molecules through aged skin. In case of neonates, the stratum corneum is only a few cell layers thick and can be considered as an impaired skin barrier, with higher permeability to drugs. Similarly, many pathological conditions of skin such as eczema or atopic dermatitis result in a compromised skin barrier. Increasing skin hydration (e.g., through occlusive dressings) can also increase skin permeability.

MODELS FOR PERCUTANEOUS ABSORPTION

Several *in vitro* and *in vivo* models have been used to study transdermal permeation of molecules. *In vitro* studies on diffusion cells can be used to estimate transdermal permeation. Human skin samples (e.g., from cadavers or tummy tuck surgery) can be obtained from a tissue bank. *In vitro* drug permeation data across human skin may be variable, however, due to a variety of factors, including thickness at which the skin was sliced/dermatomed. Skin samples may also be obtained from animals for *in vitro* studies. Rodents, such as rats and mice, have thinner skin than humans. Also, these animals have higher levels of lipids in the stratum corneum. Hairless mouse skin loses its integrity much faster than human skin and can possibly overpredict permeation. Certain penetration enhancers may also exhibit greater effects on rodent skin compared with human skin. Guinea pigs have a stratum corneum structure similar to humans, and guinea pig skin can be effectively used as a model for *in vitro* permeation studies. The postauricular skin of guinea pigs lacks hair follicles and sebaceous glands and can be used to study the role of shunt pathways. Snake skin has also been used, but it varies structurally from human skin, in lipid composition and its surface, which is covered with a layer of β-keratin. Mammalian skin models (dogs, monkeys, pigs) have also been investigated for transdermal studies. Porcine ear skin is a widely used *in vitro* skin model and resembles human skin histologically. Permeation of drugs is well predicted using this skin model [12]. Reconstructed human skin membranes or polymeric membranes such as polydimethylsiloxane can be used to compare permeation or release of drugs from different formulations. It should be noted, however, that artificial membranes do not have the complexity of living tissues and may only have limited use (e.g., to compare release from different formulations). *In vivo* permeation studies can be carried out in animal models such as rats, mice, or guinea pigs. *In vivo* studies on human volunteers are the best predictors of transdermal permeability of any drug.

DIFFUSION CELLS

Diffusion cells used for *in vitro* studies can be classified into static diffusion cells or flow-through systems. Static diffusion cells have a simpler design compared with flow-through systems, and a common design is Franz cells (**Figure 12-2**). Franz cells consist of an upper donor compartment separated by a membrane from the lower receptor compartments. The membrane used for the study can be clamped between

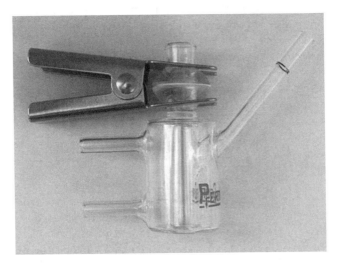

FIGURE 12-2 Vertical Franz diffusion cell. (Reproduced with permission from PermeGear.)

these compartments. For permeation studies, skin has to be mounted on the receptor compartment such that the stratum corneum side of the skin faces the donor. The receptor compartments are jacketed and connected to a water bath, which controls the temperature. Typically, the temperature of receptor is adjusted to 37°C, which results in a temperature of 32°C on the surface of skin. The diffusion area available in Franz cells can vary from 0.5 to 5 cm². Similarly, the volume of the receptor compartments can vary from 2 to 20 mL. The receptor compartments typically have a side arm from which sampling of the receptor fluid can be carried out. The receptor compartments are continuously stirred to maintain homogeneity of receptor solvent. When choosing a receptor solvent, the permeated drug should have sufficient solubility in the receptor so that sink conditions are maintained throughout the duration of the experiment, which help to maintain the concentration gradient. Franz cells can be used to study transdermal permeation from liquid as well as semisolid formulations. A variation of vertical diffusion cells is side-by-side cells where both donor and receptor compartments are continuously stirred. Flow-through diffusion cells can be used to mimic *in vivo* conditions. In this case, the receptor solvent is not stagnant and is continuously in flow. It is easier to maintain sink conditions similar to blood supply using the flow-through assembly because the receptor solvent is constantly replenished. Typical flow rates for receptor solvents in this setting are 1 to 2 mL/h.

TRANSDERMAL PATCHES

Passive transdermal drug delivery systems (TDDSs) consist of medicated adhesive patches that deliver drugs systemically when placed on the skin. A concentration gradient exists between the high concentration of the drug in the patch and the lower concentration in the skin, which serves as a driving force for passive diffusion. The diffusion of drug across the skin follows Fick's first law of diffusion, expressed as [13]:

$$J = \frac{DP\Delta C}{h}$$

where J is the flux, D the diffusion coefficient of the drug molecule, P the partition coefficient of the drug between the patch and the skin, ΔC the concentration gradient across the stratum corneum, and h the thickness of the stratum corneum.

The rate-limiting step can be either the drug release from the system or the absorption into the skin. Ideally, the TDDS should act as the rate-limiting step to ensure drug absorption occurs at a predetermined rate without introducing variability of skin between patients. Once the drug is released from the TDDS to the skin, it slowly diffuses across the stratum corneum, which acts as the rate-limiting barrier. After crossing the stratum corneum, the drug diffuses more rapidly through the remaining epidermis and is then taken up into the systemic circulation by the blood capillaries under the epidermis.

TYPES OF PATCHES

Patches currently on the market can be classified into reservoir, drug-in-adhesive (DIA), or matrix-type systems (**Figure 12-3**). A reservoir system consists of a backing membrane, reservoir, rate-controlling membrane, and adhesive. The reservoir contains either a liquid or semisolid blend of drug and polymer and any chemical permeation

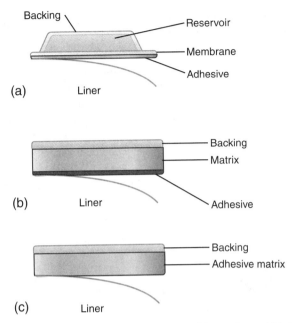

FIGURE 12-3 Types of transdermal patches: (a) reservoir, (b) matrix, and (c) drug-in-adhesive. (Reprinted with permission from Padula C, Nicoli S, Aversa V, et al. Bioadhesive film for dermal and transdermal drug delivery. *Eur J Dermatol.* Jul-Aug 2007;17(4):309-312.)

enhancers. These chemical permeation enhancers act by increasing the solubility of the drug or by disruption of the lipid structure in the skin, resulting in greater percutaneous absorption [14]. Furthermore, occlusion of the contact site with a patch hydrates the skin, subsequently enhancing absorption. The rate-controlling membrane allows the reservoir patch to achieve a true zero-order release profile. Reservoir patches have been marketed for the delivery of fentanyl, testosterone, estradiol, nitroglycerin, and clonidine (**Table 12-1**).

DIA patches consist of a drug dispersed in an adhesive polymer and sandwiched between a backing membrane and release liner. Backing membranes protect the contents of the patch and maintain proper moisture content and flexibility. The release liner temporarily protects the patch during storage and is removed before application. A matrix-type system has drug dispersed in a polymer matrix with the adhesive spread along its circumference. Pressure-sensitive adhesives are used in TDDSs to form a bond with the skin when lightly pressed on by a patient. Appropriate selection of a pressure-sensitive adhesive is critical to the design of a patch. Typically, polymers such as polyiso-butylenes, silicones, and acrylates are used in TDDSs [15]. An aqueous base, however, may sometimes be used, as in the Lidoderm patch. Because percutaneous absorption depends on the partitioning of drug between the patch and the skin, any adhesion failure will have a direct impact on permeation. Therefore, the adhesive must solubilize the drug well, be strong enough to stick to the skin during daily activity, and not cause irritation after removal.

The DIA and matrix-type patches do not provide an exact zero-order release profile because the drug in the upper region of the patch takes slightly longer to diffuse into the skin than the drug in the bottom region of the patch. This difference, however, is small, and a constant serum concentration can still be attained. The newer generation patches

TABLE 12-1 Current transdermal patches on the market

Drug	Brand Name	Manufacturer	Type	Indication	Doses Available
Buprenorphine	Butrans®	Purdue Pharma	Matrix	Continuous relief from moderate to chronic pain in patients	5, 10, and 20 µg/h
Capsaicin	Qutenza®	NeurogesX	DIA	Management of neuropathic pain associated with postherpetic neuralgia	179-mg patch (8% patch for 1 hour application) every 3 months
Clonidine	Catapres-TTS®	Boehringer Ingelheim	Reservoir	Hypertension	0.1, 0.2, and 0.3 mg/day for 7 days
	Clonidine TDS	Par Pharmaceutical	Reservoir		
Diclofenac	Flector®	IBSA Institut Biochem	DIA	Short-term pain like sprains and bruises (nonsteroidal anti-inflammatory drugs)	180-mg patch (1.3%)
Estradiol	Vivelle®/Vivelle-Dot®	Novartis/Novogyne	DIA	Menopause symptoms, postmenopausal osteoporosis associated with lowering of estrogen levels	0.025, 0.0375, 0.05, 0.075, and 0.1 mg/day
	Estraderm®	Novartis	Reservoir		0.05 and 0.1 mg/day
	Climara®	Bayer Healthcare	DIA		0.025, 0.0375, 0.05, 0.06, 0.075, and 0.1 mg/day
	Estradiol	Mylan Tech	DIA		0.025, 0.0375, 0.05, 0.06, 0.075, and 0.1 mg/day
	Alora®	Watson Pharmaceuticals	Matrix		0.025, 0.05, 0.075, and 0.1 mg/day
	Menostar®	Bayer Healthcare	DIA		0.014 mg/day
Estradiol Levonorgestrel	Climara Pro®	Bayer Healthcare	DIA	Menopausal symptoms	0.045 mg/0.015 mg/day (estradiol/levonorgestrel)
Estradiol Norethindrone acetate (NETA)	CombiPatch®	Novartis	DIA	Menopausal symptoms	0.05/0.14 and 0.05/0.25 mg/day (estradiol/NETA)
Ethinyl estradiol Norelgestromin	Ortho Evra®	Ortho-McNeil Janssen	DIA	Contraceptive	0.75/6 mg (ethinyl estradiol/norelgestromin)

Continues

Drug	Brand Name	Manufacturer	Type	Indication	Doses Available
Fentanyl	Duragesic®	Janssen (J&J)	Reservoir	Management of moderate to chronic pain	12.5, 25, 50,75 and 100 µg/h
	Fentanyl Transdermal System	Mylan Tech.	DIA		
Granisetron	Sancuso®	ProStrakan	Matrix	Antinauseant and antiemetic during chemotherapy	3.1 mg/day
Lidocaine	Lidoderm®	Endo Pharm	DIA	Local anesthetic agent	700-mg patch (5%)
Methylphenidate	Daytrana®	Noven Therapeutics	Matrix	Attention deficit hyperactivity disorder	10, 15, 20, and 30 mg/9 hours
Nicotine	Habitrol®	Novartis	Matrix	Smoking cessation	7, 14, and 21 mg/day
	Nicotine Transdermal System	Novartis, Watson Pharmaceuticals, Cardinal Health and Aveva	Matrix		
	Nicoderm CQ®	GSK	DIA		
Nitroglycerin	Transderm-Nitro®	Novartis	Reservoir	Angina pectoris	0.1, 0.2, 0.4, and 0.6 mg/h
	Nitro-Dur®	Schering/Key	DIA		0.1, 0.2, 0.3, 0.4, 0.6, and 0.8 mg/h
	Minitran ™	Graceway Pharmaceuticals	DIA		0.1, 0.2, 0.4, and 0.6 mg
	Nitroglycerin Transdermal System	Mylan Tech. and Noven Therapeutics	DIA		0.1, 0.2, 0.4, and 0.6 mg/h
Oxybutynin	Oxytrol®	Watson Lab.	Matrix	Antispasmodic and anticholinergic	3.9 mg/day
Rivastigmine	Exelon®	Novartis	Matrix	Alzheimer's disease	4.6 and 9.5 mg/day
Selegiline	Emsam®	Dey/Somerset	DIA	Antidepressant	6, 9 and 12 mg
Scopolamine	Transderm-Scop®	Novartis	DIA	Motion sickness	1.0 mg/3 days
Testosterone	Androderm®	Watson	Reservoir	Absence or low levels of endogenous testosterone	2, 2.5, 4, and 5 mg/day

are much thinner and smaller, making them more cosmetically appealing compared with reservoir patches. Commercial patches have been produced for delivery of estradiol, nicotine, and oxybutynin, to name a few (Table 12-1).

A recent TDDS is the Patchless Patch® from Acrux, which consists of an aerosol formulation of drug and chemical enhancers. A Metered Dose Transdermal Spray® applicator is loaded with the aerosol and sprayed at close range onto the skin. The spray forms a nonocclusive layer that is then rapidly absorbed into the deeper layers of the skin. Sprays for estradiol and testosterone have been marketed, whereas those for nicotine, nonsteroidal anti-inflammatory drugs, and contraceptives are in development.

CLINICAL CONSIDERATIONS

TDDSs provide several advantages, such as ease of application, bypass of first-pass metabolism, and prolonged therapeutic effect, which can all lead to greater patient compliance. Several precautions must be taken into consideration, however, when developing or using transdermal patches.

Application Site

Patches should be applied to areas of the skin that are clean, dry, and free of any hair and abrasion. Lotions or creams should not be applied before a patch because the oil reduces adhesion. Patients should be advised to rotate application sites when replacing patches to allow the previous skin site to return to its normal permeability state. In addition, the patch should be applied to the skin where rubbing or accidental removal of the patch is unlikely.

Daily Activities

Because transdermal patches are worn for days to weeks at a time, patients must be advised on how to go about daily activities during treatment. Patients should avoid excess heat because this may enhance percutaneous absorption. Patients should also seek advice from a pharmacist before taking any other medication while wearing the patch.

Removal

A patch must be removed carefully by the patient and folded with the adhesive sides facing together to prevent reuse. The TDDS can then be discarded according to the manufacturer's instructions and in a manner that is safe to others. Finally, patients should wash their hands thoroughly and cleanse the application site to remove any remaining drug.

PRODUCT DEVELOPMENT AND USAGE CONCERNS

Crystallization

Unresolved product development issues or prolonged storage of a patch may lead to formation of crystals. This can significantly reduce the amount of soluble drug available in the patch and therefore decrease drug delivery. UCB Pharma developed a rotigotine (Neupro®) patch for Parkinson's disease [16] that was recalled in 2008 due to crystallization. In 2012, the U.S. Food and Drug Administration (FDA) approved its reformulation and UCB Pharma relaunched the product. Crystallization may be circumvented by incorporating certain additives into the patch that inhibit or solubilize the crystals [17].

Adhesion

Proper adhesion of a transdermal patch is a vital factor that determines the efficacy of the patch. Poor selection of adhesive prevents a patch from uniformly adhering to the skin and thus alters the dose delivered. The Ortho Evra® contraceptive patch must be worn for a period of 7 days. Approximately 5% of users have reported improper adhesion or detachment of the patch before the completion of 7 days, thus interrupting the contraceptive cycle. Sometimes, a nonmedicated adhesive overlay can be used to make the patch stick to the skin; for example, an optional round adhesive cover included in the box can be applied directly over a clonidine patch (Catapres-TTS®) if the patch begins to separate from the skin.

Residual Drug

Because patches incorporate a saturated or near-saturated drug solution to drive diffusion, a large amount of residual drug remains after the therapeutic dose is delivered. Concerns arise for the proper disposal of patches to avoid potential abuse and provide safety to the patient and environment. For example, approximately 7% of estradiol in the Climara Pro® patch is actually delivered into the skin over a period of 7 days; thus, used patches still contain active hormones and must be disposed of with the adhesive side folded together. Recently, the FDA issued a guidance recommending manufacturers to minimize residual drug content and to provide a scientific rationale for amount of residual drug incorporated into a patch.

Skin Irritation

Both the active and inactive ingredients of a TDDS may potentially lead to skin irritation or skin sensitization. Animal models, such as the Draize rabbit test, have been used widely in the past to evaluate product safety. These tests are not always accurate, however, and are discouraged due to the adverse skin reactions that develop in the rabbits. Therefore, the 4-hour human patch test was developed to possibly replace the Draize test. This test was designed to be more reproducible and to avoid severe skin reactions [18]. Since then, other tests have been developed, and the FDA has issued a draft guidance document for skin irritation and sensitization testing of generic transdermal products in human subjects.

QUALITY CONTROL TESTING

Similar to other dosage forms, the FDA requires quality control testing for all transdermal products before they are approved for the market and patient use. Acceptable ranges for these tests are determined during the development stage for each new product. Recently, the U.S. Pharmacopeia (USP) revised a general chapter on the performance testing of topical and transdermal dosage forms. Some of the tests for quality control testing of transdermal patches are described further below.

Adhesion Testing

Peel Adhesion Test

The peel adhesion test determines if a transdermal product will properly adhere to a patient's skin (**Figure 12-4**). Specifically, it measures the force required to remove a patch from a standardized surface. The patch is peeled at a specific angle, and force measurements are recorded.

Release Liner Peel Test

The release liner peel test measures the force required to remove the release liner from an adhesive patch. An ideal release liner should be easily removable by a patient but still adhere firmly during its shelf life.

Rolling Ball Test

The rolling ball test determines how quickly an adhesive can form a bond with another surface (**Figure 12–5**). A ball rolls down a plank placed in front of a patch with the adhesive exposed. The distance the ball travels is measured and is indicative of the tackiness of the adhesive.

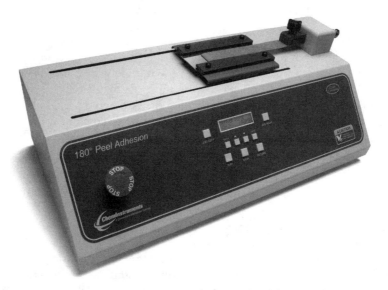

FIGURE 12-4 A 180-degree peel adhesion tester. (Reprinted with permission from Chem Instruments.)

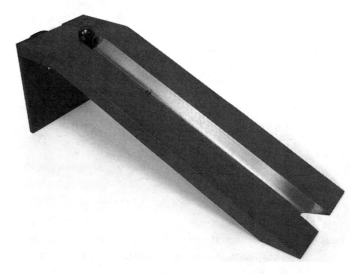

FIGURE 12-5 Rolling ball tester. (Reprinted with permission from Chem Instruments.)

In Vitro *Release Testing*

Dissolution Apparatus

The United States Pharmacopeial Convention (USP) Apparatus 5 is the paddle-over-disk dissolution apparatus used for *in vitro* release testing of transdermal patches. The assembly consists of a vessel, a rotating paddle, and a disk with a mesh screen (**Figure 12-6**). The patch is placed on the disk and held down with a mesh screen. A paddle rotates over the disk, allowing the drug to release uniformly into the vessel. This apparatus is used to determine the release kinetics of various patches *in vitro*. The USP Chapter 711 on dissolution provides guidelines on sampling times and acceptance criteria for conducting performance tests (http://www.usp.org/sites/default/files/usp_pdf/EN/USPNF/2011-02-25711DISSOLUTION.pdf).

EXAMPLES OF TRANSDERMAL DRUG DELIVERY SYSTEMS

The first transdermal patch, approved by the FDA in 1979, was Transderm Scop®, which delivered scopolamine to treat nausea associated with motion sickness. Since that time, numerous patches have come to market with improvements in both technology and design. Table 12-1 describes the design elements of transdermal patches currently on the market, with some key products detailed below.

Fentanyl

Fentanyl is a potent opioid agonist used to treat moderate to severe chronic pain. Duragesic® is a transdermal patch that can deliver fentanyl for up to 72 hours (**Figure 12-7**). It was originally marketed as a reservoir patch but later recalled in 2002 due to manufacturing issues. Breakage in the seal surrounding the patch caused fentanyl to leak out of the reservoir, leading to overdose and sometimes death for several patients. Recently, Duragesic® was redesigned as a DIA patch to avoid leakage problems. Duragesic®

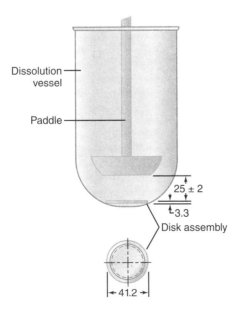

FIGURE 12-6 USP paddle-over-disk Apparatus 5 for dissolution testing of patches. (Copyright 2009 The United States Pharmacopeial Convention. Used by permission.)

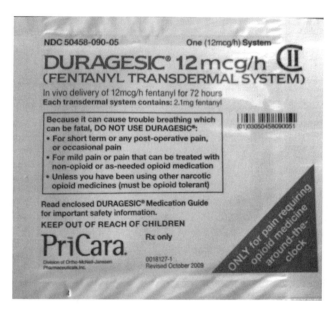

FIGURE 12-7 Duragesic® patch for delivery of fentanyl.

patches on the market range in size from 5.25 to 52 cm² and can provide a dose of 12 to 100 µg/h. Duragesic® forms a depot in the skin after application, and peak fentanyl serum concentration is achieved over 12 to 24 hours.

As a Schedule II controlled substance, fentanyl has a high potential for abuse and can lead to life-threatening conditions if not administered appropriately. Caregivers should advise patients to avoid external sources of heat such as hot baths, electric blankets, and saunas because this may lead to heat-induced increase in fentanyl release from the patch, which has been shown to be fatal [19]. The site of application must be clear of any skin abrasion, and hair may be clipped off rather than shaved off. In addition, if a new patch is to be applied, the site must be rotated. When disposing, the patch should be folded with the adhesive sides together and flushed down the toilet, thereby avoiding any potential abuse.

Nicotine

Nicotine TDDSs are available over the counter and used in smoking cessation. These patches are applied in sequentially smaller doses to reduce nicotine dependence and withdrawal symptoms. Nicoderm CQ® is a 24-hour release DIA patch available in 7-, 14-, and 21-mg strengths. Nicoderm CQ® follows a three-step program: the 21-mg patch is worn during weeks 1 to 6 (step 1), 14 mg during weeks 7 and 8 (step 2), and 7 mg during weeks 8 and 9 (step 3). Other nicotine TDDSs include Nicotrol® and Habitrol®.

Testosterone

Androderm® is a reservoir patch available for testosterone replacement therapy in men. The lower strength patch containing 12.2 mg testosterone has a contact surface area of 37 cm² and delivers 2.5 mg testosterone per day. The higher strength patch containing 24.3 mg testosterone has a contact surface area of 44 cm² and delivers 5 mg testosterone per day. Androderm® is applied to clean, dry, nonscrotal skin around 10:00 p.m. every night to mimic the natural circadian levels of testosterone in healthy men.

Estradiol

Estradiol is a potent form of estrogen used in female hormone replacement therapy as well as treatment for menopause and prevention of postmenopausal osteoporosis. Climara Pro® (Bayer Healthcare) is a DIA patch containing 4.4 mg estradiol and 1.39 mg levonorgestrel. The patch is worn on the lower abdomen, away from the waistline to avoid rubbing, and applied weekly during a 28-day cycle. Climara Pro® has a contact surface area of 22 cm² and delivers 0.045 mg estradiol/0.015 mg levonorgestrel per day. Vivelle-Dot® is another DIA patch available in five strengths ranging from 0.39 mg to 1.56 mg of estradiol content that can deliver at rates of 0.0375 mg/day to 0.1 mg/day, respectively. Vivelle-Dot® patches are smaller and thinner, with sizes of 2.5 cm² to 10.0 cm² available. This is primarily due to the novel DOT Matrix™ technology that uses specific ratios of silicone and acrylate adhesive along with a drug to achieve a controlled release over a smaller surface area. This discrete patch is worn on the lower abdomen and replaced twice weekly in rotating locations.

Contraceptive Hormones

Ortho Evra® is a combination DIA transdermal patch that contains 6 mg norelgestromin and 0.75 mg ethinyl estradiol. Unlike oral birth control pills, which must be taken daily, the Ortho Evra® patch can be worn for 7 days and replaced weekly. The Ortho Evra® patch contains a much higher concentration of active ingredients compared with oral contraceptives to maintain steady-state levels for a period of 7 days. During the application period, norelgestromin achieves a steady state of 1.17 ng/mL and ethinyl estradiol a steady state of 97.4 pg/mL. A large percentage of residual drug remains in the patch after use.

The Ortho Evra® patch has a contact surface area of 20 cm² and is applied to the abdomen, buttock, upper arm, or upper torso. Patients must be advised to strictly adhere to the patch application schedule to protect from accidental pregnancy. Each month the patch is applied on the same day each week for 3 consecutive weeks, followed by a patch-free break during the fourth week.

ACTIVE TECHNIQUES IN TRANSDERMAL DRUG DELIVERY

Macromolecules such as peptides, proteins, and DNA do not passively permeate through the skin. Several physical enhancement techniques have been developed to broaden the range of drug substances that can be delivered transdermally. These active techniques include iontophoresis, sonophoresis, microneedles, radiofrequency ablation, and laser ablation (**Table 12–2**).

IONTOPHORESIS

Iontophoresis is a noninvasive technique that involves the application of a small current to drive charged and neutral drug molecules across the skin. A transdermal iontophoretic system consists of an anode, a cathode, and a current source. A drug solution is placed under an electrode with the same polarity and is driven into the skin via the

TABLE 12-2 Current products/devices on the market and in development using active transdermal techniques[2,27]

Technique	Status	Product/Device	Manufacturer
Iontophoresis	Marketed	Companion 80™	Iomed
		Empi Action Patch™	Empi (St. Paul, MN)
		GlucoWatch® Biographer (discontinued)	Cygnus Inc. (Redwood City, CA)
		Hybresis™	Iomed
		IontoPatch®80, IontoPatch®STAT, IontoPatch®SP	Tapemark® (St. Paul, MN)
		Iontophor® II model 6111PM/DX, Microphor® model 6121	Life Tech Inc. (Stafford, TX)
		LidoSite® (discontinued)	Vyteris (Extension Fair Lawn, NJ)
		Nanoduct®	Wescor Biomedical Systems (Logan, UT)
		Trivarion®, Activadose®II, ActivaPatch®	ActivaTek™ (Salt Lake City, UT)
	Approved	Zecuity™	NuPathe® (Conshohocken, PA)
		Lidocaine IDDS System	Dharma Therapeutics (Seattle, WA)
		IONSYS®	Incline™ Therapeutics (Redwood City, CA)
Sonophoresis	Marketed	SonoPrep® (discontinued)	Echo Therapeutics (formerly Sontra Medical Corporation) (Philadelphia, PA)
Microneedles	Marketed	Dermaroller®	Dermaroller (Carson City, NV)
		Soluvia™ Prefillable Microinjection System	Becton Dickinson (Franklin Lakes, NJ), Sanofi Pasteur (Bridgewater, NJ)
	In Development	Hollow Microstructured Transdermal System (hMTS) and Solid Microstructured Transdermal System (sMTS)	3M (St. Paul, MN)

Continues

TABLE 12-2 Current products/devices on the market and in development using active transdermal techniques[2,27] (*Continued*)

Technique	Status	Product/Device	Manufacturer
		Transdermal Microprojection Delivery System	Zosano Pharma™ (Fremont, CA)
		MicroCor™	Corium (Menlo Park, CA)
		MicroPyramid Technology	NanoPass (Nes Ziona, Israel)
		Micro-Trans™	Valeritas (Bridgewater, NJ)
Radiofrequency ablation	In development	ViaDor™	Syneron (Irvine, CA)
Laser ablation	In development	P.L.E.A.S.E.®	Pantec Biosolutions (Ruggel, Leichtenstein)

Data from Banga AK. *Transdermal and Intradermal Delivery of Therapeutic Agents: Application of Physical Technologies.* Boca Raton, FL: CRC Press; 2011; and Kalluri H, Banga AK. Transdermal delivery of proteins. *AAPS PharmSciTech.* Mar 2011;12(1):431–441.

principle of *like repels like*. Thus, positively charged drugs use anodal delivery, whereas negatively charged drugs use cathodal delivery.

The transport mechanisms of iontophoresis include electromigration, electroosmosis, and passive diffusion. Electromigration is the movement of charged drug ions in response to an electrical field, and electroosmosis is the flow of solvent and neutral species induced by the movement of ions. The skin serves as a cation-permselective membrane at a physiological pH of ~7.4; thus, electroosmotic flow occurs from the anode to cathode [20].

To avoid electrolysis of water and pH shifts during iontophoresis, the use of consumable electrodes is ideal, such as the silver–silver-chloride couple, which contributes to the electrochemistry in the circuit [21]. A buffer may also be used to maintain the pH of a drug formulation; however, this may introduce competing ions and reduce drug delivery. Thus, the salt form of the drug (i.e., fentanyl hydrochloride) is preferred.

One of the key benefits of iontophoresis is the ability to control dose delivery by modulating current. Direct-current iontophoresis is the continuous flow of current from one electrode to the other, allowing continual drug delivery. Pulsed direct current periodically shuts off the current; these "off" phases can be used with varying frequency to further optimize dosing. Finally, alternating-current iontophoresis reverses the flow of current at various time scales. The current intensity and duration must be within the limits to avoid any skin irritation.

SONOPHORESIS

Sonophoresis, also known as phonophoresis, is the application of low-frequency ultrasound (20–100 kHz) to deliver drugs into the skin. Ultrasonic waves are longitudinal in nature and are transmitted through the skin via a fluid medium, such as a gel, cream, or ointment. Unlike iontophoresis, which acts on the drug, sonophoresis acts directly on the skin by enhancing its permeability to drugs. This is primarily achieved through the process of cavitation [22].

Skin tissue contains gaseous cavities that collapse when exposed to sonophoresis. In addition, application of ultrasound creates microbubbles in the coupling medium as well as possibly in the skin. These cavitation bubbles oscillate and collapse, creating shock waves that alter the surrounding skin tissue. This cavitation disrupts the lipid bilayers and forms channel-like pathways through which the drug can permeate.

Sonophoresis is typically used as a pretreatment to permeabilize the skin before drug application. After sonophoresis the skin remains permeable for several hours and then regains its barrier properties. Sonophoresis can also be applied simultaneously with the drug; however, this requires patients to wear an ultrasound device during the treatment period [23].

MICRONEEDLES

Microneedles have received a great deal of industry attention, with numerous products in development. This minimally invasive technique temporarily disrupts the stratum corneum by creating microchannels through which the drug can be delivered. A breach in the stratum corneum allows the drug to enter the pores in the skin and reach systemic circulation via passive diffusion. By penetrating only the epidermal layer of the skin, microneedles avoid nerve endings in the dermis and are virtually pain free. The microchannels formed are hydrophilic in nature due to the surrounding interstitial fluid, thus favoring delivery of hydrophilic molecules.

Microneedles can range from 50 µm up to 1,100 µm in length [2]. The entire length of a microneedle, however, will not fully penetrate due to the elasticity of the skin. To increase dose delivery capabilities, multiple microneedles may be arranged in rows to form arrays. A very large array will lead to the "bed of nails" effect in which the pressure applied to the microneedles evenly distributes, thus reducing its penetration into skin [24].

Various microneedles have been fabricated and differ in type, length, and density. Solid microneedles are composed of metal, polymer, or silicon and are inserted on the skin and removed before application of a drug solution. Coated solid microneedles are first coated with the drug solution and then inserted into the skin. Because of the dense structure of the skin, the entire length of the coated microneedle does not penetrate the skin; therefore, dose delivery may not be reproducible. Dissolving microneedles are made of a dissolvable polymer incorporated with the drug. Once inserted, the polymer dissolves and the drug diffuses into the skin. Both coated and dissolving microneedles are limited to delivering low doses. Hollow microneedles are made of glass or metal and are similar to hypodermic needles but penetrate only the epidermis and avoid nerve endings [25]. Drug solution must be infused at a low flow rate (up to 100 µL/min) to avoid the back pressure associated with compact skin tissue. Given the many microneedle options available, the method of application and incorporation of drug may be tailored depending on the therapeutic concentration desired.

RADIOFREQUENCY ABLATION

Radiofrequency ablation is another minimally invasive technique used to disrupt the barrier properties of the stratum corneum and enhance drug permeation. Microelectrodes are placed on the surface of the skin and an electrical current at high radiofrequency

(~100 kHz) is passed through the upper cell layer. Ions within the cells begin to move in response to the current, generating vibrations and frictional heat and resulting in cell necrosis and ablation. Thereafter, aqueous microchannels are formed within the stratum corneum and epidermis, facilitating drug delivery into systemic circulation [26].

LASER ABLATION

Laser ablation is a similar technique in which a laser is applied on top of the skin. The skin surface is heated and water molecules begin to evaporate, forming microchannels for drug to travel through.

SUMMARY

Transdermal delivery provides a noninvasive convenient means of administering potent drugs into the body and avoids first-pass metabolism. Only small, unionized, moderately lipophilic molecules are able to passively permeate the skin, but the scope of transdermal delivery can be expanded to delivery of hydrophilic molecules by using active transport technologies. Use of transdermal patches leads to high patient compliance because the patch can typically be worn from 1 to 7 days and provides continuous drug input during this time. Patches typically contain a drug dissolved in an adhesive at near-saturation concentration. The drug content of a patch is higher than the dose delivered; therefore, precautions should be taken to avoid intentional misuse or unintended consequences resulting from the high residual drug in patches after use. Also, application of heat should be avoided (e.g., application of heat to a fentanyl patch can result in absorption of toxic quantities of the drug, which can be fatal).

ACKNOWLEDGMENT

We thank Neha Singh for her help in the preparation of this chapter.

REVIEW QUESTIONS

1. What are some of the desired physicochemical properties of a drug that is to be incorporated into a transdermal delivery system?
2. Describe the proper handling and disposal of a transdermal patch.
3. List three counseling points for a patient using a Duragesic® transdermal fentanyl patch.
4. Describe the various active technologies available to enhance transdermal delivery.

REFERENCES

1. Naik A, Kalia YN, Guy RH. Transdermal drug delivery: overcoming the skin's barrier function. *Pharm Sci Technolo Today*. 2000;3(9):318–326.
2. Banga AK. *Transdermal and Intradermal Delivery of Therapeutic Agents: Application of Physical Technologies*. Boca Raton, FL: CRC Press; 2011.
3. Benson HA, Namjoshi S. Proteins and peptides: strategies for delivery to and across the skin. *J Pharm Sci*. 2008;97(9):3591–3610.

4. Williams AC. *Transdermal and Topical Drug Delivery from Theory to Clinical Practice*. London, UK: Pharmaceutical Press; 2004.

5. Walters KA. *Dermatological and Transdermal Formulations*. Informa Healthcare; 2002.

6. Alvarez-Roman R, Naik A, Kalia YN, Guy RH, Fessi H. Skin penetration and distribution of polymeric nanoparticles. *J Control Release*. 2004;99(1):53–62.

7. Cullander C, Guy RH. Sites of iontophoretic current flow into the skin: identification and characterization with the vibrating probe electrode. *J Invest Dermatol*. 1991;97(1):55–64.

8. Mitragotri S. Synergistic effect of enhancers for transdermal drug delivery. *Pharm Res*. 2000; 17(11):1354–1359.

9. Martanto W, Davis SP, Holiday NR, Wang J, Gill HS, Prausnitz MR. Transdermal delivery of insulin using microneedles in vivo. *Pharm Res*. 2004;21(6):947–952.

10. Prausnitz MR, Mitragotri S, Langer R. Current status and future potential of transdermal drug delivery. *Nat Rev Drug Discov*. 2004;3(2):115–124.

11. Benson HAE. Transdermal drug delivery: penetration enhancement techniques. *Curr Drug Deliv*. 2005;2:23–33.

12. Jacobi U, Kaiser M, Toll R, et al. Porcine ear skin: an in vitro model for human skin. *Skin Res Technol*. 2007;13(1):19–24.

13. Hadgraft J. Skin, the final frontier. *Int J Pharm*. 2001;224(1–2):1–18.

14. Kanikkannan N, Kandimalla K, Lamba SS, Singh M. Structure-activity relationship of chemical penetration enhancers in transdermal drug delivery. *Curr Med Chem*. 2000;7(6):593–608.

15. Wokovich AM, Prodduturi S, Doub WH, Hussain AS, Buhse LF. Transdermal drug delivery system (TDDS) adhesion as a critical safety, efficacy and quality attribute. *Eur J Pharm Biopharm*. 2006;64(1):1–8.

16. Chen JJ, Swope DM, Dashtipour K, Lyons KE. Transdermal rotigotine: a clinically innovative dopamine-receptor agonist for the management of Parkinson's disease. *Pharmacotherapy*. 2009;29(12):1452–1467.

17. Jain P, Banga AK. Inhibition of crystallization in drug-in-adhesive-type transdermal patches. *Int J Pharm*. 2010;394(1–2):68–74.

18. Basketter DA, Chamberlain M, Griffiths HA, Rowson M, Whittle E, York M. The classification of skin irritants by human patch test. *Food Chem Toxicol*. 1997;35(8):845–852.

19. Jumbelic MI. Deaths with transdermal fentanyl patches. *Am J Forensic Med Pathol*. 2010;31(1):18–21.

20. Marro D, Guy RH, Delgado-Charro MB. Characterization of the iontophoretic permselectivity properties of human and pig skin. *J Control Release*. 2001;70(1–2):213–217.

21. Gujjar M, Banga AK. Iontophoresis. In: O Heini, ed., *Encyclopedia of Pharmaceutical Science and Technology*, 4 ed. London, UK: Informa Healthcare; 2012.

22. Tang H, Wang CC, Blankschtein D, Langer R. An investigation of the role of cavitation in low-frequency ultrasound-mediated transdermal drug transport. *Pharm Res*. 2002;19(8):1160–1169.

23. Ogura M, Paliwal S, Mitragotri S. Low-frequency sonophoresis: current status and future prospects. *Adv Drug Deliv Rev*. 30 2008;60(10):1218–1223.

24. Verbaan FJ, Bal SM, van den Berg DJ, et al. Improved piercing of microneedle arrays in dermatomed human skin by an impact insertion method. *J Control Release*. 2008;128(1):80–88.

25. Prausnitz MR. Microneedles for transdermal drug delivery. *Adv Drug Deliv Rev*. 2004;56(5):581–587.

26. Sintov AC, Krymberk I, Daniel D, Hannan T, Sohn Z, Levin G. Radiofrequency-driven skin microchanneling as a new way for electrically assisted transdermal delivery of hydrophilic drugs. *J Control Release*. 2003;89(2):311–320.

27. Kalluri H, Banga AK. Transdermal delivery of proteins. *AAPS PharmSciTech*. 2011;12(1):431–441.

CHAPTER 13

PULMONARY AND NASAL DRUG DELIVERY

Nilesh Gupta, Brijeshkumar Patel, and Fakhrul Ahsan

CHAPTER OBJECTIVES

Upon completing this chapter, the reader should be able to

Review the anatomy and physiology of the respiratory system that governs drug delivery via the nasal and pulmonary routes.

- ▸ Learn the pharmaceutical and physiological factors that may affect drug deposition and absorption upon nasal and pulmonary administration.
- ▸ Know the drug formulations used for nasal and pulmonary administration.
- ▸ Be familiar with various devices used to administer drug formulations via the respiratory route.
- ▸ Know and recognize the differences among different types of nebulizers, metered dose and dry powder inhalers.
- ▸ Be knowledgeable with the recent advancement in nebulizers, metered dose and dry powder inhalers.
- ▸ Be acquainted with various spacer devices and their proper usage.

▸ Know the advantages and disadvantages of various respiratory drug delivery devices and formulations.

▸ Learn patient counseling points for inhalational devices and drug products.

CHAPTER OUTLINE

INTRODUCTION

The nose and lungs have long been used for administration of drugs for the treatment of various diseases of the respiratory system. Drug administration via nasal and oral inhalation is also collectively called the respiratory route of administration. This route has been used for administration of recreational agents since the time of ancient civilization. Over the past century, nasal and pulmonary routes have been used for delivery of drugs for the treatment of diseases that are localized in the nose and lungs such as allergic rhinitis and asthma. Over the past several decades, however, the respiratory route has been extensively studied for administration of therapeutic agents that produce systemic effects [1].

The respiratory route of drug administration offers several advantages over other routes of drug administration. This route is noninvasive and provides rapid onset of action. It reduces the total amount of drug required and hence reduces systemic side effects. It avoids first-pass metabolism and has the ability to produce both systemic and local effects. This is an environment-friendly route because it avoids disposal of

TABLE 13-1 Advantages and disadvantages of pulmonary and nasal routes of drug administration

Route	Advantages	Disadvantages
Pulmonary	Extensive surface area with rich blood supply available for drug absorption Rapid onset of action Avoidance of first pass metabolism of drug and hence reduced drug degradation Non-invasive and drugs can be self administered Can be used for both local and systemic drug delivery Reduced dose required than any other routes for the intended effect Fewer systemic side effects Enhanced patient compliant Environment friendly as no need of disposal of syringes and needles	Cost of device Complex engineering to develop devices Dose inaccuracy Not suitable for long term use Local side effects due to oropharyngeal deposition Not suitable for drugs that do not get absorbed via the pulmonary route Efficacy is limited by mucociliary clearance Lung barriers must be overcome for efficient deposition
Nasal	An alternative to parenteral route Rich vasculature and highly permeable structure Circumvents first pass metabolism Non-invasive and easily accessible route Large surface area available for drug absorption Improved patient compliance Environment friendly Can be used for systemic drug delivery Rapid onset of action Reduced risk of overdose	Not suitable for lipophilic and large molecular weight drugs Inaccuracy of dose Cost of device Performance affected in disease conditions Mucociliary clearance limits drug retention Nasal irritation Not feasible for administration of large dose

Data from Taylor G, Kellaway I. *Pulmonary Drug Delivery*. Boca Raton, FL: CRC Press. 2001:269-300; Lansley AB, Martin GP. *Nasal Drug Delivery*. Boca Raton, FL: CRC Press. 2001:237–268

needles and syringes and multiple dosing is possible without assistance from health care professionals [2]. However, one of the major limitations of this route is dose inaccuracy and dose-to-dose variability. Furthermore, many drugs do not get absorbed after delivery via the nasal or pulmonary route and exhibit premature deposition at oropharyngeal site that lead to local side effects. Some drugs may undergo enzymatic degradation in the nose and lungs or are quickly removed from the respiratory tract by mucociliary clearance mechanisms [3]. Comparative features of both routes are summarized in Table 13-1.

To understand the devices and formulations used to administer drugs via the respiratory routes, we should first know the key anatomical and physiological features of the respiratory system. Thus, below we briefly discuss the anatomy and physiology of the respiratory system.

ANATOMY AND PHYSIOLOGY OF THE RESPIRATORY SYSTEM

The respiratory tract starts at the nose and ends at the alveolar sac in the lung. In terms of anatomy, the respiratory tract is divided into three regions: nasopharyngeal, tracheobronchial, and alveolar (Figure 13-1a,b,c,d). The nasopharyngeal region is

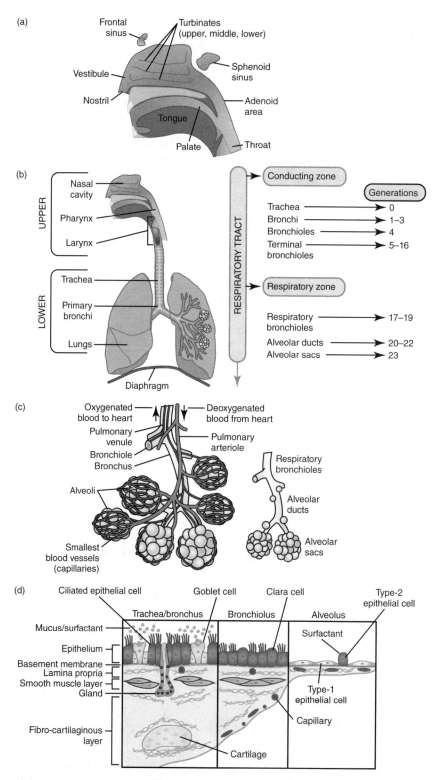

FIGURE 13-1 The human respiratory system depicting (a) the nose, (b) the lungs, (c) the alveolar region along with the vasculature, and (d) histology and cellular distribution in the airway wall.

also called the upper airways, which include airways from the nose to the larynx. The nose facilitates warming, humidifying, and filtering of inhaled air [4]. In fact, the nasal cavity functions as an air conditioner and an organ of smell. The nasal cavity, which is ~12 to 14 cm long, extends from the nostril to nasopharynx. The nostrils are guarded by hair that prevents entry of dust particles and insects. The forward section of the nasal cavity is called the vestibule. The floor of the nose and the roof of the mouth are formed by hard palatine bone, called the palate. The soft palate, which extends back to the nasopharynx, prevents lodging of food at the back of the nose. Three thin elevations are found just behind the vestibule and are called nasal conchae or turbinates (Figure 13-1a).

Although we can breathe through the mouth and nose, air inspired through the mouth is not humidified, heated, or filtered to the same extent as the air breathed through the nose. The olfactory region of the nose is located toward the roof of the nasal cavity and lined with nonciliated neuroepithelium. The large cross-sectional area and relatively low air velocity make the nasal cavity an ideal site for particle deposition [5]. The lining of the vestibule changes from skin to squamous epithelium and later to ciliated columnar secretory epithelium at the turbinates. The posterior region of the nasal cavity is covered with the epithelium, which is collectively known as the respiratory epithelium and consists of multiple types of cells. Goblet cells, scattered in the epithelium, are responsible for mucous secretion, whereas tall pseudo-stratified ciliated columnar epithelial cells contain densely packed apical cilia and are responsible for movement of the mucus. Other cells present in the posterior epithelium of nasal cavity are basal cells, present on basal membrane that serve as reserves for ciliated epithelial or goblet cells, and columnar brush cells with surface microvilli, rather than cilia, that function as sensory receptors.

The tracheobronchial region, also known as the central or conducting airways, starts at the larynx and terminates at the terminal bronchioles (Figure 13-1b). Trachea, bronchi, and bronchioles are present in this region. The alveolar region is also called respiratory airways, peripheral airways, or pulmonary region. This region is composed of the respiratory bronchioles, alveolar ducts, and alveoli (Figure 13-1c). Each branch of the trachea produces a new generation of airways; on average, two daughter branches are generated from one parent branch. Although the cross-sectional area of a single daughter branch is smaller than its parent branch, the sum of the cross-sectional area of two daughter branches is larger than their parents'. The cross-sectional area increases with the increase in distance from the mouth, which resembles the structure of a trumpet. Similarly, the surface area of airways increases with increasing generation as well as with increasing distance of the airway from the glottis. The diameter of airways decreases, however, with the increasing generation of airways [6].

The histology of the respiratory tract varies from the upper to the lower respiratory tract. The conducting airways (Figure 13-1d), starting from the trachea to bronchioles, are composed of three layers: mucosa, submucosa, and adventitia. The mucosa serves as the respiratory epithelium that is composed of pseudo-stratified, ciliated, and columnar epithelial cells. The layer below the epithelial lining, called lamina propria, is made of loose connective and lymphoid tissue and a dense layer of elastic fibers. Submucosa containing bronchial glands, elastic tissue, and cartilage is located below the lamina propria. The adventitia is composed of connective tissue that covers the airways and is supplied with arteries, veins, nerves, and lymph vessels. The cells and thickness of the respiratory tract undergo significant changes as it progresses from the conducting to respiratory airways [7].

Respiratory bronchioles and alveoli make up the respiratory zones. The respiratory bronchioles are 0.4 mm in diameter and composed of flattened squamous epithelia and a thin layer of connective tissue. Gas exchange occurs in the alveolar region, and the alveolar walls are covered with very flat squamous epithelia called typeI pneumocytes that line about 93% of the alveolar surface. On the alveolar surface, there are also cuboidal epithelial cells with microvilli called type II pneumocytes (Figure 13-1d) that constitute 7% of the alveolar surface. An important function of type II epithelial cells is to secrete lung surfactants, which mainly contain phosphatidylcholine [8]. Lung surfactants reduce surface tension and help prevent collapse of alveoli. Epithelial cells in the tracheobronchial region are almost completely covered with hair-like projections called cilia. Ciliary movement occurs in an organized manner to propel mucus along with entrapped particulate matter through airways to the throat. An important type of cells, called alveolar macrophages, reside in the alveolar region and are mainly involved in phagocytic functions to scavenge inhaled particles and subsequently transport them to the lymph nodes [6].

DRUG DELIVERY VIA THE PULMONARY ROUTE

FATE OF INHALED PARTICLES·

For administration of drugs via the respiratory route, formulations are required to be aerosolized as solid particles or liquid droplets. Aerosolized particles, administered either via oral or nasal inhalation, have to undergo a series of aerodynamic maneuvers such as changes in airflow and direction, and pass through a number of airway bifurcations and barriers before deposition in a specific region in the lungs. After deposition of particles in the nose or lungs, the drug must overcome a number of barriers before producing its pharmacological effect [9]. The undissolved particles may be cleared by the mucociliary clearance mechanism or phagocytosed by macrophages. Particles must undergo dissolution for absorption to occur. Some drugs may even undergo enzymatic degradation before they exert their pharmacological effects [10]. The fate of inhaled particles is summarized in **Figure 13-2**.

FACTORS AFFECTING PARTICLE DEPOSITION IN THE LUNGS

A number of factors, such as respiratory anatomy and physiology, formulations, and devices, may influence the deposition patterns and absorption of drugs after pulmonary administration. Formulation aspects include particle size, particle density, and type of aerosolized particles such as nebulized solutions, dry powder, and propellant-based formulations. Intended pharmacological effect may be influenced by the target disease, which may be local or systemic in origin. Physiological and pathological conditions of the lungs and drug absorption kinetics can influence the drug delivery. Because drugs arc delivered as droplets or particles, devices used to deliver drugs to the respiratory tract can have a major influence on the deposition of the particles. Drugs delivered as droplet or particles must be deposited in an appropriate lung region in sufficient quantity to produce pharmacological effects [3, 6]. Deposition of the inhaled particles is affected by several factors, categorized into physiological and pharmaceutical factors (**Table 13-2**).

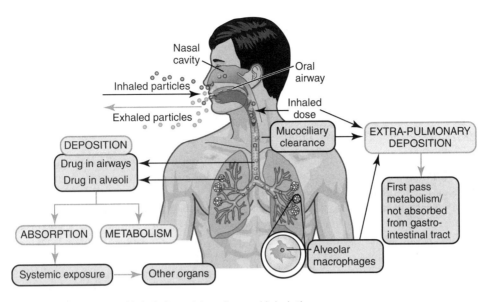

FIGURE 13-2 The fate of inhaled particles after oral inhalation.

TABLE 13-2 Factors affecting drug deposition in the lungs	
Physiological	**Pharmaceutical**
Breathing pattern	Velocity of aerosol particles
Vasculature	Aerosol properties (size, density, shape,
Lung anatomy	charge)
Mucociliary clearance	Deposition pattern
Alveolar clearance	Drug properties (solubility, lipophilicity,
Endothelial and epithelial permeability	molecular weight, stability)
Enzymatic/metabolic activity	Dose size/volume
Disease conditions	Physical stability
Coordination of aerosol generation and	Enzymatic/chemical stability
inspiration	Nature of device

Data from Yu J, Chien YW. Pulmonary drug delivery: physiologic and mechanistic aspects. *Crit Rev Ther Drug Carrier Syst.* 1997;14:395–453; Suarez S, Hickey AJ. Drug properties affecting aerosol behavior. *Respir Care.* 2000;45:652–666.

Physiological Factors

Several physiological factors, summarized in Table 13-2 and expounded on below, may affect drug deposition and consequently absorption of drugs administered via the respiratory route [2,10].

Lung Anatomy

The probability of deposition by impaction increases in each bifurcation. A decrease in airway diameter reduces the distance for particles to come in contact with the surface. A particle has to pass through a series of branching tubes with decreasing diameter and constantly change direction of flow to remain airborne. Therefore, anything that affects particle velocity or normal anatomical features of the lungs will affect particle deposition.

Route of Particle Inhalation

If an aerosol is inhaled via the nose, most particles are deposited in the nose and pharynx. For pulmonary delivery, aerosols are administered via the mouth. A formulation intended for nasal delivery should not be administered via mouth inhalation. Nasal delivery devices such as spray pumps produce larger droplets that cannot travel through the nasopharyngeal tract for efficient deposition in the lungs.

Inspiratory Flow Rate and Tidal Volume

Deposition of particles in the lungs is significantly influenced by the inspiratory flow rate (IFR); hence, patients need to adjust the IFR depending on the drug delivery device to achieve maximal drug deposition. For example, pressurized metered dose inhalers (pMDIs) are devices that use propellants to generate aerosols, and an increase in IFR will increase particle momentum and turbulence and, consequently, impaction in the proximal tracheobronchial region will increase. Hence, a slow inhalation flow rate is favored because it allows aerosolized particles to penetrate more readily to the site of action in the small peripheral airways. The effect of IFR, however, is more important for devices that require the use of energy of inspiration to generate aerosols such as dry powder inhalers (DPIs). An increase in IFR results in particles of smaller size and increase in the volume of inhaled air in a single breath, the tidal volume. Enhanced tidal volume produces greater penetration of aerosol particles into the tracheobronchial and alveolar regions.

Coordination of Aerosol Generation and Inspiration

For pMDIs, the momentum (objects mass × velocity) of aerosol particles generated depends on the device rather than the patient's IFR. The velocity of pMDI-generated particles is about 2500 to 3000 cm s^{-1}. A failure in syncing between firing of pMDI and inspiration may result in enhanced oropharyngeal deposition and reduced entry into the deep lung [2].

Breath-Holding

Breath-holding plays an important role for deposition of drugs in the respiratory tract. The time for sedimentation of particles can be extended by prolonging the interval between inspiration and exhalation. Thus, for efficient deposition, breath-holding for a period of 5 to 10 seconds after inspiration is recommended.

Disease States

The penetration and deposition of inhaled particles in the lungs and drug absorption is affected by the severity of pulmonary diseases. Bronchoconstriction and obstruction of airways may cause the airflow to divert to unobstructed airways. Narrowing of airways by mucus, inflammation, or bronchial constriction can increase linear velocities, enhance inertial deposition, and produce more deposition in the central airways [10].

Pharmaceutical Factors

Several pharmaceutical factors, summarized in Table 13-2 and explained below, may affect the deposition of particles in the airways [3, 11, 12].

Aerosol Velocity

Aerosol velocity plays an important role for efficient administration of drug using pMDIs. If aerosol droplet velocity is greater than the IFR, the aerosol droplet is likely to deposit in the oropharyngeal region. Further, the aerosol produced by nebulizers and DPIs are carried by the inhaled air, and thus the aerosol velocity for nebulizers and DPIs is controlled by the IFR.

Size, Shape, and Density of Inhaled Particles

The inhalation potential of aerosolized particles depends on a parameter called mass median aerodynamic diameter (MMAD), which is defined as the diameter of a sphere of unit density that has the same settling velocity in air as the aerosol particle in question. Because most inhalation formulations are heterodispersed, it is required by the regulatory agencies to report the MMAD, which is determined by using a piece of equipment that simulates the respiratory tract, called the cascade impactor (Figure 13-3a). For determination of MMAD, dry powder formulations are fired into the impactor using a DPI device usually at a flow rate of 28.3 L/min. The amount of particles deposited on each stage is determined and percent cumulative amount of particles deposited is plotted against an effective cut-off diameter (µm) of each stage on a semi-log graph paper to obtain the MMAD of the particles [13]. Theoretical MMAD can also be calculated from particle density and geometric diameter using the following equation:

$$MMADt = d\left[\frac{\rho}{\rho_o \cdot X}\right]^{\frac{1}{2}}$$

where d is the geometric mean diameter obtained from particle size analysis, ρ is the tapped density of inhaled particles, ρ_o is the reference density of 1 g/cm^3, and X is the shape factor, which is assumed to be 1 for spherical particles. Most micronized particles for inhalation have particle densities around 1 g/cm^3.

Physical Stability

Particles from aerosols and dry powders may interact with each other because of mutual attraction or repulsion. Particle size may also change due to hygroscopicity and solvent evaporation. For example, if particles generated from a DPI are hygroscopic, the size of such particles may increase due to absorption of moisture during their passage through the humid respiratory tract. Such an increase in size may lead to premature deposition of the drug in the lungs. Conversely, droplets size from MDIs may decrease due to solvent evaporation. During formulation, careful evaluation should be performed to avoid any changes in the particle size [12].

PARTICLE SIZE AND RESPIRABILITY

Because of the influence of various physical forces, deposition of particles is significantly affected by the particles size. The extent of deposition of inhaled particles depends on the site of deposition and size, density, and velocity of particles. As shown in Figure 13-3b, particles get deposited in different regions of the respiratory system as a function of their size. Particles that are deposited in the respiratory tract range from 1 to 10 µm. The respirable fraction is the percentage of an inhaled formulation that penetrates into the alveolar region of the lungs (10 µm). Fine particle fraction is the percentage of inhaled particles below the particle size of 5 µm. Particles larger than 5 µm impact the upper airways and are rapidly removed by coughing, swallowing, and mucociliary processes. Inhaled particles between 5 and 10 µm diameters are deposited on the tracheobronchial surface by impaction. Particles between 0.5 and 5 µm are deposited in the alveolar levels by impaction and sedimentation. About 50% of 0.5-µm particles are deposited in the alveoli by diffusion, and the rest are exhaled or may not deposit at all. Recent advancements in

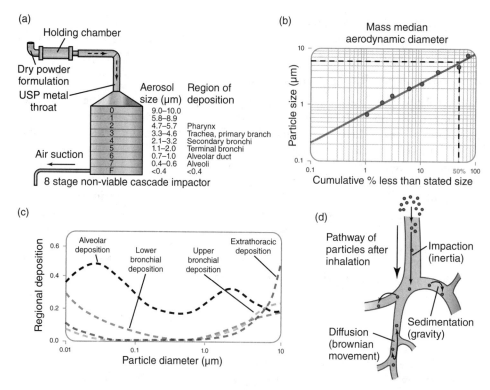

FIGURE 13-3 (a) Schematic representation of multistage Anderson cascade impactor simulating the human respiratory system. Inset demonstrates the graphical method to calculate mass median aerodynamic diameter using the cascade impactor. (b) Deposition of particles in different regions of the respiratory system as a function of particle size. (c) Three principal mechanisms by which particles deposit on the respiratory tract after inhalation.

particle technology have shown that large porous particles with a physical diameter of 20 µm and density of 0.4 g/cm³ also deposit in the lungs. Overall, inhaled particles with unit density and diameter of 1 to 5 µm exhibit efficient penetration into the lungs.

MECHANISMS INVOLVED IN DEPOSITION OF INHALED PARTICLES

As discussed above, the deposition of particles from an inhaler into the respiratory tract involves a complex interplay between particles' physical properties and the anatomy of the respiratory system. Depending on particles' aerodynamic properties and site of deposition, inhaled particles are deposited into the respiratory tract by three major mechanisms: inertial impaction, sedimentation, and diffusion [14–16]. These mechanisms are discussed below and depicted in **Figure 13-3c**.

Inertial Impaction

Particles greater than 5 µm in diameter are deposited in the respiratory tract by inertial impaction. Upon inspiration, the air changes its velocity and direction of flow throughout its passage along the respiratory tract. Larger particles or particles with higher velocity may not be able to travel in the same direction as the air stream. As a result, larger particles change their direction of flow at the airway bifurcation and consequently impact on the airways as shown in Figure 13-3c. Inertial impaction increases where airways are partially obstructed at higher airflows and by a turbulent flow in the trachea and major bronchi. Increases in particle velocity, diameter, and density can also increase deposition by inertial impaction. Because this mechanism is a velocity-dependent phenomenon, inertial deposition of particles occurs in larger airways with the highest velocity of air.

Sedimentation

Sedimentation occurs when particles fall on the surface of the respiratory tract because of the effect of gravity (Figure 13-3c). The rate of sedimentation is proportional to the square of the particle diameter and varies with the time and density of particles. Particles are deposited by sedimentation in the airways where air velocity is relatively low. Because it is a time dependent phenomenon, sedimentation occurs mainly in the regions of maximum residence time of the tidal air such as small airways and lung periphery.

Diffusion

Aerosol particles that are smaller than 0.1 μm, called ultrafine particles, are deposited by diffusion. These particles collide with gas molecules and thus change their kinetic energy, direction of motion, and move randomly on the air (Figure 13-3c). This type of deposition increases with time but decreases with decreased particle diameter. Deposition for ultrafine particles is independent of the density of the particles. Particles undergo deposition by diffusion in small airways and lung periphery.

PARTICLE CLEARANCE AND DRUG ABSORPTION FROM THE LUNGS

Drugs administered via the respiratory route have to overcome many barriers before drug absorption can occur. The three most important barriers are the mucous barrier, mucociliary clearance, and alveolar clearance. Mucus is the first barrier a drug encounters before it reaches its site of action. Drug particles in DPIs first dissolve in the mucous layer, which contains 90% to 95% water. For poorly water-soluble drugs, dissolution in the mucus may be the rate-limiting step for absorption. Highly water-soluble drugs may dissolve at the very high relative humidity in the airways. Water-soluble drugs diffuse through the mucous layer and enter the epithelium. The rate of diffusion through the mucus depends on the thickness of the mucous layer, molecular weight of the drug, and interaction between drug and mucus (i.e., binding of positively charged drugs with mucous glycoprotein). Mucocilliary clearance is a self-cleansing mechanism of the respiratory system by which the respiratory system eliminates fluid, bacteria, and particulate matter from the respiratory tract. This cleansing mechanism is the result of a close coordination among ciliary function, airway surface fluid, and mucin secretion. Particles and dissolved drug entrapped in the mucus are removed from the respiratory tract via mucociliary clearance within a few hours after deposition. Particles deposited in the alveolar region are engulfed by macrophages and are then eliminated via the lymphatic system or absorbed into the pulmonary circulation [6, 16].

The absorption of systematically active drugs is influenced by the surface area, blood supply, thickness of air–blood barriers, and permeability of the drug across the alveolar epithelium. The surface area of the airways is about 140 m², slightly larger than the small intestine. An aerosol can rapidly deliver a drug to this huge area compared with orally administered drugs, which will be delayed because of gastric emptying [17]. The thickness of the absorption barrier of the lung is much smaller compared with other routes. In the alveolar region, the thickness of absorption barrier membrane is about 0.5 μm, and hence this region makes a major contribution to the drug absorption. The lungs receive 100% of the cardiac output via a network of capillaries. The rich supply of blood facilitates drug absorption. Drugs absorbed via the lungs go directly to the heart, bypassing first-pass metabolism [18]. **Table 13-3** lists some locally and systemically active commercially available drugs administered via the nasal and pulmonary routes.

DEVICES FOR PULMONARY DRUG DELIVERY

Respiratory drug delivery systems can be used to produce local and systemic effects. Several medications such as antiallergy agents (azelastin, nedocromil), β-receptor agonists, steroids, prostaglandin analogues (iloprost), and mucolytics (n-acetyl-cysteine) can be delivered via the respiratory route for local effects. Insulin, nasal flu vaccine, calcitonin, morphine, anesthetic agents, and genetic materials have been investigated for pulmonary administration to produce systemic effects. Many other drugs are now under investigation for systemic delivery via the lungs, including low-molecular-weight

TABLE 13-3 Pulmonary and nasal drugs and devices on the market

Route	Drug	Trade name	Device type	Manufacturer
Pulmonary	Iloprost	Ventavis	Nebulizer	CoTherix, CA
	Formoterol	Foradil	DPI	Novartis,
	Mometasone	Asmanex	DPI	Switzerland
	Albuterol/	Combivent	SMI	Merck, NJ
	Ipratropium	Respimat	pMDI	BI, Germany
	Beclamethasone	QVAR	pMDI	Teva, Israel
	Fluticasone	Flovent	Nebulizer	GSK, UK
	Arformoterol	Brovana	Nebulizer	Sunovion, Japan
	Aztreonam	Cayston	DPI	Gilead, CA
	Tobramycin	TIP	Nebulizer	Novartis,
	Treprostinil	Tyvasco	DPI	Switzerland
	Insulin	Exubera		UT, MD
				Pfizer/Nektar, NY
Nasal	Sumatriptan	Optinose	Insufflator	OptiNose, PA
	Budesonide	Rhinocort	Inhaler	AstraZeneca,
	Dexamethasone	Erizas	Inhaler	Sweden
	Ketorolac	Sprix	Spray pump	Nippon-Shinyaku,
	Calcitonin	Miacalcin	Spray pump	Japan
	Oxytocin	Syntocinon	Spray pump	Luitpold, NY
	Desmopressin	Minirin	Drops	Novartis,
				Switzerland
				Defiante, Portugal
				Ferring, Sweden

DPI, dry powder inhaler; SMI, soft mist sprays; pMDI, pressurized or propellant driven metered dose inhaler; BI, Boehringer Ingelheim; GSK, GlaxoSmithKline; UT, United Therapeutics.

Data from van Drooge DJ, Hinrichs WL, Dickhoff BH, et al. Spray freeze drying to produce a stable Delta(9)-tetrahydrocannabinol containing inulin-based solid dispersion powder suitable for inhalation. *Eur J Pharm Sci.* 2005;26:231–240; Hickey AJ. Back to the future: Inhaled drug products. *J Pharm Sci.* 2013;102:1165–1172.

heparins [3]. Most currently available pulmonary drug delivery systems are concerned with drugs with local effects. As discussed above, for delivery of drugs to the lungs, an aerosol must be generated for inhalation. Devices that are commonly used to administer drugs to the lungs are nebulizers, pMDIs, and DPIs [19]. Table 13-4 summarizes the advantages and disadvantages of three commonly used devices.

Nebulizers

As a device, nebulizers transform solutions or suspensions containing drugs into aerosols that can be taken by inspiration. Solutions for nebulization are available for administration as unit doses or concentrated solutions for administration after dilution. From a design perspective, nebulizers are specialized atomizers that allow recycling of drug solution. In some nebulizers, flat plates or baffles are used to direct larger droplets toward the container. Importantly, baffles facilitate optimal size distribution of droplets for deposition of drugs in the deep lung. Based on the mechanisms of aerosol

TABLE 13-4 Comparative advantages and disadvantages of pulmonary drug delivery devices

Device type	Advantages	Disadvantages
Nebulizers	No patient coordination or specific inhalation technique required Suitable for all types of patients (children <4 years, physically challenged etc.) Variation in dose possible Potential of delivering combination of drugs Suitable in emergency like conditions Compatible with most of the drug solutions Effective with tidal breathing No release of hazardous chlorofluorocarbons Possibility as supplement of oxygen Newer technologies such as ultrasonic, static and vibrating mesh are more compact, silent and effective	Requirement of pressurized gas or electrical source Not cost effective Lack of portability Easy chances of contamination Treatment time lengthy Regular maintenance required Impreciseness in dosing Drug wastage due to drug degradation andequipment temperature rise (ultrasonic) Cumbersome in handling Not suitable for suspensions Variation in performance due to differences in operating conditions
Metered dose inhalers	Inexpensive, compact and portable Suitable for multidose regimens No wastage of drug due to degradation Reproducible performance Suitable for most drug substances Short treatment time Suitable for emergency situations No chances of contamination No requirement of drug preparation	Requirement of patient coordination and actuation Spacer necessary for children <6 years Remaining doses can not be controlled Necessary use of propellants by many devices High oropharyngeal deposition without spacer Not available for all medicinal substances Maximum 5 mg dose can be administered Possible device abuse
Dry powder inhalers	Less patient coordination required Small, portable and easy to use Actuated by breath Short treatment time Suitable for most drug substances Propellants not required	Not suitable for children <4 years Possible oropharyngeal deposition Not recommended in emergency situations Partly sensitive to humid environment Requirment of moderate to high inspiratory flow Loss of dose due to exhalation into device

Data from Dolovich MB, Dhand R. Aerosol drug delivery: developments in device design and clinical use. *Lancet.* 2011;377:1032–1045.

generations, nebulizers are classified into two major categories: air-jet and ultrasonic nebulizers [20].

Air-Jet Nebulizers: High Velocity Airstream Dispersion

This type of nebulizers uses a pressurized jet air stream delivered by a compressor that enters via a narrow tube that is forced through a constricted opening called the Venturi. The jet stream causes a pressure drop near the Venturi. The Venturi effect, named after Italian physicist Giovanni Battista Venturi, describes the phenomenon that fluid speed increases when the fluid is forced through a narrow or restricted area. The increased speed results in a reduction in pressure, which creates a vacuum effect and causes liquid drug in the reservoir to be sucked up through the liquid feeding tube. The jet stream strikes the rising liquid and breaks up into droplets of various sizes. Large droplets return to the drug holding cup or are bounced back by baffles. The air stream pushes droplets out of the nebulizer as a cloud that is taken by patients by inhalation. Air-jet nebulizers are further classified into three categories based on the output during inhalation (**Figure 13-4a**):

- **Standard unvented nebulizers** or constant output nebulizers deliver drugs during both inhalation and exhalation phases (Figure 13-4a, 1). In this type of device, an air compressor is used to continuously convert drug solution into aerosols.
- **Breath-enhanced vented nebulizers** produce a larger amount of aerosols during the inhalation phase but a reduced amount during exhalation. This device produces medicated droplets at an expedited rate during inhalation compared with unvented nebulizers (Figure 13-4a, 2).
- **Dosimetric nebulizers** produce aerosols during the inhalation phase. These nebulizers produce medicated clouds only during inhalation (Figure 13-4a, 3).

Ultrasonic Nebulizers: Ultrasonic Energy Dispersion

Ultrasonic nebulizers use a transducer of piezo-electric crystal to produce high frequency sound waves in the nebulizer solution. By traveling through the liquid, the sound wave pushes the liquid upward and thus converts the drug solution into a small fountain. Off the surface of this fountain, small particles begin to float above the liquid and appear like smoke (Figure 13-4b). The two types of ultrasonic nebulizers are **standard ultrasonic nebulizers and ultrasonic nebulizers with water interface.** In standard ultrasonic nebulizers, the drug is in direct contact with the piezo-electric transducer. This type of contact, however, increases the temperature of the drug solution, and hence this device is not recommended for thermolabile drugs. In case of ultrasonic nebulizers with water interface, a certain volume of water is used between the piezo-electric transducer and a separate drug-holding chamber. The water reduces the temperature of drug solution that tends to increase due to ultrasound.

Newer Nebulizers

Air-jet and ultrasonic nebulizers produce aerosols at a constant rate regardless of a patient's breathing phase (i.e., during exhalation, inhalation, and breath-holding). This results in huge wastage of drugs: Two-thirds of drugs are lost due to uncontrolled production of aerosol during exhalation and breath-holding. Further, with air-jet

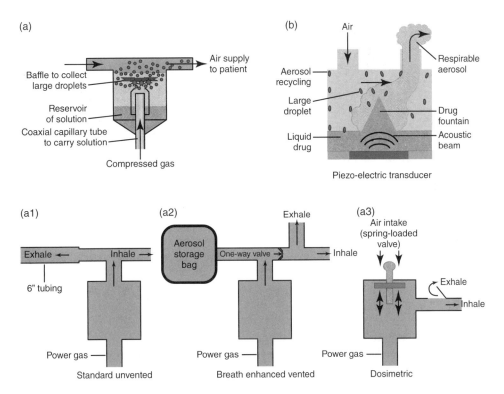

FIGURE 13-4 Different types of nebulizers in use: (a) air-jet and (b) ultrasonic nebulizers. Classification of air jet nebulizers: (a1) standard unvented, (a2) breath enhanced, and (a3) dosimetric nebulizers.

nebulizers, increase in drug concentration and crystallization of drugs may occur due to cooling of the reservoir solution and evaporation of solvents. Increase in drug concentration may result in inaccurate dosage, and subsequent crystallization may obstruct the device or produce aerosol droplets of variable size. On the other hand, with ultrasonic nebulizers, increase in solution temperature may lead to decrease in aerosol MMAD. Ultrasound-mediated increase in temperature may lead to instability to thermolabile drugs. Further, ultrasonic nebulizers cannot nebulize liquids with high viscosity [20].

Thus, to overcome the limitations of earlier nebulizers, nebulizers have been redesigned to be compact in size and battery operated. They are silent and compatible with many drug compounds. These new nebulizers are based on mesh technology and are of two types: static and vibrating mesh nebulizers (**Figure 13-5**).

Static mesh nebulizers apply sound wave to the liquid to push it through a mesh (Figure 13-5a). The ultrasonic transducer creates a wave in the liquid that pushes the droplets via a mesh, which does not undergo deformation. Unlike jet and ultrasonic nebulizers, mesh nebulizers are designed not to recycle generated droplets, which are usually in the size of (~3 μM. Micro-Air® NE-U22V (Omron Healthcare, Inc., IL) is an example of static mesh nebulizers.

Vibrating mesh nebulizers push the droplets through a mesh that undergoes deformation (Figure 13-5b). The ultrasound-producing device vibrates both mesh

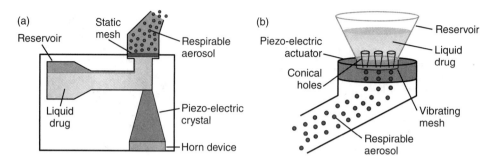

FIGURE 13-5 Recent nebulizers: (a) static and (b) vibrating mesh nebulizers.

and liquid drug, which is in contact with the mesh. As a result, mesh bends toward the drug reservoir side by forming conical holes toward the mouthpiece, as shown in Figure 13-5b. This deformation pushes the droplets out via the narrower side of conical holes into patients' mouths for inhalation. Aeroneb® Go (Aerogen, Ireland) is a vibrating mesh nebulizer.

Formulations for Nebulizers

Two types of formulations are mainly used in nebulizers: aqueous solutions and micronized suspensions. Nebulizer solutions are often available as concentrated solutions that can be used after dilution. Concentrated solutions may contain preservatives such as benzylkonium chloride. Because of reports of bronchospasm, however, unit dose, isotonic, and preservative-free solutions are preferred. For poorly water-soluble drugs, micronized suspension, cosolvents such as ethanol and propylene glycol, or micellar solubilization can be used [20].

Patient Counseling for Nebulizers

Patients should be counseled for proper use of nebulizers for maximal therapeutic benefit. Patients should be advised to wash and dry their hands thoroughly and use nebulizers under sufficient light. Nebulizers should be held upright to prevent spilling and promote nebulization. Once the mask is placed on the mouth, the patient should breathe slowly and deeply and hold the breath for up to a few seconds at the end of inhalation for better deposition of medication into the airways. Patients should be instructed not to mix any other medications with the prescribed medication for nebulization.

Pressurized Metered Dose Inhalers

MDIs allow multiple dosing using metering valves in conjunction with propellants. In pMDIs, drug is dispersed in propellants and the device facilitates aerosolization of the drug. In fact, pMDIs use conventional liquefied gas–based formulations commonly known as aerosols. An aerosol is a two-phase colloidal system that consists of a drug or any chemical substance as the dispersed phase and gas as the dispersion medium. Specifically, pharmaceutical aerosols are defined as the products containing therapeutic agents dissolved, suspended, or emulsified in a propellant mixture or a mixture of solvents and propellants. In aerosols, the drug or dispersed phase may be added as liquid, solid, or a mixture of liquid and solid. Various forces including electrical, pneumatic, and mechanical powers are used to generate aerosols from a colloidal system. In addition to administration of aerosols via the respiratory route, aerosols can be applied topically, vaginally, and rectally. Depending on the desired site of administration and design of aerosolizers, aerosols can be delivered as a mist or cloud, droplets, dry powder, combination of mist and dry powder, and foams [6, 20]. Aerosols generated by pMDIs are expelled as a fine mist.

Formulations for pMDIs

In general, an aerosol formulation for pMDIs consists of two components: a product concentrate, which is prepared by combining active ingredients with required additives such as antioxidants, surface active agents, and solvents, and a propellant, which is a liquefied gas with a vapor pressure greater than atmospheric pressure at a temperature of 40°C that pushes the product out and also acts as a solvent [2]. The propellant is the driving force or the "heart" of aerosols. Halogenated hydrocarbons, derived from methane and ethane, are used as propellants in oral and nasal inhaled formulations. Examples of propellants that have been used in aerosols for many years include dichlorodifluoromethane (propellant 12), dichlorotetrafluoromethane (propellant 114), and trichloromonofluoromethane (propellant 11). These propellants are commonly known as chlorofluorocarbon (CFC) propellants. CFC propellants reduce the amount of ozone in the atmosphere, which leads to an increased amount of ultraviolet radiation on earth. To reduce the incidence of skin cancer due to increased ultraviolet light, the use of propellants has been discouraged and prohibited for nonessential use. In recent years, use of CFCs has largely been replaced with hydrofluoroalkane propellants because the latter do not have ozone layer–depleting characteristics.

There are also propellant-free MDIs that can produce aerosols without propellants. These devices are in principle nebulizers but their application is more similar to MDIs. Respimat® (Boehringer Ingelheim, Germany) transforms aqueous solution to liquid aerosol droplets suitable for an inhaler. It is a propellant-free, multidose, handheld inhaler that can deliver a drug solution of 15 μL volume.

In CFC-containing pMDIs, micronized or spray-dried drug particles are held in suspension. Surfactants are used to disperse drug particles in suspension or lubricate the valve. Surfactants play an important role in keeping the drug in nonpolar propellants. Nonvolatile surfactants used in higher concentration may increase droplet size. Surfactant molecules may not evaporate from the surface of drug particles and may reduce the evaporation. Physical form, particle size, and dose can be controlled by metered valves. Physical form is also decided based on the intended use. For example, aerosol for inhalation therapy must produce a fine liquid mist, or finely divided solid particles and aerosols for dermatologic preparations may produce coarse particles. Medications can be easily withdrawn from the package without contamination or exposure to the remaining materials [3, 21].

Devices for pMDIs

An MDI device has three major components: container, metering valve, and spray actuator (Figure 13-6). pMDI containers, also called canisters, are made of chemically inert materials such as seamless aluminum. Plastic-coated glass containers can also be used. The metering valve hermetically seals the container and is designed to deliver a fixed volume of the product during each actuation. Each valve consists of several components made of inert materials. The metering tank contains a single dose in the range of 25 to 100 μL. When the valve is actuated by depressing the valve stem, the communication between the metering tank and the retaining cup is closed and the metering tank empties through the opening of the valve. The metered dose exits from the metering chamber under the pressure of the boiling liquid propellant. The actuator triggers the valve and makes an opening for delivering the aerosols

(a)

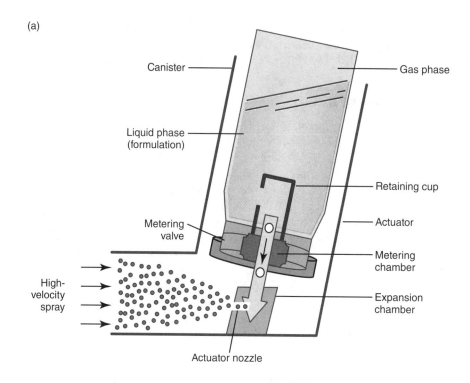

Canister

Gas phase

Liquid phase
(formulation)

Retaining cup

Actuator

Metering
valve

Metering
chamber

High-
velocity
spray

Expansion
chamber

Actuator nozzle

(b)

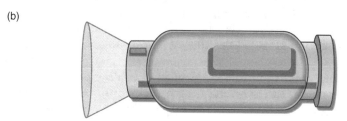

FIGURE 13-6 (a) pMDI and (b) a spacer device usually attached with pMDIs.

to the patient's mouth. Each firing of the pMDI delivers a volume of 30 to 100 μL and takes about 20 ms to produce a puff. Liquid exiting the container is converted to an aerosol due to the evaporation of propellants. As the propellant evaporates, the aerosol is released like a plume from the canister at a velocity of 15 m/s, which reduces to half of the initial velocity within 0.1 second. Although initial size of the particles produced due to flashing of propellants is ~35 μM, the particle size decreases rapidly as the distance of the plume increases from the nozzle.

Breath-actuated pMDIs are designed to reduce or eliminate hand–breath coordination. These pMDIs sense patients' inhalation through the actuator and trigger the inhaler automatically. Autohaler® (3M Pharmaceuticals, UK) and SmartMist® (Aradigm Co., CA) are examples of breath-actuated pMDIs. The Autohaler has a lever that patients have to pull to prime the device before inhalation. SmartMist® can accommodate a standard pMDI canister and automatically releases aerosols when a specific volume of the air is inspired and can record time and date of actuation.

Spacers for pMDIs

Spacers, also known as add-on devices, accessory devices, extension devices, and holding chambers, are attached to pMDIs. The add-on devices range between 20 and

750 mL (Figure 13-6b). Spacers reduce oropharyngeal deposition and increase lung deposition by increasing the distance between the point of aerosol generation and the patient's mouth. Particles generated from a pMDI often strike the spacer walls instead of the mouth. Spacers are particularly useful for pediatric patients because these accessories reduce or eliminate the coordination between actuation and inhalation. Further, spacers reduce the risk of oral candiasis and dysphonia associated with inhaled corticosteroids and diminish systemic absorption via the gastrointestinal tract.

However, spacer devices could be bulky and cumbersome to use. In some cases, electrostatic charge on the plastic surface of spacers can reduce the amount of drug delivered, but priming the chamber with the aerosol or washing with ionic detergents can reduce the electrostatic charge. A large number of spacers are available commercially, and designs vary significantly. Thus, an optimal spacer device should be chosen based on patient age and ability to self-administer medication.

Valved holding chambers and reverse flow bags are examples of two common spacer devices. **Valved holding chambers** contain a one-way valve that allows the aerosol to remain within the device until the patient inhales to open the valve. This device helps the patient prevent blowing the dose away. **Reverse flow devices** use a bag that collapses upon inhalation. It can also use a chamber with an air vent that opens during inhalation.

Patient Counseling for pMDIs

Patients should be educated about the importance of coordination between pMDI actuation and breathing and should be counseled on the correct use of the pMDI device, to breathe out first and then press down on the canister while breathing in. Breath-holding for around 10 seconds improves drug deposition in the lungs. The patient needs to shake the inhaler well before use and wait for ~1 minute between actuations, if multiple dosing is required. pMDIs are recommended to be primed several times for reproducible delivery. Without priming, the dose in the first spray may be erratic.

Dry Powder Inhalers

DPIs are pulmonary drug delivery devices containing solid drug suspended in a dry powder mix that can be fluidized when patient inhales. DPIs offer several advantages over pMDIs: They have a higher formulation stability in dry conditions and are propellant free and thus environment friendly [22].

Formulations for DPIs

Because DPIs contain powder in a static bed, the formulation in DPIs must undergo flow, fluidization, and deaggregation. Formulations of DPIs are aimed at coordinating these processes. Thus, DPI formulations are prepared in powdered form either as carrier-based formulations with large inert carrier excipients (Ventolin® Diskus®, GlaxoSmithKline) or agglomerated drug-only formulations (Pulmicort®, Astra Zeneca). Carriers are used to prevent aggregation and improve flow. Excipient can make up over 99% of the product by weight, making them an important factor for overall DPI performance. In DPIs, lactose, a crystalline substance with smooth surfaces, is the only excipient used to improve handling, dispensing, and metering of the drug. Lactose reduces cohesive forces between drug particles. Other sugars such as mannitol and glucose can also be used. However, some DPIs may not contain any excipients. For example, Pulmicort® and Turbuhaler® do not contain any excipients.

A newer type of formulation for DPIs is called large porous particles. Unlike traditional powders for inhalers, large porous particles are lighter, with a mass density of 0.4 g cm^{-3} compared with 1 g cm^{-3} for traditional powders. Because they are porous, their aerodynamic diameters are smaller than their volume diameters. Particles can be made in the respiratory aerodynamic diameter range while keeping their geometric diameter at ~20 µm. There is reduced dose requirement due to reduced aggregation and throat deposition. These particles remain longer in the alveolar region and can be prepared from lung surfactants and polymers.

Devices for DPIs

DPIs are available as either single-dose or multidose systems. In single-dose systems, patients have to refill the device with a dose before each administration, whereas in multidose systems, patients activate the dose before inhalation. Single-dose DPIs are generally capsule-based formulations such as Aerosolizer® (Novartis) and Handihaler® (Boehringer Ingelheim). Multidose DPIs are either individually packed blister units (Diskhaler® and Diskus®, GlaxoSmithKline) or metered dose powder reservoirs (Turbuhaler®, Astra Zeneca; Pulvinal®, Chiesi). Diskhaler® is an example of a multidose DPI that can accommodate reloadable disks containing sequentially numbered aluminum foil blisters containing drug formulations. The disk is placed onto a cartridge unit and slid into the outer body that has a needle and dose viewer (**Figure 13-7**). For the Diskus®, a strip of 60 blisters containing a dose in each blister is placed into the sealed plastic device during manufacturing. The device uses three wheels and an external lever to load a blister containing the dose. The wheels and needle align and pierce each blister, respectively, for aerosolization by patients' inspiratory flow (Figure 13-7). When patients inhale, air passes through the opened blister and aerosolizes the content [20, 22]. Based on the mechanisms involved in aerosolization of particles from the bulk powder bed, DPIs can be divided into two categories: passive and active DPIs.

For passive DPIs, patients use their inspiratory force to generate aerosols. Inhaled air enters the powder bed and aerosolizes the powder blend by creating shear and turbulence. The drug-carrying particles are separated from the carrier particles and are deposited into the lungs. Thus, deposition of a drug from passive DPIs depends on patients' inspiratory airflow. DPIs that use pneumatic, impact, and vibratory force to generate

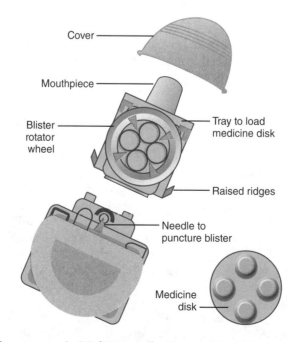

Cover

Mouthpiece

Blister rotator wheel

Tray to load medicine disk

Raised ridges

Needle to puncture blister

Medicine disk

FIGURE 13-7 Different parts of a DPI (Diskhaler®) with a medicine disk.

aerosols are known as active DPIs. Because generation of aerosols using active DPIs is independent of a patient's inspiratory force, these newer devices are likely to reduce or eliminate concerns regarding dose inaccuracy and lack of reproducibility. Further, these devices are expected to be used for efficient delivery of systemically active drugs with a narrow therapeutic window. Currently, active dispersion DPIs in development are Nektar pulmonary inhaler delivery system and Vectura Aspirair®. For both devices, small in-built pumps are used to generate compressed air to disperse the powdered drug.

Patient Counseling for DPIs

DPIs are more patient-friendly and require relatively less coordination between patient breathing and drug inhalation. Patients should be instructed to hold the device parallel to the ground to keep powder aerosolized for inhalation. Patients should be careful while puncturing the blister before using the DPI. Patients should breathe in deeply and steadily during inhalation from the device and hold their breath for a few seconds to ensure better deposition of medicine. Patients should be cautious about exposing DPIs to a humid environment [23].

STRATEGIES FOR PULMONARY DELIVERY OF LARGE MOLECULES

The pulmonary route has been used for the delivery of macromolecules and biologics for more than three decades. Because of the lack of an ideal inhalable delivery system capable of maintaining the stability and pharmacological efficacy and providing desirable release properties of encapsulated macromolecules, the success of delivering large molecules via the pulmonary route has been very limited. Furthermore, mucociliary clearance, mucus and alveolar fluid barrier, and uptake and removal by alveolar macrophages have also posed additional challenges to the success of delivering biologics via the pulmonary route. Also, controlling the aerodynamic properties of the particulate carrier system is necessary to achieve efficient deposition of the biologics in the desired region. Many particulate carrier systems such as micro- or nanoparticles, liposomes, dendrimers, and surfactant-based formulations have been investigated and successfully used to deliver large molecules via the pulmonary route [24].

Inhaled insulin, Exubera®, was the first protein drug approved by the U.S. Food and Drug Administration and commercialized as a DPI in the United States and Europe for the treatment of diabetes [25]. Because of a cumbersome delivery device and high expense, however, it failed to receive acceptance among patients and physicians, resulting in discontinuation of the product by Pfizer [26]. This failure did not stop the development of inhaled formulations of proteins, however, and many novel strategies came forward to tackle these problems. Currently, Dance Pharmaceuticals, a startup company in California, is working to address the issues related to the stability, efficacy, and untoward side effects of inhaled insulin.

DPIs are preferred devices for delivery of biologics because these devices can deliver drug formulations in a dry state. Their user-dependent interface gives them an edge over MDIs [27]. The conventional spray-drying method for preparation of inhalable dry powders for proteins and peptides suffers from instability problems. Recent advancements in the spray freeze drying technology, however, have overcome many stability problems of biologics [28]. Spray freeze drying produces spherical particles with uniform and controlled size and avoids heat or air-induced denaturation of proteins. Insulin-loaded liposomes, for example, prepared by spray freeze drying can be stored for 3 months, and intratracheal instillation of formulation resulted in about a threefold increase in bioavailability [29]. Other strategies include precipitation of particles via the solvent change method, incorporation of water-soluble cyclodextrins to prevent aggregation of proteins, and use of ink-jet devices consisting of a microheater to generate fine uniformed size droplets [24].

Recently, small interfering RNAs (siRNAs) have shown tremendous potential for the treatment of various disorders. Major obstacles to the delivery of siRNAs include susceptibility to degradation by enzymes and systemic toxicity [30]. The pulmonary route has been investigated for siRNA delivery. Liposomes, nanoparticles, cell penetrating peptide conjugates, pegylated complexes, and lipoplexes have been used as nonviral vectors for delivering siRNAs to the lungs. Lipid-based delivery carriers produce more inflammatory responses in the lungs as compared with naked siRNAs [31]. Further, *XCL1*, a critical gene associated with the pathogenesis of tuberculosis, was silenced by the intratracheal delivery of an siRNA against it, which demonstrated good potential as emerging therapy for tuberculosis [32]. The efficacy of pulmonary delivery of siRNAs and the clinical outcomes, however, are yet to be fully understood and optimized before becoming a reality.

DRUG DELIVERY VIA THE NASAL ROUTE

The nasal cavity offers a relatively large surface area for drug absorption. The rich vasculature of the nasal epithelium allows rapid absorption and onset of action after nasal administration. The nasal route avoids degradation in the gastrointestinal tract and liver and thereby avoids first-pass metabolism. Drugs can be self-administered without assistance from health care professionals. The nasal route could be used as an alternative to needle-based drug delivery. In situations when the oral route is unfeasible, such as patients with nausea, vomiting, and swallowing difficulties, the nasal route can also be used as an alternative to the oral route [4]. Nasal drug delivery is also associated with some disadvantages, such as mucociliary clearance, which reduces the retention time of drugs and thus decreases absorption. Nasal clearance, however, is not a major concern for drugs that are rapidly absorbed. Not all drugs are absorbed from the nose, especially drugs that are of large size and excessively hydrophilic. Pathological conditions of the nose such as the common cold and hay fever may limit the usefulness of the nasal route of administration. Nasal formulations may also produce irritation because the nasal epithelium is highly sensitive and fragile compared with the buccal epithelium [33].

FACTORS AFFECTING DRUG ABSORPTION VIA THE NASAL ROUTE

Both physiological factors (i.e., pathological conditions of the nose, blood supply, enzymatic activity, contact time, mucociliary clearance, immunological clearance, and mucous barrier) and pharmaceutical factors (i.e., physicochemical properties of drugs, drug concentrations, dosage forms, and delivery devices) may affect drug absorption from the nose [4]. These factors are summarized in **Table 13-5** and described further below.

Physiological Factors

Pathological Conditions

The nose can develop pathological conditions such as allergic rhinitis, polyps, and colds, and these nasal conditions are frequently associated with bleeding, excessive secretion of mucus, nasal blockage, and crusting. Increased nasal secretion, presence of polyps, and blockage by any pathological conditions may reduce absorption of nasally administered drugs. In contrast, inflammation in the nose may increase the permeability of the nasal

TABLE 13-5 Factors affecting drug absorption via nasal route

Physiological	Pharmaceutical
Rate of mucociliary clearance	Type of dosage form
Presence of pathological condition	Aerosol droplet size
(infection/allergy)	Nature of excipients
Atmospheric conditions	Physicochemical properties of drug
Nasal surface area and vasculature	Dose size/volume
Enzymatic/metabolic stability	Site of deposition
	Mechanical drug loss

Data from Lansley AB et al.

epithelium and thus increase nasal absorption. Environmental factors, including humidity, temperature, and pollution, that affect mucociliary clearance can also influence nasal absorption.

Nasal Surface Area and Blood Supply

The total surface area of the nasal cavities is favorably enhanced by the convolutions of the conchae and presence of microvilli on the surface of the nasal epithelium. The nasal surface is supplied with a dense network of blood vessels from the external and internal carotid arteries. Nasal blood flow is very sensitive to a variety of agents applied topically and systemically, which consequently can alter the size of the nasal lumen. Factors that can affect nasal blood supply include room temperature, humidity, use of vasodilating or vasconstricting agents, nasal trauma, compression of neck veins, mood swings, and exercise [33].

Mucociliary Clearance and Contact Time

As described above, mucociliary clearance is the body's defense mechanism that works by entrapping potentially hazardous substances such as dust and microorganisms within the viscoelastic mucus lining the nasal passages. At the end of the nasal septum and turbinates, the nasal mucosa is lined with ciliated epithelium. The mucus flows along with the movement of the cilia, which beats in a coordinated fashion in the sol layer, an ionic aqueous solution that facilitates ciliary movement, toward the pharynx where the entrapped particles undergo oral ingestion or expectoration as coughs. The cilia beat 10 times each second in the nasal mucosa, called the gel layer, and it takes 10 to 20 minutes for the bulk of the mucus to move from the nose to the nasopharynx.

For drug absorption to occur from the nasal epithelium, dosage forms should be in contact with the absorption site for a sufficient time to allow for drugs to cross the nasal mucosa. Contact time with nasal epithelium can vary based on the type of the dosage form. For instance, nasal gels, being viscous, remain on the nasal epithelium for a longer time compared with nasal solutions. Furthermore, the contact time of a dosage form is also affected by the mucociliary clearance rate. Depending on the region where the dosage form is deposited, the rate of clearance of the drug formulation may vary. An increased mucociliary clearance rate is likely to decrease nasal absorption. Prolonged contact time can be accomplished by increasing the viscosity of the formulations and by using bioadhesive polymer-based formulations and microspheres. Further, the mucociliary clearance rate varies depending on the distribution of ciliated epithelium in the nose. Compared with the anterior regions of the nasal cavity, the middle and posterior nasal epithelium contains more ciliated cells, and thus drugs deposited in the posterior part of the nose are cleared faster than those deposited in the anterior part of the nose. Like increased mucociliary clearance rate, permeability of the posterior nasal cavity is higher than that of the anterior segment. Considering these two factors, mucociliary clearance rate and permeability, rapidly absorbing drugs should be administered in the posterior part of the nose, and slowly absorbing drugs should be deposited in the anterior part of the nose.

Enzymatic Degradation

Nasal mucosa and secretions contain a number of enzymes that can potentially metabolize various drugs. Metabolizing enzymes that are present in the nasal epithelium include aldehyde dehydrogenase, carboxyl esterase, carbonic anhydrases, glucuronyl, sulfate transferase, and glutathione transferase. Thus, nasally administered drugs such as nasal decongestants, perfumes, anesthetics, and nicotine are reported to be metabolized by the nasal P450-dependent monooxygenase system. Progesterone, testosterone, and insulin also undergo metabolism in the nose. The metabolizing capacity of the nose is limited, however, compared with the gastrointestinal tract.

Pharmaceutical Factors

The physicochemical characteristics of the drug molecule that affect drug absorption from the nasal epithelium are similar to those affecting any transepithelial absorption, such as molecular weight, hydrophilicity, and lipophilicity of the drug molecule [4]. Lipophilic drugs are swiftly and completely absorbed from the nasal cavity, whereas absorption of hydrophilic molecules is reduced because of rapid mucociliary clearance. Furthermore, compounds with molecular weights > 1 kDa show decreased nasal absorption. Because most drugs intended to be absorbed through the nasal epithelium undergo passive diffusion, a higher drug concentration at the target site significantly increases absorption. In case of nasal spray formulations, where aerosol particles are deposited in the nasal cavity, certain dosage form characteristics, such as particle size, particle charge, and aerosol velocity, are critical parameters to affect drug absorption. Other formulation-related factors that influence drug delivery via the nose are density and viscosity of the vehicle, pH and tonicity of the dosage form, and presence of certain additives such as metabolic enzyme inhibitors, bioadhesives, and penetration enhancers. Further, considering the capacity of the human nose, the dose volume of nasal formulations should not exceed 200 μL because a human nostril can accommodate only 25 to 200 μL of drug formulations.

NASAL FORMULATIONS

Nasal formulations currently available or under development are nasal drops, nasal sprays, suspensions, powders, gels, emulsions, microspheres, and liposomes [5, 34].

Nasal solutions are the most commonly used nasal formulations. Most nasal formulations contain water as the pharmaceutical solvent. Nasal solutions may contain preservatives to prevent microbial growth; however, caution should be exercised in selecting preservatives and choosing concentrations to be added to a nasal solution because many preservatives disrupt mucociliary clearance and subsequently cause nasal irritation. Nasal solutions are quickly removed from the nose because of short contact time that can be extended by incorporating viscosity-inducing polymers into the formulations. Solutions can be administered as drops or sprays.

Suspension is not a common formulation for nasal administration. One of the major concerns for nasal suspension is the presence of particles that may produce irritation. Thus, extra caution should be exercised in the optimizing particle size of nasal suspensions. In addition to aqueous vehicles, nasal suspensions are formulated with preservatives, antioxidants, and suspending agents. Unlike nasal solutions, nasal suspensions provide prolonged residence time that is beneficial for continuous release of various drugs. Both sprayer and metering devices can be used for administration of nasal suspensions.

Nasal gels are usually water-based gels called hydrogels. Nasal gels have been developed with the assumption that, unlike solution, formulation drip and leakage will be reduced after administration. There are, however, a number of limitations in administering gels via the nose: discomfort produced by semisolid materials in the nose and possible blockage of nasal passages that may disrupt breathing. An example of a commercially available nasal gel is Nascobal® containing vitamin B12.

Powder formulations have been developed to deliver drugs via the nasal route to eliminate some important limitations of nasal solutions and suspensions. Nasal powders are more stable compared with solutions and can be prepared without preservatives. Further, because powder can easily stick to the nasal surface, they exhibit prolonged residence time compared with nasal solutions. Like nasal gels, however, nasal powder formulations may cause irritation and give a dry and gritty feeling in the nose. Both insufflators and pMDIs can be used for delivery of nasal powder. Rhinocort Turbuhaler® from Astra Zeneca is an example of a nasal powder formulation.

Nasal drops and sprays are administered as spray using squeeze bottles. Squeeze bottles, however, do not produce reproducible dosing with each administration. Nasal solutions are also available in metered dose devices, which produce more reproducible dosing. Nasal sprays are likely to deposit at the site where droplets strike first, that is, the anterior nasal cavity, a site with high airflow and slow mucociliary clearance.

Nasal solutions can also be administered as a single or multiple drops using a dropper with a flexible tip or a dropper fixed with a squeezable plastic container. Nasal drops deposit the drug into the entire nasal cavity, making it available for quick absorption because of a larger surface area. The fractions of the dose that deposit on the ciliated regions of the mucosa and the nasopharynx are eliminated by ciliary clearance and swallowing, respectively.

Nasally administered solutions are eliminated in two phases: 40% of the dose is cleared within 20 minutes followed by a second slower phase of elimination. In the second phase of elimination, the solution administered by droppers undergoes faster elimination than that administered by sprayers because most of the solution administered as spray deposits on nonciliated regions. Thus, drugs that absorb fast should be administered as drops and slow-absorbing drugs should be administered as sprays. For this reason, the bioavailability of desmopressin is greater from a nasal spray than from drops.

Nasal Drug Delivery Devices

Various nasal drug delivery devices, conventional and advanced, are summarized in **Table 13-6**, and some representative devices have been schematically presented in **Figure 13-8**.

Droppers and Squeeze Bottles

Nasal droppers and squeeze bottles are made up of a smooth plastic bottle and jet outlet. When the plastic bottle is pressed, a certain volume is atomized because of air inside the bottle. If droppers and squeeze bottles are kept uncapped, the formulations can easily get contaminated by microorganisms. For administration of decongestants, squeeze bottles have traditionally been used, although there are concerns regarding the reproducibility of the dose delivered by squeeze bottles [35].

Metered Dose Pumps

Metered dose pump sprays consist of container, pump, valve, and an actuator; these devices are used to administer potent drugs via the nose. Metered dose pumps can accurately deliver a volume ranging from 25 to 200 μL (Figure 13-8a).

TABLE 13-6 Types and subtypes of nasal drug delivery devices	
Liquid	**Vapor:** vapor inhaler **Drops:** rhinyle catheter, multi-dose dropper, unit-dose pipette **Mechanical spray pumps:** squeeze bottle, multi-dose metered-dose spray pump, single/duo- dose spray pump, bidirectional multi-dose spray pump **Gas driven spray systems/atomizers:** slow spray, nitrogen gas driven **Electrically powered nebulizers/atomizers:** pulsation membrane, hand-held, vibrating mesh
Powder	**Powder sprayers** **Breath actuated inhalers: single/duo dose, multi-dose** **Insufflators:** breath powered bidirectional

Data from van Drooge DJ, Hinrichs WL, Dickhoff BH, et al. Spray freeze drying to produce a stable delta(9)-tetrahydrocannabinol containing inulin-based solid dispersion powder suitable for inhalation. *Eur J Pharm Sci.* 2005;26:231–240.

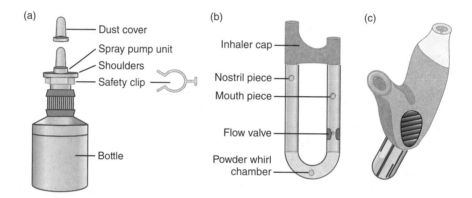

FIGURE 13-8 Some commonly used nasal drug delivery devices: (a) metered dose spray pump, (b) Directhaler®, and (c) Optinose®.

Recent Advancements in Nasal Drug Delivery Devices

Although conventional nasal spray bottles and pumps have long been used for administration of therapeutic agents via the nose, the delivery efficiency of sprayers and droppers is suboptimal. Currently used spray pumps and bottles can deliver drugs only into a portion of the nasal cavity. The size of droplets produced by spray bottles is ~50 μm, which is far above the size that can be deposited in the nose. Similarly, nebulized particles with a size below 5 μm tend to deposit in the lungs. Importantly, spraying mechanisms of current devices prevent them from delivering drugs into the upper region of the nasal cavity, which is reported to be the most effective region for drug deposition. Most drugs (~90%) that deposit in the anterior chamber of the nasal cavity are quickly eliminated or ingested. Other limitations of current nasal devices are dose inaccuracy due to variability in spray patterns, dripping of solutions, swallowing of drug formulations, and the presence of preservatives.

To overcome these limitations of current nasal drug delivery devices, a number of newer nasal drug delivery devices have emerged or their development is underway. The newer devices take into account the airflow in the nasal cavity and anatomy of the nasopharyngeal tract to minimize drug loss and maximize drug deposition and absorption after nasal instillation. Below is a summary of three devices that have shown promise in increasing absorption and deposition of drugs in the nose.

Controlled Particle Dispersion Method

Kurve Technology, Inc. (Lynnwood, WA) has developed a device that works by manipulating the natural airflow in the nose. In the human nose, inspired air flows in a parabolic fashion, and the greatest airflow is observed in the floor of the nose and decreases in the upper regions of the nasal cavity. As a result of the parabolic pattern of airflow, currently available nasal spray delivers most of the drugs to the floor of the nasal cavity. Kurve Technology produces a vortical flow and controlled dispersion of particles to disrupt the natural airflow pattern in the nose and to distribute the drug into the entire nasal cavity. Several studies have shown that the Kurve® nasal device can deliver drugs to the entire nose and reduce the amount of drug loss [36].

Bidirectional Inhalers

Similar to controlled dispersion technology, bidirectional inhalers exploit the anatomy of the nasopharyngeal tract. These devices use the principle of blowing up a balloon. When blowing up balloons, one has to exhale against the balloon wall, which closes the soft palate and separates the nasal cavity from the mouth. This mechanism cuts the communication between the cranial surface of the soft palate and the posterior margin of the nasal septum. Thus, the air entering a nostril through the sealing nozzle takes a 180-degree turn and exits through the other nostril in the opposite direction [37]. Two devices, the Directhaler® and Optinose®, use this concept to blow the air out and direct the flow of air into the nose (**Figure 13-8, b** and **c**).

The Directhaler® is a U-shaped inhaler tube with a corrugated bend. The two ends are sealed with a cap (Figure 13-8b). To use this device, patients remove the cap and place the mouth and nose pieces in the mouth and nose, respectively. When patients use this device, the air passage between the oral and nasal cavities closes, and the drug is deposited in the nasal cavity. When a patient blows air into the Directhaler® nasal device, the nasal dry powder dose is delivered into the nostril. This device can be used for both nasal and pulmonary delivery. In this single-dose device, drug powder is placed in the powder whirl chamber of the corrugated zone.

Like the Directhaler®, in Optinose®, a sealing nozzle is inserted into one nostril and the patient blows into the mouthpiece (Figure 13-8c). The blowing action closes the soft palate and creates an airflow that carries the formulation out of the device through the sealing nozzle into one nostril of the target site. This device can also be designed to incorporate existing nasal spray pumps [38].

PATIENT COUNSELING

Patients should be counseled in the proper use of nasal formulations, particularly nasal sprays. Many marketed nasal sprays require priming before use; hence, patients should be instructed to prime the device by squirting a few times away from the eyes before attempting to administer the formulation. Patients should be advised to sniff gently, not snort, in coordination with spray actuation for efficient deposition of a formulation into the nasal cavity rather than into the throat. Nasal spray containers should be stored in a safe place out of the reach of children and should not be used at a higher frequency than prescribed by the health care provider.

STRATEGIES FOR NASAL DELIVERY OF PROTEINS AND PEPTIDES

To deliver biologics via the nasal route, various approaches such as absorption enhancers, enzyme inhibitors, and mucoadhesive polymers have been investigated [24]. Traditional absorption enhancers such as bile salts, fatty acids, and surfactants induce severe irreversible damage to the nasal mucosa [39]. Because biologics are generally used for the long-term management of a disease, toxicity issues with absorption enhancers limit their use for clinical purposes. Polymeric absorption enhancers such as chitosan and carbopol have drawn attention because of their reduced toxicity both to the nasal mucosa and blood circulation [40]. Chitosan-based formulations showed no toxic effects to the nasal mucosa even after 7 days of administration [41]. The mucoadhesive property of several polymeric absorption enhancers increased the retention time of macromolecules by surpassing the mucociliary clearance [42]. Chitosan-based particulate carriers such as nano- or microparticles and liposomes have been demonstrated to increase absorption of ovalbumin with no toxic effects. Of the various derivatives of chitosan, trimethyl and thiolated forms have been shown to improve absorption and permeation of insulin and calcitonin after nasal administration. Polyethylene grafting to polymers significantly increases the solubility and compatibility profile of proteins. Other strategies to improve absorption include microemulsions, spheroid technology, and microsponges that have been used to improve the bioavailability of biologics such as human growth hormone, interferon-β, insulin, glucagon-like peptide-1 and calcitonin [43]. Over the past several years, nose to brain delivery has been a very dynamic field of research. The blood–brain barrier poses an impervious barricade for the biologics. Interestingly, the intranasal route has shown the ability to bypass the blood–brain barrier and deliver proteins directly to the central nervous system. Wang et al. [44] showed a twofold increase in availability of estradiol after nasal administration.

The nasal route has also been investigated to deliver siRNAs for various respiratory diseases such as asthma, chronic obstructive pulmonary disease, cystic fibrosis, lung cancer, and viral infections. The nasal formulations containing siRNAs have been used for the management of diseases caused by respiratory syncytial, parainfluenza, and influenza viruses without major systemic side effects [30]. In clinical trials sponsored by MedImmune, Inc. (Gaithersburg, MD), intranasal siRNA against respiratory syncytial virus has shown promising results in phase I trials and is now currently being investigated in phase II trials. In another double-blind trial conducted by Alnylam Pharmaceuticals (Cambridge, MA), siRNA against respiratory syncytial virus showed improved safety, tolerability, and pharmacokinetics as compared with naked siRNA. Currently, Nastech (Bothell, WA) and Sirna Therapeutics (San Francisco, CA) are involved in developing siRNA-based nasal formulations for various respiratory syndromes [45]. Based on the progress made over the past 5 years, it appears that nasal therapeutics involving siRNAs is proceeding at a much faster pace toward clinical use.

SUMMARY

The respiratory system, including the nose and lungs, is an important route for drug administration. Currently, the pulmonary route is mainly limited to administration of drugs for the treatment of diseases that are localized to the respiratory tract. The nasal and pulmonary routes of drug administration, however, offer tremendous opportunity for delivery of therapeutic agents that produce systemic effects. The concerns regarding the accuracy and reproducibility of respiratory drug delivery devices should be addressed by developing newer devices that can precisely control dosing and maximize the inhaled dose. Similarly, for better understanding of aerosol deposition and subsequent therapeutic effect, anatomical and physiological features of the respiratory systems such as airway geometry, airflow pattern, clearance mechanisms, respiratory disorders, and their influence on particle deposition should be further evaluated. Recent trends suggest that inhalational drug delivery is moving toward formulations and sophisticated devices that can efficiently deliver both small- and large-molecular-weight drugs and biologics to the lungs for local and systemic therapeutic interventions.

REVIEW QUESTIONS

1. Discuss the mechanisms involved and factors affecting particle deposition in the lungs.
2. Describe three major classes of devices for delivery of drugs via the pulmonary route.
3. Discuss major particle clearance mechanisms of the respiratory system.
4. Describe current pharmaceutical technologies that are used for nasal delivery of drugs.

REFERENCES

1. Hickey AJ. Back to the future: inhaled drug products. *J Pharm Sci.* 2013;102:1165–1172.
2. Hindle M. Aerosol drug delivery. In: Shayne CG, ed. *Pharmaceutical Manufacturing Handbook: Production and Processes.* Hoboken, NJ: John Wiley & Sons; 2007:683–728.
3. Taylor G, Kellaway I. *Pulmonary Drug Delivery.* Boca Raton, FL: CRC Press; 2001:269–300.
4. Thomas C, Ahsan F. Nasal delivery of peptide and nonpeptide drugs. In: Shayne CG, ed. *Pharmaceutical Manufacturing Handbook: Production and Processes.* Hoboken, NJ: John Wiley & Sons; 2007:591–650.
5. Lansley AB, Martin GP. *Nasal Drug Delivery.* Boca Raton, FL: CRC Press; 2001:237–268.
6. Traini D. Inhalation drug delivery. In: Colombo P, Taini D, Buttini F, eds. *Inhalation Drug Delivery: Techniques and Products.* Hoboken, NJ: John Wiley & Sons; 2013:1–11.
7. Klein SG, Hennen J, Serchi T, Blomeke B, Gutleb AC. Potential of coculture in vitro models to study inflammatory and sensitizing effects of particles on the lung. *Toxicol In Vitro.* 2011;25:1516–1534.
8. Burgel PR. The role of small airways in obstructive airway diseases. *Eur Respir Rev.* 2011;20:23–33.
9. Patton JS, Brain JD, Davies LA, et al. The particle has landed—characterizing the fate of inhaled pharmaceuticals. *J Aerosol Med Pulm Drug Deliv.* 2010;23(Suppl 2):S71–S87.
10. Yu J, Chien YW. Pulmonary drug delivery: physiologic and mechanistic aspects. *Crit Rev Ther Drug Carrier Syst.* 1997;14:395–453.
11. Courrier HM, Butz N, Vandamme TF. Pulmonary drug delivery systems: recent developments and prospects. *Crit Rev Ther Drug Carrier Syst.* 2002;19:425–498.
12. Suarez S, Hickey AJ. Drug properties affecting aerosol behavior. *Respir Care.* 2000;45:652–666.
13. Newman SP, Chan HK. In vitro/in vivo comparisons in pulmonary drug delivery. *J Aerosol Med Pulm Drug Deliv.* 2008;21:77–84.
14. Geiser M, Kreyling WG. Deposition and biokinetics of inhaled nanoparticles. *Part Fibre Toxicol.* 2010;7:2.
15. Darquenne C. Aerosol deposition in health and disease. *J Aerosol Med Pulm Drug Deliv.* 2012;25:140–147.
16. Stuart BO. Deposition and clearance of inhaled particles. *Environ Health Perspect.* 1976;16:41–53.
17. Patton JS, Fishburn CS, Weers JG. The lungs as a portal of entry for systemic drug delivery. *Proc Am Thorac Soc.* 2004;1:338–344.
18. Rogueda PG, Traini D. The nanoscale in pulmonary delivery. Part 1. Deposition, fate, toxicology and effects. *Expert Opin Drug Deliv.* 2007;4:595–606.
19. Dolovich MB, Ahrens RC, Hess DR, et al. Device selection and outcomes of aerosol therapy: evidence-based guidelines: American College of Chest Physicians/American College of Asthma, Allergy, and Immunology. *Chest.* 2005;127:335–371.
20. Dolovich MB, Dhand R. Aerosol drug delivery: developments in device design and clinical use. *Lancet.* 2011;377:1032–1045.
21. Traini D, Young PM. Inhalation and nasal products. In: *Inhalation Drug Delivery: Techniques and Products.* Hoboken, NJ: John Wiley & Sons; 2013:15–29.
22. Donovan MJ, Gibbons A, Herpin MJ, Marek S, McGill SL, Smyth HD. Novel dry powder inhaler particle-dispersion systems. *Ther Deliv.* 2011;2:1295–1311.

23. Melani AS, Bracci LS, Rossi M. Reduced peak inspiratory effort through the Diskus((R)) and the Turbuhaler((R)) due to mishandling is common in clinical practice. *Clin Drug Invest.* 2005;25:543–549.

24. Chung SW, Hil-lal TA, Byun Y. Strategies for non-invasive delivery of biologics. *J Drug Target.* 2012;20:481–501.

25. Lenzer J. Inhaled insulin is approved in Europe and United States. *BMJ.* 2006;332:321.

26. Klingler C, Muller BW, Steckel H. Insulin-micro- and nanoparticles for pulmonary delivery. *Int J Pharm.* 2009;377:173–179.

27. Johnson KA. Preparation of peptide and protein powders for inhalation. *Adv Drug Deliv Rev.* 1997;26:3–15.

28. van Drooge DJ, Hinrichs WL, Dickhoff BH, et al. Spray freeze drying to produce a stable delta(9)–tetrahydrocannabinol containing inulin-based solid dispersion powder suitable for inhalation. *Eur J Pharm Sci.* 2005;26:231–240.

29. Bi R, Shao W, Wang Q, Zhang N. Spray-freeze-dried dry powder inhalation of insulin-loaded liposomes for enhanced pulmonary delivery. *J Drug Target.* 2008;16:639–648.

30. Lam JK, Liang W, Chan HK. Pulmonary delivery of therapeutic siRNA. *Adv Drug Deliv Rev.* 2012;64:1–15.

31. Gutbier B, Kube SM, Reppe K, et al. RNAi-mediated suppression of constitutive pulmonary gene expression by small interfering RNA in mice. *Pulm Pharmacol Ther.* 2010;23:334–344.

32. Rosas-Taraco AG, Higgins DM, Sanchez-Campillo J, Lee EJ, Orme IM, Gonzalez-Juarrero M. Intrapulmonary delivery of XCL1-targeting small interfering RNA in mice chronically infected with Mycobacterium tuberculosis. *Am J Respir Cell Mol Biol.* 2009;41:136–145.

33. Bitter C, Suter-Zimmermann K, Surber C. Nasal drug delivery in humans. *Curr Probl Dermatol.* 2011;40:20–35.

34. Malerba F, Paoletti F, Capsoni S, Cattaneo A. Intranasal delivery of therapeutic proteins for neurological diseases. *Expert Opin Drug Deliv.* 2011;8:1277–1296.

35. Djupesland PG. Nasal drug delivery devices: characteristics and performance in a clinical perspective—a review. *Drug Deliv Transl Res.* 2013;3:42–62.

36. Craft S, Baker LD, Montine TJ, et al. Intranasal insulin therapy for Alzheimer disease and amnestic mild cognitive impairment: a pilot clinical trial. *Arch Neurol.* 2012;69:29–38.

37. Djupesland PG, Skretting A, Winderen M, Holand T. Breath actuated device improves delivery to target sites beyond the nasal valve. *Laryngoscope.* 2006;116:466–472.

38. Djupesland PG, Mahmoud RA, Messina JC. Accessing the brain: the nose may know the way. *J Cereb Blood Flow Metab.* 2013;33:793–794.

39. Cazares-Delgadillo J, Ganem-Rondero A, Kalia YN. Human growth hormone: new delivery systems, alternative routes of administration, and their pharmacological relevance. *Eur J Pharm Biopharm.* 2011;78:278–288.

40. Di Colo G, Zambito Y, Zaino C. Polymeric enhancers of mucosal epithelia permeability: synthesis, transepithelial penetration-enhancing properties, mechanism of action, safety issues. *J Pharm Sci.* 2008;97:1652–1680.

41. Aspden TJ, Mason JD, Jones NS, Lowe J, Skaugrud O, Illum L. Chitosan as a nasal delivery system: the effect of chitosan solutions on in vitro and in vivo mucociliary transport rates in human turbinates and volunteers. *J Pharm Sci.* 1997;86:509–513.

42. el Khafagy S, Morishita M, Isowa K, Imai J, Takayama K. Effect of cell-penetrating peptides on the nasal absorption of insulin. *J Control Release.* 2009;133:103–108.

43. Illum L. Nanoparticulate systems for nasal delivery of drugs: a real improvement over simple systems? *J Pharm Sci.* 2007;96:473–483.

44. Wang X, Chi N, Tang X. Preparation of estradiol chitosan nanoparticles for improving nasal absorption and brain targeting. *Eur J Pharm Biopharm.* 2008;70:735–740.

45. Thomas M, Lu JJ, Chen J, Klibanov AM. Non-viral siRNA delivery to the lungs. *Adv Drug Deliv Rev.* 2007;59:124–133.

VAGINAL DRUG DELIVERY

SANKO NGUYEN, GABRIELLA BAKI, JERRY NESAMONY, AND SAI H. S. BODDU

CHAPTER OBJECTIVES

Upon completing this chapter, the reader should be able to

▸ Identify basic anatomy and physiology of the vagina.

▸ Understand physiological and physicochemical factors that may affect vaginal absorption.

▸ Describe characteristics of the various vaginal drug delivery systems currently available on the market or in the developmental stage.

▸ Determine advantages and obstacles of vaginal drug delivery.

CHAPTER OUTLINE

INTRODUCTION

Intravaginal drug administration has been used for many years. For a long time, the primary and almost exclusive purposes of applying medications in the vagina were the local treatment of gynecological infections and contraception [1]. The vagina's absorption capacity has been recognized recently, however, and research in this field suggests that the vagina could provide a potential route for systemic drug delivery with direct entry to the bloodstream, bypassing the hepatic-gastrointestinal (GI) metabolism (also known as first-pass metabolism). As a result, the vaginal route as a novel site for drug delivery has received greater attention in the last decade. Several pharmacologically active compounds that are metabolized extensively when taken orally have been delivered intravaginally to achieve their systemic activity.

Vaginal drug administration offers a number of advantages, including the avoidance of the hepatic first-pass effect, thus enabling lower doses, and the potential to use controlled-release dosage forms. In addition, the convenience of long-term dosing regimens offered by controlled-release dosage forms may improve patient compliance. Although vaginal drug administration has many advantages, misperceptions and poor education about vaginal anatomy and physiology can lead to reluctance to use vaginal medications. By counseling and educating patients, clinicians and pharmacists can help to establish the vaginal route of drug administration as safe, effective, and convenient so that more women can experience its potential benefits.

This chapter reviews the various purposes of intravaginal drug application and the possible methods and dosage forms currently used and under development (these are referred to as advanced dosage forms). First, a short summary is provided on the anatomy and physiology of the vagina as an organ and an absorptive surface. Then, we review factors that are characteristic of the vagina with respect to vaginal drug absorption, primarily focusing on the physiological and physicochemical factors. Finally, the reader will be familiarized with the currently available dosage forms and the delivery systems of the future.

GENERAL ANATOMY AND PHYSIOLOGY OF THE HUMAN VAGINA

ANATOMICAL CHARACTERISTICS

The vagina is a slightly curved canal with an average length of about 6 to 10 cm extending from the vulva to the cervix [2, 3]. Physiologically, the vagina serves several functions, acting primarily as a receptacle during coitus, as an excretory duct for menstrual discharge, and as the lower part of the birth canal [4].

Cellular Structure

The vaginal wall is composed of four distinct layers [5] (**Figure 14-1**):

1. The vaginal lumen is lined by a nonkeratinized stratified squamous **epithelium** (often referred to as the mucosa). In the relaxed state, this epithelium forms folds called rugae. It provides an extremely large surface area for the absorption of the drugs.
2. Beneath the mucosa is the **lamina propria.** It is a thick layer that is primarily made of collagen and elastin and contains a rich supply of vascular and lymphatic channels. This layer provides elasticity for the vaginal wall. Although the epithelium itself lacks glands (it is nonsecretory), the lymph and vascular channels within the lamina propria produce a transudate seen during sexual arousal.
3. The vaginal mucosa is surrounded by an elastic **muscularis** layer consisting of layers of smooth muscle fibers arranged in both circular and longitudinal bundles. This muscular orientation allows for the tremendous vaginal distention seen in childbirth.
4. Along the rest of the vagina, the muscularis layer is surrounded by the **tunica adventitia** that consists of a loose connective tissue (elastin and collagen) and a large plexus of blood vessels as well as nerves.

Blood Supply

The human vagina has a complex and extensive network of blood vessels along its entire length. Its blood supply includes a plexus of arteries from the internal iliac artery, uterine, middle rectal, and internal pudendal arteries. Drugs absorbed from the vagina do not undergo first-pass metabolism because blood leaving the vagina enters the peripheral

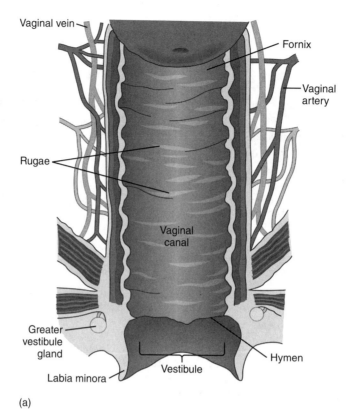

FIGURE 14-1 The anatomy (a) and histology (b) of the human vagina.

circulation via a rich venous plexus, which empties primarily into the internal iliac veins. There is some drainage to the hemorrhoidal veins as well [1].

Nervous Supply

The vagina's nerve supply comes from two sources: the **peripheral**, which primarily supplies the lower quarter of the vagina, making it a highly sensitive area; and the **autonomic,** which primarily supplies the upper three-fourths [6]. Autonomic fibers respond to stretch and are not very sensitive to pain or temperature. In addition, there are few sensory fibers in the upper vagina, making it a relatively insensitive area. This is why women rarely feel localized sensations or any discomfort when using vaginal products such as suppositories or vaginal rings and are often unaware of the presence of such items in the vagina.

PHYSIOLOGY

The physiology of the vagina is influenced by age, hormone status, pregnancy, and pH changes induced by several factors, including semen, menstruation, estrogen levels, and bacterial colonization.

Thickness of the Vaginal Wall

Changes in epithelium thickness are greatly influenced by the menstrual cycle; the change during each menstrual cycle is usually in the range of 200 to 300 μm [7]. Estrogen increases its thickness, whereas progesterone reduces it. The rate and extent of absorption of vaginally administered drugs varies with the thickness of vaginal epithelium.

Vaginal Fluid

Despite the paucity of glands, the vaginal epithelium is usually kept moist by a viscous surface film that is generally referred to as the vaginal fluid. This film is mostly transudate from vaginal and cervical cells but also contains vulvar secretions from sebaceous, sweat, Bartholin, and Skene glands; cervical mucus; endometrial and oviductal fluids; and microorganisms and their metabolic products [8]. The mucus, the principal component of vaginal fluid, plays an important role in the dissolution and absorption of drugs applied as mucoadhesive drug delivery systems because these systems are expected to come into contact with the mucus when inserted intravaginally. The mucus generally contains enzymes, proteins, carbohydrates, amino acids, aliphatic acids, immunoglobulins, and glycoproteins. Glycoproteins are the main components of the mucus and contribute greatly to the binding of mucoadhesive drugs to the vaginal wall. Glycoproteins can form a variety of bonds, including disulfide bonds, hydrogen bonds, and ionic bonds through sialic acid located at the terminal ends of the oligosaccharide chain [9]. Cyclical changes caused by hormonal influences and sexual arousal may affect the volume and composition of vaginal fluids, which can alter the drug release pattern in the vaginal delivery system. In a normal woman, mucus is produced at a rate of 20 to 60 mg/day, with as much as 1 g/day during mid-cycle. The overall volume of vaginal fluid appears to be 2 to 8 mL/day, whereas the discharge produced by postmenopausal women is reduced by 50% [10]. At the time of ovulation, vaginal fluid increases in volume.

pH

For healthy women of reproductive age, normal vaginal pH is in the range of 3.8 to 4.2 [11]. The main factor that helps maintain this acidic environment is a chemical known as lactic acid, which is produced from glycogen by the vaginal microflora. Glycogen is deposited in large amounts in the vaginal epithelium during times of high estrogen availability. Many factors can alter the vaginal pH, including the use of medicines (e.g., antibiotics and oral contraceptives), carbohydrate intake, use of feminine hygiene products, or even the presence of semen, which is slightly alkaline (pH 7.0–8.0).

Enzymes

The vaginal epithelium has a high activity of enzymes that could potentially affect short- and long-term stability of intravaginal delivery systems and devices. Some examples of enzymes are proteases, peptidase, and phosphatases [12].

Microbial Flora

The vaginal lumen is a nonsterile area inhabited by a variety of microorganisms, mainly *Lactobacillus, Bacteroides,* and *Staphylococcus epidermidis,* as well as potentially pathogenic aerobes [13]. When the normal pH balance of the vagina is disturbed (e.g., after the use of antibiotics), the pathogenic bacteria may overgrow and cause discomfort and symptoms of vaginal infection. Lactobacilli are beneficial for vaginal health because they compete with exogenous microbes for nutrients. The protective role is facilitated by the production of lactic acid and hydrogen peroxide. Hydrogen peroxide is toxic to other microorganisms that produce little or no hydrogen peroxide–scavenging enzymes. Thus, hydrogen peroxide–producing lactobacilli regulate the growth of other vaginal microbes, making the environment less hospitable to others, such as *Escherichia coli,* group B *Streptococcus,* and even HIV [14]. The existence of potentially harmful microbes and their metabolites may also have a detrimental effect on the intravaginal stability of a vaginal drug delivery device.

FACTORS AFFECTING THE VAGINAL ABSORPTION OF DRUGS

The absorption of a drug from the vaginal delivery systems occurs in three main steps: (1) drug release from the delivery system, (2) drug dissolution in vaginal lumen, and (3) penetration through the vaginal wall [12]. Absorption depends on numerous factors that are usually categorized into two main classes, namely physiological and physico-chemical factors.

PHYSIOLOGICAL FACTORS

Throughout the lifetime of a woman, a number of interrelated changes take place in vaginal physiology, which ultimately can affect the absorption of drugs. Before puberty, the vaginal epithelium is relatively thin; thus, vaginal absorption of drugs will be easier. After puberty, the thickness of vaginal epithelium increases, leading to the decrease in the absorption of drugs. The menstrual cycle, sexual arousal, and menopause can also potentially affect drug release because significant changes can be observed in the pH, epithelium thickness, and composition and viscosity of the vaginal fluids.

Normal Menstruation

The thickness of the vaginal epithelium, pH, and viscosity and composition of the vaginal fluid are highly affected by ovarian hormones. During the follicular phase (first part of a menstrual cycle, i.e., time between the end of menstruation and the day of ovulation) estradiol levels increase, resulting in the epithelium increasing in thickness, slightly decreased pH, and thinner mucus. During the luteal phase (second part of a menstrual cycle, i.e., time after ovulation until menstruation), the thickness of the vaginal epithelium decreases, pH increases slightly within the normal range, and vaginal fluids become thicker [15].

Menopause

The natural aging process results in significant changes in the vagina, including a decrease in vaginal size, loss of elasticity, loss of vascularity, and a thinning of the mucosa. Glycogen is very low or completely absent, contributing to the change in vaginal microbiology and pH. Vaginal secretions become scant and watery, and the pH increases from 4.5–5.5 to 7.0–7.4. Resistance to bacterial and fungal infections is reduced due to the lower population of acidophilic organisms [16].

The mucus present in the vagina helps to keep mucoadhesive drug delivery forms attached to the vaginal wall for a longer period of time. Too large an amount and rapid turnover of the mucus, however, can also present a barrier and remove a drug from the site of delivery. Dosage forms can undergo different absorption due to the differing dissolution patterns in vaginal fluid. A comparison of vaginal inserts versus creams showed that creams have a longer contact time in the vagina [12]. The enzyme activity of the vaginal fluid is also a considerable factor in the design of vaginal drug delivery systems.

PHYSICOCHEMICAL FACTORS OF THE DRUG/DOSAGE FORM

The important physicochemical factors that can influence vaginal drug absorption include the molecular weight and size, lipophilicity, ionization, surface charge, chemical nature, and local action of the active ingredient. The transport mechanism of most vaginally absorbed substances is simple diffusion. Lipophilic substances are absorbed through the intracellular (or transcellular) pathway, whereas hydrophilic substances are absorbed through the intercellular (or paracellular) pathway or across aqueous pores present in the vaginal mucosa [17]. Also, receptor-mediated transport mechanisms can be involved in the absorption of some substances.

Because vaginal fluid contains a large amount of water, any drug intended for vaginal delivery requires a certain degree of water solubility. Regarding the size and molecular weight, it is generally accepted that low-molecular-weight lipophilic drugs are more likely to penetrate the vaginal wall and be absorbed than are large-molecular-weight lipophilic or hydrophilic drugs [18]. Because many drugs are weak electrolytes, vaginal pH may change their degree of ionization and affect the absorption of drug [19].

The characteristics of the dosage forms applied in the vagina also contribute to their residence time and the absorption of the active ingredient. Solutions and many of the conventional tablets and suppositories usually leak from the vaginal cavity shortly after application. This is due to the low viscosity of the dispersion that forms in the vaginal cavity after dissolution and/or disintegration of the dosage form. Bioadhesion is recognized as a great asset to increase the contact time between the dosage form and the vaginal wall, thus avoiding leakage. The shape of dosage forms is another factor that has significant influence on the drug absorption. The larger surface area a dosage form provides, the faster absorption is offered for the drug; absorption, of course, depends on many of the above-mentioned factors as well. All these attributes reflect the complex interrelationship between vaginal physiology and physicochemical properties of the drug/dosage form that must be considered when developing a vaginal delivery system.

CONVENTIONAL VAGINAL DOSAGE FORMS

Traditionally, solutions, suppositories, gels, foams, and tablets have been used as vaginal formulations for the treatment of local diseases. Ideally, a vaginal drug delivery system that is intended for local effect should distribute uniformly throughout the vaginal cavity. To achieve this, a semisolid or fast–dissolving solid system is preferred. A more modern type of vaginal dosage form is the vaginal ring, intended for systemic delivery of female hormones. A few vaginal ring products are available on the market. Table 14-1 gives some examples of the currently available vaginal dosage forms.

TABLE 14-1 Examples of currently available vaginal dosage forms				
Dosage Form	**Therapeutic Drug**	**Brand Name**	**Intended Use**	**Availability**
Solution (douche)	0.3% povidone-iodine	Summer's Eve Special Care Medicated Douche®	Minor vaginal irritation or itching	OTC
Cream	2% miconazole nitrate	Monistat 3-day Vaginal Cream®	Vaginal yeast infections (candidiasis)	OTC
Gel	0.75% metronidazole 4% or 8% gel of progesterone	MetroGel-Vaginal® Crinone®	Bacterial vaginosis Progesterone supplementation or replacement for infertile women with progesterone deficiency	Rx only Rx only
Foam	12.5% nonoxynol-9	VCF Vaginal Contraceptive Foam®	Contraception, spermicide	OTC
Suppository	20 mg dinoprostone per suppository 100 mg nonoxynol-9 per insert	Prostin E2® Encare Vaginal Contraceptive Inserts®	Termination of pregnancy from 12th to 20th gestational week Contraception, spermicide	Rx only OTC
Tablet	10.3 μg estradiol hemihydrate (=10 μg estradiol) per tablet	Vagifem®	Atrophic vaginitis due to menopause	Rx only
Capsule	600 mg fenticonazole nitrate per capsule	Gynoxin 600-mg Vaginal Capsule®	Vulvovaginal candidiasis	Rx only (Europe)
Vaginal ring	120 μg etonogestrel + 15 μg ethinyl estradiol per day 2 mg estradiol	Nuvaring® Estring®	Contraception Hormone replacement therapy	Rx only Rx only

OTC, over the counter; Rx prescription.

VAGINAL SOLUTIONS

Douching is the irrigation of vagina with a liquid possessing either cosmetic or medicinal actions. This cleaning technique has been practiced for some time, mainly for the treatment of inadequate vaginal hygiene, restoring the normal vaginal pH after vaginal infections, or simply cleaning [20]. This technique provides a number of cosmetic benefits, such as improving vaginal hygiene through mechanical cleansing action, soothing and refreshing the vaginal vault, and deodorizing. The common ingredients in douches are purified water and components that provide an acidic pH, including citric acid, sodium citrate, acetic acid (known as vinegar), lactic acid, sodium lactate, or boric acid [21]. Medicated douches may contain active ingredients as well, such as antimicrobial agents (cetylpyridinium chloride), spermicides (octoxynol-9), and antiseptics (povidone-iodine) [22]. These cleaning solutions for cosmetic or medicinal purposes are generally supplied in prefilled plastic containers with an applicator head.

Theoretically, douching is an advantageous technique that helps normalize vaginal pH and microflora; however, some concerns have arisen in the last decade. Because of the large volume of fluid, douches may wash away a variety of the vaginal defenses and can promote colonization of bacteria or alter vaginal pH, allowing pathogenic bacteria and yeast to proliferate. Douching has been associated with many adverse outcomes, including pelvic inflammatory disease, bacterial vaginosis, cervical cancer, low birth weight, preterm birth, HIV transmission, sexually transmitted infections (STIs), ectopic pregnancy, recurrent vulvovaginal candidiasis, and infertility [23]. The near-universal medical view is that douching is not needed for routine vaginal hygiene [24]. The current notion is that douching should not be practiced for normal vaginal hygiene because the vagina is naturally self-cleaning. Women with vaginal symptoms such as odor and yellow vaginal discharge should consult with a pharmacist or other health care professional to identify an underlying infection requiring treatment and a visit to the physician [23].

VAGINAL CREAMS, GELS, AND FOAMS

Many cosmetic and over-the-counter products are available as vaginal creams, gels, and foams, for example, antimicrobial agents, spermicides, and ingredients for the treatment of postmenopausal symptoms. These vaginal dosage forms can also contain hormones used as labor inducers; however, they are marketed as prescription-only medications.

Vaginal spermicide products are placed in the vagina before sexual intercourse to prevent pregnancy. Currently, the only safe and effective vaginal spermicide is nonoxynol-9. Products containing this ingredient function by two methods. First, they present a physical barrier to prevent sperms from entering the uterus. Second, they destroy sperm through their actions as nonionic surfactants [25]. The treatment of vaginal infections involves the application of nonprescription ingredients such as clotrimazole, miconazole, and butoconazole [26] and ingredients only available by prescription (e.g., metronidazole and clindamycin) [27]. The products are usually available in 1-, 3-, or 7-day formulations and are usually supplied with an applicator for convenient use. Labor inducers are used to assist in cervical ripening; examples include oxytocin, dinoprostone, and misoprostol [12].

Most vaginal dosage forms are messy to apply, might cause irritation and a burning sensation, and are sometimes embarrassing when they leak into undergarments. Furthermore, it is believed that creams and gels may not provide an exact dose because of non-uniform distribution and leakage. More recently, however, hydrogel-based controlled-release systems have received more attention. These hydrogels, when placed in an aqueous environment, swell and retain large volumes of water and release the drug in a controlled fashion. The use of controlled-release systems should reduce the occurrence of leakage and the number of applications [28].

VAGINAL SUPPOSITORIES, TABLETS, CAPSULES, AND INSERTS

A large number of vaginal medications are available in the form of tablets or suppositories. The terms "insert," "tablet," "suppository," and "capsule" are often used interchangeably; however, they are not exactly the same. Tablets are made of compressed powders (similarly to oral tablets) and are designed to disintegrate and dissolve in the vaginal fluids. They usually have oblong (**Figure 14–2, a** and **b**), round (**Figure 14–2c**), ovule (**Figure 14–2d**), or other (**Figure 14–2e**) shapes to ease administration. Vaginal capsules contain the active ingredient(s) in a gelatin shell that dissolves in the vaginal fluid. Vaginal tablets and capsules are also called inserts. The name refers to the method of application, that is, the dosage form is inserted into the vagina [29]. Vaginal suppositories are lipid-based formulations designed to melt in the vaginal cavity and release the drug for several hours. An important characteristic of vaginal suppositories that should be emphasized is their shape. For easier application, these suppositories usually have an almond-like shape (**Figure 14–2f**), unlike torpedo-shaped rectal suppositories. Vaginal inserts and suppositories are usually supplied with a plastic applicator that assists in the insertion of the dosage form; an applicator for Vagifem® vaginal tablet is shown in **Figure 14–3**.

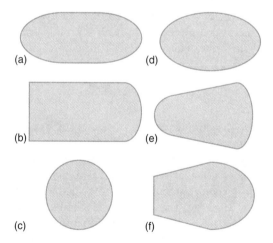

FIGURE 14-2 Different shapes of available vaginal tablets and suppositories: (a and b) oblong, (c) round, (d) ovule, (e) other, and (f) almond-like shape.

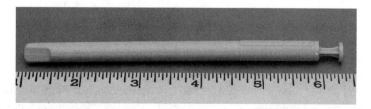

FIGURE 14-3 A plastic disposable applicator for the insertion of Vagifem® vaginal tablet (length in inches). To release the tablet from the applicator after insertion, the plunger (right end) needs to be pushed gently until a clicking sound is heard.

The most common use of vaginal inserts and suppositories is for the treatment of vaginal infections, similarly to the vaginal creams. A recent application of suppository systems is to induce cervical ripening before childbirth. Vaginal inserts and suppositories containing different species of lactobacilli are available for restoring normal pH and microbial balance. Vaginal suppositories containing dinoprostone are indicated for termination of pregnancy; this medication can only be used from the 12th through the 20th gestational week.

Vaginal inserts, suppositories, and some creams are marketed in kits in the pharmacies for the treatment of vaginal yeast infections. These kits consist of several cooling wipes for the genital area; the actual dosage form that contains the active ingredient, which should be inserted into the vagina using the applicator; and a cream for external use (i.e., outside the vagina).

As in the case of the semisolid preparations (vaginal creams and gels), the main disadvantages are leakage and relatively short contact time. These negative effects can be significantly improved by using mucoadhesive excipients, a more detailed discussion of which can be found under Recent Advances in Vaginal Drug Delivery, below.

VAGINAL RINGS

Vaginal rings are flexible, thin, and circular-shaped devices that are capable of releasing pharmacologically active agents into the systemic circulation in a controlled manner over an extended period of time (**Figure 14-4**). These devices are constructed to be self-inserted and placed around the upper part of the vagina (i.e., the cervix). It is important that the ring is in contact with the vaginal epithelium for the drugs to be absorbed into the systemic circulation. Vaginal rings are primarily used to deliver hormonal steroids as a modern method for contraception or for hormone therapy in postmenopausal women [30, 31]. A major advantage of using vaginal rings over oral administration of drugs is

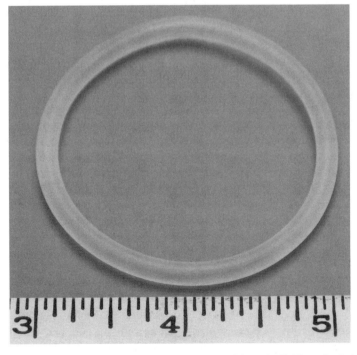

FIGURE 14-4 The intravaginal ring used for contraception (Nuvaring®). The ruler is in inches.

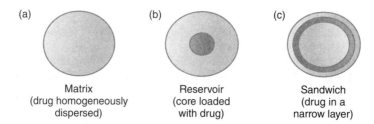

FIGURE 14-5 The different types of vaginal rings.

the improved adherence associated with the rings. Hormones delivered orally require intake on a daily basis. Vaginal rings, however, are able to rapidly attain peak plasma drug concentration and maintain a stable therapeutic level for several weeks, contributing to a more convenient dosing regimen for the patient. This leads to increased therapeutic efficacy and improved patient compliance. For contraceptive applications, the vaginal rings are normally kept in the vagina for 3 consecutive weeks and removed for a week to allow menstrual flow. An example is Nuvaring®, which contains a combination of two active ingredients, ethinyl estradiol and etonogestrel. Vaginal rings designed for hormone replacement therapy are placed in the vagina once every 3 months. Marketed products are Femring® and Estring®, both for the intravaginal delivery of estrogen.

The material for making vaginal rings is usually polymeric in nature. Traditionally, silicone elastomers, notably polydimethylsiloxane, have been used due to their biocompatible properties. Alternative materials such as thermoplastic elastomers, particularly poly(ethylene vinyl acetate), have recently emerged to ease the ring manufacturing process. There are three different types of vaginal ring devices: matrix, reservoir, and sandwich [30] (**Figure 14-5**). They can be distinguished by the method of drug incorporation and the release mechanism from the device. Vaginal rings of the matrix type contain drug homogeneously dispersed throughout the polymer matrix. Drug molecules near the surface are released faster than the ones located in the inner region of the matrix. This often creates an initial burst release. As time progresses, the pathway of the inner drug molecules diffusing through the polymer increases, leading to a decreased amount of drug released. The rate of drug release from matrices thus depends on both the amount of drug loaded in the matrix and the surface area of the device. To obtain a more constant release of drug, reservoir and sandwich rings have been developed. The reservoir-type devices are designed to consist of an outer polymer membrane encapsulating a core loaded with drug. The release of the drug can be controlled by varying the thickness of the rate-limiting membrane. In sandwich-type vaginal rings, the drug is incorporated in a narrow layer positioned between a nonmedicated central core and a thin, nonmedicated outer membrane. The close location of the drug to the surface is advantageous for drugs with poor polymer diffusion properties. Lower drug loading may also minimize side effects and be more cost-effective compared with matrix systems.

ADVANTAGES AND LIMITATIONS

The predominant advantage of vaginal delivery over oral delivery is that drugs do not undergo GI degradation and hepatic first-pass metabolism. Bypassing presystemic elimination is especially advantageous for progesterone and estrogen, because these steroids are rapidly metabolized after oral administration, leading to decreased bioavailability [32]. Avoiding the oral route also reduces the incidence and severity of GI side effects, so that intravaginal administration is preferable for drugs that produce GI irritation (for example, indomethacin).

In the therapy of vaginal disorders, localized treatment is most often desirable. Vaginal dosage forms allow drug delivery at the targeted site of action with minimal systemic absorption. This enhances the local therapeutic effect and reduces unfavorable side effects. The choice of vaginal treatment over oral treatment is especially important in pregnant women. In recurrent conditions, such as vaginal fungal infections, repeated therapy is necessary. In such cases, local vaginal treatment is therefore highly recommended during pregnancy.

The vaginal tract offers a large surface area, rich blood supply, and high permeability for low-molecular-weight drugs. These anatomical factors promote improved drug bioavailability and make the vaginal route a good alternative for systemic absorption of drugs. For instance, therapeutic proteins and peptides are prone to degradation in the GI tract. Although proteins and peptide drugs are of high molecular weight, vaginal delivery offers another option to oral administration in maintaining their systemic effects.

Vaginal delivery is also a favorable alternative to the parenteral route for certain drugs, such as calcitonin, oxytocin, luteinizing hormone–releasing hormone agonists, human growth hormones, and bromocriptine. Drug delivery by the vaginal route circumvents the inconvenience caused by pain, tissue damage, and possible infection associated with this invasive method. Moreover, vaginal dosage forms are easy to administer and allow the possibility of self-insertion and removal of the devices.

The vagina as the targeted site of drug delivery offer several advantages for drug therapy. Certain drawbacks, however, are associated with the physiological nature of the vagina that may challenge drug delivery. Factors such as cyclic variations, thickness and porosity of the epithelium, and volume, viscosity, and pH of the vaginal fluid affect the absorption process across the vaginal epithelium. Physiological changes in the intravaginal environment lead to considerable variability in the rate and extent of absorption of vaginally administered drugs. The most common problem with vaginal drug delivery is the premature discharge of the dosage forms so that sufficient therapeutic effect is not obtained. Low pH, microbial flora, and enzymatic activity in the vagina can affect the stability of the intravaginal delivery systems or devices. The permeability of the vaginal membrane depends on estrogen concentrations. This may influence the pharmacokinetics of drugs designed for systemic absorption. The inherent gender specificity with the delivery method is also an important perspective when designing vaginally administered drugs for systemic action. Other factors that need to be considered when developing vaginal dosage forms are local irritation of vaginal mucosa, cultural sensitivity and acceptability, personal hygiene, age, and the influence on sexual intercourse.

RECENT ADVANCES IN VAGINAL DRUG DELIVERY

New developments in vaginal drug delivery strive to overcome the disadvantages associated with conventional products, for example, by the use of bioadhesive systems. Traditionally, the vaginal route of drug delivery has been used for local treatment. The new trend observed in the past decade is the exploration of the vaginal cavity as a new route of administration for systemic effect of drugs, in particular, drugs subjected to extensive first-pass metabolism. One area of rigorous research in vaginal drug delivery is the prevention of HIV or other STIs. HIV infection is a significant health problem worldwide. Statistics on the HIV/AIDS epidemic from the World Health Organization estimates the number of people living with HIV in 2011 at 34.0 million, the number of new HIV infections at 2.5 million, and deaths due to AIDS at 1.7 million [33]. Despite sustained efforts, it has been estimated that no safe and effective HIV vaccine will be readily available in the near future [34, 35]. Obviously, there is a major need to develop other prophylactic methods to prevent and eradicate transmission of HIV.

BIOADHESIVE DRUG DELIVERY SYSTEMS FOR VAGINAL ADMINISTRATION

Common drawbacks to conventional vaginal formulations are low retention to the vaginal epithelium, leakage, and messiness, thereby causing inconvenience to the user and poor patient compliance. To overcome these problems, bioadhesive drug delivery systems have been developed. Bioadhesion has been defined as a state wherein two materials, one of them biological matter, are attached to each other for a prolonged time period [36]. One type of bioadhesion widely referred to in pharmaceutical sciences is mucoadhesion, in which the adhesion is to mucus or a mucosal membrane. The vaginal epithelium is considered a mucosal site and can therefore be exploited to improve the residence time of intravaginal drug delivery systems. Although the mechanism of mucoadhesion has been explained by a number of different theories, the general description of the mucoadhesion process is divided into two steps [36]. The initial step is the intimate contact between the mucoadhesive agent and the mucosal membrane (wetting), followed by a consolidation stage wherein the bond is strengthened by various physicochemical interactions. For this purpose, biocompatible polymers with mucoadhesive properties have been investigated extensively in novel intravaginal formulations. Polymers are able to swell when they come into contact with an aqueous environment and thereby exhibit controlled drug release. The chains of the polymer structure can interpenetrate the mucosal surface (physical entanglements), providing intimate contact and prolonging the vaginal residence. Mucoadhesive materials include polymers of synthetic, semisynthetic, and natural origin. Typically, these polymers are hydrophilic in nature with high molecular weights. The different types of polymers that have been investigated in vaginal delivery systems are listed in Table 14–2 [37].

Mucoadhesive polymers have been used in gels and tablets to increase the vaginal retention of the dosage forms. Bioadhesive vaginal tablets have been studied in the treatment of vaginal infections to provide a long-term effect at the site of infection,

TABLE 14-2 Mucoadhesive polymers tested in vaginal formulations	
Origin	**Polymer**
Synthetic	Poly(acrylic acid) derivatives (polycarbophil) Poly(ethylene glycol)
Semisynthetic	Cellulose derivatives (hydroxy methylcellulose, hydroxypropyl methylcellulose, carboxy methylcellulose)
Natural	Carrageenan Chitosan Gelatin Hyaluronic acid and derivatives Na alginate Pectin Starch Sulfated polysaccharides Tragacanth

allowing a reduction in dose and dose frequency. Moreover, local treatment is favorable to minimize the systemic side effects associated with oral antibacterial and antifungal formulations. In a randomized and placebo-controlled trial with 116 patients, Voorspoels and colleagues [38] found that a single application of metronidazole bioadhesive vaginal tablet was a valid alternative to oral administration in the treatment of bacterial vaginosis. The bioadhesive component consisted of synthetic polyacrylic acid.

Natural polymers have also been explored in vaginal formulations. The biopolymer chitosan exhibits several favorable properties, such as biocompatibility, mucoadhesivity, biodegradability, antibacterial activity, and nontoxicity, and has therefore often been investigated as a carrier system in vaginal tablets [39, 40]. Furthermore, polymers have been modified to improve the mucoadhesive properties with the introduction of thiol groups to their structure [39, 41]. Kast and colleagues [39] found that thiolated chitosan remained on vaginal mucosa for a longer period compared with the unmodified polymer. They explained the increased adhesion with the formation of disulfide bonds between the thiomer and the mucosal tissue.

A recent innovation in vaginal tablets combines the key concepts of bioadhesion and osmosis [42]. Tablets that release drugs based on osmotic principles are called osmotic pump tablets [43]. These devices consist of a semipermeable membrane that coats a core containing the active material. Water from bodily fluids enters the core through the membrane, generating an osmotic pressure in the core to induce the release of the drug substance through a predrilled orifice. Osmotic pump tablets thus have the ability to deliver drugs at a controlled manner (zero-order release rates) for prolonged periods. Based on this approach, Rastogi et al. [42] explored the use of osmotic pumps for the delivery of antiretrovirals to the vaginal mucosa. The core comprised the active substance together with the bioadhesive polymer hydroxypropyl cellulose. When water flowed through the membrane, the polymer swelled and created a drug-loaded gel that extruded through the orifice and slowly released the drug in the vaginal canal. In this way, the osmotic pump tablet was able to deliver the drug for several days after a single application—a duration that ranges between that of gels and intravaginal rings. The development of osmotic pump technology for vaginal antiretroviral therapy is a promising strategy as was demonstrated by positive results in a sheep model. This approach has great potential for further elaborate investigations.

The development of bioadhesive vaginal gels has brought about a few products on the market. Crinone® is a vaginal gel with sustained release of progesterone to promote fertility. A number of studies have shown that Crinone® gel exhibits the same effect as other progesterone preparations (capsules and intramuscular injection); however, reduced dosing intervals and less vaginal discharge were reported for Crinone® gels [44, 45]. These superior attributes are due to the retentive properties of the polymer carbophil. Another intravaginal gel on the market containing carbophil is Replens®, a vaginal moisturizer used by postmenopausal women to relieve discomfort related to vaginal atrophy, such as vaginal dryness and pain. Replens®, however, does not contain any hormonal agents. Several studies have evaluated the efficacy of Replens® and reported that the product is a good drug-free alternative to hormone replacement therapy [46–48].

Bioadhesive vaginal gel products are under investigation for several other applications [28]. Most promising are vaginal gels as microbicides. Microbicides are chemical agents used to protect against STIs, including HIV. A microbicidal vaginal gel can inactivate genital pathogens and offer a mechanism to prevent or reduce the transmission of STIs. Several microbicidal gels have been developed: Carraguard® contains carrageenan derived from seaweed, BufferGel® is a polyacrylic acid–based gel, and Pro 2000® contains synthetic naphthalene sulfonate polymer. Although these topical microbicides are considered nonirritating to vaginal mucosa and safe for use, clinical trials have failed to show efficacy at preventing HIV infection [49–51]. Studies have reported promising results with antiretroviral drugs (tenofovir, dapivirine) formulated as gels [52]. An important consideration of using gel formulations is the social aspect associated with a woman's ability to control the administration of the medications. Women may have limited ability to protect themselves due to social, economic, and legal factors. Although gel products are made for short-term use, women have an option to easily protect themselves without high costs or a partner's cooperation.

A novel bioresponsive hydrogel for microbicides has been described by Gupta and colleagues [53]. The so-called smart system is both temperature and pH sensitive. The hydrogel appears as a liquid at room temperature for easy application and gels when approaching body temperature. The increased viscosity improves the retention of the gel inside the vagina. Furthermore, the formulation exploits the pH difference between the vagina (pH 4–5) and semen (pH ~7.5). The hydrogel released entrapped content in response to a pH change, which is when the environmental pH changed from vaginal pH to the pH of semen, allowing for a semen-triggered release of the microbicide. Drug release and cytotoxicity studies were performed under simulated physiological conditions [53]. Promising results were reported; however, further investigations in a clinical setting are needed.

An acceptable alternative to gels and tablets in the prevention and treatment of vaginal problems is the use of vaginal films. Vaginal films are solid dosage forms designed to quickly dissolve in contact with vaginal fluids. They are most commonly square shaped with soft surfaces and edges that can be folded for insertion into the vagina without the need of an applicator. Film dosage forms for vaginal applications have been approved and mostly marketed as spermicidal products [54]. In recent years there has been a growing interest in vaginal film formulations for contraceptive, antimicrobial, and microbicidal purposes due to the female-controlled and user-friendly aspect of the dosage form [55]. Vaginal films are often preferred over other dosage forms due to patient comfort, portability, and ease of application, storage, and handling. Especially for microbicidal indication, effective prophylaxis requires products that women are likely to use. Moreover, the film manufacturing method is relatively mild, facilitating the incorporation of heat-sensitive drugs. Modern vaginal films use bioadhesive polymers in their formulations. This allows for the fabrication of thin, flexible strips that can prolong intravaginal retention by immediately forming a viscous, bioadhesive gel after film disintegration. The most common polymers used are polyacrylates, polyethylene glycol (PEG), polyvinyl alcohol, and cellulose derivatives. Despite several advantages associated with vaginal films, difficulties with film administration (sticking of the films to fingers) and complex manufacturing processes are issues that have limited their success as vaginal drug delivery systems.

In summary, bioadhesive polymeric systems allow for a relatively easy application of formulations directly to vaginal mucosa and retain the formulations at the site of action for sufficient absorption and bioavailability. This is an acceptable, feasible, and low-cost method for patients that reduces the discomfort and messiness associated with conventional systems. Until recently, only synthetic polymers have been included in marketed intravaginal products; however, more and more research is being conducted on natural polymers. These biopolymers can be expected to enter the market in modern bioadhesive vaginal applications.

NEW DEVELOPMENTS IN VAGINAL RINGS

Vaginal delivery to prevent HIV or other STIs has received strong interest over the past decade as a new route of administration of microbicides and antiretrovirals. Formulations of bioadhesive gels for vaginal delivery have been previously mentioned. Another strategy to combat the HIV/AIDS epidemic is by the use of vaginal rings. New ring designs have evolved through the need for improving the permeation of high-molecular-weight and/or relatively hydrophilic drugs such as HIV microbicides and antiretroviral agents. Dapivirine is a non–nucleoside reverse transcriptase inhibitor that has been incorporated in a vaginal ring formulation. Both matrix- and reservoir-type rings have been loaded with the drug and clinically evaluated [56]. Both types of rings were found to be safe and equally well tolerated for 28 days of use in eight women. The matrix ring was, however, able to deliver a larger amount of drug per unit mass of drug loaded.

More sophisticated multicomponent ring designs have been proposed [57]. One type is the coated pod-insert vaginal ring (**Figure 14-6a**). This device consists of a polymer-coated solid core of drug incorporated into a silicone elastomer ring. The drug cores are coated with layers of semipermeable poly(lactic acid) polymers. By changing the amount and composition of the polymer coating of the drug core and the number of drug pods in each ring, the amount of drug released from each ring can be adjusted. This structure makes it possible for release of multiple drugs of varying solubilities from the ring. Another type is called a rod- or tablet-insert vaginal ring (**Figure 14-6b**). These rings comprise one or more polymeric solid dosage forms, lyophilized polymer gel rods, and directly compressed tablets inserted into a silicone elastomer ring. The ring body acts mainly as a holder for insertion and retention of the solid dosage forms. The lyophilized gel rod inserts are potentially useful for incorporation of peptide- and protein-based drugs, as the dried product serves to stabilize the active ingredient.

NANOPARTICULATE DRUG DELIVERY SYSTEMS TO THE VAGINA

Nanoparticulate drug delivery systems are structures in the nanoscale size range, typically 10 to 200 nm, that are used to carry, transport, and deliver pharmaceuticals to their sites of action. Because of their extremely small size, nanoparticulate systems possess unique physical and chemical properties. The high surface area to volume ratio is especially important in the context of drug delivery. A large surface area of particles can increase drug solubility and absorption, hence improving drug bioavailability while reducing the dose and potential side effects. Nanoparticles also offer the ability to control and target drug delivery. The incorporation of therapeutic compounds in nanoparticles may also protect them from degradation and increase *in vitro* and/or *in vivo* stability.

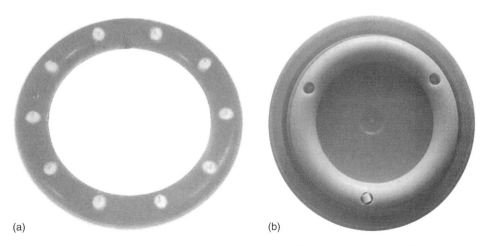

(a)   (b)

FIGURE 14-6 A coated pod-insert vaginal ring (a) and a tablet-insert vaginal ring (b). (Reprinted from *Antiviral Research*, 88S, Malcolm RK, Edwards KL, Kiser P, Romano J, Smith TJ, Advances in microbicide vaginal rings, S30–S39, 2010, with kind permission from Elsevier.)

The size, shape, surface charge, and chemical composition of nanoparticles are parameters that determine the biological fate of the drug.

The use of nanoparticles in drug delivery has been investigated for various routes of administration, including the vaginal route. Cu and collaborators [58] prepared poly(lactide-co-glycolic acid) (PLGA) polymer nanoparticles intended for vaginal delivery of potential antiviral drugs. The PLGA nanoparticles were also modified with the protein, avidin, or the polymer, PEG, on their surfaces to investigate the retention and penetration abilities of the nanoparticles in the vaginal tract. PLGA and PEG are well-studied materials approved by the U.S. Food and Drug Administration for use in pharmaceutical formulations. The researchers found that PEG-modified PLGA nanoparticles penetrated the vaginal epithelium faster and more efficiently than other nanoparticle formulations. They proposed that this type of polymer vehicle could be used for intravaginal delivery to enhance the transport through mucus and facilitate entry of potential antiviral agents or vaccinogens into cells.

More advanced intravaginal drug carrier systems have been explored by Yoo and colleagues [59], who investigated the vaginal delivery of pH-sensitive nanoparticles. These particles were developed to dissolve and release their loaded content in response to a pH change, from acidic pH in the vaginal cavity (pH 4) to physiological pH in vaginal epithelial cells (pH 7.4). The polymer Eudragit S-100, composed of methacrylic acid and methyl methacrylate, was chosen as the pH-sensitive material. The low pH of the vaginal cavity provides a hostile and harsh environment for acid labile compounds, such as peptide and protein drugs. Vaginal absorption may also be hindered by enzymatic degradation by various peptidases present in the vagina. The rationale for preparing pH-sensitive nanoparticles was to protect the drug from such degradation in the vaginal cavity and control the release of loaded drug in vaginal epithelial cells with tunable surface properties. The nanoparticles contained model drugs of both hydrophilic and hydrophobic characters. The *in vitro* experiments showed that both types of model compounds remained stable in the nanoparticles at vaginal pH but were rapidly released from the particles at a physiological pH [59]. Cellular uptake of nanoparticles by vaginal cells with no sign of cytotoxic activity was also revealed [59].

Zhang and collaborators [60] prepared a blend of PLGA and Eudragit S-100 nanoparticles as the platform to exhibit a pH-sensitive and sustained release of antiretrovirals. Tenofovir, an HIV reverse transcriptase inhibitor, was loaded in nanoparticles. The results from this study demonstrated the potential of a sustained-release and semen-triggered delivery system. The best formulation in terms of drug loading, *in vitro* release, and safety, however, exhibited only 24% encapsulation efficiency. Solid lipid nanoparticles have also been used to encapsulate tenofovir [61]. The idea of using solid lipid nanoparticles was to explore the lipidic nature of the nanoparticles to enhance penetration and, thus, cellular uptake of the hydrophobic drug. Still, relatively low encapsulation efficiency was observed. Future studies will likely concentrate on optimizing nanoparticles by improving encapsulation efficiency and proving the safety and efficacy of such nanoformulations.

One special type of pharmaceutical carrier that is widely recognized in the nanotechnology domain is liposomes. Liposomes are lipids, typically phospholipids, that spontaneously form spherical bilayer structures in the presence of an aqueous environment. Liposomes have been popular as nanocarriers because they are capable of incorporating a variety of hydrophilic and hydrophobic drugs. They are biocompatible and easy to prepare and design for a specific purpose. The use of liposomes in vaginal delivery has been explored for local treatment. The antifungal agents, clotrimazole and metronidazole, were loaded in liposomes for the local treatment of vaginal infections [62, 63]. The entrapment efficiency was found to be rather high for the lipophilic drug clotrimazole (64–71%); however, low entrapment was found for metronidazole (5–7%), which generally has low solubility in both lipophilic and hydrophilic media. The drug-loaded liposomes were further incorporated in a bioadhesive gel made of the polymer carbopol. It was shown that this vehicle improved the stability of the liposomes in simulated vaginal conditions and contributed to sustained release of the drugs.

More recently, a dual-sensitive liposome-based gel containing arctigenin was developed [64]. Arctigenin is a bioactive agent extracted from burdock fruit (*Fructus arctii*) that is commonly used in traditional Chinese medicine and reported to have antioxidant, anti-HIV, antitumor, and anti-inflammatory activity and therefore chosen to treat vaginal fungal infections. Arctigenin was incorporated into liposomes to improve its solubility. The liposomes were modified with the polymer methoxy-PEG 2000-hydrazone cholesteryl hemisuccinate. This material is stable at pH 7.4 but degrades under acidic vaginal conditions (pH 5.5). These pH-sensitive liposomes were further incorporated in a thermosensitive gel composed of poloxamers. Poloxamers are nonionic triblock copolymers composed of a central hydrophobic chain of poly(propylene oxide) flanked by two hydrophilic chains of poly(ethylene oxide). The mechanism of the formulation was to form a thermoresponsive gel at body temperature that retains the entrapped liposomes at the delivery site where the acidic environment will degrade the liposomes to release arctigenin. The entrapment efficiency of arctigenin in pH-sensitive liposomes was determined to be above 90% by Chen and colleagues [64]. The researchers showed that the *in vitro* release of the dual-sensitive liposome gel was constant at pH 5.0 for 3 days. Moreover, the liposome-based formulation was less toxic *in vitro* when compared with administration of the free drug as determined by a cell viability assay. The researchers suggested that this complex formulation could be used in developing effective formulations of hydrophobic drugs for vaginal delivery [64].

INTRAVAGINAL SMALL INTERFERING RNA DELIVERY

The ability of small interfering RNA (siRNA) molecules to knock down a gene of interest and thereby interfere with the expression of that gene has generated research in the prevention and treatment of therapeutically challenging diseases, such as neurodegenerative diseases, cancers, and viral infections. The mechanistic principles behind RNA interference and siRNA gene silencing is complex and beyond the scope of this chapter. Comprehensive reviews on this topic can be found elsewhere [65,66]. With regard to the therapeutic modalities for vaginal delivery, siRNA can be used as a novel, potent microbicidal agent. Studies have demonstrated its potential in the prophylaxis of viral infections caused by HIV, herpes simplex virus, and human papillomavirus. Therapeutic siRNA can suppress the viral life cycle by silencing specific viral genes, resulting in the prevention of viral entry into cells or the establishment of productive infections [67].

A significant hindrance to realizing siRNA-based therapy is the difficulty of delivering the effector molecules *in vivo*. Because of the physical and chemical barriers present in the vaginal environment, naked siRNA cannot be administered directly into the vaginal tract. To resolve problems such as poor stability and cellular uptake, nontargeted biodistribution, and low endosomal escape efficiency, the priority has been to develop drug delivery systems capable of transporting siRNA through extracellular and intracellular roadblocks. Two types of delivery systems have been proposed: viral and nonviral vectors. Viral vectors, including retrovirus, lentivirus, and adenovirus, have shown to be an efficient delivery strategy; however, the method is associated with the stimulation of undesirable immune reactions. Because of safety concerns, research efforts have been directed toward the engineering of nonviral vectors.

The development of nonviral platforms for intravaginal siRNA delivery is focused on three main structures: liposome-based cationic transfection agents, macromolecule conjugates, and polymeric nanoparticles. It has been shown that cationic siRNA–lipoplexes electrostatically interact with cell membranes promoting the intracellular transport of therapeutic siRNA and protecting mice from lethal herpes simplex virus type 2 infection [68]. The protection was short-lived, however, and the transfection lipid itself could enhance viral infection. Consequently, this led to the search for other transfection complexes. Wu et al. [69] coupled siRNA with cholesterol forming a neutral macromolecule that could deliver siRNA intracellularly through active transport mechanisms without eliciting an inflammatory response. The encapsulation of siRNA in nanoparticles also provided several advantages, in particular, physical protection of the siRNA molecules and the possibility of controlled drug release. Woodrow and coworkers [70] prepared PLGA nanoparticles for the vaginal delivery of siRNA and demonstrated the silencing of gene expression for at least 2 weeks after a single dose. Although this finding was considered a milestone, the PLGA nanoparticles exhibited low encapsulation efficiency and poor mucous penetration ability, resulting in decreased drug dose at the administered site. To overcome these hurdles, strategies such as surface modification of the nanoparticles to prevent hydrophobic interactions with mucin [71] and complexation of siRNA with the polycation polyethylenimin to decrease leakage from the nanoparticles [72] have been explored. Overall, significant success in *in vitro* and *in vivo* preclinical studies have been reported for the nonviral-based systems; however, major improvements are still needed to ensure the efficacy and safety of the siRNA-based therapeutics.

NOVEL DISPOSABLE INTRAVAGINAL DEVICE FOR STRESS URINARY INCONTINENCE

Stress urinary incontinence (SUI) is defined as loss of urine without bladder contraction and affects many women over the age of 50. The unintentional urine output is often induced by sneezing, coughing, lifting, or exercise and negatively influences the quality of life of these women. Pharmaceutical interventions and various vaginal and urethral inserts have been used in the nonsurgical treatment of SUI. Limited efficacy and poor patient compliance, however, especially in patients with mild to moderate SUI, are concerns related to the current therapies. In an attempt to find a well-tolerated, noninvasive, and effective alternative, a novel disposable intravaginal device has been developed for treating SUI. The device resembles a tampon and is comprised of a core, cover, and applicator (Figure 14-7).

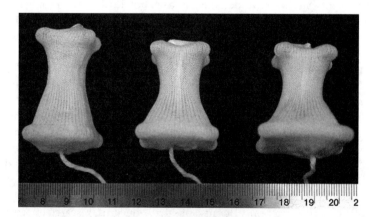

FIGURE 14-7 The tampon-like intravaginal device for urinary stress incontinence. (Adapted with kind permission from *Bentham Open: The Open Women's Health Journal*, 5, Farage MA, Aronstein WS, Miller KW, Karram M, Katz M, Hertzman B, A disposable intravaginal device for the management of stress urinary incontinence, 16–21, 2011.)

The core is made of resin designed to prevent the device from moving within the vagina. The cover around the core is made of soft, biocompatible nylon mesh that acts as a tension-free sling without obstructing urinary flow. A cotton string is attached to the distal end of the cover for removal of the device. The core and the cover are contained within a smooth applicator for easy self-insertion into the vagina. The safety and efficacy of the tampon-like device have been evaluated by several researchers [73, 74]. The studies reported that the device is easy to use, well tolerated, and effective in reducing SUI. Despite no content of therapeutic components, this novel device illustrates a different application of vaginal dosage forms in the treatment of local conditions.

SUMMARY

Applications of vaginal drug delivery systems have primarily been targeted to prevent or treat local and gynecological conditions such as vaginal infections, contraception, and postmenopausal symptoms. Drug candidates for vaginal administration are antimicrobials (metronidazole, clotrimazole, clindamycin), antiretrovirals (dapivirine, tenofovir), hormonal steroids (progesterone, estrogen), spermicidal agents for fertility control (nonoxynol-9, octoxynol-9), prostaglandins for cervical ripening and induction of labor, and an abortifacient and therapeutic proteins/peptides (gonadotropin-releasing hormones, calcitonin, and luteinizing hormone-releasing hormone). The vagina has been explored as an alternative route of administration because of the constraints of extensive first-pass metabolism with oral delivery. Recently, vaginal drug delivery in the prevention of HIV and other STIs has been intensively studied.

An ideal vaginal dosage form should be easy to administer and should distribute evenly and retain drug in the vaginal tract; it should also resist the acidic vaginal environment without being cytotoxic, exhibiting mucosal irritation, or imparting stains or offensive odors to the user. The vaginal conditions, including the viscosity, volume, and pH of the vaginal fluid; enzymatic activity and presence of microbial flora; and the thickness and porosity of the vaginal epithelium, can vary greatly from day to day; therefore, developing an ultimately accepted and advantageous dosage form is very challenging. Great efforts have been made to optimize the conventional dosage forms; however, no perfect vaginal dosage form has yet been developed. Apart from physiological constraints, physicochemical properties of the drug and/or the dosage form are factors that can be readily altered to address these challenges. Emerging knowledge in polymer science, nanotechnology, and biotechnology allow for more advanced approaches to circumvent the formulation obstacles. The use of bioadhesive systems and nanoparticulate structures are promising innovations in future perspectives of vaginal drug delivery. The efficacy and safety of these formulations remain to be proven in the clinic, however, before successful product development can be achieved.

ACKNOWLEDGMENTS

We gratefully acknowledge Erin Klorer at OB/GYN in the University of Toledo Physicians Group and Gabor Balazs for their invaluable assistance in the acquisition and preparation of the figures. We also thank Charisse Montgomery for her editorial assistance.

REVIEW QUESTIONS

1. List the advantages of vaginal drug delivery.
2. Give a general overview of the structure of the vagina.
3. Name some physicochemical factors that influence vaginal drug absorption.
4. What are vaginal rings? What are the benefits of vaginal rings over oral administration of drugs?
5. What are the challenges with vaginal drug delivery?
6. What are the advantages of nanosized particles for vaginal drug delivery?

REFERENCES

1. Hussain A, Ahsan F. The vagina as a route for systemic delivery. *J Control Release.* 2005;103:301–313.
2. Woolfson A, Malcolm RK, Gallagher, R. Drug delivery by the intravaginal route. *Crit Rev Ther Drug Carrier Syst.* 2000;17:509–555.
3. Washington N, Washington C, Wilson CG. *Vaginal and Intrauterine Drug Delivery.* London: Taylor and Francis; 2001.
4. Kistner R. The human vagina. In: *Physiology of the Vagina.* New York: North Holland Publishing; 1978:109–120.
5. Martini FH, Nath JL, Bartholome EF. The reproductive system. In: *Fundamentals of Anatomy and Physiology,* 9th ed. Upper Saddle River, NJ: Pearson Education; 2012:1061.
6. Alexander NJ, Baker E, Kaptein M, Karck U, Miller L, Zampaglione E. Why consider vaginal drug administration? *Fertil Steril.* 2004;82(1):1–12.
7. Sjoberg I, Cajander S, Rylander E. Morphometric characteristics of the vaginal epithelium during the menstrual cycle. *Gynecol Obstet Invest.* 1988;26(2):136–144.
8. Paavonen J. Physiology and ecology of the vagina. *Scand J Infect Dis* 1983;40(Suppl):31–35.
9. Horvat B, Multhaupt HAB, Damjanov I. Glycoproteins of mouse vaginal epithelium: differential expression related to estrous cyclicity. *J Histochem Cytochem.* 1993;41(9):1351–1357.
10. Bergh PA. Vaginal changes with aging. In: Breen JL, ed. *The Gynecologist and the Older Patient.* Gaithersburg, MD: Aspen Publishers; 1988:299–311.
11. Herbst AL, Mishell DR, Stenchever MA, Droegemueller W. *Comprehensive Gynecology,* 2nd ed. St. Louis, MO: Mosby-Year Book; 1992.
12. Chien YW, Lee CH. Drug Delivery: Vaginal route. In: Swarbrick J, ed. *Encyclopedia of Pharmaceutical Technology.* Vol. 1, 3rd ed. New York, NY: Marcel Dekker; 2002:1339–1361.
13. Sparks RA, Purrier BG, Watt PJ, Elstein M. The bacteriology of the cervix and uterus. *Br J Obstet Gynaecol.* 1977;84(9):701–704.
14. Martin HL, Richardson BA, Nyange PM, et al. Vaginal lactobacilli, microbial flora, and risk of human immunodeficiency virus type 1 and sexually transmitted disease acquisition. *J Infect Dis.* 1999;180(6):1863–1868.
15. Richardson JL, Illum L. The vaginal route of peptide and protein drug delivery. *Adv Drug Deliv Rev.* 1992;8(2–3):341–366.
16. Brown W. Microbial ecology of the normal vagina. In: Hafez ESE, Evans TN, eds. *The Human Vagina.* Amsterdam: North Holland Publishing; 1978:407–422.
17. Sassi AB, McCullough KD, Cost MR, Hillier SL, Rohan LC. Permeability of tritiated water through human cervical and vaginal tissue. *J Pharm Sci.* 2004;93(8):2009–2016.
18. Brannon-Peppas L. Novel vaginal drug release applications. *Adv Drug Deliv Rev.* 1993;11(1–2):169–177.
19. Hwang S, Owada E, Suhardja L, Ho NFH, Flynn GL, Higuchi WI. Systems approach to vaginal delivery of drugs. IV: Methodology for determination of membrane surface pH. *J Pharm Sci.* 1977;66(6):778–781.
20. Simpson T, Merchant J, Grimley Diane M, Oh MK. Vaginal douching among adolescent and young women: more challenges than progress. *J Pediatr Adolesc Gynecol.* 2004;17(4):249–255.
21. Zhang J, Hatch M, Zhang D, Shulman J, Harville E, Thomas AG. Frequency of douching and risk of bacterial vaginosis in African-American women. *Obstet Gynecol.* 2004;104(4):756–760.

22. Pray WS. *Nonprescription Product Therapeutics*, 2nd ed. Philadelphia, PA: Lippincott Williams and Wilkins; 2006:397–410.

23. Cottrell BH. An updated review of evidence to discourage douching. *Am J Maternal Child Nurs.* 2010;35(2):102–107.

24. Martino JL, Vermund SH. Vaginal douching: evidence for risks or benefits to women's health. *Epidemiol Rev.* 2002;24(2):109–124.

25. Smith JM, Huggins GR. Birth control. In: Barker LR, Burton JR, Zieve PD, eds. *Ambulatory Medicine*, 5th ed. Baltimore, MD: Williams & Wilkins; 1999:1423–1434.

26. Lipsky MS, Waters T. The "prescription-to-OTC switch" movement. Its effects on antifungal vaginitis preparations. *Arch Family Med.* 1999;8(4):297–300.

27. duBouchet L, McGregor JA, Ismail M, McCormack WM. A pilot study of metronidazole vaginal gel versus oral metronidazole for the treatment of *Trichomonas vaginalis* vaginitis. *Sex Transm Dis.* 1998;25(3):176–179.

28. Das Neves J, Bahia M. Gels as vaginal drug delivery systems. *Int J Pharm.* 2006;318(1):1–14.

29. Shitut NR, Rastogi SK, Singh S, Kang F, Singh J. Rectal and vaginal routes of drug delivery. In: Ghosh TK, Jasti BR, eds. *Theory and Practice of Contemporary Pharmaceutics.* Boca Raton, FL: CRC Press; 2005:455–478.

30. Malcolm RK. The intravaginal ring. *Drugs Pharm Sci.* 2003;126:775–790.

31. Kerns J, Darney P. Vaginal ring contraception. *Contraception.* 2011;83(2):107–115.

32. Adlercreutz H, Martin F. Biliary excretion and intestinal metabolism of progesterone and estrogens in man. *J Steroid Biochem.* 1980;13(2):231–244.

33. WHO. Global summary of the HIV/AIDS epidemics, December 2011. Available at: http://www.who.int/hiv/data/en/. Accessed October 30, 2013.

34. Girard MP, Osmanov S, Assossou OM, Kieny M-P. Human immunodeficiency virus (HIV) immunopathogenesis and vaccine development: a review. *Vaccine.* 2011;29(37):6191–6218.

35. Koff WC. HIV vaccine development: challenges and opportunities towards solving the HIV vaccine-neutralizing antibody problem. *Vaccine.* 2012;30(29):4310–4315.

36. Smart JD. The basics and underlying mechanisms of mucoadhesion. *Adv Drug Deliv Rev.* 2005;57(11):1556–1568.

37. Valenta C. The use of mucoadhesive polymers in vaginal delivery. *Adv Drug Deliv Rev.* 2005;57(11):1692–1712.

38. Voorspoels J, Casteels M, Remon JP, Temmerman M. Local treatment of bacterial vaginosis with a bioadhesive metronidazole tablet. *Eur J Obstet Gynecol Reprod Biol.* 2002;105(1):64–66.

39. Kast CE, Valenta C, Leopold M, Bernkop-Schnürch A. Design and in vitro evaluation of a novel bioadhesive vaginal drug delivery system for clotrimazole. *J Control Release.* 2002;81(3):347–354.

40. Perioli L, Ambrogi V, Pagano C, Scuota S, Rossi C. FG90 chitosan as a new polymer for metronidazole mucoadhesive tablets for vaginal administration. *Int J Pharm.* 2009;377(1):120–127.

41. Baloglu E, Ay Senyıgıt Z, Karavana SY, et al. In vitro evaluation of mucoadhesive vaginal tablets of antifungal drugs prepared with thiolated polymer and development of a new dissolution technique for vaginal formulations. *Chem Pharm Bull.* 2011;59(8):952–958.

42. Rastogi R, Teller RS, Mesquita PM, Herold BC, Kiser PF. Osmotic pump tablets for delivery of antiretrovirals to the vaginal mucosa. *Antiviral Res.* 2013;100(1):255–258.

43. Herrlich S, Spieth S, Messner S, Zengerle R. Osmotic micropumps for drug delivery. *Adv Drug Deliv Rev.* 2012;64(14):1617–1627.

44. Tavaniotou A, Smitz J, Bourgain C, Devroey P. Comparison between different routes of progesterone administration as luteal phase support in infertility treatments. *Hum Reprod Update.* 2000;6(2):139–148.

45. Simunic V, Tomic V, Tomic J, Nizic D. Comparative study of the efficacy and tolerability of two vaginal progesterone formulations, Crinone 8% gel and Utrogestan capsules, used for luteal support. *Fertil Steril.* 2007;87(1):83–87.

46. Nachtigall LE. Comparative study: Replens versus local estrogen in menopausal women. *Fertil Steril.* 1994;61(1):178–180.

47. Bygdeman M, Swahn M. Replens versus dienoestrol cream in the symptomatic treatment of vaginal atrophy in postmenopausal women. *Maturitas.* 1996;23(3):259–263.

48. Gelfand M, Wendman E. Treating vaginal dryness in breast cancer patients: results of applying a polycarbophil moisturizing gel. *J Women's Health.* 1994;3(6):427–434.

49. Skoler-Karpoff S, Ramjee G, Ahmed K, et al. Efficacy of Carraguard for prevention of HIV infection in women in South Africa: a randomised, double-blind, placebo-controlled trial. *Lancet.* 2008;372(9654):1977–1987.

50. McCormack S, Ramjee G, Kamali A, et al. PRO2000 vaginal gel for prevention of HIV-1 infection (Microbicides Development Programme 301): a phase 3, randomised, double-blind, parallel-group trial. *Lancet.* 2010;376(9749):1329–1337.

51. Karim SSA, Richardson BA, Ramjee G, et al. Safety and effectiveness of BufferGel and 0.5% PRO2000 gel for the prevention of HIV infection in women. *AIDS.* 2011;25(7):957–966.

52. Adams JL, Kashuba ADM. Formulation, pharmacokinetics and pharmacodynamics of topical microbicides. *Best Pract Res Clin Obstet Gynaecol.* 2012;26(4):451–462.

53. Gupta KM, Barnes SR, Tangaro RA, et al. Temperature and pH sensitive hydrogels: an approach towards smart semen-triggered vaginal microbicidal vehicles. *J Pharm Sci.* 2007;96(3):670–681.

54. Garg S, Goldman D, Krumme M, Rohan LC, Smoot S, Friend DR. Advances in development, scale-up and manufacturing of microbicide gels, films, and tablets. *Antiviral Res.* 2010;88:S19–S29.

55. Machado RM, Palmeira-De-Oliveira A, Martinez-De-Oliveira J, Palmeira-De-Oliveira R. Vaginal films for drug delivery. *J Pharm Sci.* 2013;102(7):2069–2081.

56. Nel A, Smythe S, Young K, et al. Safety and pharmacokinetics of dapivirine delivery from matrix and reservoir intravaginal rings to HIV-negative women. *J Acquired Immune Defic Syndr.* 2009;51(4):416–423.

57. Malcolm RK, Edwards KL, Kiser P, Romano J, Smith TJ. Advances in microbicide vaginal rings. *Antiviral Res.* 2010;88:S30–S39.

58. Cu Y, Booth CJ, Saltzman WM. In vivo distribution of surface-modified PLGA nanoparticles following intravaginal delivery. *J Control Release.* 2011;156(2):258–264.

59. Yoo JW, Giri N, Lee CH. pH-sensitive Eudragit nanoparticles for mucosal drug delivery. *Int J Pharm.* 2011;403(1):262–267.

60. Zhang T, Sturgis TF, Youan BBC. pH-Responsive nanoparticles releasing tenofovir intended for the prevention of HIV transmission. *Eur J Pharm Biopharm.* 2011;79(3):526–536.

61. Alukda D, Sturgis T, Youan BBC. Formulation of tenofovir-loaded functionalized solid lipid nanoparticles intended for HIV prevention. *J Pharm Sci.* 2011;100(8):3345–3356.

62. Pavelić Ž, Škalko-Basnet N, Schubert R. Liposomal gels for vaginal drug delivery. *Int J Pharm.* 2001;219(1):139–149.

63. Pavelić Ž, Škalko-Basnet N, Jalšenjak I. Characterisation and in vitro evaluation of bioadhesive liposome gels for local therapy of vaginitis. *Int J Pharm.* 2005;301(1):140–148.

64. Chen D, Sun K, Mu H, et al. pH and temperature dual-sensitive liposome gel based on novel cleavable mPEG-Hz-CHEMS polymeric vaginal delivery system. *Int J Nanomed.* 2012;7:2621–2630.

65. Boutros M, Ahringer J. The art and design of genetic screens: RNA interference. *Nat Rev Genet.* 2008;9(7):554–566.

66. Whitehead KA, Langer R, Anderson DG. Knocking down barriers: advances in siRNA delivery. *Nat Rev Drug Discov.* 2009;8(2):129–138.

67. Yang S, Chen Y, Ahmadie R, Ho EA. Advancements in the field of intravaginal siRNA delivery. *J Control Release.* 2013;167(1):29–39.

68. Palliser D, Chowdhury D, Wang Q-Y, et al. An siRNA-based microbicide protects mice from lethal herpes simplex virus 2 infection. *Nature.* 2005;439(7072):89–94.

69. Wu Y, Navarro F, Lal A, et al. Durable protection from herpes simplex virus-2 transmission following intravaginal application of siRNAs targeting both a viral and host gene. *Cell Host Microbe.* 2009;5(1):84–94.

70. Woodrow KA, Cu Y, Booth CJ, Saucier-Sawyer JK, Wood MJ, Saltzman WM. Intravaginal gene silencing using biodegradable polymer nanoparticles densely loaded with small-interfering RNA. *Nat Mater.* 2009;8(6):526–533.

71. Yu T, Wang Y-Y, Yang M, et al. Biodegradable mucus-penetrating nanoparticles composed of diblock copolymers of polyethylene glycol and poly (lactic-co-glycolic acid). *Drug Deliv Transl Res.* 2012;2(2):124–128.

72. Patil Y, Panyam J. Polymeric nanoparticles for siRNA delivery and gene silencing. *Int J Pharm.* 2009;367(1):195–203.

73. Ziv E, Stanton SL, Abarbanel J. Efficacy and safety of a novel disposable intravaginal device for treating stress urinary incontinence. *Am J Obstet Gynecol.* 2008;198(5):594.e591–594.e597.

74. Farage MA, Aronstein WS, Miller KW, Karram M, Katz M, Hertzman B. A Disposable Intravaginal Device for the Management of Stress Urinary Incontinence. *Open Women's Health J.* 2011;5:16–21.

15

DRUG DELIVERY TO THE CENTRAL NERVOUS SYSTEM: BREAKING DOWN THE BARRIER

MOHAMED ISMAIL NOUNOU, CHRIS E. ADKINS, TORI B. TERRELL-HALL, KACI A. BOHN, AND PAUL R. LOCKMAN

CHAPTER OBJECTIVES

Upon completing this chapter, the reader should be able to

▶ Describe the structure of the blood–brain barrier (BBB) and explain its functions, importance, significance, and drawbacks.

▶ Explain anatomical, physiological, and pharmacological mechanisms through which the BBB protects the central nervous system (CNS).

▸ Explain CNS drugs' physicochemical criteria governing their uptake into the brain across the BBB.

▸ Understand the major effect of lipophilicity on CNS penetration.

▸ Describe Lipinski's "rule of five" and its importance.

▸ Describe the different current strategies for CNS drug delivery.

▸ Explain interstitial drug delivery methods and their pros and cons.

▸ Describe the different chemical modification strategies to enhance CNS drug delivery.

▸ Enumerate various currently investigated targeting moieties that can enhance CNS drug delivery, and explain their mechanism of action and the reasoning behind using them.

▸ Enumerate novel drug delivery systems and their functions, mechanisms, importance, and advantages.

▸ Understand the flexibility of novel drug delivery systems, and how they can be tailor-designed to enhance CNS drug delivery.

▸ Define prodrugs, lipidization strategy, liposomes, solid lipid nanoparticles, targeting moieties, transferrin, OX26, and influx and efflux transporters.

CHAPTER OUTLINE

INTRODUCTION

On an anatomical level, the central nervous system (CNS) consists of the brain and the spinal cord, with some classifications including the retina and the cranial nerves. Our CNS creates and represents most of what we can associate with being a human. The CNS is the main control of our reality and entity. It coordinates the activity of all parts of the body of animals by interpreting, analyzing, and reacting to the different and overwhelming amount of information and actions through the various input sensory organs [1, 2].

The first known components of the CNS were the meninges, the external surface of the brain, the cerebrospinal fluid (CSF), and the intracranial pulsations, which were detailed in the Ancient Egyptian medical text entitled Edwin Smith Papyrus [3–7], which is dated 1500 BC to Dynasties 16 and 17 of the Second Intermediate Period in Ancient Egypt. In this papyrus the word "brain" appeared for the first time in any written language [8, 9].

The CNS is actually multiple organs that include the brain, spinal cord, and the CSF. The brain plays a central role in the regulation and control of most body functions, including awareness, movements, sensations, thoughts, speech, and memory. The spinal cord is connected to the brain through the brainstem and runs through the spinal canal. The leptomeninges surround the brain and the spinal cord. The CSF surrounds the brain and the spinal cord and also circulates within the cavities of the CNS. It circulates between two meningeal layers called the pia mater and the arachnoid. The outer, thicker layer serves the role of a protective shield and is called dura mater (Figure 15-1).

The basic unit of the CNS is the neuron (nerve cell). Billions of neurons allow different parts of the body to communicate with each other via the brain and the spinal

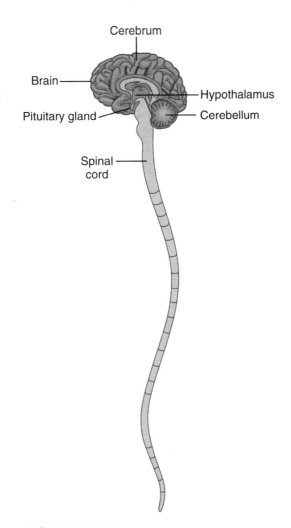

FIGURE 15-1. The central nervous system.

cord. A fatty material called the "myelin" coats nerve cells to insulate them and to facilitate rapid communication.

The brain and the spinal cord are securely shielded within the cranial skull bones. Further, the CNS is safeguarded against potentially toxic and harmful substances by the presence of two barrier systems: the blood–brain barrier (BBB) and the blood–CSF barrier [10].

Although these mechanisms protect the CNS against the entry of undesirable chemicals, these barriers also represent a hurdle to efficient therapeutic drug delivery. In spite of research efforts to overcome these barriers, patients suffering from fatal and/or debilitating CNS diseases, such as brain tumors, Parkinson's and Alzheimer's diseases, HIV encephalopathy, epilepsy, cerebrovascular diseases, and neurodegenerative disorders, far outnumber those dying of systemic cancers or heart disease [11, 12].

The global market for CNS drugs is now one of the largest, high-selling, money-making therapeutic sectors, with sales estimated at almost $92 billion in 2007 [13–15]. In spite of the financial and therapeutic potential, commercialization of CNS drugs is difficult because of poor delivery methods and the inability of therapeutic agents to cross the BBB. The BBB has a structurally unique vasculature compared with peripheral blood vessels in the rest of the body, which limits passive diffusion of many therapeutic agents into the brain [16, 17]. Therefore, the development of successful methods to enhance drug delivery to the brain across the BBB is paramount to the treatment of various CNS disorders.

Presently, there are two general strategies to move drugs across the BBB. Invasive techniques rely primarily on disrupting BBB integrity by direct intracranial drug delivery through intracerebroventricular, intracerebral, or intrathecal administration. In comparison, noninvasive methods include modification of a drug's molecular structure (i.e., lipophilic analogues, prodrugs, chemical drug delivery systems, carrier-mediated drug delivery, receptor/vector mediated drug delivery, and intranasal drug delivery) [18].

BLOOD–BRAIN BARRIER

The BBB restricts the passive diffusion of hydrophilic and charged compounds from inside the capillary into the brain [19]. The BBB has a unique anatomical structure compared with other blood vessels. One of the hallmark structural features of the BBB is the near-complete sealing of the luminal vascular endothelial cells by tight junction protein complexes (Figure 15-2). These complexes are made up of multiple proteins, including occludin, claudins [20], and intercellular junctional adhesion molecules [21]. The sealing of the luminal endothelial cells of the BBB is so effective that transendothelial electrical resistance (a measure of how tight a capillary is sealed) is orders of magnitude higher than that of the peripheral capillaries [22]. Further, unlike peripheral capillaries, brain capillaries generally lack fenestrations [23, 24] and have a relatively low pinocytic activity. Taken together, if a drug is to cross the BBB, it typically has to dissolve or diffuse through the endothelial cell membrane on the luminal side of the BBB (cell next to the blood). In addition to the endothelial cell, astrocytic foot processes, pericytes, and the presence of neurons provide even more restriction for paracellular diffusion [25–27].

In addition to the physical barriers found at the BBB, there are also efflux transport proteins ("pumps") and enzymatic proteins in the BBB vascular endothelia [28–30] that limit drug penetration into the brain. Efflux transporters actively move molecules from the endothelia back into blood. These pumps are ubiquitous at the BBB and limit the entry of a broad range of anticancer, antiviral, antibacterial, antiepileptic, and analgesic drugs into

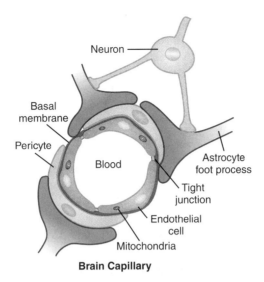

Brain Capillary

FIGURE 15-2. A cross-section of a brain capillary, which represents the structure of the blood–brain barrier (BBB). The BBB does not represent a distinct organ but rather is a functional concept.

the CNS [31, 32]. The primary efflux protein transporters implicated at limiting drug entry into the brain are P-glycoprotein (ABCB1), breast cancer resistant protein (ABCG2), multidrug resistant proteins (ABCC1–6), and organic anion transporter. In addition, other transporters implicated in this category are organic anion transporter polypeptide, equilibrative nucleoside transporter, and concentrative nucleoside transporter [33]. The BBB also has a high expression of numerous enzymes that break down or "inactivate" several drug molecules before they can reach the brain parenchyma [34–36]. Overcoming efflux transporters and inactivation enzymes is a current focal point of research.

Although there are restrictions for compounds to gain access to brain, there are mechanisms that can be exploited to facilitate brain penetration. The BBB has a high number of proteins that can shuttle small nutrient-based molecules from blood to brain [24, 37]. The major endogenous influx transporters at the BBB are broadly classified into two categories:

1. Influx transporters, which translocate various polar nutrients (glucose, amino acids, monocarboxylic acids), vitamins, or hormones from blood into the brain across the BBB [38–40]
2. Receptor mediated transporters, which transport various macromolecules into the brain (e.g., insulin, leptin, transferrin, etc.) [41, 42]

In summary, the BBB highly regulates the entry and exit of compounds in and out of the brain by a multitude of efflux and influx transporters that can be found both on the luminal (blood side) and abluminal membranes (brain side) of the capillary endothelium.

DRUG DELIVERY TO THE CNS

IMPORTANCE

The global demand for CNS medications has risen remarkably and stands to rise farther because over 1.5 billion people around the world are likely to suffer from at least one or more CNS diseases in the future [43]. The marked increase in the number of people aged over 65 years (the "baby boomer" effect) is a leading reason for an increased demand of more safe and effective medicines for CNS disorders. Further, the incidence of primary and metastatic brain tumors has dramatically increased over the past decade. More than 600,000 people, approximately 209 out of every 100,000, in the United States are currently living with a brain tumor. An estimated 66,290 new cases of primary brain tumors were expected to be diagnosed in 2012. Additionally, brain tumors are the second leading cause of cancer-related deaths in people under the age of 20 and in men aged 20 to 30 and the fifth leading cause of cancer-related deaths in women aged 20 to 39 [44]. Also, advances in understanding the causes and treatment approaches to CNS disorders have fueled the pharmaceutical interest in this field [10].

BBB AND DRUG DEVELOPMENT

In spite of the increasing need for efficient and safe CNS therapeutic agents, the problem of getting drugs through the BBB has significantly limited development of drugs. The physicochemical features of CNS drugs that govern their ability to penetrate the BBB were extensively reviewed in 1989 by Gupta [45]. The Hansch approach was one of the first techniques that tried to quantify BBB penetration by using quantitative structure-activity relationship (QSAR) equations to correlate biological activity of CNS drugs to variations in the drugs' physical and/or structural properties [46, 47]. A large number of parameters were included in Hansch QSAR equations such as lipophilicity, area, molecular volume and flexibility, charge, permeability, pharmacokinetic parameters, metabolic stability, protein binding, and metabolic liability.

The molecules degree of lipophilicity is crucial for CNS penetration [18, 45]. The log P value (the octanol–water partition coefficient, P) is a common measure of lipophilicity because it shows where the molecule prefers to exist in either the aqueous (blood) and lipid membrane environments. The role of log P has been shown to be the governing factor for CNS penetration for anesthetics, barbiturates, and benzodiazepines [48]. Hansch and Leo [49] demonstrated BBB penetration is optimal when log P values range from 1.5 to 2.7, with a mean value of 2.1.

Typically, CNS drugs have smaller molecular weights compared with other drugs. The reduced size allows better passive diffusion across the BBB, notably when the molecular mass is below 500 Da [50]. Hydrogen bonding (polar surface area, hydrogen bond donor, and acceptor counts) also affects CNS penetration. Increasing hydrogen bonding decreases BBB penetration. On average, the current commercially available CNS drugs have oxygen and nitrogen atom counts of 4.32, a polar surface area of 16.3%, 2.12 hydrogen bond acceptors, and 1.5 hydrogen bond donors [51].

Based on these factors, a "rule of five" was developed by Lipinski et al. [52] to correlate a drug candidate's physicochemical parameters with its absorption, permeability, and pharmacologic efficacy. According to Lipinski's "rule of five," a desirable absorption and BBB penetrance is likely if

- Molecular weight ≤500
- Oil–water distribution coefficient (log P) ≤5
- Number of hydrogen bond donors ≤5 (expressed as the sum of OHs and NHs)
- Number of hydrogen bond acceptors ≤10 (expressed as the sum of Ns and Os)
- Number of rotatable bonds ≤10

The "rule of five" was not originally developed to predict CNS activity; instead, it aimed to provide a general rule for almost all oral drugs to correlate a drug candidate's physicochemical parameters with its absorption, permeability, and pharmacological efficacy. This rule was further modified by Lipinski [53] for good CNS penetration using a set of 1,500 drugs that were filtered from the U.S. Adopted Name or Nonproprietary Names databases. The modified rule stated that CNS penetration is expected if

- Molecular weight ≤400
- Log P ≤5
- Number of hydrogen bond donors ≤3
- Number of hydrogen bond acceptors ≤7

Pajouhesh and Lenz [48] reviewed and summarized all factors that can contribute to successful CNS therapy. These attributes are summarized in **Table 15-1**.

DRUG CLASSES THAT PENETRATE THE CNS AND RESULT IN SIDE EFFECTS

Beta-blockers (e.g., propranolol) are good examples of a class of drugs that have the potential to generate CNS side effects. Beta-blockers are widely used, well tolerated, and provide efficient treatments for a variety of cardiovascular and noncardiovascular disorders. Propranolol, however, is a small-molecular-weight lipophilic beta-blocker [54] shown both in animals and humans to readily cross the BBB and produce the CNS effects of insomnia, nausea, depression, vivid dreaming, and memory loss [55, 56]. Atenolol, which is less hydrophobic than propranolol, does not pass through the BBB to a large extent and therefore has very few CNS side effects [57].

H_1 antihistamines represent a second example of a drug class with a therapeutic target outside the CNS but induce CNS side effects. Antihistamines have been categorized

TABLE 15-1 Factors governing successful CNS therapeutic drugs

Factors	Recommended Values
Potency	Subnanomolar level
Molecular weight	<450
Hydrophilicity and log P	Minimal hydrophobicity (clog P < 5)
Hydrogen bonding	Number of H-bond donor < 3 Number of H-bond acceptor < 7 Number of rotatable bonds < 8 H-bonds < 8
Charge	pKa, neutral or basic with pKa 7.5–10.5 (excluding acidic moieties)
Polar surface area	<60–70 Å^2
Metabolic stability	P-450 enzyme cytochrome inhibition < 50% at 30 μM Should not be a potent CYP3A4 inducer Should not be metabolized by CYP2D6 Should not be an efficient P-glycoprotein substrate (*in vivo*)
Protein binding	Should not have a high affinity to serum albumin (Kd < 10 μM)
Aqueous solubility	>60 μg/mL
Effective permeability	>1 × 10^{-6} cm/s

into first- and second-generation drugs according to their pharmacokinetic properties, structural characteristics, and side effects. The effects exerted on the CNS by these therapeutic agents are primarily determined by their capacity to cross the BBB and bind to the central H_1 receptors [58–60]. First-generation antihistamines (e.g., astemizole [Hismanal®], fexofenadine [Allegra®], and diphenhydramine [Benadryl®]) are lipid soluble, which provides an enhanced ability to cross the BBB and then exert the typical central side effects such as drowsiness and loss of coordination. Unlike first-generation antihistamines, second-generation antihistamines (e.g., loratidine [Claritin®]) are more lipophobic and therefore lack the ability to appreciably cross the BBB, thus failing to produce adverse effects in the CNS [18, 59, 60].

CURRENT STRATEGIES FOR CNS DRUG DELIVERY

Systemic drug administration, intrathecal or intraventricular administration, and polymer implantation are the most common CNS drug delivery techniques that are currently used (**Figure 15-3**) [61–63]. The most typical route of administration to the CNS is systemic delivery. Unfortunately, this drug delivery approach suffers from systemic toxicity, nontargeted delivery, and the inability to penetrate the BBB. On the other hand, diffusion-dependent methods such as intrathecal or intraventricular administration along with polymer implantation also suffer from nontargeted distribution, non-uniform drug dispersion, and ineffective volumes of distribution [64].

INTERSTITIAL DELIVERY

Interstitial delivery is an invasive technique that involves administration of therapeutic agents directly into the brain interstitium. This delivery strategy helps a drug to bypass the BBB and will theoretically yield high intracranial drug concentrations while reducing systemic toxicity.

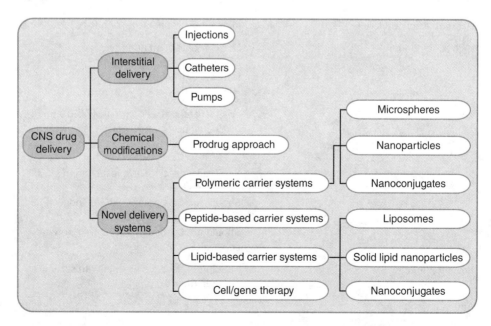

FIGURE 15-3 Schematic flow chart of current CNS drug delivery techniques.

The MiniMed PIMS® pump system represents one example of an interstitial drug delivery to the CNS. It uses a solenoid (coil wound into a tightly packed helix) pumping mechanism. Another example is the Medtronic SynchroMed™ pump system, which delivers drugs via a peristaltic mechanism. Creating and maintaining a continuous pressure gradient during interstitial drug infusion is the key factor to effective drug delivery to the CNS [65–68]. The resulting pressure gradient establishes fluid convection through the brain interstitium and, therefore, facilitates efficient drug delivery [69, 70].

Cranial catheters can be important tools for delivering drugs and imaging agents to the brain. This approach has been widely tested for timed-release chemotherapy to deliver drug directly to the tumor through a catheter implanted in the brain that is connected to a drug reservoir placed underneath the scalp [67, 71]. Currently, some companies such as NexGen™ are developing advanced cranial catheters such as their EViTAR™ neurotrauma device for monitoring and treating patients with traumatic head injury. It is designed to be a multifunctional single-catheter–based system offering drug delivery, CSF drainage, intracranial pH, pressure and metabolic monitoring, and high-resolution tissue perfusion imaging [72].

A more recent technique for interstitial drug delivery is the use of polymeric biodegradable implants. Intracranially implanted polymeric drug formulations bypass the BBB and locally release a therapeutic agent to establish a sustained concentration in the brain [73, 74]. An early example of polymeric implants in the brain is carmustine (BCNU) [75]. Brem and Gabikian [74] showed the carrier system had a protective effect to BCNU by slowing down its degradation kinetics. Compared with systemic delivery, the interstitial delivery extended BCNU half-life by orders of magnitude. Moreover, it provided sustained drug delivery over 2 to 3 weeks and higher local concentrations in the brain. The main drawback to this approach is the invasive nature of a surgical craniotomy [73–75].

CHEMICAL MODIFICATIONS

Chemical drug delivery systems are a novel approach to target delivery of therapeutic agents to the CNS, thus enabling them to circumvent the BBB. Prodrugs represent the main premise for chemical drug delivery systems. The term "prodrug" was first introduced in 1958 to describe compounds that undergo biotransformation before exerting their therapeutic activity [76]. Prodrugs involve chemically transforming the active drug, which does not have the ability to cross the BBB, to an inactive chemical derivative through chemical modifications. The prodrug should be generally comparable in size with the original molecule and facilitate its passage through the BBB. Finally, when the prodrug reaches its target site, it should be easily broken down or metabolized to its active compound through multistep enzymatic and/or chemical transformations [77] (Figure 15-4).

The design of a successful prodrug to circumvent the BBB involves one of these strategies [77–79]:

- Lipidization strategy
- Use of endogenous transporters in the CNS prodrug design
- Use of receptor-mediated prodrug delivery
- Use of antibodies in CNS prodrug design

The lipidization strategy involves the introduction of a lipophilic moiety that facilitates BBB penetrance and the trapping of drugs in the brain. One of the best examples of the lipidization approach is the diacetylated form of morphine, also known as heroin. Heroin, the lipophilic prodrug of morphine, exhibits a permeability coefficient that is 100-fold higher than morphine [80]. Dihydrotrigonelline (1,4-dihydro-*N*-methylnicotinic acid)

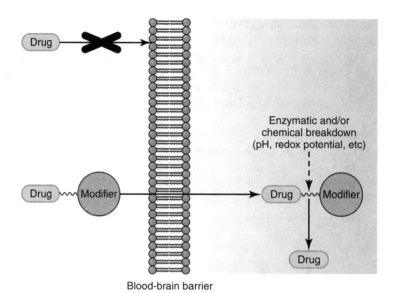

FIGURE 15-4 A representative illustration of the prodrug concept. The drug modifier is generally pharmacologically inactive. Enzymatic or chemical activity break down the drug-modifier prodrug to free the active drug based on the physiological conditions of the target tissue (reduced pH, high redox potential, degradative enzymes, etc.).

uses bioremovable lipophilic-targeting moieties that result in a prodrug that crosses the BBB more efficiently due to its lipophilic nature. Pop et al. [81] chemically conjugated penicillinase-resistant semisynthetic penicillins through esterification of the penicillin's hydroxyl group with the dihydrotrigonelline carrier to produce a prodrug that is more lipophilic than the parent drug. This prodrug improved the parent compound penetration into the CNS in rat and rabbit [81]. The use of lipidization approaches in the design of CNS-targeted prodrugs has been investigated with a wide variety of hydroxy- and amino-containing drugs [81–84]. This approach has successfully increased brain targeting for different drug moieties such as ganciclovir [85] and estradiol [86].

The second approach is the use of endogenous transporters in the design of prodrugs for CNS delivery. Several specific endogenous influx transporters, mainly nutrients, amino acids, glucose, and vitamins, have been identified at the BBB [87]. This approach involves the conjugation of an endogenous transporter substrate to the active drug molecule. The large neutral amino acid transporter LAT1 is an efficient transporter for L-amino acids. L-dopa, an α-amino acid derivative of dopamine, readily crosses the BBB via LAT1. The glucose transporter GLUT1 is another influx transporter used in the prodrug approach. GLUT1 transports glucose through the BBB with one of the highest transport capacities of all transporters in the BBB [88, 89]. This renders GLUT1 an extremely attractive transporter for prodrug delivery. Glycosylation strategies are also used to increase permeability of dopamine across the BBB through the use of a galactose dopamine conjugate [90, 91].

Receptor-mediated CNS drug delivery also takes advantage of the endogenous receptors located at the BBB. This strategy involves coupling of BBB receptor–specific substrates to therapeutic molecules. The anti-rat transferrin receptor antibody OX26 has been widely used in receptor-mediated transcytosis becasue the transferrin receptor is highly expressed on brain capillaries [92]. Saito et al. [92] used this approach to deliver ^{125}I-labeled β-amyloid peptide through the BBB to image Alzheimer's disease amyloid structures.

NOVEL CNS DELIVERY SYSTEMS

Most of the current novel CNS delivery carrier systems are colloidal based. Such systems include liposomes, nanoparticles, microspheres, nanospheres, nanotubes, micelles, and nanoconjugates. The chemical composition of these systems is lipid, peptide, or polymer–based. Each system has pros and cons when it comes to its formulation techniques, stability, versatility, ability to scale-up the formulation, and cost. The common advantages of these novel carrier systems are their ability to change or "hide" the physicochemical parameters of the active drug, enhance tissue specificity and "targetability" with proper targeting moieties, and protect the active drug from degradation and enzymatic inactivation [93]. Such new physicochemical characteristics can be tailored based on the proper design of the colloidal carrier system, which is illustrated in **Figure 15-5**.

Figure 15-5 shows the versatility of novel colloidal carrier systems. As illustrated, colloidal carrier systems can be surface grafted with polyethylene glycol (PEG) or triethylene glycol chains (PEGylation) with various sizes and chemical compositions. PEGylation improves the pharmacokinetic and pharmacodynamic profiles by increasing water solubility and half-life, decreasing plasma clearance, protecting it from enzymatic degradation, reducing renal clearance, and limiting immunogenic and antigenic reactions [94]. PEGylation provides a protective sheath around the colloidal carrier system, which hides it from the harsh external environment. This formulation also protects the carrier system from the removal of the system from circulation by the reticuloendothelial

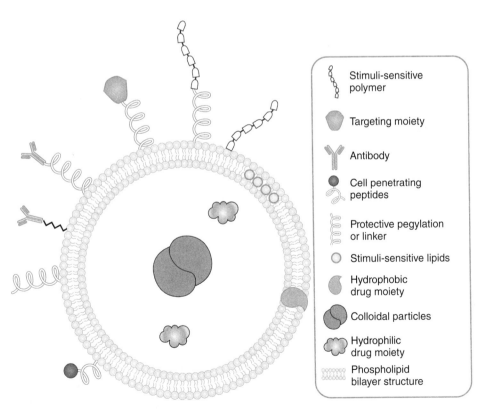

FIGURE 15-5 Liposomes as a novel colloidal drug delivery system. Liposomes can be tailor designed to adopt diverse grafting strategies on their surfaces or modifications within the liposomal composition to provide tissue specificity and targetability.

system and consequently leads to pharmacokinetic and pharmacodynamic parameter improvement [95].

In addition to PEGylation, colloidal carrier systems can be surface grafted with specific antibodies, targeting moieties, cell penetration peptides, and stimuli-sensitive moieties [96–99]. Colloidal carrier systems grafted with stimuli-sensitive moieties are considered "smart" carrier systems, which alter and modify their chemical structure or configuration based on a change in the biological environment. Such technology is used to target diseased tissues by using cues specific to the targeted tissue or cell. For example, pH changes, temperature, light, redox potential, or ionic strength represent some of the currently used triggers to design smart stimuli-sensitive bioresponsive colloidal carrier systems [100–102].

Targeting Centers and Receptors

An additional way to circumvent the BBB is to allow drugs to be taken up past the BBB endothelia by receptor-mediated endocytosis. Receptor-mediated endocytosis targeting can be achieved by direct coupling of a targeting ligand to a drug molecule or to a delivery carrier system. The targeting ligand binds to a receptor on the vascular endothelium of the BBB, which shuttles the drug and targeting ligand across the BBB. Some widely used mechanisms include the transferrin receptor, the insulin receptor, the low-density-lipoprotein receptor, and the diphtheria toxin receptor [103]. This mechanism has high capacity and has been shown to move large molecules or nanoparticles grafted across brain endothelial cells [103–105]. After endocytosis, transcytosis takes place to transport the drug molecules of the carrier system to the abluminal side (brain parenchyma perivascular space).

Holotransferrin

Neuronal survival requires the nutrient iron, which is predominantly delivered to the brain by transferrin. The transferrin receptor is a widely studied receptor for brain endothelial cell targeting. Transferrin is an iron-binding blood plasma glycoprotein that governs the level of free iron in biological fluids. Transferrin binds to iron reversibly but very tightly. Transferrin is the major source of iron delivery to neurons and satisfies the iron requirements for maintaining myelination. The transferrin receptor is a transmembrane glycoprotein consisting of two linked 90-kDa subunits that can each bind a transferrin molecule. The receptor is highly expressed on endothelial cells of the BBB, immature erythroid cells, placental tissue, hepatocytes, and rapidly dividing normal and malignant cells [12, 66, 106]. Cellular iron uptake from transferrin is initiated by the binding of holotransferrin, or a transferrin grafted drug carrier system, to the transferrin receptor, followed by endocytosis [107, 108].

Bruce et al. [109] explored the use of transferrin as a targeting moiety in chemotherapy for glioblastoma multiform. In this study, a transferrin-modified paclitaxel conjugate–loaded micelle was used and showed a significant ability to cross the BBB, antiglioma activity, and less toxicity *in vitro* and *in vivo* compared with nontargeted paclitaxel conjugates.

Olivi et al. [110] studied the potential of targeted bifunctional liposomes as a high-efficiency, low-toxicity gene delivery system for the treatment of CNS disorders. The liposomal delivery system combined transferrin-mediated receptor targeting and poly-L-arginine for facilitated cell penetration. Although there are many successful *in vitro* studies for the use of transferrin for BBB targeting, this application is limited *in vivo* because of the high endogenous levels of transferrin, which results in the saturation of transferrin receptors [107, 108].

OX26

To overcome the limitations of using transferrin as a targeting ligand *in vivo*, antibodies directed against the transferrin receptor (e.g., OX26) have been developed and used. OX26 binds selectively to an epitope of the rat TfR that is different from the transferrin-binding site [111].

Because OX26 only binds to the rat transferrin receptor, other antibodies, 8D3 and RI7217, were developed to target mice [112]. In addition, Walter et al. [113] used transferrin antibodies to surface graft novel nanoparticles for CNS targeted drug delivery systems made of hyperbranched polyglycerol conjugated poly(lactic-co-glycolic acid) (PLGA). In this study, OX26 achieved better *in vivo* analgesic effects compared with other groups based on the rat model of chronic constriction injury of the sciatic nerve.

Another example of the use of OX26 as a novel drug carrier was formulated by Phillips et al. [114]. Poly(ethylene glycol)-poly(epsiloncaprolactone) polymersomes were formulated and conjugated with mouse anti-rat monoclonal antibody OX26. The optimized OX26 had increased BBB permeability and the percentage of injected dose per gram brain compared with unconjugated drug. These results indicate that OX26-PO is a promising carrier for peptide brain delivery.

Angiopep-2

One of the predominant receptors found on BBB endothelium is the low-density lipoprotein receptor–related protein. The β-amyloid precursor protein can bind to the low-density-lipoprotein receptor-related protein. The critical binding region is a sequence called the Kunitz protease inhibitor domain [115, 116]. Several other proteins, including aprotinin and bikunin, contain a similar Kunitz protease inhibitor domain. Alignment of the amino acid sequence of aprotinin with the Kunitz domains helped identify a family of peptides, named Angiopeps by Schenk et al. [117]. The peptides, and in particular Angiopep-2 (19-mer peptide, TFFYGGSRGKRNNFKTEEY), have a high transcytosis capacity and can accumulate in brain parenchyma compared with aprotinin. The Kunitz-derived peptides are continuing to be explored as drug carriers that can bypass the BBB [117, 118].

There have been other attempts to target brain cancer by using Angiopep-2 conjugated to paclitaxel [118]. The Angiopep-2–paclitaxel conjugate was shown to enter the brain significantly better than paclitaxel alone. It was hypothesized that not only did the drug have greater brain penetration because it underwent receptor-mediated endocytosis, but this mechanism also allowed paclitaxel to bypass P-glycoprotein at the BBB [118]. Further enhancement and chemical modifications of Angiopep-2 for the treatment of primary and secondary brain cancers were investigated by Allen and Hogg [119], who reported the synthesis and preliminary biological characterization of two modified chemical entities of Angiopep-2, ANG1007 and ANG1009. ANG1007 consists of three doxorubicin molecules conjugated to Angiopep-2. ANG1009 has a similar structure except that three etoposide moieties are conjugated to Angiopep-2. ANG1007 and ANG1009 exhibited dramatically higher BBB penetrance than unconjugated doxorubicin and etoposide [119]. Angiopep-2 has also been extensively investigated and tested as a BBB targeting ligand for dendrimers [120] and nanoparticles [121].

COG133

Cholesterol represents an essential compound for all cells in the human body. Apolipoprotein E is a 34-kDa protein complex consisting of both very-low-density lipoprotein and high-density lipoprotein that transports cholesterol and other lipids across the BBB [122–126]. The apolipoprotein E complex uses specific receptors at the

BBB, including the low-density-lipoprotein receptor and the low-density-lipoprotein receptor–related protein. To take advantage of this, grafting nanoparticles or drug molecules with apolipoprotein E could be used for brain targeting [127, 128]. Apolipoprotein E, however, is a large complex that could theoretically limit its usefulness as a drug carrier to the CNS [129–131]. Further studies identified that the critical region of apolipoprotein E for interaction with the low-density-lipoprotein receptor is located between amino acid residues 140 and 160 [129]. Based on that data, Vemuri and Rhodes [131] derived a peptide from amino acids 133 to 149 that mimics apolipoprotein E, named COG133 (LRVRLASHLRKLRKRLL). COG133 retains biological activity in the low-density-lipoprotein receptor critical binding region of apolipoprotein E *in vitro* and *in vivo*.

CRM197

Cross-reacting material 197, known as CRM197, a nontoxic mutant of diphtheria toxin, contains a single point mutation at position 52, and can act as a diphtheria toxin receptor–specific carrier protein. CRM197 is nontoxic and retains the ability to bind heparin-binding epidermal growth factor, which is expressed in various regions of the brain and helps deliver drugs across the BBB [132]. Ulshafer et al. [133] investigated the capability of CRM197-grafted polybutylcyanoacrylate nanoparticles to transport zidovudine across the BBB. An increase in the grafting quantity of CRM197 enhanced the permeability coefficient of zidovudine across the BBB and the uptake quantity of zidovudine-loaded nanoparticles by human brain-microvascular endothelial cells.

Carrier Systems

Nanoparticles and vesicular liposomal formulations are two widely explored CNS drug delivery systems. Liposomes are small vesicles comprising one or more concentric bilayers of phospholipids separated by aqueous compartments. Although liposomes have been reported to enhance the uptake of certain drugs into the brain after intravenous injection, the application of liposomes as therapeutic devices started in the mid-1950s with the work of Friedman and Freedman [124]. Liposomes (lipid vesicles) are sealed sacs dispersed in an aqueous environment with sizes ranging from 10 nm to 2 μm [131]. Liposomal preparations can be used to improve the therapeutic index of drugs by targeting the active ingredient to the appropriate site of action and modulating drug release from the vehicle. The wall of the sac is composed of suitable amphiphilic molecules. The nature of these bilayers ensures the formation of internal aqueous compartments, which can differ from the outside medium. The presence of two different environments in the carrier, the aqueous "milieu interne" and the membrane, makes liposomes a unique model for studying biological membranes and a versatile carrier for a broad spectrum of hydrophilic, amphipathic, and hydrophobic agents. The vesicles consist of one or more concentric spheres of lipid bilayers separated by water or aqueous buffer compartments [130, 131, 134–136]. Many studies use liposomes as drug carriers in treating diseases of the CNS.

Compared with synthetic liposomes, conventional unmodified liposomes consisting of naturally occurring phospholipids and cholesterol suffer from high systemic plasma clearance. They are generally cleared from the systemic circulation after administration by immune system macrophages of the reticuloendothelial system [137]. Numerous strategies have been adopted to overcome the short half-life of liposomes in the circulation, such as grafting the liposomes with gangliosides [138] or PEG [139, 140]. Conventional liposomes grafted with a PEG layer are considered to be sterically stable and safe from degradation. Moreover, this PEGylated layer prevents liposomes from binding to opsonins and subsequently prevents their clearance by phagocytotic cells [141]. The sterically stabilized liposomes also offer a drastic change in pharmacokinetic parameters. A 50-fold decrease in plasma volume of distribution (from 200 to ~4 L), a 200-fold decrease in systemic plasma clearance (from 22 to 0.1 L/h), and a nearly 20-fold increase in half-life (~90 hours) were observed with PEGylated liposomes compared with conventional liposomes [142–144].

Grafting liposomes with different targeting peptides or antibodies for targeting strategies has been a successful tool in drug and gene delivery. Huwyler et al. [145] presented the first preclinical trial to use liposomal drug delivery to target the brain. They used PEGylated liposomes conjugated to the OX26 monoclonal antibody to successfully enter the brain via transferrin receptor-mediated endocytosis. Similarly, peptide grafted liposomes facilitated a sixfold increase in ferulic acid uptake into the brain [146].

Solid lipid nanoparticles (SLNs) are also a major lipid-based drug carrier system. SLNs, developed in the 1990s as alternatives to emulsions, liposomes, and polymeric nanoparticles, are spherical solid particles of a lipid core matrix that can solubilize lipophilic molecules. The lipid core is stabilized by surfactants (emulsifiers). SLNs range in size from 10 to 500 nm. SLNs were designed, developed, and formulated to take advantage of the liposomal vesicular systems such as surface functionalization, neutral lipid characteristics, and nanoscale particle size. These factors can effectively facilitate transport of therapeutic agents such as biologically active agents, pharmaceutically active agents, magnetically active agents, and imaging agents to the CNS. Formulation of SLNs provides improved drug loading and protein stability, targeting, and controlled drug release. Furthermore, SLN lipophilic features provide multiple advantages such as incorporation of lipid-soluble drugs with high drug loading, thus targeting them to the CNS by an endocytotic mechanism. Patel et al. [147] formulated risperidone into SLNs and showed brain uptake via the olfactory route. Montenegro et al. [148] demonstrated the *in vitro* permeation of idebenone-loaded SLNs across an MDCKII-MDR1 cell monolayer.

In addition to lipid-based delivery systems, other components have been used in the construction of nanoparticles used for CNS delivery. PLGA copolymer is one of the most widely used copolymers in the formulation of nano- and microparticles. PLGA-block-PEG nanoparticles coated with polysorbate 80 loaded with atorvastatin were effectively internalized within the endothelial cells and were able to penetrate the BBB [149]. In another example, Kirthivasan et al. [150] developed magnetic nanoparticles for brain targeting. The nanoparticle's matrix was prepared by single-emulsion solvent evaporation of PLGA and methoxy poly(ethyleneglycol)–poly(lactic acid) polymers. The nanoparticle matrix was coated with oleic acid to generate the final oleic acid magnetic nanoparticles that were loaded with the water-soluble P-glycoprotein substrate rhodamine 123. The magnetic nanoparticles efficiently transported the rhodamine 123 into the brain, which would normally be inhibited by P-glycoprotein.

Polybutyl cyanoacrylate polymers have been used to formulate nanoparticles that move by rapid transport across the BBB [151]. It appears, however, that this formulation requires a coating of polysorbate 80 to move across the BBB. Gulyaev et al. [152] showed significant amounts of doxorubicin could accumulate in the brain with polysorbate 80–coated polybutyl cyanoacrylate nanoparticles. Nanoparticles consisting of polycyanoacrylate that were grafted with PEG, however, could only overcome the BBB if the BBB was defective and had become more permeable [152]. The mechanism by which polysorbate 80–coated polybutyl cyanoacrylate nanoparticles facilitated drug entry into the brain is hypothesized to be related to apolipoprotein E. Plasma proteins, especially apolipoprotein E, adsorb on the surface of the coated nanoparticles. Such apolipoprotein

E–coated nanoparticles are thought to be mistaken for low-density-lipoprotein particles by the BBB endothelium and are internalized by the low-density-lipoprotein uptake system [153–155].

Polyethylenimine is considered to be the gold standard for polymeric nonviral gene delivery systems based on its efficacy [156–159]. Such efficacy is due to the high cationic charge density on the surface of the polymeric chains [160–162].

Chitosan is a natural polymer classified as a linear polysaccharide composed of randomly distributed β-(1-4)-linked D-glucosamine and N-acetyl-D-glucosamine. Chitosan has a positive charge under acidic conditions coming from protonation of its free amino groups. Aktaş et al. [163] used chitosan nanoparticles grafted with PEG using avidin–biotin technology for uptake across the BBB.

Regarding the mechanism of action of drug delivery by polymeric/lipid carrier systems across the BBB, a number of possibilities and hypotheses can explain the delivery mechanism [10]. The main possibility includes the increased retention of the carrier system in brain capillaries along with sustained adsorption of the capillary walls, creating a higher concentration gradient that would enhance the transport of drug across the endothelial cell layer and, as a result, its delivery to the brain. Most nanoparticle systems involve the use of surfactants, which could aid in the solubilization of endothelial cell membrane lipids, leading to membrane fluidization and enhanced drug permeability at the BBB. Furthermore, the carrier system could facilitate an opening of the tight junctions between the endothelial cells. The drug could then permeate through the tight junctions either in free form or together with the nanoparticles. One possibility is the engulfment of the whole carrier system into the cell. The nanoparticles may be endocytosed by the endothelial cells followed by the sustained and/or controlled release of the drug within these cells.

The use of novel drug carrier systems for drug targeting to brain is a promising alternative to conventional CNS therapy. The currently used polymers, peptides, or lipids used in these carrier systems are nontoxic, biodegradable, and biocompatible. The carrier systems have a particle size ranging from 10 to 100 nm. Particle size should be restricted to 200 nm to enable it to be used intravenously. These carriers, especially polymeric nanoparticles and SLNs, are physically stable *in vivo* and *in vitro*. Moreover, surface modification allows escape from the phagocytosis by the reticuloendothelial system, thus prolonging the blood circulation time. Further, surface modifications can also allow the attachments of targeting ligands, which facilitate CNS targeted delivery through receptor-mediated transcytosis.

SUMMARY

The global CNS pharmaceutical market is expected to grow significantly, overtaking the cardiovascular therapeutics market in the next 10 years [10, 164]. Although much work has been devoted to finding drugs that can cross the BBB into the brain, no single approach has worked for all drugs. The lack of technology to effectively cross the BBB or the blood–tumor barrier prevents researchers from providing effective therapeutics for most patients with brain disorders. Further research is required to take brain targeting and CNS delivery systems from bench to bedside and to overcome the hurdles facing the successful development of an effective formulation. There are challenges ahead to resolve the question of delivery of the drugs to the CNS. More research is required and in progress to address these challenges and to resolve the question of delivery of the drugs across the BBB. We have a long way to go, however, to optimize and evaluate these methods before potential clinical application.

REVIEW QUESTIONS

1. What is the BBB and what are its functions?
2. What defense mechanisms does the BBB have in controlling the trafficking of various chemical moieties into and out of the brain?
3. What are the CNS drug's physicochemical criteria governing its uptake into the brain across the BBB?
4. What are current strategies for CNS drug delivery?
5. What are the current novel drug delivery carrier systems used in CNS delivery?
6. How are novel drug delivery carrier systems beneficial in CNS drug delivery?

REFERENCES

1. Packer RJ, Macdonald T, Vezina G. Central nervous system tumors. *Hematol Oncol Clin North Am.* 2010;24(1):87–108.
2. Mineta K, Nakazawa M, Cebria F, Ikeo K, Agata K, Gojobori T. Origin and evolutionary process of the CNS elucidated by comparative genomics analysis of planarian ESTs. *Proc Natl Acad Sci USA.* 2003;100(13):7666–7671.
3. Sullivan R. The identity and work of the ancient Egyptian surgeon. *J R Soc Med.* 1996;89(8):467–473.
4. Stiefel M, Shaner A, Schaefer SD. The Edwin Smith Papyrus: the birth of analytical thinking in medicine and otolaryngology. *Laryngoscope.* 2006;116(2):182–188.
5. Bugyi B. [The Edwin Smith papyrus]. *Orv Hetil.* 1972;113(20):1079–1080.
6. Cunha F. The Edwin Smith surgical papyrus. *Am J Surg.* 1949;77(6):793–795.
7. Jex HS. The Edwin Smith Surgical Papyrus: first milestone in the march of medicine. *Merck Rep.* 1951;60(2):20–22.
8. Atta HM. Edwin Smith Surgical Papyrus: the oldest known surgical treatise. *Am Surg.* 1999;65(12):1190–1192.
9. Kamp MA, Tahsim-Oglou Y, Steiger HJ, Hanggi D. Traumatic brain injuries in the Ancient Egypt: insights from the Edwin Smith Papyrus. *Cent Eur Neurosurg.* 2011;72(S01):e25.
10. Pathan SA, Iqbal Z, Zaidi SM, et al. CNS drug delivery systems: novel approaches. *Recent Pat Drug Deliv Formul.* 2009;3(1):71–89.
11. Norman P. The challenges of CNS drug discovery. *IDrugs.* 2003;6(4):297–301.
12. Costantino L, Tosi G, Ruozi B, Bondioli L, Vandelli MA, Forni F. Colloidal systems for CNS drug delivery. *Prog Brain Res.* 2009;180:35–69.
13. Celanire S, Campo B. Recent advances in the drug discovery of metabotropic glutamate receptor 4 (mGluR4) activators for the treatment of CNS and non-CNS disorders. *Exp Opin Drug Discov.* 2012;7(3):261–280.
14. Pritchard JF. Risk in CNS drug discovery: focus on treatment of Alzheimer's disease. *BMC Neurosci.* 2008;9(Suppl 3):S1.
15. Palmer AM, Stephenson FA. CNS drug discovery: challenges and solutions. *Drug News Perspect.* 2005;18(1):51–57.
16. Introduction. *Recent Pat CNS Drug Discov.* 2012;7(1):1–2.
17. Toth A, Veszelka S, Nakagawa S, Niwa M, Deli MA. Patented in vitro blood-brain barrier models in CNS drug discovery. *Recent Pat CNS Drug Discov.* 2011;6(2):107–118.
18. Kazantsev AG, Outeiro TF. Drug discovery for CNS disorders: from bench to bedside. *CNS Neurol Disord Drug Targets.* 2010;9(6):668.
19. Abbott NJ, Patabendige AA, Dolman DE, Yusof SR, Begley DJ. Structure and function of the blood-brain barrier. *Neurobiol Dis.* 2010;37(1):13–25.
20. Ballabh P, Braun A, Nedergaard M. The blood-brain barrier: an overview: structure, regulation, and clinical implications. *Neurobiol Dis.* 2004;16(1):1–13.
21. Nitta T, Hata M, Gotoh S, et al. Size-selective loosening of the blood-brain barrier in claudin-5-deficient mice. *J Cell Biol.* 2003;161(3):653–660.
22. Butt AM, Jones HC, Abbott NJ. Electrical resistance across the blood-brain barrier in anaesthetized rats: a developmental study. *J Physiol.* 1990;429:47–62.
23. Neuwelt EA. Mechanisms of disease: the blood-brain barrier. *Neurosurgery.* 2004;54(1):131–140; discussion 141–132.

24. Smith QR. A review of blood-brain barrier transport techniques. *Methods Mol Med.* 2003;89:193–208.

25. Huber JD, Egleton RD, Davis TP. Molecular physiology and pathophysiology of tight junctions in the blood-brain barrier. *Trends Neurosci.* 2001;24(12):719–725.

26. Abbott NJ, Ronnback L, Hansson E. Astrocyte-endothelial interactions at the blood-brain barrier. *Nat Rev Neurosci.* 2006;7(1):41–53.

27. Hawkins BT, Davis TP. The blood-brain barrier/neurovascular unit in health and disease. *Pharmacol Rev.* 2005;57(2):173–185.

28. Begley DJ. ABC transporters and the blood-brain barrier. *Curr Pharm Des.* 2004;10(12):1295–1312.

29. Deeken JF, Loscher W. The blood-brain barrier and cancer: transporters, treatment, and Trojan horses. *Clin Cancer Res.* 2007;13(6):1663–1674.

30. Gong T, Huang Y, Zhang ZR, Li LL. Synthesis and characterization of 9-[P-(N, N-dipropyl sulfamide)] benzoylamino-1,2,3,4-4H-acridine—a potential prodrug for the CNS delivery of tacrine. *J Drug Target.* 2004;12(3):177–182.

31. Loscher W, Potschka H. Role of drug efflux transporters in the brain for drug disposition and treatment of brain diseases. *Prog Neurobiol.* 2005;76(1):22–76.

32. Smith QR. Drug delivery to brain and the role of carrier-mediated transport. *Adv Exp Med Biol.* 1993;331:83–93.

33. Begley DJ, Brightman MW. Structural and functional aspects of the blood-brain barrier. *Prog Drug Res.* 2003;61:39–78.

34. Minn A, Ghersi-Egea JF, Perrin R, Leininger B, Siest G. Drug metabolizing enzymes in the brain and cerebral microvessels. *Brain Res Brain Res Rev.* 1991;16(1):65–82.

35. Witt KA, Gillespie TJ, Huber JD, Egleton RD, Davis TP. Peptide drug modifications to enhance bioavailability and blood-brain barrier permeability. *Peptides.* 2001;22(12):2329–2343.

36. Brownlees J, Williams CH. Peptidases, peptides, and the mammalian blood-brain barrier. *J Neurochem.* 1993;60(3):793–803.

37. Smith QR. Brain perfusion systems for studies of drug uptake and metabolism in the central nervous system. *Pharm Biotechnol.* 1996;8:285–307.

38. Oldendorf WH. Brain uptake of radiolabeled amino acids, amines, and hexoses after arterial injection. *Am J Physiol.* 1971;221(6):1629–1639.

39. Tamai I, Tsuji A. Transporter-mediated permeation of drugs across the blood-brain barrier. *J Pharm Sci.* 2000;89(11):1371–1388.

40. Tsuji A, Tamai II. Carrier-mediated or specialized transport of drugs across the blood-brain barrier. *Adv Drug Deliv Rev.* 1999;36(2–3):277–290.

41. Pardridge WM. Re-engineering biopharmaceuticals for delivery to brain with molecular Trojan horses. *Bioconjug Chem.* 2008;19(7):1327–1338.

42. Karkan D, Pfeifer C, Vitalis TZ, et al. A unique carrier for delivery of therapeutic compounds beyond the blood-brain barrier. *PLoS One.* 2008;3(6):e2469.

43. Pardridge WM. Why is the global CNS pharmaceutical market so under-penetrated? *Drug Discov Today.* 2002;7(1):5–7.

44. American Brain Tumor Association. American Brain Tumor Association offers "top ten" brain tumor facts. Available at: http://www.abta.org/news/press-releases/american-brain-tumor-6.html. Retrieved May 2, 2012.

45. Gupta SP. QSAR studies on drugs acting at the central nervous system. *Chem Rev.* 1989;89(2):1765–1800.

46. Topliss JG. A manual method for applying the Hansch approach to drug design. *J Med Chem.* 1977;20(4):463–469.

47. Kubinyi H. Quantitative structure-activity relationships. 2. A mixed approach, based on Hansch and Free-Wilson Analysis. *J Med Chem.* 1976;19(5):587–600.

48. Pajouhesh H, Lenz GR. Medicinal chemical properties of successful central nervous system drugs. *NeuroRx.* 2005;2(4):541–553.

49. Hansch C, Leo A. *Substituent Constants for Correlation Analysis in Chemistry and Biology.* New York: Wiley; 1979.

50. Hansch C, Bjorkroth JP, Leo A. Hydrophobicity and central nervous system agents: on the principle of minimal hydrophobicity in drug design. *J Pharm Sci.* 1987;76(9):663–687.

51. van de Waterbeemd H, Kansy M. Hydrogen bonding capacity and brain penetration. *Chimia.* 1992;46:299–303.

52. Lipinski CA, Lombardo F, Dominy BW, Feeney PJ. Experimental and computational approaches to estimate solubility and permeability in drug discovery and development settings. *Adv Drug Deliv Rev.* 2001;46(1–3):3–26.

53. Lipinski C. Lead- and drug-like compounds: the rule-of-five revolution. *Drug Discov Today Technol.* 2004;1:337–341.

54. McCown TJ. The future of epilepsy treatment: focus on adeno-associated virus vector gene therapy. *Drug News Perspect.* 2010;23(5):281–286.

55. Gelfand JM, Nolan R, Schwartz DM, Graves J, Green AJ. Microcystic macular oedema in multiple sclerosis is associated with disease severity. *Brain.* 2012;135(Pt 6):1786–1793.

56. Yemisci M, Gursoy-Ozdemir Y, Caban S, Bodur E, Capan Y, Dalkara T. Transport of a caspase inhibitor across the blood-brain barrier by chitosan nanoparticles. *Methods Enzymol.* 2012; 508:253–269.

57. Mondin V, Ferlito A, Devaney KO, Woolgar JA, Rinaldo A. A survey of metastatic central nervous system tumors to cervical lymph nodes. *Eur Arch Otorhinolaryngol.* 2010;267(11):1657–1666.

58. Cerami A. Beyond erythropoiesis: novel applications for recombinant human erythropoietin. *Semin Hematol.* 2001;38(3 Suppl 7):33–39.

59. Cerami A, Brines ML, Ghezzi P, Cerami CJ. Effects of epoetin alfa on the central nervous system. *Semin Oncol.* 2001;28(2 Suppl 8):66–70.

60. Muraro PA, Martin R, Lassmann H, Gambi D. Plaques, T cells and beyond: report on an international meeting on the immunological basis of multiple sclerosis held at the University of Chieti, Italy. *J Neuroimmunol.* 1999;96(2):251–254.

61. Su Y, Sinko PJ. Drug delivery across the blood-brain barrier: why is it difficult? how to measure and improve it? *Expert Opin Drug Deliv.* 2006;3(3):419–435.

62. Kabanov AV, Batrakova EV. New technologies for drug delivery across the blood brain barrier. *Curr Pharm Des.* 2004;10(12):1355–1363.

63. Illum L. Is nose-to-brain transport of drugs in man a reality? *J Pharm Pharmacol.* 2004;56(1):3–17.

64. Gabathuler R. Approaches to transport therapeutic drugs across the blood-brain barrier to treat brain diseases. *Neurobiol Dis.* 2010;37(1):48–57.

65. Mehta AI, Choi BD, Ajay D, et al. Convection enhanced delivery of macromolecules for brain tumors. *Curr Drug Discov Technol.* 2012;9(4):305–310.

66. Krauze MT, Forsayeth J, Yin D, Bankiewicz KS. Convection-enhanced delivery of liposomes to primate brain. *Methods Enzymol.* 2009;465:349–362.

67. Ferguson SD, Foster K, Yamini B. Convection-enhanced delivery for treatment of brain tumors. *Expert Rev Anticancer Ther.* 2007;7(12 Suppl):S79–S85.

68. Bobo RH, Laske DW, Akbasak A, Morrison PF, Dedrick RL, Oldfield EH. Convection-enhanced delivery of macromolecules in the brain. *Proc Natl Acad Sci USA.* 1994;91(6):2076–2080.

69. Luther N, Karampelas I, Souliopoulos EP, Edgar MA, Boockvar JA, Souweidane MM. Interstitial infusion of erlotinib in the rodent brain. *J Exp Ther Oncol.* 2009;8(2):79–84.

70. Kroll RA, Pagel MA, Muldoon LL, Roman-Goldstein S, Neuwelt EA. Increasing volume of distribution to the brain with interstitial infusion: dose, rather than convection, might be the most important factor. *Neurosurgery.* 1996;38(4):746–752; discussion 752–744.

71. Ferguson S, Lesniak MS. Convection enhanced drug delivery of novel therapeutic agents to malignant brain tumors. *Curr Drug Deliv.* 2007;4(2):169–180.

72. NexGen. EViTAR cell & drug delivery device. 2012. Available at : http://nexgenmedsystem.com/our-products/evitar-neurological-products/.

73. Langer R. Biodegradable polymers for drug delivery to the brain. *ASAIO Trans.* 1988;34(4):945–946.

74. Brem H, Gabikian P. Biodegradable polymer implants to treat brain tumors. *J Control Release.* 2001;74(1–3):63–67.

75. Olivi A, Brem H. Interstitial chemotherapy with sustained-release polymer systems for the treatment of malignant gliomas. *Recent Results Cancer Res.* 1994;135:149–154.

76. Albert A. Chemical aspects of selective toxicity. *Nature.* 1958;182(4633):421–422.

77. Rautio J, Laine K, Gynther M, Savolainen J. Prodrug approaches for CNS delivery. *AAPS J.* 2008;10(1):92–102.

78. Vytla D, Combs-Bachmann RE, Hussey AM, McCarron ST, McCarthy DS, Chambers JJ. Prodrug approaches to reduce hyperexcitation in the CNS. *Adv Drug Deliv Rev.* 2012;64(7): 666–685.

79. Springer CJ, Niculescu-Duvaz II. Antibody-directed enzyme prodrug therapy (ADEPT): a review. *Adv Drug Deliv Rev.* 1997;26(2–3):151–172.

80. Oldendorf WH, Hyman S, Braun L, Oldendorf SZ. Blood-brain barrier: penetration of morphine, codeine, heroin, and methadone after carotid injection. *Science.* 1972;178(4064):984–986.

81. Pop E, Wu WM, Bodor N. Chemical delivery systems for some penicillinase-resistant semisynthetic penicillins. *J Med Chem.* 1989;32(8):1789–1795.

82. Bodor N, Buchwald P. Recent advances in the brain targeting of neuropharmaceuticals by chemical delivery systems. *Adv Drug Deliv Rev.* 1999;36(2–3):229–254.

83. Pop E, Bodor N. Chemical systems for delivery of antiepileptic drugs to the central nervous system. *Epilepsy Res.* 1992;13(1):1–16.

84. Pop E, Wu WM, Shek E, Bodor N. Chemical delivery systems for drugs containing an amino group: synthesis and properties of some pyridine derivatives of desipramine. *Drug Des Deliv.* 1989;5(2):93–115.

85. Brewster ME, Raghavan K, Pop E, Bodor N. Enhanced delivery of ganciclovir to the brain through the use of redox targeting. *Antimicrob Agents Chemother.* 1994;38(4):817–823.

86. Estes KS, Brewster ME, Simpkins JW, Bodor N. A novel redox system for CNS-directed delivery of estradiol causes sustained LH suppression in castrate rats. *Life Sci.* 1987;40(13):1327–1334.

87. Pardridge WM, Oldendorf WH. Transport of metabolic substrates through the blood-brain barrier. *J Neurochem.* 1977;28(1):5–12.

88. Cornford EM, Hyman S, Pardridge WM. An electron microscopic immunogold analysis of developmental up-regulation of the blood-brain barrier GLUT1 glucose transporter. *J Cereb Blood Flow Metab.* 1993;13(5):841–854.

89. Farrell CL, Pardridge WM. Blood-brain barrier glucose transporter is asymmetrically distributed on brain capillary endothelial lumenal and ablumenal membranes: an electron microscopic immunogold study. *Proc Natl Acad Sci USA.* 1991;88(13):5779–5783.

90. Fernandez C, Nieto O, Fontenla JA, Rivas E, de Ceballos ML, Fernandez-Mayoralas A. Synthesis of glycosyl derivatives as dopamine prodrugs: interaction with glucose carrier GLUT-1. *Org Biomol Chem.* 2003;1(5):767–771.

91. Fernandez C, Nieto O, Rivas E, Montenegro G, Fontenla JA, Fernandez-Mayoralas A. Synthesis and biological studies of glycosyl dopamine derivatives as potential antiparkinsonian agents. *Carbohydr Res.* 2000;327(4):353–365.

92. Saito Y, Buciak J, Yang J, Pardridge WM. Vector-mediated delivery of 125I-labeled beta-amyloid peptide A beta 1–40 through the blood-brain barrier and binding to Alzheimer disease amyloid of the A beta 1–40/vector complex. *Proc Natl Acad Sci USA.* 1995;92(22):10227–10231.

93. Kreuter J, Kreuter K, Kreuter J. *Colloidal Drug Delivery Systems.* Philadelphia, PA: Taylor & Francis; 1994.

94. Milla P, Dosio F, Cattel L. PEGylation of proteins and liposomes: a powerful and flexible strategy to improve the drug delivery. *Curr Drug Metab.* 2012;13(1):105–119.

95. Pasut G, Veronese FM. State of the art in PEGylation: The great versatility achieved after forty years of research. *J Control Release.* 2012;161(2):461–472.

96. Baker JR, Jr. Dendrimer-based nanoparticles for cancer therapy. *Hematol Am Soc Hematol Educ Progr.* 2009:708–719.

97. Yellepeddi VK, Kumar A, Palakurthi S. Surface modified poly(amido)amine dendrimers as diverse nanomolecules for biomedical applications. *Expert Opin Drug Deliv.* 2009;6(8):835–850.

98. Roy EJ, Gawlick U, Orr BA, Kranz DM. Folate-mediated targeting of T cells to tumors. *Adv Drug Deliv Rev.* 2004;56(8):1219–1231.

99. Douglas SJ, Davis SS, Illum L. Nanoparticles in drug delivery. *Crit Rev Ther Drug Carrier Syst.* 1987;3(3):233–261.

100. Torchilin V. Multifunctional and stimuli-sensitive pharmaceutical nanocarriers. *Eur J Pharm Biopharm.* 2009;71(3):431–444.

101. Na K, Sethuraman VT, Bae YH. Stimuli-sensitive polymeric micelles as anticancer drug carriers. *Anticancer Agents Med Chem.* 2006;6(6):525–535.

102. Pluta J, Karolewicz B. [Hydrogels: properties and application in the technology of drug form. I. The characteristic hydrogels]. *Polim Med.* 2004;34(2):3–19.

103. Jones AR, Shusta EV. Blood-brain barrier transport of therapeutics via receptor-mediation. *Pharm Res.* 2007;24(9):1759–1771.

104. Mizisin AP, Kalichman MW, Myers RR, Powell HC. Role of the blood-nerve barrier in experimental nerve edema. *Toxicol Pathol.* 1990;18(1 Pt 2):170–185.

105. Davidson BL, Bohn MC. Recombinant adenovirus: a gene transfer vector for study and treatment of CNS diseases. *Exp Neurol.* 1997;144(1):125–130.

106. Ricci M, Blasi P, Giovagnoli S, Rossi C. Delivering drugs to the central nervous system: a medicinal chemistry or a pharmaceutical technology issue? *Curr Med Chem.* 2006;13(15):1757–1775.

107. Mamelak AN. Locoregional therapies for glioma. *Oncology.* 2005;19(14):1803–1810; discussion 1810, 1816–1817, 1821–1802.

108. Nguyen TT, Pannu YS, Sung C, et al. Convective distribution of macromolecules in the primate brain demonstrated using computerized tomography and magnetic resonance imaging. *J Neurosurg.* 2003;98(3):584–590.

109. Bruce JN, Falavigna A, Johnson JP, et al. Intracerebral clysis in a rat glioma model. *Neurosurgery.* 2000;46(3):683–691.

110. Olivi A, Grossman SA, Tatter S, et al. Dose escalation of carmustine in surgically implanted polymers in patients with recurrent malignant glioma: a New Approaches to Brain Tumor Therapy CNS Consortium trial. *J Clin Oncol.* 2003;21(9):1845–1849.

111. Kong Q, Kleinschmidt-Demasters BK, Lillehei KO. Intralesionally implanted cisplatin cures primary brain tumor in rats. *J Surg Oncol.* 1997;64(4):268–273.

112. Menei P, Benoit JP, Boisdron-Celle M, Fournier D, Mercier P, Guy G. Drug targeting into the central nervous system by stereotactic implantation of biodegradable microspheres. *Neurosurgery.* 1994;34(6):1058–1064; discussion 1064.

113. Walter KA, Cahan MA, Gur A, et al. Interstitial taxol delivered from a biodegradable polymer implant against experimental malignant glioma. *Cancer Res.* 1994;54(8):2207–2212.

114. Phillips PC, Levow C, Catterall M, Colvin OM, Pastan I, Brem H. Transforming growth factor-alpha-Pseudomonas exotoxin fusion protein (TGF-alpha-PE38) treatment of subcutaneous and intracranial human glioma and medulloblastoma xenografts in athymic mice. *Cancer Res.* 1994;54(4):1008–1015.

115. Ko YT, Bhattacharya R, Bickel U. Liposome encapsulated polyethylenimine/ODN polyplexes for brain targeting. *J Control Release.* 2009;133(3):230–237.

116. Umezawa F, Eto Y. Liposome targeting to mouse brain: mannose as a recognition marker. *Biochem Biophys Res Commun.* 1988;153(3):1038–1044.

117. Schenk JL, Amann RP, Allen CH. Effects of extender and insemination dose on postthaw quality and fertility of bovine sperm. *J Dairy Sci.* 1987;70(7):1458–1464.

118. Allen CR. A new generation of drug diverters. *Am Pharm.* 1987;NS27(9):42–45.

119. Allen CA, Hogg N. Association of colorectal tumor epithelium expressing HLA-D/DR with CD8-positive T-cells and mononuclear phagocytes. *Cancer Res.* 1987;47(11):2919–2923.

120. Allen CK, Allen RE. Cognitive disabilities: measuring the social consequences of mental disorders. *J Clin Psychiatry.* 1987;48(5):185–190.

121. Price GJ, Jones CJ, Charlton RA, Allen CM. A combined approach to the assessment of neurological dysphagia. *Clin Otolaryngol Allied Sci.* 1987;12(3):197–201.

122. Caird D, Klinke R. Processing of binaural stimuli by cat superior olivary complex neurons. *Exp Brain Res.* 1983;52(3):385–399.

123. Friedman LL. Tumors of the pleura. *Dis Chest.* 1950;17(6):756–763.

124. Friedman AP, Freedman D. Amyotrophic lateral sclerosis. *J Nerv Ment Dis.* 1950;111(1):1–18.

125. Friedman V, Brown JE, Jr., Turner EV. A case of proven systemic histoplasmosis with apparent recovery. *Ohio Med.* 1950;46(1):44–46.

126. Frank HA, Fine J, Friedman E, Glotzer P, Jacob S, Schwartz A. Adrenal cortical therapy and hepatic vascular resistance: two aspects of an inquiry into the pathologic physiology of experimental hemorrhagic shock. *Surg Forum.* 1950:522–529.

127. Bonnekoh B, Mahrle G. [Cutaneous administration of liposomes—a review of the literature with special reference to findings from keratinocyte cultures, animal experiments and clinical studies]. *Z Hautkr.* 1990;65(1):99–105.

128. Meure LA, Foster NR, Dehghani F. Conventional and dense gas techniques for the production of liposomes: a review. *AAPS Pharm Sci Tech.* 2008;9(3):798–809.

129. Yang K, Clifton GL, Hayes RL. Gene therapy for central nervous system injury: the use of cationic liposomes: an invited review. *J Neurotrauma.* 1997;14(5):281–297.

130. Riaz M. Review article: stability and uses of liposomes. *Pak J Pharm Sci.* 1995;8(2):69–79.

131. Vemuri S, Rhodes CT. Preparation and characterization of liposomes as therapeutic delivery systems: a review. *Pharm Acta Helv.* 1995;70(2):95–111.

132. Ulshafer RJ, Allen CB, Nicolaissen B, Jr., Rubin ML. Scanning electron microscopy of human drusen. *Invest Ophthalmol Vis Sci.* 1987;28(4):683–689.

133. Ulshafer RJ, Spoerri PE, Allen CB, Kelley KC. Scanning electron microscopic observations on differentiation and maintenance of photoreceptor cells in vitro. *Scanning Microsc.* 1987;1(1):241–246.

134. Bangham AD. Lipid bilayers and biomembranes. *Annu Rev Biochem.* 1972;41:753–776.

135. Matteucci ML, Thrall DE. The role of liposomes in drug delivery and diagnostic imaging: a review. *Vet Radiol Ultrasound.* 2000;41(2):100–107.

136. Kaye SB, Richardson VJ. Potential of liposomes as drug-carriers in cancer chemotherapy: a review. *Cancer Chemother Pharmacol.* 1979;3(2):81–85.

137. Frank MM. The reticuloendothelial system and bloodstream clearance. *J Lab Clin Med.* 1993;122(5):487–488.

138. Allen TM, Chonn A. Large unilamellar liposomes with low uptake into the reticuloendothelial system. *FEBS Lett.* 1987;223(1):42–46.

139. Papahadjopoulos D, Allen TM, Gabizon A, et al. Sterically stabilized liposomes: improvements in pharmacokinetics and antitumor therapeutic efficacy. *Proc Natl Acad Sci USA.* 1991;88(24):11460–11464.

140. Uster PS, Allen TM, Daniel BE, Mendez CJ, Newman MS, Zhu GZ. Insertion of poly(ethylene glycol) derivatized phospholipid into pre-formed liposomes results in prolonged in vivo circulation time. *FEBS Lett.* 1996;386(2–3):243–246.

141. Moghimi SM, Patel HM. Opsonophagocytosis of liposomes by peritoneal macrophages and bone marrow reticuloendothelial cells. *Biochim Biophys Acta.* 1992;1135(3):269–274.

142. Gabizon A, Shmeeda H, Barenholz Y. Pharmacokinetics of pegylated liposomal Doxorubicin: review of animal and human studies. *Clin Pharmacokinet.* 2003;42(5):419–436.

143. Gabizon AA. Pegylated liposomal doxorubicin: metamorphosis of an old drug into a new form of chemotherapy. *Cancer Invest.* 2001;19(4):424–436.

144. Gabizon A, Martin F. Polyethylene glycol-coated (pegylated) liposomal doxorubicin. Rationale for use in solid tumours. *Drugs.* 1997;54(Suppl 4):15–21.

145. Huwyler J, Wu D, Pardridge WM. Brain drug delivery of small molecules using immunoliposomes. *Proc Natl Acad Sci USA.* 1996;93(24):14164–14169.

146. Qin J, Chen D, Hu H, Qiao M, Zhao X, Chen B. Body distribution of RGD-mediated liposome in brain-targeting drug delivery. *J Pharm Soc Jpn.* 2007;127(9):1497–1501.

147. Patel S, Chavhan S, Soni H, et al. Brain targeting of risperidone-loaded solid lipid nanoparticles by intranasal route. *J Drug Target.* 2011;19(6):468–474.

148. Montenegro L, Trapani A, Latrofa A, Puglisi G. In vitro evaluation on a model of blood brain barrier of idebenone-loaded solid lipid nanoparticles. *J Nanosci Nanotechnol.* 2012;12(1):330–337.

149. Allen CB, Ulshafer RJ, Ellis EA, Woodard JC. Scanning electron microscopic analysis of intraocular ossification in advanced retinal disease. *Scanning Microsc.* 1987;1(1):233–239.

150. Kirthivasan B, Singh D, Bommana MM, Raut SL, Squillante E, Sadoqi M. Active brain targeting of a fluorescent P-gp substrate using polymeric magnetic nanocarrier system. *Nanotechnology.* 2012;23(25):255102.

151. Kreuter J. Nanoparticulate systems for brain delivery of drugs. *Adv Drug Deliv Rev.* 2001;47(1):65–81.

152. Gulyaev AE, Gelperina SE, Skidan IN, Antropov AS, Kivman GY, Kreuter J. Significant transport of doxorubicin into the brain with polysorbate 80–coated nanoparticles. *Pharm Res.* 1999;16(10):1564–1569.

153. Wilson B. Brain targeting PBCA nanoparticles and the blood-brain barrier. *Nanomedicine.* 2009;4(5):499–502.

154. Olivier JC, Fenart L, Chauvet R, Pariat C, Cecchelli R, Couet W. Indirect evidence that drug brain targeting using polysorbate 80-coated polybutylcyanoacrylate nanoparticles is related to toxicity. *Pharm Res.* 1999;16(12):1836–1842.

155. Kreuter J, Ramge P, Petrov V, et al. Direct evidence that polysorbate-80-coated poly(butylcyanoacrylate) nanoparticles deliver drugs to the CNS via specific mechanisms requiring prior binding of drug to the nanoparticles. *Pharm Res.* 2003;20(3):409–416.

156. Perez-Martinez FC, Guerra J, Posadas I, Cena V. Barriers to non-viral vector-mediated gene delivery in the nervous system. *Pharm Res.* 2011;28(8):1843–1858.

157. Sun X, Zhang N. Cationic polymer optimization for efficient gene delivery. *Mini Rev Med Chem.* 2010;10(2):108–125.

158. Schatzlein AG. Non-viral vectors in cancer gene therapy: principles and progress. *Anticancer Drugs.* 2001;12(4):275–304.

159. Abdallah B, Sachs L, Demeneix BA. Non-viral gene transfer: applications in developmental biology and gene therapy. *Biol Cell.* 1995;85(1):1–7.

160. Eliyahu H, Barenholz Y, Domb AJ. Polymers for DNA delivery. *Molecules.* 2005;10(1):34–64.

161. Demeneix B, Behr JP. Polyethylenimine (PEI). *Adv Genet.* 2005;53:217–230.

162. Lungwitz U, Breunig M, Blunk T, Gopferich A. Polyethylenimine-based non-viral gene delivery systems. *Eur J Pharm Biopharm.* 2005;60(2):247–266.

163. Aktas Y, Yemisci M, Andrieux K, et al. Development and brain delivery of chitosan-PEG nanoparticles functionalized with the monoclonal antibody OX26. *Bioconjug Chem.* 2005;16(6):1503–1511.

164. Olivier JC. Drug targeting to brain with targeted nanoparticles. *NeuroRx.* 2005;2:108–119.

16

GENE DELIVERY: AN ESSENTIAL COMPONENT FOR SUCCESSFUL GENE THERAPY

MOHAMMAD AL SAGGAR AND DEXI LIU

CHAPTER OBJECTIVES

Upon completing this chapter, the reader should be able to

▶ Explain the rationale for gene therapy approaches and the limitations toward their applications in clinical practice.

▶ Compare and contrast various types of viral vectors and the current technologies to derive viral vectors from wild-type viruses.

▶ Identify the challenges associated with viral vectors and the increasing need for nonviral methods of gene transfer.

▶ Explain the mechanism of polymer- and liposome-based gene delivery systems.

▸ Compare and contrast various physical methods of gene transfer as alternatives to viral and chemical methods.
▸ Recognize the remaining challenges for efficient *in vivo* gene transfer and current research in overcoming these challenges.
▸ Apply the theories of gene delivery systems to design a clinical trial to treat human diseases using gene therapy approaches

CHAPTER OUTLINE

INTRODUCTION

The concept of human gene therapy emerged in the 1960s as a consequence of advancing research in molecular genetics [1]. Earlier experiments show that the Shope papilloma virus is capable of inducing arginase activity in infected cells of rabbits [2] and the tobacco mosaic virus is effective in expressing viral genome along with the added sequence in tobacco leaves after infection [3]. Therefore, it was suggested that viral genomes can be used to deliver therapeutic effects mediated by viral endogenous or added genes.

Initially, this idea was applied clinically in the first human gene therapy trial conducted in 1970 with the intention of treating arginase deficiency using Shope papilloma viruses [4]. Three German siblings with severe arginase deficiency received systemic injections of purified Shope papilloma virus as a means of supplementation for the missing enzyme activity. Unfortunately, the study failed to provide any benefit to the patients, largely due to flaws in the experimental design, an incomplete understanding of the disease mechanism, and the lack of gene expression. Nevertheless, this study provided a direct path toward the use of viruses as a gene carrier in disease treatment. In September 1990, the first approved clinical trial for gene therapy using retroviral vectors was conducted in the treatment of severe combined immunodeficiency disease (SCID) caused by adenosine deaminase deficiency [5]. Although the trial was considered a great success and inspired significant efforts in applying the gene therapy concept to the treatment of other diseases, it was later realized that retroviral vectors used in the protocol had a tendency to activate the oncogene through insertional mutagenesis and induced leukemia in four of nine patients treated [6]. This finding raised a serious concern about the safety of viral vectors and welcomed efforts in improving them and developing non-viral alternatives. Since then, many methods of gene delivery have been developed.

METHODS OF GENE DELIVERY

The site of gene expression is in a cell's nucleus. Since nuclear acid sequences encoding a therapeutic gene in the form of either RNA or DNA are polyanion and nonpermeable through cell membranes, the primary objective of gene delivery is to apply the principles of cell biology, chemistry, and physics to facilitate gene transfer from the site of administration to the nuclei of intended cells. Three systems have been studied in the past. The first system uses the power of viral infection as a means for gene delivery. The second, takes advantage of the cellular function of endocytosis to facilitate gene internalization, whereas the third system simply uses physical force to overcome membrane barriers and allow gene-coding sequences to enter the cells.

VIRUS-BASED GENE DELIVERY

Gene transfer using viral vectors has evolved as an advanced technology for efficient gene delivery. Preparation of viral vectors follows a common procedure, summarized in **Figure 16-1**. Virus-based gene delivery aims to harness the natural viral infection

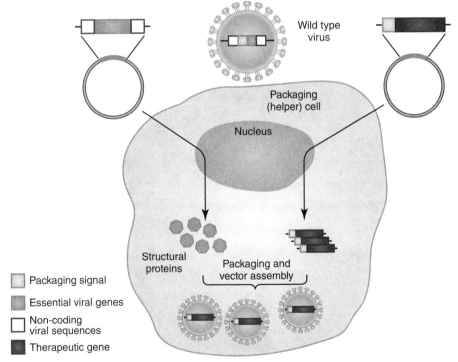

FIGURE 16-1 Production of viral vectors. For safety reasons (see text), viral vector production involves two unrelated DNA contexts: the first context aims to produce viral structural proteins while lacking their packaging signal, and the second one aims to generate viral RNA or DNA harboring the transgene of interest. The helper (packaging) cell is co-transfected with two plasmids intended for each purpose. Viral proteins and RNA are generated independently. Viral structural proteins recognize the vector (having packaging signal) but not the helper nucleic acid, resulting in packaging of the vector genome into a particle along with the transgene.

pathway for efficient gene delivery while avoiding the subsequent expression of viral genes associated with replication and toxicity, an approach achieved using replication-deficient viruses harboring the gene of interest, with viral virulent genes deleted [7]. Current viral vectors found in research and clinical use are based on RNA and DNA viruses that have different genomic structures and host ranges. Table 16-1 summarizes the main features of commonly used viral vectors.

Retroviral (RNA-Based) Vectors

Efficient integration of the viral genome into host DNA is a key feature of the retroviral life cycle, creating replication–deficient retroviral vectors for sustained expression of transgenes in target cells [6]. Retroviral vectors have been the second most commonly used gene delivery vehicles after adenoviral vectors [8], and their therapeutic potential has been demonstrated impressively in clinical gene therapy of SCID using an *ex vivo* approach [9–12]. Retroviruses are enveloped viruses with capsid encapsulating viral genome and two key enzymes: *reverse transcriptase* generates DNA from viral RNA and *integrase* incorporates DNA into the host genome [13].

The retroviral genome contains four genes (*gag*, *pol*, *pro*, and *env*) that encode structural and envelope proteins, as well as *cis*-acting sequences such as long terminal repeats and the viral packaging signal (ψ). Long terminal repeats contain elements required to drive expression, reverse transcription, and integrate into the host genome, whereas the packaging signal (ψ) sequence interacts with viral proteins, allowing specific packaging of viral RNA [14]. With a genome size of 8 through 11 kb, retroviral vectors can harbor exogenous gene inserts of 7 through 10 kb [13].

As noted in Table 16-1, retroviral vectors have shown high transduction efficiency and long-term gene expression, with relatively lower immunogenic potential than

TABLE 16-1 Summarized features of most commonly used viral vectors

Vector	Genetic Material	Capacity (kb)	Titer	Vector Genome	Immune Induction	Limitations	Advantages
ORV	ss-RNA	8	10^6	Integrated	Low	Random integration, efficient for dividing cells only	High transduction efficiency
LV	ss-RNA	8	10^8	Integrated	Low	Random integration	Efficient and sustained gene expression in nondividing and dividing cells
FV	ss-RNA	9	10^3	Integrated	Low	Random integration, low titer	Efficient and sustained gene expression in dividing cells
Ad	ds-DNA	8–10	10^{12}	Episomal	High	Transient gene expression, highly immunogenic	High transduction in dividing and nondividing cells
HDAV	dsDNA	35	10^{10}	Episomal	High	Significant immunogenicity	High transduction, enhanced safety
AAV	ss-DNA	4-5	10^6	Both	Low	Low loading capacity	Nonpathogenic, low immunogenicity
HSV	ds-DNA	30	10^{10}	Episomal	High	Immunogenicity, transient expression in nonneuronal cells	High loading capacity, highly efficient in neuronal gene delivery

ORV, oncoretrovirus; LV, lentivirus; FV, foamy virus; HDAV, helper-dependent adenovirus; ss, single strand; ds, double strand.

most DNA viruses. Importantly, they lead to stable gene transfer due to integration of the viral genome into chromosomes of target cells. Retroviruses exploited for gene delivery include oncoretroviruses, lentiviruses, foamy viruses, and spumaviruses. Oncoretroviruses, like the murine leukemia virus, were the first to be used as vectors for gene transfer, and their efficiency was demonstrated in several clinical trials. However, transduction of these vectors is limited to dividing cells [7]. Lentiviral vectors, another group of retroviruses, have been most commonly used for gene delivery because of their ability to transduce nondividing cells [15], due to the additional proteins they have to facilitate transport through the nuclear membrane and eliminate the need for membrane breakage during mitosis to get into nucleus [16]. Lentiviral vectors showed an enhanced safety profile compared with oncoretroviruses [17, 18]. In addition, they have demonstrated huge successes and much promise in several clinical trials [19–22].

Adenoviral Vectors

Adenoviruses (Ad) evolved as highly effective gene expression vectors in the early 1980s [23]. By 2007, Ad became the most commonly used DNA-viral vector in clinical trials, accounting for almost 25% of clinical gene therapy trials [8]. In fact, the use of Ad has significantly increased as an alternative to retroviruses because of their unique set of attributes: highly efficient gene transduction in dividing and nondividing cells, high titer (10^{12}–10^{13} virus particles/mL) of recombinant viruses can be produced, can accept up to 8 kb of exogenous sequence, and lacks insertional oncogenesis associated with retroviruses [24, 25].

Ad are un-enveloped, double-stranded DNA viruses with an icosahedral protein capsid of 70 to 100 nm in diameter encasing a viral genome of 36 kb [26]. The Ad genome consists of nine major transcription units termed as early (E1–E4) and late (L1–L5) transcription units relative to the onset of viral DNA replication and inverted terminal repeat sequences (ITRs) located at each end of the genome. E1 products, subdivided into E1A and E1B, play essential roles in viral replication, with E1A proteins serving to activate all remaining viral transcription units [27].

Ad infection involves capsid protein interaction with multiple host cell receptors, including coxsackie and the Ad receptor [28, 29], CD46 [30], and sialic acid [31]. These interactions promote sequential steps in cell entry, including attachment and receptor-mediated internalization followed by endosomal escape [32]. After escaping to the cytosol, the viral capsid migrates toward the nuclear membrane for disassembly. Nuclear entry is completed upon dissociation of the capsid and release of the viral genome within the nucleus where it is episomally transcribed and replicated. Similar to retroviral vectors, production of recombinant Ad vectors involves the viral DNA construct containing the exogenous gene replacing E1 and E3 genes and packaging cells expressing the viral proteins. Deletion of the E1 region essential for replication and the nonessential E3 region allows cloning of the exogenous gene insert with size up to 8.2 kb [33]. E1, E3-deleted Ad vectors, referred to as first-generation vectors, have shown high levels of transient gene expression and have been widely used in gene transfer *in vitro* and *in vivo*, including preclinical studies on different animal models and clinical trials in human patients [24, 34]. The use of first-generation Ad vectors, however, was limited by strong immune and inflammatory responses to the vector itself resulting in vector loss [35, 36].

Deletion of all viral coding sequences was the next logical improvement in enhancing the safety profile of Ad vectors. Indeed, helper-dependent or "gutless" Ad vectors were developed, having all viral sequences deleted except the ITR and packaging signal, allowing accommodation of up to 35 kb of exogenous genes. Products of deleted genes are supplied from the replication incompetent (helper) viruses in packaging cells. Gutless vectors have shown reduced immunogenicity and more sustained gene expression [37, 38].

Adeno-Associated Viral Vectors

Adeno-associated virus (AAV) is a nonpathogenic human parvovirus that has attracted considerable interest in gene therapy applications where sustained gene expression is required as a gene transfer vector over the past several years [39]. The therapeutic value of AAV vectors has been attributed to many features, including the lack of pathogenicity and minimal immunogenicity of the virus as well as efficient and sustained gene expression in dividing and nondividing cells [40]. AAV has the ability to specifically integrate to establish latent infection. Current AAV vectors do not have this ability, and this site-specific integration would ensure long-term transgene expression in tissues with a minimal risk of insertional mutagenesis.

AAV is an un-enveloped parvovirus with a capsid of 22 nm in diameter, packaging a single-stranded DNA of 4 to 5 kb. The AAV genome consists of two major genes, *rep* and *cap*, encoding proteins *Rep40, Rep52, Rep68, Rep78, and VP1, VP2, VP3*, respectively. The two genes are flanked by palindromic sequences (ITR) at each end. These ITRs are essential for AAV DNA replication, genome packaging and transcription, and site-specific integration [41]. AAV vectors are naturally replication-deficient because viral promoters are inactive in the absence of the helper virus. Viral replication can be facilitated by proteins derived from Ad or herpes simplex virus (HSV) genomes [42]. Production of AAV vectors involves co-transfection of packaging cells with the AAV vector plasmid where the exogenous gene replaces viral *rep/cap* genes and flanked by ITRs and helper plasmids express AAV *rep/cap* proteins. The adenoviral helper function is provided by superinfecting packaging cells with Ad or transfection with a third plasmid expressing Ad proteins required to facilitate AAV replication [43]. After infection, most of the AAV genome remains in episomal form in the host cell nucleus with almost 10% integrated into host DNA [44]. AAV vectors are increasingly used in gene transfer applications, and its efficacy has been demonstrated in clinical trials [45–48], suggesting AAV as a reliable gene transfer vector, particularly in cases where sustained gene expression is needed.

Other Types of Viral Vectors

Although most gene-transfer studies and gene therapy applications involve the previously mentioned viral vectors, many other viruses have been considered and have successfully demonstrated potential in gene delivery. HSV, a double-stranded DNA virus with theoretical loading capacity of >100 kb [49], has been an attractive vehicle for gene delivery, particularly in studies including gene transfer to neuronal tissues using neurotropic features of HSV [50]. HSV vectors have been successfully used in clinical trials for gene therapy of brain tumors, chronic pain, and other neuronal disorders [50–52]. Other viral vectors that are being developed and used in gene transfer studies include, but are not limited to, vaccinia virus [53], baculovirus [54], members of alphavirus genus [55], and others. More advanced vectors contain selected components of different viruses to yield hybrid viral vectors possessing the advantages of the original viruses. An example of a hybrid viral vector is Ad/AAV, an Ad vector containing the transgene flanked by AAV ITRs, Ad packaging signals, and Ad ITRs. AAV ITRs added the feature of integration to Ad vectors [56]. Alternative hybrid viral vectors include HSV/AAV and HSV/Epstein-Barr virus [57].

CHEMICAL-BASED GENE DELIVERY SYSTEMS

Chemical methods (also called nonviral vectors) for gene transfer using synthetic compounds began in the 1960s when diethylaminoethyl dextran was first shown to enhance the transfer of RNA into mammalian cells in culture [58]. The rationale of this approach is to formulate DNA into particles to protect DNA from nuclease–mediated degradation and to facilitate DNA internalization by endocytosis. Being synthetic, chemical carriers are generally less immunogenic and safer than viral vectors. They are also amenable for modifications and inclusion of desirable features such as target specificity and controlled release of DNA. The most studied nonviral carriers are cationic liposomes.

Cationic Liposomes

Liposomes were first described as a model of cell membranes in the 1960s [59] and became increasingly used as a vehicle for delivery of drugs and nutrients. Efficient gene delivery using cationic liposomes was first demonstrated in 1987 using *N*-(2,3-dioley loxypropyl)-*N*,*N*,*N*-trimethylamonium chloride [60]. Cationic liposomes spontaneously interact with negatively charged DNA to form stable DNA–liposome complexes (lipoplexes) (**Figure 16-2**). Liposomes have shown significant transfection efficiency and minimal toxicity in animal studies and clinical trials [61]. Cationic liposome formulations with varying lipid structures and chemical compositions are now commercially available. Among many, lipofectamine appears to be the most commonly used as a transfection reagent *in vitro*.

Cationic Polymers

Cationic polymers are also shown to be effective in gene delivery. Similar to cationic liposomes, highly water-soluble polycations form complexes with DNA (polyplexes) (Figure 16-2) by means of electrostatic interaction, condensing both DNA and the cationic polymers. Polyplexes have comparable *in vivo* efficiency to lipoplexes; however, they tend to have a higher risk of toxicity. Polyethyleneimines emerged as efficient chemical carriers in 1995 and became the most extensively used cationic polymers in

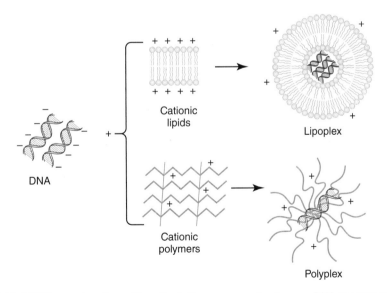

FIGURE 16-2 DNA complexation with cationic liposomes and polymers. DNA spontaneously makes complexes with cationic species like cationic lipids and polymers. The purpose for this complexation is to protect DNA from serum and tissue nuclease enzymes. DNA forms these complexes by means of electrostatic interactions with oppositely charged lipids and polymers to produce lipoplexes and polyplexes, respectively.

gene transfer experiments [62]. Efficiency of polyethyleneimines as a delivery vehicle is a function of molecular weight. Lower-molecular-weight polyethyleneimines are associated with higher efficiency and lower toxicity [63]. Different polymers have been used as gene carriers, including dendrimers, polyallylamines, polyamidoamines, cationic peptides, and chitosan, as well as many others [64].

Other Chemical Methods

Alternative nonviral carriers have been developed for over 30 years. For example, small insoluble Ca^{2+}-DNA precipitates, now called calcium phosphate nanoparticles, are effective in delivering plasmid into cells *in vitro* [65]. Nanoparticles prepared from metal-like gold or inorganic salts—like carbonate salts of magnesium or calcium have also demonstrated a promising potential for efficient and safe gene delivery [66]. Efforts have been made to combine polymers with liposomes for better transfection activities.

PHYSICAL METHODS OF GENE DELIVERY

Physical methods of gene delivery have emerged recently as a simpler and safer approach for gene transfer using mechanical forces (pressure, sound waves, shocks, or electric pulses) to overcome the physical barriers of cells and tissues. These methods facilitate gene delivery to cells or tissues by inducing transient injuries or defects on cell membranes without the aid of cellular functions like endocytosis or pinocytosis.

Needle Injection

The simplest way to deliver genetic material is the direct injection of DNA into target tissues. Gene expression was achieved *in vivo* by direct injection of reporter plasmids into the skeletal muscles of mice [67] as well as other tissues. The mechanism of DNA uptake is not clear, but data collected so far suggest that the physical damage induced by needle penetration plays an important role. Due to its low transfection efficiency, applications of direct needle injection are limited to DNA vaccination [68] where small amounts of gene product produced are sufficient to stimulate an immune response. It is worth noting that microinjection using glass micropipettes to deliver genetic material into living cells is the most commonly used method for creating transgenic animals [69].

Gene Gun

Another physical approach is the use of a gene gun, also called ballistic DNA transfer or DNA-coated particle bombardment [70]. Gene gun is mostly applied in gene transfer to exposed tissue like skin and mucosa or to tissues surgically exposed like liver and muscle [71]. DNA is deposited on the surface of spheres made from gold or tungsten, and these DNA-coated particles are propelled against tissues and cells by the aid of accelerating forces such as pressurized inert gas (helium) or high-voltage electronic discharge. Particles penetrate a few millimeters deep into the tissue and release DNA into cells on the path. Due to limited gene expression achieved, gene gun–based gene transfer has been used in vaccination [72, 73] and immune therapy [74].

Electroporation

Electroporation is based on the fact that the application of a pulsed electrical field into living cells enhances the permeability of cell membranes by creating transient pores across the membrane, resulting in cellular uptake of DNA. Electroporation has been introduced as an efficient method of gene transfer for *in vitro* experiments in 1982 [75] and later became a versatile method extensively used for *in vivo* gene transfer to skin, muscle, and other tissues [76]. The efficiency of gene transfer is a function of voltage, pulse duration, and number of cycles from two electrodes applied. Electroporation has gained increased attention for applications in DNA vaccination [77] and is currently involved in clinical trials for treatment of various cancers and infectious diseases [78]. *In vivo* application of electroporation is challenged by its limited effective range of ~1 cm between the electrodes and the need for surgery to place the electrodes deep into the internal organs [79].

Sonoporation

Application of an ultrasound to cells for gene delivery (sonoporation) was reported initially in 1990 for plant cell transfection [80]. Mechanistically, ultrasound waves applied to cells create plasma membrane defects by cavitation-induced bilayer disordering [81]. Sonoporation applied in gene transfer experiments was reported to significantly enhance transfection efficiency of plasmid DNA both *in vitro* and *in vivo* [82]. The presence of gas-filled microbubbles has been suggested to enhance gene transfer efficiency upon ultrasound exposure [83].

Photoporation

Photoporation is a laser-assisted method of gene delivery resembling that of electroporation and sonoporation mechanistically. Laser pulses serve as a physical force to create transient pores in cell membranes, allowing DNA to enter [84]. This method has demonstrated a significant potential for gene transfer [85] and has been successfully used in *in vitro* gene transfer to human hepatocarcinoma cells [86]. Additional efforts are needed, however, for further optimization of various parameters involved.

Magnetofection

Magnetofection uses magnetic nanoparticles made of iron oxide with or without coupling with nonviral [87] or viral vectors [88] to enhance gene transfer into target cells or tissues in the presence of an external magnetic field [89]. Magnetofection has been successfully applied to gene transfer studies *in vitro* and *in vivo* and has successfully delivered small interfering RNA to tumors in a mouse model [90]. However, there is an increased safety concern regarding the fate of iron oxide in the cell, especially when multidosing is needed. It is worth noting that success in magnetofection-mediated gene transfer requires endocytosis. Magnetofection can be considered as a modified procedure for viral and chemical methods of gene delivery with an advantage of trapping gene carriers at the tissue where the magnetic field is applied.

Hydrodynamic Gene Delivery

Hydrodynamic gene delivery is the most efficient method developed so far for gene delivery *in vivo*. In 1999, it was reported as a simple and effective method of gene transfer [91, 92] using a tail vein injection of plasmid DNA. It has become one of the most commonly used methods for liver gene delivery in rodents. DNA transfer is mediated by a rapid injection of a large volume of DNA solution into the tail vein, resulting in subsequent structural defects of vascular endothelia (fenestrations) and cell membranes of nearby hepatocytes [93]. The efficiency of hydrodynamic gene delivery has been demonstrated impressively in delivering various types of nucleic acid–based and protein-based therapeutics [55] and was approved as an efficient cell delivery technique for the establishment of a metastatic tumor model in mice [94]. Since its development, hydrodynamic delivery has gone through several improvements, bridging the achieved success in animal models to real application in the clinic. A computer-controlled injection device has been developed for hydrodynamic gene delivery in large animals [95] with great success in gene transfer to pig livers, kidneys, and muscles. Further improvement was made in combining this device with an image-guided catheterization technique, allowing lobe-specific gene delivery to the liver of pigs [96] and offering great promise for a method of choice for human gene therapy without using viral or nonviral vectors.

REMAINING CHALLENGES IN GENE DELIVERY

In practice, success of gene therapy is largely dependent on the amount of protein expressed toward the desired therapeutic outcome, which in turn depends on the quantity of therapeutic gene that is successfully delivered to target cells. Each method developed thus far has advantages and disadvantages and faces a series of challenges that limit its applications in research and clinical applications. Therefore, the development of a delivery system that effectively and safely delivers therapeutic genes into target cells is in an urgent need. Future efforts need to focus on the following aspects depending on the method of delivery.

VIRAL GENE DELIVERY

Viral vectors have the advantage of achieving highly efficient gene transfer *in vivo*. Although replication-deficient vectors are used, viral vectors still pose significant safety concerns. Induction of an immune response is the main obstacle associated with viral vectors, and it greatly limits the application of viral vectors in successful human gene therapy. Ad is the most potent immunogenic vector among all viral vectors. Ad induces multiple components of the immune response. Cytotoxic T-lymphocyte responses can be induced against viral proteins, transgene products that are expressed by transduced cells, and/or against the viral capsid itself. Humoral virus-neutralizing antibody responses and potent cytokine-mediated systemic inflammatory responses are also induced against Ad vectors and, to a lesser degree, other viral vectors [44, 97]. Integration into a host genome is the hallmark for long-term expression obtained with retroviral vectors. Random integration of retroviral vectors, however, can result in inactivation of tumor suppressor genes or activation of oncogenes, both of which are associated with tumorogenesis. Indeed, incidences of T-cell leukemia were reported after retroviral gene therapy for SCID [98, 99], and the uncontrolled proliferation of T cells were attributed to expression deregulation of (LMO2) oncogene as a consequence of retroviral integration [100, 101].

NONVIRAL GENE DELIVERY

For gene delivery with nonviral carriers, DNA complexes with cationic lipids and polymers significantly protect DNA against nucleases. The colloidal stability of these lipoplexes and polyplexes in extracellular environments, however, is a major problem to be solved. Aggregation of these complexes is frequently observed with most systems involving complexes prepared near charge neutrality [102, 103]. The (+/−) charge ratio of the cationic polymer/liposomes to DNA greatly affects the size and structural geometry of the complexes, and larger size aggregates have been observed with lower charge ratios. An excess positive charge further increases the colloidal stability of complexes in serum as a result of interactions with negatively charged serum proteins that compete for pDNA binding to cationic complex [104]. Introduction of these systems into biological compartments is accompanied by an increased ionic strength of the media that significantly affects the physical stability and increases the tendency for aggregation of these complexes [97]. Increased ionic strength decreases electrostatic interactions between polycation and DNA while shielding interparticulate electrostatic repulsive forces, resulting in aggregation of complexes. Physical stability of these systems was improved by shielding the particle surface with hydrophilic, uncharged polymers such as polyethylene glycol (PEG). Surface PEG coating sterically hinders aggregation and the interaction and binding of serum components with the complex surface [105, 106]. It has been reported that cationic polymers with high charge densities are most resistant to polyanion-mediated particle disintegration. Indeed, serum polyanion-mediated instability of lipoplexes was significantly improved by incorporation of helper lipids like 1,2-dioleoylphosphatidyl-ethanolamine and cholesterol [107]. Furthermore, these helper lipids stabilize complexes against interactions and fusion with erythrocytes in case of intravenous administration [108}.

An additional challenge in nonviral carrier-mediated gene delivery is associated with the interaction between the DNA complexes and blood components that triggers their clearance from blood and uptake by the reticuloendothelial system (Figure 16-3). Binding of plasma proteins (opsonization) is the major mechanism for the reticuloendothelial system in recognizing circulating particulate substances and consequently clearing them from the circulation [109]. Macrophages, such as the Kupffer cells in the liver and histiocytes in spleen and lymph nodes, recognize the opsonized nanoparticles via the

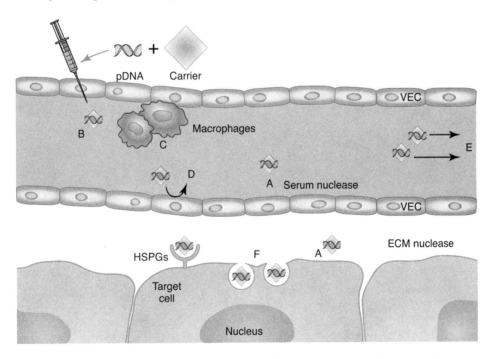

FIGURE 16-3 Extracellular barriers of gene transfer. DNA is delivered as naked plasmid or in complex with the carrier system. Transfer of DNA is challenged with serum and extracellular matrix (ECM) nucleases (a), physical stability of the DNA complex in the biological compartment (b), reticuloendothelial uptake by macrophages and organs of reticuloendothelial system (c), extravasation across vascular endothelial cells (VEC) (d), distribution and nonspecific targeting (e), and interactions with cell surface and subsequent internalization (f). (Data from Nishikawa M. et al. *Adv Drug Deliv Rev.* 2005;57:657–688.)

scavenger receptor. Escape from the reticuloendothelial system is currently achieved by coating particulate systems with PEG to counteract opsonization of these systems by blood proteins and minimize their macrophage recognition and uptake [110, 111].

Extravasation of gene-carrying particles through capillary walls is controlled by several biological factors, such as regional differences in capillary structure and disease state of the tissue as well as physicochemical properties of macromolecules like size, shape, and permeability through the vascular walls they encounter. The transfer of DNA complexes through capillary walls into target tissues **(Figure 16-4)** after systemic administration is another challenge in efficient gene transfer, because it limits deposition of DNA complexes in target tissues and greatly affects the bioavailability and distribution of these complexes in the body. Blood capillaries in most tissues have continuous endothelium acting as a barrier for macromolecules, and those materials of up to 6.0 nm in diameter can extravasate. On the other hand, liver and tissue of the reticuloendothelial system have fenestrated and discontinuous endothelium with fenestrations of up to 150 nm, and particles of 100 nm in diameter can pass through [112]. Tumor endothelium has a leaky and discontinuous vasculature structure, allowing easier extravasation in the tumor region, an effect known as enhanced permeability and retention [113]. Direct tissue injection of DNA complexes can overcome the extravasation barrier by direct deposition of complexes in target tissue [114].

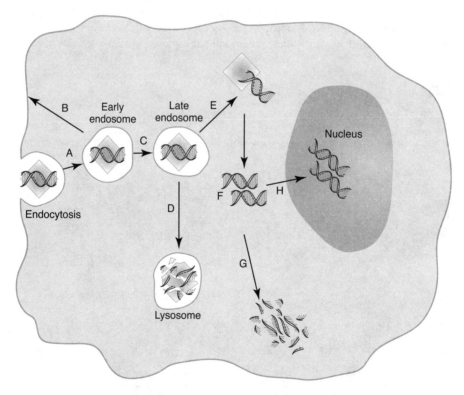

FIGURE 16-4 Intracellular trafficking of DNA. After internalizing the DNA complex via endocytosis, the complex is trafficked into an early endosome (a), which may be recycled to the cell surface (b), or proceed to late endosome (c); this results in either trafficking of the complex to the lysosome for degradation (d) where DNA degradation takes place, or escape of the DNA with or without the carrier (e) into the cytoplasm. DNA becomes free in cytoplasm (f), which might be degraded by the cytoplasmic nuclease (g). Free DNA is then transported into the nucleus (h).

Targeted gene delivery is a most desirable method for gene therapy. It seeks to concentrate therapeutic gene delivery systems in the tissues of interest while reducing the relative concentration of these systems in the remaining tissue, aiming to improve efficacy while reducing side effects. Systemically administered gene carriers are distributed throughout the body through the systemic blood circulation, and a small portion of these systems reaches the desired tissue. Biodistribution of DNA complexes is a function of morphological properties of complexes like size, shape, and charge. Therapeutic effects can be specified for target tissue through two strategies: targeted gene delivery, where gene delivery system is preferentially deposited in target tissues and taken up by target cells, and targeted gene transcription, where gene transcription takes place only in target cells despite gene delivery to several tissues and cell types [115]. Strategies to achieve tissue-specific gene delivery include conjugation of DNA complexes with targeting ligands of receptors overexpressed on target cells, like conjugation of DNA lipoplexes with folate to specifically targeting cells overexpressing folate receptors, or using synthetically modified complexes capable of releasing DNA content under specific stimuli providing means of spatial and temporal release control [116]. Table 16-2 summarizes some of these strategies. Targeted gene transcription is achieved using synthetic promoters that are activated by signaling factors abundant in target cells, like specific targeting of colon cancers using promoters activated by β-catenin and T-cell factor; both are highly abundant in colon cancer cells [117].

TABLE 16-2 Strategies currently used to achieve target specific gene delivery

Strategy		Principle	Example	Reference
Conjugation with targeting ligand		Complex binds to target cells expressing receptors for the ligand	EGF to target cancer cells overexpressing EGFR	141
Coating with antibody against cancer-specific antigens		Complex recognizes target cells by antibody binding to antigens on target cell surface	Antibody against tumor cell surface nucleosomes	142
Stimuli-responsive DNA complexes	pH-Sensitive complexes	Acid-sensitive complex that disassembles at certain pH values of tissue environment	Tumor-specific gene delivery using pH-sensitive polymer	143
	Thermosensitive complexes	Enhanced aggregation and endosomal escape of DNA complexes and DNA release	Enhanced gene transfer after heat application	144
	Redox-sensitive complexes	Change in complex architecture under different redox potentials with controlled DNA release	Enhanced DNA release in tumor-relevant redox environment	145

EGF, epidermal growth factor; EGFR, epidermal growth factor receptor.

At the cellular level, internalization of therapeutic genes is one of the most critical steps for successful gene delivery. For chemical carrier-mediated gene delivery, DNA complexes are taken up by cells through endocytosis (Figure 16-4). The fate of internalized materials is either to be returned to the cell surface, like in the case of recycling endosomes, or proceed via late endosomes with a progressive increase of acidity to lysosomes to be degraded in enzymatic-degrading environment [118]. In both cases, failure of the DNA complex to escape from the endosome results in a significant reduction in intracellular bioavailability of DNA, which greatly affects the efficiency of therapeutic gene delivery and subsequent gene expression. Therefore, efficient endosomal escape is critical for efficient gene delivery and successful gene therapy.

DNA lipoplexes possess enhanced endosomal escape and DNA release as a result of lipid mixing between endosomal and cationic lipid membranes, which results in membrane disruption of endosome and DNA release into cytoplasm [119]. The escape and release of DNA complexed with cationic polymers are mediated by interactions of cationic polymers with negatively charged lipids of the endosomal membrane to form neutral ion pairs that destabilize and promote disassembly of the endosomal membrane and consequent release of DNA [120]. Polymers with ionizable amine groups, like polyethyleneimine, have enhanced endosomal escape and DNA release. Protonation of these amine groups in acidic environments within the endosome is associated with the extensive inflow of protons, ions, and water into the endosomal lumen that leads to the rupture of the endosomal membrane and release of the entrapped components; this process is known as the proton sponge effect [62].

Destabilization of the endosomal membrane was also achieved by stimuli–responsive lipids or polymer derivatives that are responsive to sulfhydryl reduction [121] and enzymatic cleavage [122]. Endosomal enzymes and/or a reducing environment activate these derivatives to fuse with the endosomal membrane and, finally, release the entrapped cargo. Lysosomotropic agents that accumulate preferentially in the lysosomes of cells, like chloroquine and polyvinylpyrolidone, are commonly used in conjunction with plasmid vectors, viral vectors, and in combination with polymeric systems to improve the efficiency of gene delivery. It is believed that chloroquine inhibits endosomal DNA degradation by preferential accumulation and protonation in lysosomes and subsequent ions and water influx and raising pH within lysosomes, thereby providing a suboptimal pH environment for enzymatic degradation of DNA [123]. In addition, being large in molecular weight and negatively charged, DNA was reported to have minimal association with the cell membrane as a result of electrostatic repulsion with negatively charged components that cover the cell surface, namely heparin sulfate proteoglycans (HSPGs) that possess negative charges [97]. Neutralization of the negative charge of DNA by means of complexation with cationic lipids and polymers enhances cellular association and internalization of DNA by increasing interactions between positively charged DNA complexes with HSPGs. Therefore, efficiency of gene transfection is greatly dependent on the expression level of HSPGs on the cell surface, and reduced expression of these HSPGs was associated with reduced levels of transgene expression [124]. Increased DNA complex binding with HSPGs helps induce internalization of DNA complexes by different processes of endocytosis like adsorptive endocytosis [125], clathrin-mediated endocytosis [126], phagocytosis [127], and, rarely, macropinocytosis [128].

Efficient delivery of DNA from the cytosol to the nucleus, where the transcription takes place, is another area that needs additional work. The DNA complex dissociation seems to occur in the endosomal compartment to release DNA into the cytosol [129]. Therefore, after endosomal escape, DNA should make its way through the cytosol to reach the nucleus. The cytoplasm is crowded with organelles, solutes, soluble macromolecules, and a network of skeletal proteins that maintain cell structure like microtubules and actin filaments, and this crowding significantly hinders diffusion of macromolecules through the cytoplasmic compartment [130, 131]. Diffusion of noncomplexed DNA in the cytoplasm is significantly lower than in water, with a diffusion coefficient <1% of that in water for DNA >2000 bp [132]. Smaller plasmids are preferred for higher transfection efficiency, because the diffusion coefficient inversely correlates to the size of the plasmid.

Metabolic instability of DNA in the cytoplasm is another challenge in gene delivery [133]. Cytosolic calcium-sensitive nucleases rapidly degrade microinjected DNA, with a half-life of 50 to 90 minutes [134, 135]. Encapsulation of microinjected plasmids into stabilized lipid particles delays the degradation of DNA with enhanced efficiency [134]. The nuclear envelope is the ultimate barrier to the nuclear entry of plasmid DNA. Evidence of inefficient nuclear uptake of plasmid DNA from the cytoplasm was further demonstrated when compared with the transfection efficiency of microinjected plasmid DNA either into the cytosol or the nucleus [136]. It has been suggested that possible routes through which DNA can translocate to the nucleus include passive (or active) transport through nuclear pores, physical association with chromatin during mitosis, or traverse nuclear envelope; the last seems less likely as it lacks experimental evidence [97].

Nuclear pores embedded in the nuclear envelope allow passage of particles <26 nm [137] but do not allow typical nonviral gene delivery complexes. In dividing cells, the nuclear envelope disassembles and breaks down during mitosis; nuclear translocation can occur at this stage after the permeability barrier is eliminated. In nondividing cells, developing mechanisms of DNA nuclear transport is of critical importance. Nuclear translocation of DNA was improved by attachment with nuclear localization signal peptides (or sequences), which tags cargo for import into the cell nucleus by nuclear transport. Nuclear localization signal peptides bind to cytoplasmic receptors known as importins; together, the complex moves through the nuclear pore. The most well-known and popularly used nuclear localization signal is from the large tumor antigen of simian virus 40; plasmids cloned with the simian virus 40 enhancer region showed significant nuclear localization. Some DNA sequences themselves have nuclear import activity based on their ability to bind to cell-specific transcription factors, such as the SMGA promoter and flk-1 promoter [138].

Physical Gene Delivery

Physical methods were designed to overcome barriers of gene transfer by means of physical forces that create defects in cell membranes and essentially enforce cellular uptake of DNA. Physical methods of gene transfer are generally well tolerated. Results reported on cell or tissue toxicity are inconsistent. Targeted cell type, type of physical force used, and physical parameters of the procedure (pulse strength and frequency, acoustic pressure, exposure duration, etc.) are the key determinants of the degree of cytotoxicity, and local tissue damage may be associated with this procedure [139].

Physical methods have some practical issues that limit their applicability in gene therapy trials, along with relatively lower *in vivo* efficiency compared with viral and nonviral methods. Microinjection, for example, is challenged by its fastidious technique that requires a skilled person to do injections one by one to individual cells. The gene gun uses a special device that is quickly and easily operated; however, *in vivo* efficiency is limited by the shallow penetration of particles into biological tissue. Electroporation-mediated gene transfer, on the other hand, is limited to the area where the electrodes were positioned. These issues are also encountered by other methods of gene transfer. Other challenges associated with most physical methods include the requirement of special hardware to run the procedure. This hardware adds an extra challenge regarding the technical aspects of these devices. Improving the efficiency of physical methods for gene transfer, while minimizing the collateral damage to the tissue being treated, represents the major focus for future development.

CASE STUDIES

CASE STUDY 1: GENE THERAPY FOR ADA-SCID USING RETROVIRAL VECTOR

Background

This case study was extracted from Gaspar et al. [140]. Adenosine deaminase-deficient (ADA) SCID is a fatal disorder of purine metabolism that results in abnormal T, B, and natural killer cell development and immunodeficiency. A child with ADA-SCID who showed a poor response to PEG-ADA enzyme replacement was enrolled in the clinical gene therapy study. Autologous CD34$^+$ bone marrow cells transduced with a retroviral vector contained the ADA gene were introduced into the child with SCID after nonmyeloablative conditioning with melphalan. Enzyme-replacement therapy was withdrawn 1 month prior to infusion of the cells. Cessation of PEG-ADA and use of chemotherapy are necessary prerequisites for successful engraftment and proliferation of gene modified cells.

Rationale for Conducting This Study

Criteria for entry into the gene therapy trial were (1) confirmation of ADA-SCID by identification of the genetic defect or biochemical abnormality associated with disease (like dATP serum level), (2) lack of an HLA-matched donor for hematopoietic stem cell transplantation, and (3) failure of enzyme replacement therapy.

Results

Two years after the procedure, immunological and biochemical correction has been maintained with a progressive increase in lymphocyte numbers, reinitiation of thymopoiesis, and systemic detoxification of ADA metabolites. Sustained vector marking with detection of polyclonal vector integration sites in multiple cell lineages and detection of ADA activity in red blood cells suggests transduction of early hematopoietic progenitors. No serious side effects were seen, either as a result of the conditioning procedure or due to retroviral insertion.

Conclusion

Gene therapy with nonmyeloablative conditioning is a promising approach for all patients with SCID due to ADA deficiency who lack an HLA-matched donor. This study suggests that gene therapy, in combination with appropriate conditioning regimens, could be successfully extended for the treatment of other congenital disorders.

CASE STUDY 2: GENE THERAPY FOR METASTATIC MELANOMA USING LIPOPLEXES SYSTEM

Background

This case study was extracted from Stopeck et al. [61]. Melanoma is a highly malignant cancer that became resistant to most current treatment strategies, including chemotherapy and radiation. It has been reported that melanoma cells have reduced expression of the MHC class I protein, and this mechanism is responsible for tumor escape of immunosurveillance. In this clinical trial, gene therapy was considered as the immunotherapy approach to treat melanoma by direct intratumoral injections of lipoplexes (plasmid DNA–cationic lipids complex) having genes for allogeneic expression of MHC class I protein, HLA-B7 and β_2-microglobulin of MHC-I.

Rationale for Conducting This Study

- Reintroduction of MHC-I expression in tumor cells using the gene therapy approach would induce immune response against and suppress growth of tumor.
- Expression of a foreign and highly immunogenic cell surface protein like HLA-B7 and replacement of β_2-microglobulin would increase expression of the patient's own MHC-I.
- Preclinical studies on mice have shown that direct gene transfer of an allogeneic MHC-I gene induces a specific cellular immune response and the subsequent rejection of tumor cells.
- Phase I study using direct gene transfer into patients resulted in partial success.

Results

Treatment was safe and well tolerated, with mild to moderate adverse events including ecchymosis, pruritus and discomfort at the injection site, and pneumothoraxes. Injected lesions regressed in nine patients, with one complete response, three partial responses, and five minor responses. An overall response rate was 4% (two partial responses), and nine patients (18%) maintained the stable disease for at least 11 weeks. Six patients remained alive 25.1 to 39.4 months from first injection, including two patients with local (injected tumor) responses and one patient with an overall disease partial response.

Conclusion

This study demonstrates the potential of gene therapy as an efficient and safe alternative to current anticancer strategies. Despite the need for further improvements, lipoplexes systems have impressive potential to be applied in human gene therapy.

SUMMARY

The potential and promise for gene therapy in treating diseases have grown exponentially, paralleling advances in molecular biology that offer powerful tools to address the very basis of disease pathogenesis. One can think of genes that may ultimately be used as other small molecule drugs. When given as simple intravenous injections, gene transfer vehicles seek out target cells for stable and regulated gene expression. Delivery of transgenes in target cells is currently achieved using three different strategies: viral vectors, nonviral vectors, and physical methods. So far, viral vectors remain the most prevalent in human clinical trials despite the increased safety concerns associated with their *in vivo* applications. Synthetic or nonviral vectors, on the other hand, offer safer, though less efficient, alternatives to viral vectors. Physical methods use physical forces to enforce cellular uptake of DNA. With the exception of hydrodynamic gene transfer, *in vivo* efficiency of physical methods has not been fully demonstrated thus far. Current research is devoted to the engineering of more efficient, safer, and targeted systems for gene delivery and is aimed at overcoming challenges associated with current methods of gene delivery. What diseases will ultimately be curable by gene therapy and which strategies will be developed and successfully applied remain to be seen. At this point, with the progression of science, it seems safe to predict that gene therapy and DNA-based therapeutics will account for a large part of our next generation tools to fight against human diseases, prominently cancers and genetic disorders.

REVIEW QUESTIONS

1. Which cell type would not be a direct target for gene therapy?
   a. Endothelial cells
   b. White blood cells
   c. Red blood cells
   d. Muscle cells
   e. Liver cells
2. Among the physical methods of gene transfer, what is the simplest and most effective method to achieve *in vivo* gene transfer in the liver?
   a. Gene gun
   b. Needle injection
   c. Electroporation
   d. Hydrodynamic gene transfer
   e. Sonoporation
3. Successful gene therapy requires efficient gene transfer in target cells. What are the barriers encountered for gene delivery into target cells?
4. Explain how the physical methods of gene transfer eliminate the need for gene carriers (i.e., viral and nonviral vectors) to achieve gene transfer in target cells.
5. Cystic fibrosis is a genetic disorder affecting many organs, primarily the lungs and intestines. Your job is to design a gene therapy strategy for disease treatment.
   a. What is the genetic cause of the disease?
   b. What are the points to be considered to justify disease candidacy for gene therapy? What is your strategy to cure the disease?
   c. You have decided that cystic fibrosis is a good candidate for gene therapy. Now you need to select a gene delivery system to deliver therapeutic genes into lung tissue. Vectors available for use in your facility are the herpes simplex virus, adenovirus, adeno-associated virus, and liposome–DNA systems. What vector would be your choice? Why? Explain why the other types would not be good choices.
6. Taqi is a graduate student working on a muscle dystrophy mice model. Muscle dystrophy is a genetic disorder that occurs when a gene on the X chromosome fails to make an essential muscle protein, dystrophin. Taqi hypothesized that overexpression of dystrophin in muscle fibers should cure the disease, so he transfected the mice with the dystrophin gene using a retrovirus vector. However, no disease improvement was observed with the treatment. As a result, Taqi concluded that

his hypothesis was wrong. Do you agree with his conclusion? Why? What would be your strategy instead?

REFERENCES

1. Cotrim AP, Baum BJ. Gene therapy: some history, applications, problems, and prospects. *Toxicol Pathol.* 2008;36(1):97–103.
2. Rogers S. Induction of arginase in rabbit epithelium by the Shope rabbit papilloma virus. *Nature.* 1959;183(4678):1815–1816.
3. Rogers S, Pfuderer P. Use of viruses as carriers of added genetic information. *Nature.* 1968; 219(5155):749–751.
4. Friedmann T. Stanfield R. Insights into virus vectors and failure of an early gene therapy model. *Mol Ther.* 2001;4(4):285–288.
5. Scollay R. Gene therapy: a brief overview of the past, present, and future. *Ann NY Acad Sci.* 2001;953:26–30.
6. Yi Y, Noh MJ, Lee KH. Current advances in retroviral gene therapy. *Curr Gene Ther.* 2011; 11(3):218–228.
7. Kay MA, Glorioso JC, Naldini L. Viral vectors for gene therapy: the art of turning infectious agents into vehicles of therapeutics. *Nat Med.* 2001;7(1):33–40.
8. Edelstein ML, Abedi MR, Wixon J. Gene therapy clinical trials worldwide to 2007—an update. *J Gene Med.* 2007;9(10):833–842.
9. Blaese RM, Culver KW, Miller AD, et al. T lymphocyte-directed gene therapy for ADA- SCID: initial trial results after 4 years. *Science.* 1995;270(5235):475–480.
10. Hacein-Bey-Abina S, Le Deist F, Carlier F, et al. Sustained correction of X-linked severe combined immunodeficiency by *ex vivo* gene therapy. *N Engl J Med.* 2002;346(16):1185–1193.
11. Aiuti A, Cattaneo F, Galimberti S, et al. Gene therapy for immunodeficiency due to adenosine deaminase deficiency. *N Engl J Med.* 2009;360(5):447–458.
12. Gaspar HB, Cooray S, Gilmour KC, et al. Hematopoietic stem cell gene therapy for adenosine deaminase-deficient severe combined immunodeficiency leads to long-term immunological recovery and metabolic correction. *Sci Transl Med.* 2011;3(97):97–80.
13. Barquinero J, Eixarch H, Perez-Melgosa M. Retroviral vectors: new applications for an old tool. *Gene Ther.* 2004;11(Suppl 1):S3–S9.
14. Hu WS, Pathak VK. Design of retroviral vectors and helper cells for gene therapy. *Pharmacol Rev.* 2000;52(4):493–511.
15. Naldini L, Blomer U, Gallay P, et al. *In vivo* gene delivery and stable transduction of nondividing cells by a lentiviral vector. *Science.* 1996;272(5259):263–267.
16. Lewis PF, Emerman M. Passage through mitosis is required for oncoretroviruses but not for the human-immunodeficiency-virus. *J Virol.* 1994;68(1):510–516.
17. Matrai J, Chuah MK, Vanden Driessche T. Recent advances in lentiviral vector development and applications. *Mol Ther.* 2010;18(3):477–490.
18. Kumar P, Woon-Khiong C. Optimization of lentiviral vectors generation for biomedical and clinical research purposes: contemporary trends in technology development and applications. *Curr Gene Ther.* 2011;11(2):144–153.
19. Levine BL, Humeau LM, Boyer J, et al. Gene transfer in humans using a conditionally replicating lentiviral vector. *Proc Natl Acad Sci USA.* 2006;103(46):17372–17377.
20. D'Costa J, Mansfield SG, Humeau LM. Lentiviral vectors in clinical trials: current status. *Curr Opin Mol Ther.* 2009;11(5):554–564.
21. Kaiser J. Gene therapy: beta-thalassemia treatment succeeds, with a caveat. *Science.* 2009; 326(5959): 1468–1469.
22. Cartier N, Hacein-Bey-Abina S, Bartholomae CC, et al. Hematopoietic stem cell gene therapy with a lentiviral vector in X-linked adrenoleukodystrophy. *Science.* 2009;326(5954):818–823.
23. Berkner KL. Development of adenovirus vectors for the expression of heterologous genes. *BioTechniques.* 1988;6(7):616–629.
24. Kovesdi I, Brough DE, Bruder JT, Wickham TJ. Adenoviral vectors for gene transfer. *Curr Opin Biotechnol.* 1997;8(5):583–589.
25. Imperiale MJ, Kochanek S. Adenovirus vectors: biology, design, and production. *Curr Top Microbiol Immunol.* 2004;273:335–357.
26. Goncalves MA, de Vries AA. Adenovirus: from foe to friend. *Rev Med Virol.* 2006;16(3):167–186.

27. Flint J, Shenk T. Viral transactivating proteins. *Annu Rev Genet*. 1997;31:177–212.
28. Bergelson JM, Cunningham JA, Droguett G, et al. Isolation of a common receptor for Coxsackie B viruses and adenoviruses 2 and 5. *Science*. 1997;275(5304):1320–1323.
29. Roelvink PW, Lizonova A, Lee JG, et al. The coxsackievirus-adenovirus receptor protein can function as a cellular attachment protein for adenovirus serotypes from subgroups A, C, D, E, and F. *J Virol*. 1998;72(10):7909–7915.
30. Gaggar A, Shayakhmetov DM, Lieber A. CD46 is a cellular receptor for group B adenoviruses. *Nat Med*. 2003;9(11):1408–1412.
31. Arnberg N, Kidd AH, Edlund K, Nilsson J, Pring-Akerblom P, Wadell G. Adenovirus type 37 binds to cell surface sialic acid through a charge-dependent interaction. *Virology*. 2002;302(1):33–43.
32. Leopold PL, Crystal RG. Intracellular trafficking of adenovirus: many means to many ends. *Adv Drug Deliv Rev*. 2007;59(8):810–821.
33. Mizuguchi H, Kay MA, Hayakawa T. Approaches for generating recombinant adenovirus vectors. *Adv Drug Deliv Rev*. 2001;52(3):165–176.
34. Walther W, Stein U. Viral vectors for gene transfer: a review of their use in the treatment of human diseases. *Drugs*. 2000;60(2):249–271.
35. Worgall S, Wolff G, Falck-Pedersen E, Crystal RG. Innate immune mechanisms dominate elimination of adenoviral vectors following *in vivo* administration. *Hum Gene Ther*. 1997;8(1):37–44.
36. Jooss K, Chirmule N. Immunity to adenovirus and adeno-associated viral vectors: implications for gene therapy. *Gene Ther*. 2003;10(11):955–963.
37. Jozkowicz A, Dulak J. Helper-dependent adenoviral vectors in experimental gene therapy. *Acta Biochim Pol*. 2005;52(3):589–599.
38. Segura MM, Alba R, Bosch A, Chillon M. Advances in helper-dependent adenoviral vector research. *Curr Gene Ther*. 2008;8(4):222–235.
39. Coura R dos S, Nardi NB. The state of the art of adeno-associated virus-based vectors in gene therapy. *Virol J*. 2007;4:99.
40. Hildinger M, Auricchio A. Advances in AAV-mediated gene transfer for the treatment of inherited disorders. *Eur J Hum Genet*. 2004;12(4):263–271.
41. Daya S, Berns KI. Gene therapy using adeno-associated virus vectors. *Clin Microbiol Rev*. 2008; 21(4):583–593.
42. Geoffroy MC, Salvetti A. Helper functions required for wild type and recombinant adeno-associated virus growth. *Curr Gene Ther*. 2005;5(3):265–271.
43. Ayuso E, Mingozzi F, Bosch F. Production, purification and characterization of adeno-associated vectors. *Curr Gene Ther*. 2010;10(6):423–436.
44. Thomas CE, Ehrhardt A, Kay MA. Progress and problems with the use of viral vectors for gene therapy. *Nat Rev Genet*. 2003;4(5):346–358.
45. Manno CS, Chew AJ, Hutchison S, et al. AAV-mediated factor IX gene transfer to skeletal muscle in patients with severe hemophilia B. *Blood*. 2003;101(8):2963–2972.
46. McPhee SW, Janson CG, Li C, et al. Immune responses to AAV in a phase I study for Canavan disease. *J Gene Med*. 2006;8(5):577–588.
47. Moss RB, Rodman D, Spencer LT, et al. Repeated adeno-associated virus serotype 2 aerosol-mediated cystic fibrosis transmembrane regulator gene transfer to the lungs of patients with cystic fibrosis: a multicenter, double-blind, placebo-controlled trial. *Chest*. 2004;125(2):509–521.
48. Wagner JA, Nepomuceno IB, Messner AH, et al. A phase II, double-blind, randomized, placebo-controlled clinical trial of tgAAVCF using maxillary sinus delivery in patients with cystic fibrosis with antrostomies. *Hum Gene Ther*. 2002;13(11):1349–1359.
49. Epstein AL. Progress and prospects: biological properties and technological advances of herpes simplex virus type 1-based amplicon vectors. *Gene Ther*. 2009;16(6):709–715.
50. Manservigi R, Argnani R, Marconi P. HSV recombinant vectors for gene therapy. *Open Virol J*. 2010;4:123–156.
51. Friedman GK, Pressey JG, Reddy AT, Markert JM, Gillespie GY. Herpes simplex virus oncolytic therapy for pediatric malignancies. *Mol Ther*. 2009;17(7):1125–1135.
52. Glorioso JC, Fink DJ. Herpes vector-mediated gene transfer in the treatment of chronic pain. *Mol Ther*. 2009;17(1):13–18.
53. Thorne SH. Next-generation oncolytic vaccinia vectors. *Methods Mol Biol*. 2012;797:205–215.
54. Hu YC. Baculoviral vectors for gene delivery: a review. *Curr Gene Ther*. 2008;8(1):54–65.
55. Kamimura K, Suda T, Zhang G, Liu D. Advances in gene delivery systems. *Pharm Med*. 2011; 25(5):293–306.
56. Lieber A, Steinwaerder DS, Carlson CA, Kay MA. Integrating adenovirus-adeno-associated virus hybrid vectors devoid of all viral genes. *J Virol*. 1999;73(11):9314–9324.

57. Oehmig A, Fraefel C, Breakefield XO, Ackermann M. Herpes simplex virus type 1 amplicons and their hybrid virus partners, EBV, AAV, and retrovirus. *Curr Gene Ther.* 2004;4(4):385–408.

58. Pagano JS, Vaheri A. Enhancement of infectivity of poliovirus RNA with diethylaminoethyl-dextran (DEAE-D). *Arch Gesamte Virusforsch.* 1965;17(3):456–464.

59. Bangham AD, Standish MM, Watkins JC. Diffusion of univalent ions across the lamellae of swollen phospholipids. *J Mol Biol.* 1965;13(1):238–252.

60. Felgner PL, Gadek TR, Holm M, et al. Lipofection: a highly efficient, lipid-mediated DNA-transfection procedure. *Proc Natl Acad Sci USA.* 1987;84(21):7413–7417.

61. Stopeck AT, Jones A, Hersh EM, et al. Phase II study of direct intralesional gene transfer of allo-vectin-7, an HLA-B7/beta2-microglobulin DNA-liposome complex, in patients with metastatic melanoma. *Clin Cancer Res.* 2001;7(8):2285–2291.

62. Boussif O, Lezoualc'h F, Zanta MA, et al. A versatile vector for gene and oligonucleotide transfer into cells in culture and *in vivo*: polyethylenimine. *Proc Natl Acad Sci USA.* 1995; 92(16): 7297–7301.

63. Fischer D, Bieber T, Li Y, Elsasser HP, Kissel T. A novel non-viral vector for DNA delivery based on low molecular weight, branched polyethylenimine: effect of molecular weight on transfection efficiency and cytotoxicity. *Pharm Res.* 1999;16(8):1273–1279.

64. Al-Dosari MS, Gao X. Nonviral gene delivery: principle, limitations, and recent progress. *AAPS J.* 2009;11(4):671–681.

65. Roy I, Mitra S, Maitra A, Mozumdar S. Calcium phosphate nanoparticles as novel non-viral vectors for targeted gene delivery. *Int J Pharm.* 2003;250(1):25–33.

66. Sokolova V, Epple M. Inorganic nanoparticles as carriers of nucleic acids into cells. *Angew Chem Int Ed Engl.* 2008;47(8):1382–1395.

67. Wolff JA, Malone RW, Williams P, et al. Direct gene transfer into mouse muscle *in vivo*. *Science.* 1990;247(4949 Pt 1):1465–1468.

68. Prausnitz MR, Mikszta JA, Cormier M, Andrianov AK. Microneedle-based vaccines. *Curr Top Microbiol Immunol.* 2009;333:369–393.

69. Auerbach AB. Production of functional transgenic mice by DNA pronuclear microinjection. *Acta Biochim Pol.* 2004;51(1):9–31.

70. Klein RM, Wolf ED, Wu R, Sanford JC. High-velocity microprojectiles for delivering nucleic acids into living cells. *Nature.* 1987;327(6117):70–73.

71. Yang NS, Burkholder J, Roberts B, Martinell B, McCabe D. *In vivo* and *in vitro* gene transfer to mammalian somatic cells by particle bombardment. *Proc Natl Acad Sci USA.* 1990;87(24):9568–9572.

72. Kim D, Hoory T, Monie A, Ting JP, Hung CF, Wu TC. Enhancement of DNA vaccine potency through coadministration of CIITA DNA with DNA vaccines via gene gun. *J Immunol.* 2008; 180(10):7019–7027.

73. Roberts LK, Barr LJ, Fuller DH, McMahon CW, Leese PT, Jones S. Clinical safety and efficacy of a powdered Hepatitis B nucleic acid vaccine delivered to the epidermis by a commercial prototype device. *Vaccine.* 2005;23(40):4867–4878.

74. Cassaday RD, Sondel PM, King DM, et al. A phase I study of immunization using particle-mediated epidermal delivery of genes for gp100 and GM-CSF into uninvolved skin of melanoma patients. *Clin Cancer Res.* 2007;13(2 Pt 1):540–549.

75. Neumann E, Schaefer-Ridder M, Wang Y, Hofschneider PH. Gene transfer into mouse lyoma cells by electroporation in high electric fields. *EMBO J.* 1982;1(7):841–845.

76. Heller LC, Ugen K, Heller R. Electroporation for targeted gene transfer. *Expert Opin Drug Deliv.* 2005;2(2):255–268.

77. Sardesai NY, Weiner DB. Electroporation delivery of DNA vaccines: prospects for success. *Curr Opin Immunol.* 2011;23(3):421–429.

78. Bodles-Brakhop AM, Heller R, Draghia-Akli R. Electroporation for the delivery of DNA-based vaccines and immunotherapeutics: current clinical developments. *Mol Ther.* 2009;17(4): 585–592.

79. Gao X, Kim KS, Liu D. Nonviral gene delivery: what we know and what is next. *AAPS J.* 2007;9(1):E92-E104.

80. Zhang LJ, Chen LM, Yuan J, Jia SR, Xu N, Zhao NM. Ultrasonic direct gene transfer - establishment of a high-efficiency genetic transformation system for tobacco. *Sci Agri Sin.* 1990;23(5):88–90.

81. Mitragotri S, Edwards DA, Blankschtein D, Langer R. A mechanistic study of ultrasonically-enhanced transdermal drug delivery. *J Pharm Sci.* 1995;84(6):697–706.

82. Hosseinkhani H, Aoyama T, Ogawa O, Tabata Y. Ultrasound enhances the transfection of plasmid DNA by non-viral vectors. *Curr Pharm Biotechnol.* 2003;4(2):109–122.

83. Shen ZP, Brayman AA, Chen L, Miao CH. Ultrasound with microbubbles enhances gene expression of plasmid DNA in the liver via intraportal delivery. *Gene Ther.* 2008;15(16):1147–1155.

84. Zeira E, Manevitch A, Khatchatouriants A, et al. Femtosecond infrared laser—an efficient and safe *in vivo* gene delivery system for prolonged expression. *Mol Ther.* 2003;8(2):342–350.

85. Yao CP, Zhang ZX, Rahmanzadeh R, Huettmann G. Laser-based gene transfection and gene therapy. *IEEE trans Nanobioscience.* 2008;7(2):111–119.

86. He H, Kong SK, Lee RK, Suen YK, Chan KT. Targeted photoporation and transfection in human HepG2 cells by a fiber femtosecond laser at 1554 nm. *Opt Lett.* 2008;33(24):2961–2963.

87. Kievit FM, Veiseh O, Bhattarai N, et al. PEI-PEG-chitosan copolymer coated iron oxide nanoparticles for safe gene delivery: synthesis, complexation, and transfection. *Adv Funct Mater.* 2009;19(14):2244–2251.

88. Sapet C, Pellegrino C, Laurent N, Sicard F, Zelphati O. Magnetic nanoparticles enhance adenovirus transduction *in vitro* and *in vivo*. *Pharm Res.* 2012;29(5):1203–1218.

89. Plank C, Zelphati O, Mykhaylyk O. Magnetically enhanced nucleic acid delivery. Ten years of magnetofection-progress and prospects. *Adv Drug Deliv Rev.* 2011;63(14–15):1300–1331.

90. Namiki Y, Namiki T, Yoshida H, et al. A novel magnetic crystal-lipid nanostructure for magnetically guided *in vivo* gene delivery. *Nat Nanotechnol.* 2009;4(9):598–606.

91. Liu F, Song Y, Liu D. Hydrodynamics-based transfection in animals by systemic administration of plasmid DNA. *Gene Ther.* 1999;6(7):1258–1266.

92. Zhang G, Budker V, Wolff JA. High levels of foreign gene expression in hepatocytes after tail vein injections of naked plasmid DNA. *Hum Gene Ther.* 1999;10(10):1735–1737.

93. Zhang G, Gao X, Song YK, et al. Hydroporation as the mechanism of hydrodynamic delivery. *Gene Ther.* 2004;11(8):675–682.

94. Li J, Yao Q, Liu D. Hydrodynamic cell delivery for simultaneous establishment of tumor growth in mouse lung, liver and kidney. *Cancer Biol Ther.* 2011;12(8):737–741.

95. Suda T, Suda K, Liu D. Computer-assisted hydrodynamic gene delivery. *Mol Ther.* 2008;16(6):1098–1104.

96. Kamimura K, Suda T, Xu W, Zhang G, Liu D. Image-guided, lobe-specific hydrodynamic gene delivery to swine liver. *Mol Ther.* 2009;17(3):491–499.

97. Wiethoff CM, Middaugh CR. Barriers to nonviral gene delivery. *J Pharm Sci.* 2003;92(2):203–217.

98. Kohn DB, Sadelain M, Glorioso JC. Occurrence of leukaemia following gene therapy of X-linked SCID. *Nat Rev Cancer.* 2003;3(7):477–488.

99. Hacein-Bey-Abina S, von Kalle C, Schmidt M, et al. A serious adverse event after successful gene therapy for X-linked severe combined immunodeficiency. *N Engl J Med.* 2003;348(3):255–256.

100. Hacein-Bey-Abina S, Von Kalle C, Schmidt M, et al. LMO2-associated clonal T cell proliferation in two patients after gene therapy for SCID-X1. *Science.* 2003;302(5644):415–419.

101. McCormack MP, Rabbitts TH. Activation of the T-cell oncogene LMO2 after gene therapy for X-linked severe combined immunodeficiency. *N Engl J Med.* 2004;350(9):913–922.

102. Gustafsson J, Arvidson G, Karlsson G, Almgren M. Complexes between cationic liposomes and DNA visualized by cryo-TEM. *Biochim Biophys Acta.* 1995;1235(2):305–312.

103. Narang AS, Thoma L, Miller DD, Mahato RI. Cationic lipids with increased DNA binding affinity for nonviral gene transfer in dividing and nondividing cells. *Bioconj Chem.* 2005;16(1):156–168.

104. Oupicky D, Konak C, Dash PR, Seymour LW, Ulbrich K. Effect of albumin and polyanion on the structure of DNA complexes with polycation containing hydrophilic nonionic block. *Bioconj Chem.* 1999;10(5):764–772.

105. Hong K, Zheng W, Baker A, Papahadjopoulos D. Stabilization of cationic liposome-plasmid DNA complexes by polyamines and poly(ethylene glycol)-phospholipid conjugates for efficient in vivo gene delivery. *FEBS Lett.* 1997;400(2):233–237.

106. Lee M, Kim SW. Polyethylene glycol-conjugated copolymers for plasmid DNA delivery. *Pharm Res.* 2005;22(1):1–10.

107. Ruponen M, Yla-Herttuala S, Urtti A. Interactions of polymeric and liposomal gene delivery systems with extracellular glycosaminoglycans: physicochemical and transfection studies. *Biochim Biophys Acta.* 1999;1415(2):331–341.

108. Sakurai F, Nishioka T, Saito H, et al. Interaction between DNA-cationic liposome complexes and erythrocytes is an important factor in systemic gene transfer via the intravenous route in mice: the role of the neutral helper lipid. *Gene Ther.* 2001;8(9):677–686.

109. Li SD, Huang L. Stealth nanoparticles: high density but sheddable PEG is a key for tumor targeting. *J Control Release.* 2010;145(3):178–181.

110. Dufort S, Sancey L, Coll JL. Physico-chemical parameters that govern nanoparticles fate also dictate rules for their molecular evolution. *Adv Drug Deliv Rev.* 2012;64(2):179–189.

111. Martina M-S, Nicolas V, Wilhelm C, Ménager C, Barratt G, Lesieur S. The *in vitro* kinetics of the interactions between PEG-ylated magnetic-fluid-loaded liposomes and macrophages. *Biomaterials.* 2007;28(28):4143–4153.

112. Takakura Y, Mahato RI, Hashida M. Extravasation of macromolecules. *Adv Drug Deliv Rev.* 1998;34(1):93–108.

113. Seymour LW. Passive tumor targeting of soluble macromolecules and drug conjugates. *Crit Rev Ther Drug Carrier Syst.* 1992;9(2):135–187.

114. Pouton CW, Seymour LW. Key issues in non-viral gene delivery. *Adv Drug Deliv Rev.* 2001; 46(1-3):187–203.

115. Boeckle S, Wagner E. Optimizing targeted gene delivery: chemical modification of viral vectors and synthesis of artificial virus vector systems. *AAPS J.* 2006;8(4):E731-E742.

116. Upadhyay KK, Agrawal HG, Upadhyay C, et al. Role of block copolymer nanoconstructs in cancer therapy. *Crit Rev Ther Drug Carrier Syst.* 2009;26(2):157–205.

117. Lipinski KS, Djeha HA, Gawn J, et al. Optimization of a synthetic beta-catenin-dependent promoter for tumor-specific cancer gene therapy. *Mol Ther.* 2004;10(1):150–161.

118. Nguyen J, Szoka FC. Nucleic acid delivery: the missing pieces of the puzzle? *Acc Chem Res.* 2012.

119. Xu YH, Szoka FC. Mechanism of DNA release from cationic liposome/DNA complexes used in cell transfection. *Biochemistry.* 1996;35(18):5616–5623.

120. Zhang ZY, Smith BD. High-generation polycationic dendrimers are unusually effective at disrupting anionic vesicles: membrane bending model. *Bioconj Chem.* 2000;11(6):805–814.

121. West KR, Otto S. Reversible covalent chemistry in drug delivery. *Curr Drug Discov Technol.* 2005;2(3):123–160.

122. Hatakeyama H, Akita H, Kogure K, et al. Development of a novel systemic gene delivery system for cancer therapy with a tumor-specific cleavable PEG-lipid. *Gene Ther.* 2007;14(1):68–77.

123. Ciftci K, Levy RJ. Enhanced plasmid DNA transfection with lysosomotropic agents in cultured fibroblasts. *Int J Pharm.* 2001;218(1-2):81–92.

124. Mislick KA, Baldeschwieler JD. Evidence for the role of proteoglycans in cation-mediated gene transfer. *Proc Natl Acad Sci USA.* 1996;93(22):12349–12354.

125. Pratten MK, Cable HC, Ringsdorf H, Lloyd JB. Adsorptive pinocytosis of polycationic copolymers of vinylpyrrolidone with vinylamine by rat yolk sac and rat peritoneal macrophage. *Biochim Biophys Acta.* 1982;719(3):424–430.

126. Zuhorn IS, Kalicharan R, Hoekstra D. Lipoplex-mediated transfection of mammalian cells occurs through the cholesterol-dependent clathrin-mediated pathway of endocytosis. *J Biol Chem.* 2002;277(20):18021–18028.

127. de Semir D, Petriz J, Avinyo A, et al. Non-viral vector-mediated uptake, distribution, and stability of chimeraplasts in human airway epithelial cells. *J Gene Med.* 2002;4(3):308–322.

128. Basner-Tschakarjan E, Mirmohammadsadegh A, Baer A, Hengge UR. Uptake and trafficking of DNA in keratinocytes: evidence for DNA-binding proteins. *Gene Ther.* 2004;11(9):765–774.

129. Cornelis S, Vandenbranden M, Ruysschaert JM, Elouahabi A. Role of intracellular cationic liposome-DNA complex dissociation in transfection mediated by cationic lipids. *DNA Cell Biol.* 2002;21(2):91–97.

130. Luby-Phelps K. Cytoarchitecture and physical properties of cytoplasm: volume, viscosity, diffusion, intracellular surface area. *Int Rev Cytol.* 2000;192:189–221.

131. Verkman AS. Solute and macromolecule diffusion in cellular aqueous compartments. *Trends Biochem Sci.* 2002;27(1):27–33.

132. Lukacs GL, Haggie P, Seksek O, Lechardeur D, Freedman N, Verkman AS. Size-dependent DNA mobility in cytoplasm and nucleus. *J Biol Chem.* 2000;275(3):1625–1629.

133. Lechardeur D, Lukacs GL. Intracellular barriers to non-viral gene transfer. *Curr Gene Ther.* 2002; 2(2):183–194.

134. Lechardeur D, Sohn KJ, Haardt M, et al. Metabolic instability of plasmid DNA in the cytosol: a potential barrier to gene transfer. *Gene Ther.* 1999;6(4):482–497.

135. Pollard H, Toumaniantz G, Amos JL, et al. Ca2+-sensitive cytosolic nucleases prevent efficient delivery to the nucleus of injected plasmids. *J Gene Med.* 2001;3(2):153–164.

136. Capecchi MR. High efficiency transformation by direct microinjection of DNA into cultured mammalian cells. *Cell.* 1980;22(2 Pt 2):479–488.

137. Mattaj IW, Englmeier L. Nucleocytoplasmic transport: the soluble phase. *Annu Rev Biochem.* 1998; 67:265–306.

138. Dean DA, Strong DD, Zimmer WE. Nuclear entry of nonviral vectors. *Gene Ther.* 2005; 12(11):881–890.

139. Mehier-Humbert S, Guy RH. Physical methods for gene transfer: improving the kinetics of gene delivery into cells. *Adv Drug Deliv Rev.* 2005;57(5):733–753.

140. Gaspar HB, Bjorkegren E, Parsley K, et al. Successful reconstitution of immunity in ADA-SCID by stem cell gene therapy following cessation of PEG-ADA and use of mild preconditioning. *Mol Ther.* 2006;14(4):505–513.

141. Lee H, Hu M, Reilly RM, Allen C. Apoptotic epidermal growth factor (EGF)-conjugated block copolymer micelles as a nanotechnology platform for targeted combination therapy. *Mol Pharm.* 2007;4(5):769–781.

142. Lukyanov AN, Gao Z, Torchilin VP. Micelles from polyethylene glycol/phosphatidylethanolamine conjugates for tumor drug delivery. *J Control Release.* 2003;91(1–2):97–102.

143. Sethuraman VA, Na K, Bae YH. pH-Responsive sulfonamide/PEI system for tumor specific gene delivery: an *in vitro* study. *Biomacromolecules.* 2006;7(1):64–70.

144. Zintchenko A, Ogris M, Wagner E. Temperature dependent gene expression induced by PNIPAM-based copolymers: potential of hyperthermia in gene transfer. *Bioconj Chem.* 2006;17(3):766–772.

145. Cai X, Dong C, Dong H, et al. Effective gene delivery using stimulus-responsive catiomer designed with redox-sensitive disulfide and acid-labile imine linkers. *Biomacromolecules.* 2012;13(4):1024–1034.

CHAPTER 17

PEPTIDE AND PROTEIN DRUG DELIVERY

CHRIS KULCZAR, WYATT ROTH, STEPHEN CARL, OLAFUR GUDMUNDSSON, AND GREGORY KNIPP

CHAPTER OBJECTIVES

Upon completing this chapter, the reader should be able to

▸ Understand the physicochemical differences between small molecule and protein/peptide drugs.

▸ Understand the physiological and chemical barriers that protein/peptide drugs face for different methods of delivery.

▸ Explain why parenteral delivery is most often used with protein/peptide drugs.

▸ Distinguish the advantages and disadvantages of different alternative routes for delivering protein/peptide drugs.

▸ Understand the challenges faced when formulating a protein/peptide drug for oral delivery.

▸   Discuss the intricacies of insulin that make nonparenteral delivery challenging.

▸   Describe different novel techniques for delivering protein/peptide drugs and understand the challenges they help overcome.

CHAPTER OUTLINE

INTRODUCTION

The pharmaceutical biotechnology field is rapidly expanding, with sales of biologics reaching $163 billion in 2012 and projected to reach $253 billion by 2017 [1]. The combined therapeutic protein and monoclonal antibody market sales were $130.3 billion in 2012 and projected to reach $203.3 billion in 2017, representing 56% growth over the 5-year period. Clearly, such a large growth rate in the generation of these peptide/protein-based agents requires an increased understanding of the rate-determining steps associated with their production, handling, and utility in the clinic.

For clarity purposes, we define peptide and protein drugs as those that include monoclonal antibodies, hormones, recombinant proteins, small and large oligopeptide-based agents, and related compounds. Peptide and protein drugs are often sought after because of their high specificity and potency. This may lead to the clinical utility of lower doses and potentially reduce off-target side effects [2]. Scientists face a number of potential issues, however, when attempting to scale up peptide and protein drugs and develop quality formulations that ensure chemical and physical stability of the peptide and protein drugs. This is largely due to the physicochemical properties associated with these agents. In this chapter, we discuss some of the differences between small molecule and protein/peptide drugs, the challenges these differences present, and methods for overcoming them.

PHYSICOCHEMICAL DIFFERENCES BETWEEN PEPTIDE/PROTEINS AND SMALL MOLECULES

Peptides and proteins represent a heterogeneous polymer of 20 common amino acids and several other noncommonly occurring analogues, as presented in Table 17-1. It is important to note that the individual amino acid side chains vary in charge, lipophilicity/hydrophilicity, size, and rigidity, which all contribute to higher order structure of peptides and proteins. We briefly highlight below the importance of these side chains in determining the structure and function of peptides and proteins. For additional detail on their importance, a biochemistry or biophysics textbook should be consulted [3, 4].

The physicochemical properties of proteins and peptides are quite different from those of small molecules, particularly with respect to chemical and physical structure, molecular weight, functional group diversity, lipophilic/hydrophilic balance that influences the polar surface area, and ionization. For example, small molecule drugs generally possess molecular weights of less than 800 Da, whereas some protein therapeutics can reach up to 150 kDa. As discussed below, these changes in size can greatly influence the ability of a molecule to permeate a cellular membrane [5].

STRUCTURE

Four different orders of structure are found in peptides and proteins: primary, secondary, tertiary, and quaternary. A number of forces are involved in maintaining the different levels of peptide and protein structure:

- Covalent amide bonds that hold the peptide backbone together and disulfide bonds between neighboring cysteine residues.

TABLE 17-1 Amino acid classification				
Aliphatic, Unsubstituted Acyclic (Apolar)	Aliphatic, Substituted Acyclic (Polar)	Aliphatic, Substituted Acyclic (Apolar)	Cyclic (Apolar/Polar)	Representative Uncommon (Apolar/Polar*)
Glycine (Gly, G)	Serine (Ser, S)	Cysteine (Cys, C)	Proline (Pro, P)	Hydroxyproline (Hyp, O)
Alanine (Ala, A)	Threonine (Thr, T)	Methionine (Met, M)	Phenylalanine (Phe, F)	Homocysteine (Hcy)
Valine (Val, V)	Aspartic acid (Asp, D)		Tyrosine (Tyr, Y)*	Homoserine (Hse)*
Leucine (Leu, L)	Glutamic acid (Glu, E)		Histidine (His, H)*	Homohistidine (Hhs)*
Isoleucine (Ile, I)	Asparagine (Asn, N)		Tryptophan (Trp, W)*	Ornithine (Orn)*
	Glutamine (Gln, Q)			Citrulline (Cit)*
	Lysine (Lys, K)			Thyroxine (Thx)*
	Arginine (Arg, R)			

- Electrostatic interactions, which are generally subdivided under charge–charge or dipolar interactions. For example, ionic interactions analogous to those found in salts can occur between amino acid side chains (called salt bridges). Dipolar interactions are also important forces that are classified as follows:
  - Charge–dipole interactions between an ion and a dipole on a neighboring functional group but are weaker than ionic interactions.
  - Keesom forces, which occur between neighboring oppositely charged dipoles.
  - Debye forces, which occur between a neighboring permanent dipole interacting with and inducing a dipole on another molecule.
  - London forces, which occur between neighboring molecules where there exists a dipole-induced dipole interaction. London forces commonly stabilize hydrophobic regions of proteins.
- Polar interactions can also form between π electron orbitals and include aromatic-aromatic interactions as well as oxygen or sulfur electron lone pair interactions with an aromatic residue. These interactions are dipolar in nature but are often separated out when discussing protein structure.
- Solvation is the last primary force commonly found in large molecules and consists of hydration or hydrogen bonding with the media. Hydrogen bonding arises from a net dipole in water and could be classified in both sections.

There may be other forces involved as well, but this list is fairly comprehensive. These forces vary greatly in energy. Depending on the energy balance in a peptide or a protein, it may range from being very stable to being highly susceptible to physical denaturation. Understanding the forces that govern protein-folding energy is critical before manufacturing, because shear and stress induced from unit operations and scale up varies and can dramatically influence physical and chemical stability [2].

The primary structure of a peptide or protein consists of its covalent alignment of amino acids in the single chain. The covalent amide bond is formed between the carbonyl of the first residue and the nitrogen of the second residue. The electron withdrawing capability of the oxygen in the carbonyl draws the lone pair of electrons on the nitrogen across the carbon–nitrogen bond, providing a partial double-bond–like character, and results in a net dipole formed between the δ^+ nitrogen and the δ^- oxygen. The double-bond–like character of the amide bond conformationally locks the rotation around into the sterically favored *trans* conformation. This becomes important in higher orders of structure, particularly the secondary structure. The amino acids in the primary structure are numbered from the amino terminus, and the sequence must be defined and fixed. Simple changes in the amino acid sequence of the primary structure can result in distinctly different higher order folding and functional properties. For example, an oligopeptide containing a sequence of YPGDV may not possess the same folding properties as YPDGV. These are two distinct peptides and must be characterized as such, even though the amino acid composition is identical.

In general, the secondary structure describes the steric relation of the neighboring amino acids related to the conformation of the peptide or protein region. Steric interactions between neighboring amino acids in the peptide or protein control the formation of the most energetically favored regional conformations. There are three rotational (dihedral) angles along the amino acid backbone [5, 6–8]: (1) The ω angle describes rotation around the carbonyl carbon to the amine (amide) bond, which is normally locked in the *trans* conformation; (2) the phi (φ) angle arises from rotation amine to the alpha carbon (Cα) bond; and (3) the psi (ψ) angle defines the rotation around the Cα to carbonyl carbon bond. The primary rotational angles around the

ϕ and ψ dihedral angles fall into energetically favored patterns that lead to our ability to classify the main types of secondary structure, which goes beyond the scope of this text. Disulfide bonds forming in close proximity can be considered part of the secondary structure. Conventionally, proteins were viewed as ball and stick figures representing the individual atoms and bonds of every amino acid along the backbone. It was difficult, however, to determine where the backbone resided compared with the side chains and what local secondary structures were present in various regions of a globular protein. To overcome this difficulty and obtain a better understanding of the secondary structural regions found in peptides and proteins, ribbons with arrows were used to represent the backbone of an α-helix and two antiparallel helices (discussed below) to clearly illustrate the orientation of the secondary structure were adapted (**Figure 17-1**) [6–8]. The common different regularly ordered secondary structural patterns arising from steric interactions found in peptides and proteins include the α-helix, β-sheet, and β-turn and in constrained conditions a γ-turn. We briefly review these secondary structural motifs below.

Helices are a common, secondary structural type. Several varieties of helices are found in proteins. We restrict ourselves to the discussion of a 3.6_{13} helix (α-helix), but there are a number of other helices, including the constrained 3.0_{10} helix and different helix-like structures that are found in collagen. A 3.6_{13} helix has 13 atoms and 3.6 residues per turn and possesses the following features:

- Hydrogen bonding along the backbone between the carbonyl of residue i and the amine of residue i+4 provides the stabilization of α-helices.
- There are 13 atoms in the backbone that are within the hydrogen bonded loop.
- A net macrodipole that runs along the helix also acts to stabilize the structure [6].
- Ala, Glu, Leu, and Met are favored α-helix formers.
- Gly, Pro, Tyr, and Ser are very poor α-helix formers.

Helical wheels are often used to determine amphipathicity (**Figure 17-2**) because α-helices often align themselves and can have polar residues align on one half helix and the other half could contain hydrophobic residues. This is very important for a helix to form stable multiple helix regions that are commonly found in helix bundle tertiary structures. They are also a good tool for finding regions of instability and have been used to improve the melting temperature of common proteins.

β-Sheets are one of the most common forms of secondary structure found in proteins that can form extended β-regions oriented in the parallel (a series of neighboring β-sheets

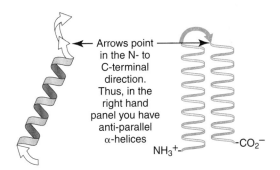

FIGURE 17-1 Representative ribbon structure for the α-helix (left) and for two antiparallel α-helices (right) in a protein. In the ball and stick diagrams, you could not decipher where the helices where based on the functional groups in the side chains and potentially obfuscating tertiary structure.

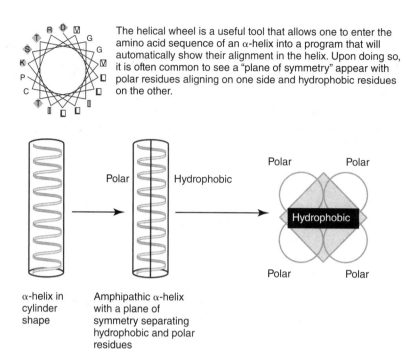

The helical wheel is a useful tool that allows one to enter the amino acid sequence of an α-helix into a program that will automatically show their alignment in the helix. Upon doing so, it is often common to see a "plane of symmetry" appear with polar residues aligning on one side and hydrophobic residues on the other.

α-helix in cylinder shape

Amphipathic α-helix with a plane of symmetry separating hydrophobic and polar residues

FIGURE 17-2 A helical wheel is presented at the top of the figure. There are helical wheel programs that can be used to enter the amino acid sequence from the start of the helix until the end. Upon close inspection, it is common to find that polar residues align on one side of the helix and apolar residues on the other. This is illustrated below in the cylinder representation of the α-helix. As illustrated, in a cytoplasmic protein the hydrophobic regions of the α-helices would all associate in the core. In contrast, the hydrophilic residues would be on the external surface and would more favorably interact with the aqueous environment. The opposite alignment would be expected for membrane bound proteins (see Figure 17-3 with the influx and efflux transporters). Finally, it should be noted that the helical wheels can be aligned and destabilizing residues (e.g., a charged amino acid like Lys) in a hydrophobic core region can be readily identified and potentially replaced by a technique like site-directed mutagenesis to increase the stability of the protein. This should only be performed if the substitution does not alter the protein function.

running in the same backbone orientation, e.g., N- to C-terminus) and antiparallel (a series of neighboring β-sheets running in the opposite backbone orientation, e.g., N- to C-terminus neighboring a β-sheet in the C- to N-terminus) directions [7, 8]. Both parallel and antiparallel β-sheets are held together by intramolecular hydrogen bonds from the CO of the first peptide backbone strand to the NH of the next strand. The parallel and antiparallel β-sheets are held together by differing hydrogen bonding patterns between the peptide backbones. Weaker forces, as described above, also act to stabilize the sheets.

Turns can play an important role in enabling tertiary structures to form may be important for facilitating protein functions, and may also possess other significance as well. A β-turn is a four amino acid bend in the peptide backbone that occurs in proteins when different regions fold back on themselves. β-Turns can occur in small peptides and can be critical to the activity of the peptide or protein. Several different types of β-turns can occur in proteins and are distinguished from one another by the φ and ψ dihedral angles. A γ-turn is a three amino acid bend in the peptide backbone that is more constrained and less common than a β-turn. A γ-turn usually occurs where there is a need for a tight turn for a protein to fold back upon itself. These structures are well defined elsewhere [7, 8] for the reader to gain further insight into their properties.

Tertiary structure arises from the coalescence of the many different secondary structural domains within a single covalently bonded amino acid oligomer (primary structure) that comprises the peptide or protein. Disulfide bonds, hydrogen bonding between domains, hydration, ionic interactions, and dipolar and hydrophobic forces all occur to provide the driving forces for folding into a more compact globular conformation and stabilization of the final tertiary structure. The tertiary structure can fold into a number of different patterns including all helix bundles, all β-sheet rolls or barrels, mixes between α-helices and β-sheets, and several other domains.

Briefly, quaternary structure describes the intermolecular interactions of the neighboring tertiary structural elements of two or more proteins. Quaternary structure can be in any form of multimer from a dimer, trimer, tetramer, up to larger aggregates. Quaternary structure can occur naturally, for example, insulin actually forms a hexamer in the presence of zinc *in vivo*. The formation of quaternary structure can also be essential for the function of many proteins and can also form to increase solubility or stability of certain proteins. For example, many receptors dimerize to perform a function like signaling across a membrane when a ligand binds. Although there are benefits to quaternary structure formation, there are also a significant number or problems as well. Association into complexes can serve as nucleation points for aggregate growth and even precipitation, which could result in a less efficacious dose of a drug administered and possibly an insoluble particle being injected into an artery or vein of a patient. This is a critical point, and care needs to be taken when working with proteins that tend to form quaternary structure. It should also be noted that aggregation is believed to be one of the major causes of immunogenicity reactions observed with therapeutic peptides and proteins.

Because of the zwitterionic properties of amino acids and the functional diversity of their side chains, ionization of a peptide or protein also plays a key role in governing several aspects of performance, including stability, conformation, and permeability [2, 9]. Changes in charge can lead to unfolding, aggregate formation, a potential loss of solubility, changes in chemical stability, reduced potency, or even safety if an epitope is exposed, leading to immunogenicity [2, 10]. Although ionization is also critical for small molecules, it is often more easily controlled. Finally, the chemical instability for peptide and protein drugs is more complex to elucidate, may occur at several different reaction sites simultaneously, and can result in denaturation, which makes it much harder to study than for small molecule drugs. In fact, peptides and proteins do not adhere to simple Arrhenius kinetics because of the number of different concurrent reactions that occur. Care and handling of peptides and proteins based on the manufacturer's guidelines must be strictly maintained.

A number of different experiments must be performed to determine the physicochemical properties of a peptide or protein based therapeutic. Although some techniques used to determine these properties overlap with methodology used to characterize small molecule drugs, peptide and protein molecules necessitate their own characterization techniques for measuring quality, safety, and efficacy based on their structural diversity. Some of these techniques include Western blotting, isoelectric focusing, reverse phase high-performance liquid chromatography, ultraviolet absorbance, circular dichroism, nuclear magnetic resonance imaging, mass spectrometry, epitope mapping, differential scanning calorimetry, and accelerated/long-term stability [2, 11]. Although the techniques themselves are outside the scope of this chapter, their use allows physicochemical analysis to produce the same efficacious protein/peptide formulation in every dosage form.

PHYSIOLOGICAL BARRIERS TO PEPTIDE AND PROTEIN DELIVERY

Similar to small molecule drugs, peptide and protein drugs must cross a number of barriers to reach their site of action. The amount of barriers depends on both the method of delivery and the site of action. Although these barriers are the same for both small molecule and peptide/protein drugs, the route of permeation may be very different [12]. Peptides and proteins can traverse cellular barriers via essentially four general pathways: (1) passive paracellular (between the cells) diffusion, (2) passive transcellular (lipophilic diffusion across the membrane) routes, (3) facilitative or active transport, and/or (4) endocytosis [5]. **Figure 17-3** provides a general illustration of the primary routs of permeation across the intestinal epithelium, and it should be noted that endocytosis is not a major route of oral absorption for peptides and proteins. The main physicochemical properties that influence the route of passage across a cell barrier are polarity/charge, size, conformation, and hydrophobicity. Tight epi- and endothelial barriers largely restrict paracellular diffusion because of the presence of tight junctions [13]. Therefore, only small peptides may cross these barriers via the paracellular route, because tight junctions have finite pore radii that exclude the permeation of larger peptides and proteins [5]. Likewise, polarity/charge and size restricts the passive transcellular permeation of most peptides and proteins across both tight and "leaky" cell barriers because this would require diffusion across a hydrophobic, liquid crystalline lipid bilayer [14, 15].

Therefore, based on the size, charge, and conformation of the peptide or protein, the passive routes may not be feasible, with the exception of organs perfused by leaky (fenestrated or discontinuous) endothelia [16]. Hence, most peptides and proteins rely

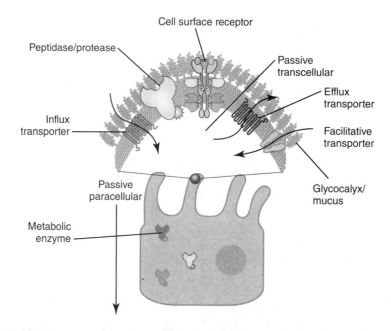

FIGURE 17-3 Various general peptide and protein absorption and metabolism routes across the GI epithelial cell. It should be noted that endocytosis is not readily observed along the GI tract, with the potential exception of M-cells. A comprehensive discussion of these cells is not presented here.

on facilitative, active, or endocytic routes of transcellular permeation for absorption and distribution [17]. Facilitative permeation occurs when a peptide or a protein interacts with a transporter that can transport the peptide or protein across the cell membrane using a concentration gradient. Active transporters require energy, normally derived directly or indirectly from ATP, to transport a peptide or a protein across a cell membrane [5, 18]. A number of active and facilitative transporters are capable of transporting a peptide into the cell (influx) and out of the cell (efflux), and a review of their properties is beyond the scope of this chapter.

Endocytosis occurs via an adsorptive or receptor mediated mechanism [18]. In adsorptive endocytosis, the peptide or protein nonspecifically adsorbs to the surface of the cell and is generally absorbed by endolysosomal trafficking pathways. A number of strategies, including the attachment of cell-penetrating peptides, can be used to enhance membrane adsorption and potentially penetration of peptide and protein drugs and drug delivery systems like liposomes to increase adsorptive endocytosis [19]. Receptor mediated endocytosis is a highly specific process where either the peptide or protein drug is designed to interact with a cell surface protein and then is absorbed by endolysosomal trafficking pathways. This approach can also be applied to drug delivery systems, where the drug delivery system is conjugated to a specific targeting moiety for absorption into or across cells [18]. A number of different approaches used to enhance either adsorptive or receptor mediated endocytosis are beyond the scope of this chapter to review.

Upon administration *in vivo*, the amideide bonds of the peptide or protein therapeutic are subject to peptidase and protease-based digestion that has evolved to cleave dietary and recycle endogenous proteins. Hence, the half-life of peptide or protein drugs are often much lower than traditional small molecules [20].

ORAL ROUTE

Peptide and protein therapeutics represent a growing proportion of drugs in preclinical development, the vast majority of which are delivered parenterally and formulated as solutions, suspensions, or lyophilized products for reconstitution [21, 22]. Interestingly, for long-term indication compounds such as these, the delivery route has a significant impact on both their commercial success and market potential, which may not be maximized because of the requirement for repeated injections [23, 24]. Although a large variety of alternate delivery approaches are currently under investigation [19, 25–27], it is abundantly clear that development of safe and effective oral delivery systems designed specifically to meet the many difficulties inherent to biopharmaceutical compound delivery is required [25, 29].

Traditionally, peroral delivery of peptide and protein therapeutics has been particularly challenging [23, 25, 26, 29]. The proteinaceous nature of these compounds limits their peroral bioavailability due to chemical susceptibility to gastrointestinal (GI) pH shifts and proteolytic degradation, as well as charge, size, and chemical limitations inherent to permeating the highly restrictive GI epithelium [2, 16, 25]. Furthermore, these compounds tend to be extremely potent molecules, and many exhibit a narrow therapeutic index, further complicating the potential of oral delivery. These issues notwithstanding, oral delivery of biopharmaceutical therapeutics is still the most sought after route of administration for many of the same reasons as for traditional pharmaceutical compounds.

As of the time at which this book chapter was written, there are only two approved orally delivered peptide pharmaceuticals, cyclosporine and desmopressin. Cyclosporine, due to its unique physicochemical properties and lipid-based formulation, exhibits an oral bioavailability of approximately 30%, whereas the oral bioavailability of desmopressin is much more in line with what one would expect from an orally delivered peptide at 0.1% [28]. Although the lack of agency-approved, orally delivered peptides is certainly in part due to the difficulties discussed, it is also a function of the higher manufacturing costs associated with delivering a compound with inherently low bioavailability. To this end, active pharmaceutical ingredient (API) manufacturing techniques should be sufficiently low to enable the higher dosages inherent to these low bioavailability compounds, thus negating this cost of goods issue.

Irrespective of the compound of interest, it is clear that because of the physico-chemical nature of therapeutic peptides and proteins, delivery strategy includes two primary points: protect the peptide from proteolytic degradation and include a strategy, in the form of excipients or otherwise, to facilitate transport across the GI epithelium, the defining barrier limiting absorption of these important molecules. In the case of cyclized peptides or derivatized peptides, such as those that include a combination of cyclization and/or racemization, or N-linked substituents, like polyethylene glycol (PEG) and acyl groups, these changes are clearly designed to meet each of these needs, although inclusion of secondary excipients to facilitate transport has also been demonstrated to be helpful. To this end, a number of companies have been founded based on technologies that increase proteolytic resistance by derivatization in some form.

Aileron Therapeutics' stapled peptides are one such contemporary example of a peptide design strategy to both increase proteolytic resistance while simultaneously increasing the compound's gut permeation potential [30, 31]. Briefly, Aileron's stapled peptides are a class of molecule where the α-helical secondary structure is stabilized by ring-closing metathesis via side chain or backbone functionalities [30]. The result is a store of stabilized, proteolytically resistant peptides designed to traverse biological membranes, not only enabling peroral absorption but peptides that can also hit intracellular targets. Commensurate with the underlying factors affecting membrane permeation, however, bioavailability of Aileron's stapled peptides is still limited primarily due to size restrictions but also to a lesser extent charge, lipophilicity, and so on. Significant works describing the molecular mechanisms controlling cyclic peptide prodrug permeation have been published [32–36], and for the most part it is clear that compound design will only get you so far in terms of creating an orally bioavailable peptide. In short, oral bioavailability in the absence of formulation strategies, independent of compound design, is not enough to make a marketable, orally delivered peptide drug.

This has been evident for a number of clinical development programs. One such example is Biocon's IN-105, a human insulin ortholog that has been chemically derivatized with a short-chain methoxy-PEG to lysine 29 residue of the β-chain [37]. The PEG modified active is then orally delivered in a formulation containing the fatty acid salt sodium caprate as a permeation enhancer. Although a dose ranging study found plasma IN-105 at 352.5 ± 279.3 mU/L with a respective change in 2-hour postprandial glucose of 53.06 ± 47.27 mg/dL upon peroral administration of 30 mg IN-105 (doses ranged from 10 to 30 mg) [38], the company reported in 2010 that a large multicenter phase III clinical trial conducted in India failed to meet its primary endpoint. Although they are continuing development of IN-105, the clinical failure to date of Biocon's (and others) oral insulin products may not simply be a function of poor oral absorption but also a function of pharmacokinetic (PK) variability.

This case is a good example of the difficulties inherent to oral peptide and protein delivery. Biocon attempted to derivatize their molecule to increase its proteolytic resistance, in addition to including a permeation enhancer in their formulation. Although this system did generate appreciable IN-105 plasma levels, it still failed to meet the primary endpoint in the clinic, which may be due to the special case that is orally delivered insulin. Merrion Pharmaceuticals (http://www.merrionpharma.com) has an oral formulation enabling platform technology, termed GIPET™, based on a library of combinations of salts of food-grade medium-chain fatty acids, such as the sodium caprate used by Biocon, prepared in enterically coated capsules or tablets. Merrion claims the primary mechanism of action to be mixed micelle formation with freely available GI bile acids, which facilitate passive transcellular permeation.

Clinical studies investigating the pharmacokinetic profile of various strength Mer–101 tablets (GIPET™ enhanced zoledronic acid) in postmenopausal women indicated significant food and diurnal effects on absorption [39]. It is unclear if these effects are due to enteric coating or, more likely, to an additional result of the mechanism by which GIPET™ enhances bioavailability. Preclinical results demonstrated modest GIPET™ mediated enhancement effects for this compound, which was replicated in humans, where a low 10-mg dose resulted in 7.2% bioavailability and a high 20-mg dose showed only 5.3%, relative to intravenous formualtions [40]. These results clearly indicate that not only does the formulation itself suffer from a lack of dose linearity, but minute changes in the formulation components, as one might see with different dosages, clearly effects bioavailability and variability.

Although most GIPET™ enhanced oral formulation products under development at Merrion appear to be small molecule based, others include MER–102 (ultra-low-molecular-weight heparin) and MER–104 (acyline, a decapeptide gonadotropin releasing hormone antagonist with five D-amino acids: Ac-D2Nal-D4Cpa-D3Pal-Ser-4Aph(Ac)-D4Aph(Ac)-Leu-ILys-Pro-DAla-NH2). Of their self-funded pipeline, MER–104 appears to be the only peptide-based agent in development. Oral delivery of MER–104 was investigated in eight healthy men at 10-, 20-, and 40-mg doses administered at weekly intervals. Pharmacokinetic data for six of the eight volunteers demonstrated a positive, although nonlinear, dose response increase in acyline plasma levels [41]. Maximum concentration values ranged from under 5 ng/mL to approximately 55 ng/mL for the 10- and 40-mg doses, respectively. Interestingly, the pharmacokinetic profiles for the 20- and 40-mg doses appeared biphasic with respect to maximum concentration.

Although Merrion appears to have had some modest success in early phase clinical studies with a peptide, the two companies furthest along in oral macromolecule delivery are clearly Unigene Laboratories (currently Enteris Biopharma)(Boonton, NJ) and Emisphere (Cedar Knolls, NJ). Both companies have studied oral delivery of salmon calcitonin in phase III clinical studies but with different levels of success. Although Unigene's single phase III study met its primary endpoint (study conducted by Unigene's partner Tarsa Therapeutics), studies conducted by Novartis using Emisphere's oral delivery technology failed to meet primary endpoints in a single osteoarthritis study and two osteoporosis studies. The differences in efficacy of salmon calcitonin could be due to the differences in delivery strategy between Unigene and Emisphere's delivery platforms.

The basis for Unigene's oral delivery technology capitalizes on the apparently synergistic effects of a combination of two excipients to effectively deliver peptide therapeutics: (1) an organic acid in sufficient quantities to decrease the microenvironment pH in the small intestinal lumen, thereby lowering the pH sufficiently out of the pH_{max} for GI proteases, ultimately inhibiting their activity, and (2) a cationic acylcarnitine permeation enhancer, which transiently opens tight junctional complexes, allowing for increased passive paracellular permeation. The direct compression core was isenterically coated to protect the active form from longer term exposure to the acidic, pepsin-rich gastric environment. Interestingly, this description is a newer version of Unigene's oral peptide delivery platform, compared with that used by Tarsa in phase III investigations, which did not use the acylcarnitine permeation enhancer. When using the acylcarnitine enhancer, Unigene also announced positive phase

II clinical results for a parathyroid hormone analogue and 16% absolute bioavailability of Cara Therapeutics' κ-opioid agonist, CR845, in a phase I clinical study (both by corporate press release available at http://www.caratherapeutics.com/cr845-phase1-complete-release .shtml). An interesting corporate development at Unigene (Enteris Biopharma) is the fairly recent announcement that Enteris Biopharma is now externalizing their oral delivery technology to licensing partners, whereas before the technology was only used for internal therapeutic programs. This news is a boon in terms of oral macromolecule development because this is the only delivery technology that has demonstrated positive phase III results and API derivatization is not a prerequisite for the system's utility, because it is specifically designed to protect against proteolytic degradation.

In contrast, Emisphere maintains a library of permeation enhancers, termed Eligen. Two Emisphere permeation enhancers have gained certain prevalence in their repertoire, sodium 8-(2-hydroxybenzoyl) amino caproate (scalprazolate sodium [SNAC]) and 8-(N-2-hyroxy-5-chlorobenzoyl) amino caproate. The latter was the enhancer included in Novartis' phase III clinical trials for peroral salmon calcitonin delivery. Emisphere, either individually or through partners, has also sponsored phase II clinical studies for insulin and heparin as well as recent phase I studies for glucagon-like peptide-1 (GLP-1), parathyroid hormone (PTH), peptide YY (PYY), growth hormone, and the small molecules acyclovir and gallium. Although the final drug product is not enterically coated, the physicochemical nature of Eligen enhancers causes a coprecipitate with the active form in the acidic gastric environment, thereby protecting the molecule in the stomach [42, 43]. This literature suggests that as the GI luminal pH rose due to subsequent bicarbonate release in the small intestine, the gastric complex dissolved but did not dissociate, and the Eligen molecule then acted to passively chaperone the active transcellularly. Moreover, it was further argued that any respective changes in membrane fluidity did not alter the overall barrier functionality of the targeted GI epithelial cells [42, 43]. Indeed, other reports indicate that not only does SNAC (at permeation enhancing concentrations) have lytic effects [44–46], as determined by both intracellular component leakage and trypan blue exclusion, but that the compound does not directly chemically interact with the drug moiety [44]. Moreover, these reports indicate that mechanistically SNAC decreases membrane anisotropy similar to benzyl alcohol but is apparently less potent [44]. Taken together with the clinical data, these studies suggest Eligen technology is limited not only by its gastric protective mechanism, which would limit the theoretical amount of peptide available for absorption and increase potential variability, but that the undefined permeation mechanism, whether indeed by chaperoning, micelle formation, epithelial lytic effects, and so on, is each subject to dilutive effects, which would again highly limit the system's real-world application.

Although no oral delivery technology has yet been approved by a regulatory body for widespread commercial use, the success of Enteris Biopharma's, formerly Unigene, (Tarsa) salmon calcitonin product should lead to approval in the near future. Other delivery systems not mentioned here but in various stages of preclinical and clinical development include sodium caprylate suspended in an oil phase (Chiasma Pharma), aromatic alcohols used in concert with various bile salts (Bone Medical), pharmaceutical films used to disperse and immobilize nanocarriers (MonosolRx), perorally delivered, bioadherent wafers (Entrega), and numerous particulate-based delivery systems. It is also interesting that for the most part, clinical investigations tend toward a few well-known hormones, such as salmon calcitonin, PTH analogues, GLP-1 analogues, and insulins. Because the industry has realized that not only is oral delivery of peptide molecules feasible, however, the range of compounds being studied has also increased to human growth hormone, erythropoietin (EPO), various tumor necrosis factors, and potentially even orally delivered vaccines.

ALTERNATIVE ROUTES OF DELIVERY

The peroral route of drug delivery is usually preferred by drug manufacturers, but for active ingredients such as peptides and proteins there is considerable difficulty in the formulation and obtaining reproducible plasma levels via delivery systems developed for oral delivery. The stomach is an acidic environment filled with enteric enzymes and microbes designed to break down peptides and proteins [29]. Moreover, there are regional differences throughout the GI tract, where the epithelial barrier possesses tight junctions to form a barrier against paracellular transport of larger peptide- and protein-based molecules and largely restricts absorption to occur via the transcellular route [29, 47]. Moreover, regional differences do exist throughout the segments of the GI tract that can act as additional confounding variables for protein absorption, including mucus/glycocalyx, which can accumulate insulin and lead to increased proteolysis [48, 49]. Because of these barriers, peptide and protein formulations are most often designed to use alternative routes of delivery.

PARENTERAL

The parenteral route is by far the most common method of delivery for proteins and peptides, because direct injection avoids many of the barriers and enzymatic activity of other routes of delivery. The parenteral route, however, is not without its downfalls. As with other drug substances, compliance for parenteral dosing is low [50].

Proteins and peptides are some of the most expensive APIs on the market. Therefore, getting the best bioavailability possible is of great importance to the pharmaceutical industry. By injecting proteins and peptides intravenously, intramuscularly, or subcutaneously, the API is placed into a comparatively neutral and enzyme-free environment [51]. Although the blood is slightly basic, enzymatic activity does occur, and difficulties can arise from protein binding, these challenges can be met no matter the route because the blood will likely be responsible for final distribution throughout the body. This increased bioavailability can often be the only way to get above the minimum effective concentration for peptide and protein formulations [52].

Although the disadvantages of other routes often force industry's hand into taking the parenteral route, the parenteral route has its own disadvantages. Compliance is often problematic. Administration of peptides and proteins requires a trained professional [53]. Because proteins have relatively short half-lives, this can mean frequent visits to a doctor. Even when peptide and protein drugs can be formulated for intramuscular or subcutaneous delivery, needles must still be used, which can be painful to the patient [50]. Furthermore, immunogenicity is often an issue when delivering peptides and proteins intravenously. High concentrations of APIs are delivered to one site upon injection. This can cause precipitation of API, leading to phlebitis, inflammation of the vein, and an immune response [54]. This is especially detrimental when using proteins or peptides found in the human body, causing an immune response against the body's endogenous source of these molecules [55].

EPO is an endogenous protein produced by the body to induce erythropoiesis, the production of red blood cells. EPO is found in low levels in patients suffering from kidney disease, leading to anemia. It was hypothesized that dosing recombinant EPO would increase erythropoiesis and eliminate the symptoms of anemia. Although the recombinant protein was successful with many patients, a handful of patients experienced immune reactions to the protein. Antibodies formed against the recombinant protein and rendered it ineffective. These patients stopped the EPO regimen; however, they shortly experienced pure red cell aplasia, a complete loss of red blood cells [55].

It was found that patients' immune systems not only recognized and eliminated the recombinant EPO but also their own endogenous EPO. Thankfully, a synthetic form of EPO, darbepoetin, which reconfigured this antigenic site, was formulated. This change significantly reduces the potential for autoimmunogenicity [55].

PULMONARY

The lungs have been exploited for API delivery for many decades. Often, these drugs are used for local delivery for ailments of the lungs such as asthma. Systemic delivery, however, is also possible. More recently, the lungs have become one of the most targeted areas for delivery of peptides and protein delivery [56]. Under ideal circumstances, delivery to the lungs only requires normal breathing or one quick inhalation, making administration relatively easier than parenteral delivery.

The advantages of delivery through the lung greatly lie in its function of gas exchange. For gases to be quickly and easily exchanged with the environment, the body supplies the lungs with a large supply of blood. The capillaries coating the enormous surface area of the lung's alveoli, the final site for absorption, are attached by a submicron layer of cells. This blood is then moved directly back to the heart for systemic circulation [57]. Clearly, this approach offers a considerable advantage for peptide and protein drug delivery. As an API molecule enters the lung, it has a huge surface area in which to diffuse through. It then must only diffuse through a handful of cell layers before it reaches the blood. Once the peptide or protein therapeutic reaches systemic circulation, it is routed directly to the heart and pumped throughout the body, bypassing first-pass metabolism [58]. Unlike the stomach and the upper small intestine, the lungs also have a relatively neutral pH and a low level of metabolizing enzymes. This microenvironment can provide added physical and chemical stability that leads to an increased half-life compared with oral delivery [59].

Once at the site of absorption, the lungs provide one of the best environments for peptide and protein absorption; however, reaching this location can be difficult. The lung epithelium is one of the largest surface areas of the body that is consistently exposed to the external environment through respiration. Upon inhalation of air, many foreign objects may also enter the lungs and potentially confound drug access to the pulmonary alveoli. To counteract these particles, the lungs have a series of barriers. The first of these is a thick mucous layer that traps particles as they move through the lung [60]. The lungs also have cilia to clear this mucus away from the lung and possess moderate enzymatic activity that can degrade therapeutically delivered peptides and proteins. Finally, even if peptides and proteins traversed these physiological barriers to reach the alveoli membrane for absorption, macrophages are present in the basal compartment to assist in their proteolytic elimination [60].

Pulmonary delivery is noninvasive and well tolerated by many subpopulations, but formulation for pulmonary delivery can be challenging [57]. Because of the difficulty of getting APIs to the alveoli for delivery in the lungs, much research has gone into developing strategies for increased deposition to the site of absorption. A considerable portion of this research focused on delivery systems and the effects of particle size. The lungs are formed by a series of branched tubes of decreasing size. To accomplish high yields in the alveoli for absorption, particles must have certain aerodynamic properties, that is, each particle must have a certain size, shape, and speed [56].

NASAL

Similar to other routes for alternative peptide and protein delivery, the nasal mucosa is often targeted due to its mild environment when compared with the GI tract [29, 48, 61]. In many ways the benefits and downfalls of nasal delivery are similar to those of pulmonary delivery. Delivery to the nasal cavity is noninvasive and is generally accomplished by using a nozzled device to eject a spray or mist onto the mucosa [62]. Similar to the lungs, the nasal passages contain a thick mucous layer that is cleared by the cilia of the nasal epithelium [63]. This mucous layer is also variable depending on disease state, which can decrease API half-life, residence time, and complicate administration. If, however, peptide and protein API molecules can reach the epithelium, the microenvironment is inviting with minimal, though still active, enzymatic clearance [64].

One of the major drawbacks for nasal delivery lies in its small surface area. The surface area of the nasal cavity is much smaller than those encountered in the GI tract or the alveoli of the lungs. This limits the amount of drug that can be administered, which in turn limits the dose. This is less of a factor for peptide and protein molecules because a comparatively low dose is often needed; however, it cannot be overlooked when developing a dosage form [65]. Even though the surface area is small, the nasal epithelium consists of wider tight junctions, which can allow increased passive permeability, especially with peptide and protein APIs. Also, similar to the lungs, proteins and peptides that are able to permeate the nasal mucosa enter the systemic circulation, bypassing first-pass metabolism [61].

Many epithelial properties of the nasal mucosa have been well characterized for years. Only recently, however, has the potential for peptide and protein drug delivery across the nasal mucosa been realized as offering a strategic advantage, particularly for central nervous system acting and highly potent analogues. For example, there is growing interest in the fact that the olfactory sensing cells in the nose may also offer a significant target for enhancing macromolecular drug delivery like peptides and proteins. Although presenting only a relatively small part of the nasal epithelium surface, the olfactory cells are responsible for endocytosis and translocation of sensory molecules to the olfactory region of the brain. This pathway bypasses the blood–brain barrier, allowing direct access to the central nervous system. As more and more focus is put on diseases of the brain, permeation through the blood–brain barrier has proved to be very difficult. Circumnavigating this defense by using nasal delivery, potentially targeted to olfactory cells, may soon be seen as a valuable asset for the growing trend of needed central nervous system delivery [66].

TRANSDERMAL

Transdermal delivery of peptides and proteins has traditionally been investigated for peptide and protein drug delivery, although overcoming the dermal epithelium has been rate limiting because of its physiology, as discussed elsewhere [29]. Recent developments in technology, however, have made this route increasingly attractive based on the development of novel drug delivery formulation and permeation strategies that can overcome the dermal epithelium because of its inherent advantages over other routes of administration. A number of factors contribute to making transdermal drug delivery attractive, including bypassing the hydrolytic acidic pH of the stomach and the proteolytic enzymes of the GI tract, which rapidly denature and metabolize orally administered peptides and proteins as part of the natural digestion process. Moreover, transdermal drug delivery is noninvasive and has been used extensively in controlled-release applications. The latter statement is particularly advantageous for peptide and protein drug delivery because many peptides and proteins possess short biological half-lives, which lead to repeated administration to maintain therapeutic levels in the plasma [67]. Therefore, a dosage form that has the ability to eliminate repeated administration through continuous delivery (i.e., transdermal) should improve patient compliance for biopharmaceutical administration.

In theory, transdermal delivery of peptides and proteins is quite similar to transdermal delivery of traditional small molecule APIs. In both situations the transdermal delivery system (e.g., patch, topical ointment, etc.) is placed in direct contact with the skin and the drug must penetrate and absorb through the skin to achieve systemic circulation. The rate and extent of absorption depend on the physicochemical properties of the drug (e.g., molecular weight, lipophilicity, pKa, solubility etc.) and the physiological properties of the skin (epidermal and dermal permeability, epidermal and dermal thickness, blood perfusion, etc.). Skin thickness varies significantly with location on the body (0.5 mm on the eyelids to 4.0 mm on the heel) [68], which plays a large role in determining drug absorption.

Despite the similarities discussed above, transdermal delivery of peptides and proteins does present some unique challenges not often encountered with transdermal delivery of small molecule APIs. Because of their large molecular weight, adequate absorption of peptides and proteins through the skin is much more difficult to obtain than for small molecule APIs. For this reason, formulations that rely on simple diffusion of the protein through the skin have been largely unsuccessful. The use of both chemical and physical penetration enhancers in second- and third-generation formulations, however, may enable a more widespread use of transdermal protein delivery [69]. Balancing these confounding factors is the fact that many peptide- and protein-based drugs can be highly potent based on their high affinity for targets, therefore leading to lower dose levels. The most common formulation strategy to overcome the dermal barrier and increase transdermal absorption is the addition of chemical penetration enhancers such as alcohols and surfactants. These enhancers function by solubilizing and fluidizing the lipid components in the stratum corneum [29]. Physical penetration enhancers are also being widely investigated to improve transdermal protein delivery. Physical penetration enhancement is most commonly performed through microporation, or the creation of micron-sized holes in the skin that allow the passage of proteins [70, 71]. Other techniques investigated to improve transdermal delivery of proteins include iontophoresis, sonophoresis, electroporation, and thermal ablation [70]. Of more recent interest has been the rapid development of microneedle applications, which are minimally invasive and offer the potential to deliver peptides or proteins beneath the outer stratum corneum [72].

BUCCAL

Similar to transdermal delivery, research into buccal delivery of peptides and proteins is becoming increasingly important as pharmaceutical companies explore alternatives to parenteral administration. Buccal delivery is noninvasive, provides easy and accurate administration, allows for the treatment of both local and systemic conditions, and avoids many of the disadvantages of oral drug delivery such as exposure of the drug to acidic and enzymatic conditions associated with the GI tract and hepatic first-pass metabolism. The buccal mucosa is also highly vascularized and has a much greater permeability than that of skin because of differences in the epithelial structure [29], which may result in increased exposure compared with transdermal delivery [73]. Furthermore, buccal delivery has the potential to allow for prolonged and/or continuous administration, which would reduce repeated administration and increase patient compliance.

In many respects buccal delivery is quite similar to transdermal delivery except the dosage form is placed directly on the buccal mucosa where mucoadhesive strategies can be used in contrast to the skin. The rate and extent of absorption depend on the physicochemical properties of the drug (molecular weight, lipophilicity, pKa, solubility, etc.)

and the physiological properties of the buccal mucosa (e.g., mucosal permeability, mucosal thickness, mucous layer thickness, etc.). The average buccal mucosa thickness ranges from approximately 500 to 800 μm [74]. Despite the reduced thickness of the buccal mucosa compared with skin, absorption across the buccal mucosa has been limited to peptides with a molecular weight of less than 1000 Da and has been demonstrated to occur through passive diffusion [59, 75]. Permeation enhancers are frequently used to increase the absorption of peptides greater than 1000 Da. The function of these permeation enhancers is very similar to those used in transdermal delivery and includes altering membrane fluidity of buccal epithelium, reducing the viscosity of the mucous layer, and altering intercellular junctions [76].

Another disadvantage of buccal delivery for peptides and proteins is the potential for inadvertently swallowing the dosage form, which would result in the exposure of the peptide or protein to the harsh acidic and enzymatic conditions of the GI tract. Additionally, there is also limited residence time of the dosage form on the buccal mucosa. To reduce both of these problems, mucoadhesive delivery systems can be formulated that adhere to the inner cheek and increase the contact time with the buccal mucosa [77]. These systems incorporate water-soluble polymers into a mucoadhesive patch that adheres very quickly to the buccal mucosa upon hydration. Absorption is enhanced by increased contact time of the peptide with the buccal mucosa. Other formulation strategies studied to increase peptide absorption across the buccal mucosa include incorporation of the peptide or protein into liposomes, conjugating the peptide or protein to lipophilic polymers, and inclusion of enzyme and/or transporter inhibitors [76].

ORAL INSULIN: EXPECTATIONS VERSUS CHALLENGES

Insulin is a 5.8-kD hormone used to treat patients with diabetes. The development of oral insulin has long been regarded as the Holy Grail of drug delivery. An oral insulin product would have tremendous patient benefit to a large number of diabetic patients by reducing or eliminating the need for injection and potentially reducing the incidence of side effects. Furthermore, it is likely that a successful product with low variability would have a blockbuster capability in terms of sales [78–81].

The variability in onset and duration of action after insulin absorption is the biggest confounder of efforts to mimic physiological insulin secretion. Hypoglycemia is the most common adverse effect associated with insulin therapy [82]. It would be highly advantageous if insulin could be delivered orally, because oral administration could mimic the physiological pathway in which absorption of the insulin from the GI tract would enter into the portal vein and target the liver. Hence, oral insulin would not only reduce the need for subcutaneous delivery but by targeted delivery could also provide better glucose homeostasis [78].

The oral administration of peptides and proteins, as previously discussed, is not an easy task. Their poor bioavailability originates both from enzymatic degradation of the molecules in the GI tract and the difficulty in transporting these relatively large polar molecules across the intestinal barrier. The GI tract and liver are designed to break down proteins and peptides into smaller, more easily absorbable fragments, and insulin is no exception to this. The second problem is that the GI tract possesses very few carrier systems for absorption of peptides that are much larger than three to four amino acids. For insulin, oral administration is then further confounded by the narrow therapeutic index; other issues are listed in Table 17-2 [78, 81].

Design and formulation of drug delivery systems for insulin to the GI tract has been a formidable challenge because of its unfavorable properties of enzymatic degradation and poor membrane permeability [78]. To date, most approaches have applied the use of some method to reduce the enzymatic degradation (Table 17–3) and/or excipients to increase the permeability (Table 17–4) of insulin across the GI tract. Insulin absorption across the GI barrier has been postulated to occur mainly by the transcytosis pathway, thus making drug absorption possible as long as the insulin can be delivered to the site of absorption [78, 81]. Permeability can then be further enhanced with the use of various permeation enhancers or the use of a carrier system. The delivery to the membrane is, however, both site and time dependent because of the rapid enzymatic degradation of insulin. Because of enzymatic degradation, only a small fraction of the drug administered is available for permeation. Furthermore, the enzymatic degradation in general leads to large inter- and intravariability between subjects. Insulin delivery, with low reproducible variability, can therefore best be achieved if the activity of the enzymes is significantly reduced or eliminated [78, 81].

In recent years there has been a great deal of interest in exploring noninvasive oral delivery technologies for insulin delivery and their development by the pharmaceutical industry. All these strategies have focused on maximizing the oral bioavailability of insulin and developing safe and effective oral insulin therapies [78, 81]. Table 17–5 presents a summary of some of the more recent efforts to develop an oral insulin delivery system

TABLE 17-2 Considerations in developing oral insulin drug delivery systems

Narrow therapeutic index
Variability: gastric emptying, gastroparesis
Food effect: high-fat meal
Meal-time glucose control (short-acting) vs. basal insulin (long-acting)

Insulin has been reported to accumulate in the glycocalyx

Implications of deviations from instructions

TABLE 17-3 Pros and cons of potential strategies for increasing the oral and/or systemic delivery of peptide- and protein-based therapeutics

Strategy	Pro/Method	Con
Enzyme inhibition	Coadministration of the peptide with protease inhibitors	Interfere with digestion, dilution effect, toxicity on chronic administration
Sequestration	Enteric coating technology, biodegradable polymers escapes stomach and upper GI tract digestion/chemical instability	Safety (non-Generally Regarded as Safe [GRAS] excipients), low encapsulation alters efficiency, complex scale-up and manufacturing
Site-specific targeting	Target areas like colon, oral cavity with low protein degradation	Limited area for absorption, low BA
Structure modification	Alter chemical structure to enable the drug to escape proteolytic enzyme cleavage	Creating a new protein that has different properties and potential immunogenicity

TABLE 17-4 Pros and cons of potential formulation strategies for increasing the oral and/or systemic delivery of peptide- and protein-based therapeutics

Strategy	Pro/Method	Con
Absorption enhancers	Formulation additives to open tight-junctions: surfactants, chelators, bile acids/salts	Toxicity/local irritation, reproducibility, sensitivity to food, toxins, more effective for smaller peptides
Carriers	Nonspecific drug delivery	Safety of carriers, high carrier-to-drug ratio, variability, food effect on absorption
Mucoadhesive excipients	Adherence to GI wall, intimate contact with GI, prolong residence time at site of absorption	Mucous lining turnover, local irritation due to high drug and polymer concentration
Targeted receptors	Peptide prodrugs that have receptor binding ligands, vesicular transport for large-molecular-weight proteins	New molecular entity (NME), low efficiency/capacity of transport mechanism

TABLE 17-5 Companies currently performing clinical testing on oral insulin products

Company	Technology/Mechanism	Clinical Stage	Product Name
Diabetology/Proxima Concepts	Enhancer, cosolvent, uses access technology to increase intestinal absorption	Phase II	Capsulin
Biocon/Nobex Tech	Nobex: alkyl-PEG insulin prodrugs	Phase III completed	
Emisphere	Eligen carriers (oral capsule using nonacetylated amino acids as carriers)	On hold after phase II	
OraMed	Protease and permeability enhancers formulation (enteric coated capsules containing protease inhibitors, bile salts and fish oil)	Phase II in India	ORMD-0801
Merrion/Novo	Enhancer formulation	Phase I completed	NN-1952

and provides insight into what is known about their current clinical status (see also www.clinicaltrials.gov). Various approaches have been used to try to both increase absorption of insulin and to protect it from enzymatic degradation in the GI tract. Despite multiple strategies over the last several decades, difficulties in achieving adequate blood insulin levels with low variability have been elusive. Therefore, to date the inability to achieve safe, low variability oral insulin blood levels has kept this modality from being clinically used as an oral drug delivery therapy.

Because of the narrow therapeutic index and stringent quantitative and temporal dosing requirements of insulin, its delivery via the GI tract is unlikely to ever replace the need for subcutaneous administration due to bioavailability constraints. It is possible, however, that an oral insulin delivery could serve as supplementary insulin dosing to parenteral regimens. The oral dosing could then potentially reduce the frequency and thus offer some advantages to improve patience compliance and reduce side effects from frequent administration of insulin parenterally.

NOVEL PEPTIDE- AND PROTEIN-BASED DELIVERY TECHNOLOGY

Because of the vast promise of peptide- and protein-based therapeutic drugs, new technologies are continually being pursued to overcome some of their poor properties. Whereas previous parts of this chapter discussed the current use of strategies for various routes of delivery, this section is focused on improving delivery through these routes by using new formulation strategies. Although some of these technologies have been previously associated with small molecule drugs, they have also shown the ability to improve patient care and reduce morbidity. These techniques include the use of enteric polymers, long-acting parenteral formulations, targeted drug delivery, and the PowderJect.

As previously discussed, one of the main downfalls of peptide delivery through the oral route is the breakdown of proteins and peptides in the stomach through biological proteolysis [83]. However, previous small molecule drugs have been formulated to bypass this proteolysis through a process known as enteric coating. Enteric coating involves the process of coating particles in a pH-sensitive polymer. The polymer does not dissolve at low pH and protects the drug molecules until they reach the less extreme environment in the small intestine. Although the technique is just getting started with protein/peptide drugs, results show it may be feasible for stable protein/peptide drugs with higher therapeutic indices [83].

Another technique looks to improve patient compliance by increasing the time needed between injections. Because of the low half-life and narrow therapeutic indices of most protein/peptide drugs, injections may often be needed daily or weekly. By using new formulations, however, patients are able to extend the time between injections to monthly or biannually in some cases. This is done through a number of ways, including PEGylation, hyperglycosylation, and nanoparticle carriers [84]. PEGylation is the process of adding different lengths of polyethylene glycol chains to a protein or peptide. This addition allows the protein/peptide drug to reduce clearance by the kidneys because of an increase in size [85]. Hyperglycosylation is similar to PEGylation in that a large moiety is conjugated to the molecule. Hyperglycosylation, however, involves the addition of large oligosaccharide chains. These chains also reduce renal clearance through increased size, but they also increase stability by reducing aggregation [86]. Finally, as opposed to modifying the protein/peptide itself, much work has been done using nanocarriers for the drug. Many times these involve nanoparticles made of biodegradable polymer matrices. These nanoparticles circulate in the bloodstream and are slowly degraded by enzymatic activity. As the nanoparticles are degraded, the protein/peptide is slowly released from the polymer matrix over time [87].

Targeted drug delivery has long been the gold standard in pharmaceutical research. Targeted drug delivery, however, is no longer thought of as the "magic bullet" cure-all. Scientists are now focused on synthesizing and formulating drugs for higher affinity for their site of action. This gives the opportunity for doctors to give lower doses because of the increased local concentrations given by the targeted drug. Lower doses can often lead to lower side effects and decreases in patient morbidity. Targeting can be done in a number of ways but is most often accomplished by using nanoparticles with their surfaces coated in site-specific moieties [88]. For instance, oral vaccines show promise due to M-cells located in the GI tract that deliver absorbed molecules directly into the lymph system. Vaccine nanoparticles have been formulated to target uptake by these M-cells for better efficacy [89].

Finally, new devices are being produced to improve patient compliance, such as the PowderJect (PowderJect Pharmaceuticals PLC, Oxford, UK). The PowderJect is enticing because it delivers powders to the epidermal layer of the skin without using a needle. Because of the high incidence of patients' fear of needles, the PowderJect may be a useful technology for drug delivery, especially for pediatric vaccinations. Early studies have shown that vaccines given with the PowderJect are able to produce an antibody response and protective immunity [90].

Although these novel ideas show promise, basic formulation of protein/peptide drugs for common parenteral delivery is difficult in itself. New technologies often must be used on a case-by-case basis. Few protein/peptide drugs have high bioavailability even in the milder environment of the small intestine. Long-acting parenteral formulations run the risk of overdose because of the large amount of drug that is given at once, and control of release often proves difficult for drugs with a low therapeutic index. Although targeted drug delivery has shown some improvement in increasing local concentrations, the level of improvement *in vivo* is often much lower than expected. Finally, even when new drug delivery systems are introduced, they still may have their own issues. For instance, even though the PowderJect uses no needle, some patients find the pain more intense than simple needle injections [90].

SUMMARY

Peptide and protein drugs are becoming extremely important for treating various forms of disease. These drugs are most often given parenterally through various kinds of injections. Although oral delivery would provide many benefits to the patient, the physicochemical nature of proteins and peptides makes peroral delivery almost impossible. Much work has been done to alleviate the issues with peroral peptide and protein drug delivery; however, the more common method is to avoid the route all together. Because of the more mild nature of various alternative routes of administration, these methods of delivery have shown some promise. Future work will act to alleviate the physiochemical challenges that face protein/peptide delivery.

REVIEW QUESTIONS

1. What are three physicochemical differences between peptide- and protein-based drugs versus small molecules?
2. What are four challenges for the oral delivery of insulin?
3. How does particle size influence the delivery of protein/peptide formulations to the lungs?
4. Choose one alternative method of delivery and discuss its advantages and weaknesses compared with peroral delivery of protein/peptide drugs.
5. What route is most common for the delivery of peptide and protein drugs and why?
6. Choose one challenge facing the delivery of protein/peptide drugs and discuss a novel strategy to circumvent this challenge.

REFERENCES

1. Highsmith J. Biologic therapeutic drugs: technologies and global markets. *BCC Research Biotechnology Report Brochure*. 2013. Available at: http://www.bccresearch.com/market-research/biotechnology/biologic-therapeutic-drugs-markets-bio079b.html. Accessed June 25, 2013.

2. Carl SM, Lindley DJ, Knipp GT, et al. Biotechnology-derived drug product development. In: Gad SC, ed. *Pharmaceutical Manufacturing Handbook: Production and Processes*. Hoboken, NJ: John Wiley & Sons; 2008.

3. Alberts B, Johnson A, Lewis J, Raff M, Roberts K, Walter P. *Proteins. Molecular Biology of the Cell*, 4th ed. New York, NY: Garland Science; 2002.

4. Whitford D. *Proteins: Structure and Function*. Chichester, UK: John Wiley & Sons; 2005.

5. Carl SM, Herrera-Ruiz DR, Bhardwaj RK, Gudmundsson OS, Knipp GT. Mammalian oligopeptide transporters. In: You G, Morris M, eds. *Drug Transporters: Molecular Characterization and Role in Drug Disposition*. New York, NY: John Wiley & Sons; 2007:105–146.

6. Wada A. The alpha-helix as an electric macro-dipole. *Adv Biophys*. 1976:1–63.

7. Richardson JS. The anatomy and taxonomy of protein structure. *Adv Prot Chem*. 1981;34:167–339.

8. Richardson JS, Richardson DC. Principles and patterns of protein conformation. In: Fasman GD, ed. *Prediction of Protein Structure and the Principles of Protein Conformation*. New York, NY: Plenum Press; 1990:1–98.

9. Bontempo JA. Parenteral formulation for peptides, proteins, and monoclonal antibodies drugs: a commercial development overview. In: Wang B, Siahaan, TJ, Soltero, RA, eds. *Drug Delivery: Principles and Applications*. Hoboken, NJ: Wiley & Sons; 2005:321–339.

10. Jitendra PK et al. Noninvasive routes of proteins and peptides drug delivery. *Ind J Pharm Sci*. 2011; 73(4):367–375.

11. Falconer RJ, Jackson-Matthews D, Mahler SM. Analytical strategies for assessing comparability of biosimilars. *J Chem Technol Biotechnol*. 2011;86(7):915–922.

12. Catnach SM, Fairclough PD, Hammond SM. Intestinal absorption of peptide drugs: advances in our understanding and clinical implications. *Gut*. 1994;35(4):441–444.

13. Hebden JM, et al. Regional differences in quinine absorption from the undisturbed human colon assessed using a timed release delivery system. *Pharm Res*. 1999;16(7):1087–1092.

14. Wang W. Oral protein drug delivery. *J Drug Target*. 1996;4(4):195–232.

15. Renukuntla J, et al. Approaches for enhancing oral bioavailability of peptides and proteins. *Int J Pharm*. 2013;447(1-2):75–93.

16. Washington N, Washington C, Wilson CG. *Physiological Pharmaceutics: Barriers to Drug Absorption*, 2nd ed. Philadelphia: Taylor & Francis; 2001.

17. Kwan KC. Oral bioavailability and first-pass effects. *Drug Metab Dispos*. 1997;25(12):1329–1336.

18. Russell-Jones GJ. The potential use of receptor-mediated endocytosis for oral drug delivery. *Adv Drug Deliv Rev*. 2001;46(1-3):59–73.

19. Khafagy el-S, Morishita M. Oral biodrug delivery using cell-penetrating peptide. *Adv Drug Deliv Rev*. 2012;64(6):531–539.

20. Lee HJ. Protein drug oral delivery: the recent progress. *Arch Pharm Res*. 2002;25(5):572–584.

21. Frokjaer S, Otzen DE. Protein drug stability: a formulation challenge. *Nat Rev Drug Discov*. 2005; 4(4):298–306.

22. Niu CH, Chiu YY. FDA perspective on peptide formulation and stability issues. *J Pharm Sci*. 1998; 87(11):1331–1334.

23. Goldberg M, Gomez-Orellana I. Challenges for oral delivery of macromolecules. *Nat Rev Drug Discov*. 2003;2(4):289–295.

24. Glowka E, Sapin-Minet A, Leroy P, Lulek J, Maincent P. Preparation and *in vitro-in vivo* evaluation of salmon calcitonin-loaded polymeric nanoparticles. *J Microencapsul*. 2009;27(1):25–36.

25. Langer R. Drugs on target. *Science*. 2001;293(5527):58–59.

26. Mustata G, Dinh SM. Approaches to oral drug delivery for challenging molecules. *Crit Rev Ther Drug Carrier Syst*. 2006;23(2):111–135.

27. Bariya SH, Gohel MC, Mehta TA, Sharma OP. Microneedles: an emerging transdermal drug delivery system. *J Pharm Pharmacol*. 2012;64(1):11–29.

28. Maher S, Leonard TW, Jacobsen J, Brayden DJ. Safety and efficacy of sodium caprate in promoting oral drug absorption: from *in vitro* to the clinic. *Adv Drug Del Rev*. 2009;61(15):1427–1449.

29. Hamman JH, Enslin GM, Kotze AF. Oral delivery of peptide drugs: barriers and developments. *BioDrugs*. 2005;19(3):165–177.

30. Sawyer TK. Aileron Therapeutics. *Chem Biol Drug Des*. 2009;73(1):3–6.

31. Wolfson W. Aileron staples peptides. *Chem Biol*. 2009;16(9):910–912.

32. Ouyang H, Tang F, Siahaan TJ, Borchardt RT. A modified coumarinic acid-based cyclic prodrug of an opioid peptide: its enzymatic and chemical stability and cell permeation characteristics. *Pharm Res*. 2002;19(6):794–801.

33. Ouyang H, Chen W, Andersen TE, Steffansen B, Borchardt RT. Factors that restrict the intestinal cell permeation of cyclic prodrugs of an opioid peptide (DADLE). Part I. Role of efflux transporters in the intestinal mucosa. *J Pharm Sci.* 2009;98(1):337–348.

34. Ouyang H, Chen W, Andersen TE, Steffansen B, Borchardt RT. Factors that restrict intestinal cell permeation of cyclic prodrugs of an opioid peptide (DADLE). Part II. Role of metabolic enzymes in the intestinal mucosa. *J Pharm Sci.* 2009;98(1):349–361.

35. Nofsinger R, Fuchs-Knotts T, Borchardt RT. Factors that restrict the cell permeation of cyclic prodrugs of an opioid peptide, part 3: synthesis of analogs designed to have improved stability to oxidative metabolism. *J Pharm Sci.* 2012;101(9):3486–3499.

36. Nofsinger R, Borchardt RT. Factors that restrict the cell permeation of cyclic prodrugs of an opioid peptide, part 4: characterization of the biopharmaceutical and physicochemical properties of two new cyclic prodrugs designed to be stable to oxidative metabolism by cytochrome P-450 enzymes in the intestinal mucosa. *J Pharm Sci.* 2012;101(9):3500–3510.

37. Hazra P, Adhikary L, Dave N, et al. Development of a process to manufacture PEGylated orally bioavailable insulin. *Biotechnol Prog.* 2010;26(6):1695–1704.

38. Khedkar A, Iyer H, Anand A, et al. A dose range finding study of novel oral insulin (IN-105) under fed conditions in type 2 diabetes mellitus subjects. *Diabetes Obes Metab.* 2010;12(8):659–664.

39. Leonard TW, McHugh C, Madigan K, Walsh A, Fox JS. Studies of bioavailability and food effects of MER-101 zoledronic acid tablets in post-menopausal women. Presented at the ASCO Breast Cancer Symposium, San Francisco, October 2009, Poster 317. Available at: http://www.merrionpharma.com/archive/portfolio/Oct2009ASCOBCPoster.pdf.

40. Leonard TW, McHugh C, Adamczyk B, Walsh A. MER-101 tablets: a pilot bioavailability study of a novel formulation of zoledronic acid. Presented at the AACR-NCI-EORTC International Conference on Molecular Targets and Cancer Therapeutics, San Francisco, October 2007. Available at: http://www.merrionpharma.com/archive/portfolio/Oct2007EORTCPoster.pdf.

41. Amory JK, Bremmer WJ, Page ST, et al. MER-104: a dose ranging study of an oral formulation of gonadotropin-releasing hormone antagonist, acyline. Presented at the AACR-NCI-EORTC International Conference on Molecular Targets and Cancer Therapeutics, San Francisco, October 2007. Available at: http://www.merrionpharma.com/archive/MER-104.pdf.

42. Ding X, Rath P, Angelo R, et al. Oral absorption enhancement of cromolyn sodium through non-covalent complexation. *Pharm Res.* 2004;21(12):2196–2206.

43. Malkov D, Angelo R, Wang HZ, Flanders E, Tang H, Gomez-Orellana I. Oral delivery of insulin with the Eligen technology: mechanistic studies. *Curr Drug Deliv.* 2005;2(2):191–197.

44. Alani AW, Robinson JR. Mechanistic understanding of oral drug absorption enhancement of cromolyn sodium by an amino acid derivative. *Pharm Res.* 2008;25(1):48–54.

45. Wu SJ. *Mechanistic Studies on the Enhanced Mucosal Transport of Human Growth Hormone by Certain Amino Acid Derivatives.* Madison, WI: University of Wisconsin–Madison, 1999.

46. Li B. Non-covalent carrier enhanced protein absorption-cellular and subcellular mechanistic studies. (Ph.D. dissertation.) Madison, WI: University of Wisconsin–Madison, 2001.

47. Knipp GT, Vander Velde D, Siahaan TJ, Borchardt RT. The effect of β-turn structure on the passive diffusion of peptides across Caco-2 monolayers. *Pharm Res.* 1997;14:1332–1340.

48. Kimura T, Higaki K. Gastrointestinal transit and drug absorption. *Biol Pharm Bull.* 2002;25:149–164.

49. Aoki Y, Morishita M, Asai K, Akikusa B, Hosoda S, Takayama K. Region-dependent role of the mucous/glycocalyx layers in insulin permeation across rat small intestinal membrane. *Pharm Res.* 2005;22:1854–1862.

50. Pettit DK, Gombotz WR. The development of site-specific drug-delivery systems for peptide and protein biopharmaceuticals. *Trends Biotechnol.* 1998;16(8):343–349.

51. Lu YJ, Yang J, Sega E. Issues related to targeted delivery of proteins and peptides. *AAPS J.* 2006;8(3):E466–E478.

52. Antosova Z, et al. Therapeutic application of peptides and proteins: parenteral forever? *Trends Biotechnol.* 2009;27(11):628–635.

53. Agrawal H, Thacker N, Misra A. Parenteral delivery of peptides and proteins. In: A Misra, *Challenges in Delivery of Therapeutic Genomics and Proteomics.* New York, NY: Elsevier; 2011:531–622.

54. Makarewicz PA, Freeman JB, Fairfullsmith RF. Prevention of superficial phlebitis during peripheral parenteral-nutrition. *Am J Surg.* 1986;151(1):126–129.

55. Casadevall N, et al. Pure red-cell aplasia and antierythropoietin antibodies in patients treated with recombinant erythropoietin. *N Engl J Med.* 2002;346(7):469–475.

56. Clark AR, et al. The application of pulmonary inhalation technology to drug discovery. *Annu Rep Med Chem.* 2006;41:383–393.

57. Smith PL. Peptide delivery via the pulmonary route: a valid approach for local and systemic delivery. *J Control Release.* 1997;46(1-2):99–106.

58. Sanders N, et al. Extracellular barriers in respiratory gene therapy. *Adv Drug Deliv Rev.* 2009;61(2):115–127.
59. Patton JS. Pulmonary delivery of drugs for bone disorders. *Adv Drug Deliv Rev.* 2000;42(3):239–248.
60. Kirch J, et al. Mucociliary clearance of micro- and nanoparticles is independent of size, shape and charge—an ex vivo and in silico approach. *J Control Release.* 2012;159(1):128–134.
61. Turker S, Onur E, Ozer Y. Nasal route and drug delivery systems. *Pharm World Sci.* 2004;26(3):137–142.
62. Behl CR, et al. Effects of physicochemical properties and other factors on systemic nasal drug delivery. *Adv Drug Deliver Rev.* 1998;29(1-2):89–116.
63. Romeijn SG, et al. The effect of nasal drug formulations on ciliary beating in vitro. *Int J Pharm.* 1996;135(1-2):137–145.
64. Deshpande VS, et al. Characterization of lidocaine metabolism by rat nasal microsomes: implications for nasal drug delivery. *Eur J Drug Metab Pharmacokinet.* 1999;24(2):177–182.
65. Pontiroli AE. Peptide hormones: review of current and emerging uses by nasal delivery. *Adv Drug Deliv Rev.* 1998;29(1-2):81–87.
66. Lochhead JJ, Thorne RG. Intranasal delivery of biologics to the central nervous system. *Adv Drug Deliv Rev.* 2012;64(7):614–628.
67. Herwadkar A, Banga AK. Transdermal delivery of peptides and proteins. In: Van Der Walle C, ed. *Peptide and Protein Delivery.* London, UK: Academic Press; 2011:69–86.
68. Tortora GJ, Derrickson B. The integumentary system. In: GJ Tortora, SR Grabowski, eds. *Principles of Anatomy and Physiology,* 11th ed. Hoboken, NJ: John Wiley & Sons; 2002:144–170.
69. Prausnitz MR, Langer R. Transdermal drug delivery. *Nat Biotechnol.* 2008;26(11):1261–1268.
70. Kalluri H, Banga AK. Transdermal delivery of proteins. *AAPS PharmSciTech.* 2011;12(1):431–441.
71. Kim J, Jang JH, Lee JH, et al. Enhanced topical delivery of small hydrophilic or lipophilic active agents and epidermal growth factor by fractional radiofrequency microporation. *Pharm Res.* 2012;29(7):2017–2029.
72. Singh N, Kalluri H, Herwadkar A, Badkar A, Banga AK. Transcending the skin barrier to deliver peptides and proteins using active technologies. *Crit Rev Ther Drug Carrier Syst.* 2012;29(4):265–298.
73. Squier CA, Cox P, Wertz PW. Lipid content and water permeability of skin and oral mucosa. *J Invest Dermatol.* 1991;96:123–126.
74. Wertz PW, Squier CA. Cellular and molecular basis of barrier function in oral epithelium. *Crit Rev Ther Drug Carrier Syst.* 1991;8:237–269.
75. Merkle HP, Wolany GJM. Buccal delivery for peptide drugs. *J Control Release.* 1992;21:155–164.
76. Veuillex F, Kalia YN, Jacques Y, Deshusses J, Buri P. Factors and strategies for improving buccal absorption of peptides. *Eur J Pharm Biopharm.* 2001;51:93–109.
77. Khutoryanskiy VV. Advances in mucoadhesion and mucoadhesive polymers. *Macromol Biosci.* 2011;11(6):748–64.
78. Khafagy E-S, Morishita M, Onuki Y, Takayama K. Current challenges in non-invasive insulin delivery systems: a comparative review. *Adv Drug Deliv Rev.* 2007;59(15):1521–46.
79. Gowthamarajan K, Kulkarni G. Oral insulin: fact or fiction? *Resonance.* 2003;8(5):38–46.
80. Korythowski M. When oral agents fail: practical barriers to starting insulin. *Int J Obes Relat Metab Disord.* 2002;26(3):S18–S24.
81. Liu P, Dinh S. Oral delivery of protein/peptide therapeutics. In: Hu M, Li X, eds. *Oral Bioavailability, Basic Principles, Advanced Concepts and Applications.* Hoboken, NJ: John Wiley & Sons; 2011:371–380.
82. DeWitt DE, Hirsch IB. Outpatient insulin therapy in type 1 and type 2 diabetes mellitus: scientific review. *JAMA.* 2003;289(17):2254–64.
83. Toorisaka E, et al. An enteric-coated dry emulsion formulation for oral insulin delivery. *J Control Release.* 2005;107(1):91–96.
84. Pisal DS, Kosloski MP, Balu-Iyer SV. Delivery of therapeutic proteins. *J Pharm Sci.* 2010;99(6):2557–2575.
85. Caliceti P, Veronese FM. Pharmacokinetic and biodistribution properties of poly(ethylene glycol)-protein conjugates. *Adv Drug Deliv Rev.* 2003;55(10):1261–1277.
86. Gregoriadis G, et al. Improving the therapeutic efficacy of peptides and proteins: A role for polysialic acids. *Int J Pharm.* 2005;300(1–2):125–130.
87. Mi FL, et al. Chitin/PLGA blend microspheres as a biodegradable drug delivery system: a new delivery system for protein. *Biomaterials.* 2003;24(27):5023–5036.
88. Salmaso S, et al. Nanotechnologies in protein delivery. *J Nanosci Nanotechnol.* 2006;6(9-10):2736–2753.
89. Rajapaksa TE, et al. Claudin 4-targeted protein incorporated into PLGA nanoparticles can mediate M cell targeted delivery. *J Control Release.* 2010;142(2):196–205.
90. Giudice EL, Campbell JD. Needle-free vaccine delivery. *Adv Drug Deliv Rev.* 2006;58(1):68–89.

DRUG METABOLOMICS AND PROTEOMICS ANALYSIS IN DRUG DELIVERY AND DISCOVERY

RAVINDER EARLA AND ASHIM K. MITRA

CHAPTER OBJECTIVES

Upon completing this chapter, the reader should be able to

▸ Comprehend proteomics and proteomic-based mass spectrometric analysis, including sample preparation, isolation, and purification techniques.

▸ Describe mass spectrometry instrumentation and ionization techniques.

▸ Understand top-down protein and bottom-up (shotgun) peptide sequencing.

▸ Apply mass spectrometry in quantitative proteomics of phosphorylation, glycosylation post-translational modifications.

CHAPTER OUTLINE

INTRODUCTION

Tandem mass spectrometry (MS/MS) is a widely used fundamental technique in pharmaceutical and biomedical research for metabolomics and proteomics to characterize cellular functions. Exogenous compounds such as drug and protein molecules undergo metabolism when they are exposed to xenobiotics in all living systems to facilitate their consumption and/or elimination.

The xenobiotics either affect positively or negatively by generating metabolites by various pathways of native molecules that have led to several discoveries in modern biomedical research. In modern drug discovery and drug delivery, the major enzymes responsible for the biotransformation of most of the molecules that generate bioactive chemicals lead to beneficial or harmful pharmacological effects by various interactions. The study of biotransformation of xenobiotics for toxicological research can improve our strategies on chemical-induced toxicity and carcinogenesis. For example, tobacco/smoke contains mainly nicotine that forms many xenobiotic compounds. Nicotine is metabolized to cotinine (75%), nornicotine, and other metabolites. Cotinine is further metabolized to cotinine N-oxide, norcotinine, *trans* 3'-hydroxycotinine, and other minor metabolites [1]. Some of these compounds are further metabolized to precarcinogenic compounds such as nicotine-derived nitrosamine ketone [2].

Similarly, macromolecules such as proteins and peptides undergo xenobiotic metabolism. The proteins and peptides are biochemical compounds made up of amino acid residues that are chemically formed by the formation of an amide link between the α-carboxyl groups of one amino acid attached to the α-amino group of an adjacent amino acid. These amino acid moieties are essential building blocks of plants, microbes, animals, and humans. Each amino acid is primarily made of carbon, hydrogen, oxygen, and nitrogen, which are required to form a polypeptide or protein. A peptide that is composed of less than 50 amino acid residues [3] is called an *oligopeptide*. Each peptide contains an amine and a carboxyl terminus unless it is cyclic and absorbs ultraviolet light within wavelengths of 190 to 230 nm. The smallest peptide is a dipeptide that can be formed by dehydration or condensation [4]. A functional group of $-C-(=O)-NH-$ in a peptide or protein is called a peptide link, as shown in **Figure 18-1**. A polypeptide chain that contains more than 50 amino acid residues is known as a protein. The molecular weight of proteins usually ranges between 5,500 and 220,000 kDa. Proteins plays a key role in essential processes in the cell including signaling, immune responses, cell adhesion, division, and replication.

Proteomics is the study of proteins and their fragments, including peptides and free amino acids. Proteomics is an essential aspect of biological research in investigating

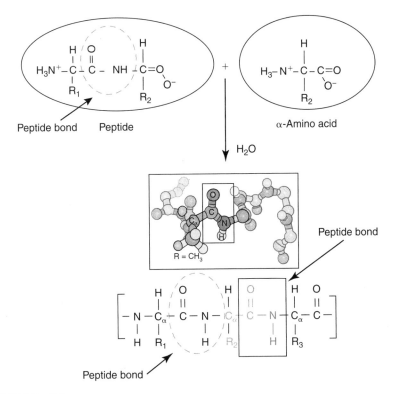

FIGURE 18-1 Peptide.

post-translational protein modifications such as phosphorylation and glycosylation. The stable isotope labeling by amino acids in cell culture (SILAC) is a commonly used approach for the proteomics study described in this chapter. The SILAC technique is used to measure the abundance of a protein in normal versus diseased clinical samples using mass spectrometry (MS). This approach provides fundamental information on cellular regulatory mechanisms [5].

In addition, proteomics is considered one of the most important techniques to identify potential targets that may lead to effective drug therapy [6–8]. It is quite difficult to use. Proteomics research requires a high cost per sample and has limited quantitative precision. However, this approach is used in finding clinical biomarkers. Therefore, there is a need to study the proteomics to establish systematic protocols for day-to-day clinical applications [9, 10].

MS is one of the most widely used technologies for proteomics research. The MS multiple reactions monitoring (MRM) technique is commonly used for quantitative biomarker analysis. MRM generates data that are reliable, precise, and accurate [11]. However, challenges remain, because of its sensitivity and the samples contain low protein expressions [11].

HISTORY OF MS

MS is a well-established technology that was first developed in 1897 by a Joseph John Thomson, who won a Nobel Prize in 1906 for his discoveries of electrons and isotopes. Arthur J. Dempster and Francis William Aston developed more sensitive MS technology in 1918 and 1919, respectively. In 2002, John Bennett Fenn, and Koichi Tanaka developed electrospray ionization (ESI) along with a novel method for the analysis of biological macromolecules with a tandem MS technique [12–15]. The various built-in MS technologies include single MS, tandem MS (MS/MS), and the quadrupole linear ion trap (QTrap MS/MS. These types of MS systems are ultimate tools for qualitative and quantitative proteomics. The basic principle of MS is based on the mass-to-charge (m/z) ratio of a compound [16]. Here, m is the mass and z is the charge of a compound. For example, for peptide MH^+, z = 1; MH_2^{2+}, z = 2, MH_2^{3+}, z = 3, MH^-, z = 1; MH^{2-}, z = 2. Commonly, MS generates ions with adducts such as proton (H^+), sodium (Na^+), potassium (K^+), and calcium (Ca^{2+}). In addition to proteomics, MS is also applied to biochemical and clinical research including pharmacokinetics, pharmacodynamics, forensics, environmental science, basic cell biology, and drug testing and screening [17].

MS IONIZATION TECHNIQUES

ELECTROSPRAY IONIZATION

ESI generates ions from macro- and micro-molecules that in turn increases the ionization of a compound at atmospheric pressure. ESI produces an electron from a molecule to generate a positively charged ion by applying potential difference (3–6 kV) in a capillary through which analyte solution flows in a process known as infusion. The ion source produces a 10^6 V/m electric field that causes charge buildup at the surface of a liquid solution, thereby splitting to form highly charged cluster droplets. These droplets are declustered into tiny droplets and then dried to one or more (typically not more than six) charge units. An electron from a target molecule (M) is ejected during this collision with an electron beam, thereby converting the molecule to a positive charge radical cation [$M^{+\cdot}$] with an odd number of electrons. The molecule can form with the addition or subtraction of a proton like [M+H]$^{+\cdot}$ and [M–H]$^{+\cdot}$. In case of multiple charged ions it can form either [M+nH]$^{n+\cdot}$ and [M–nH]$^{n+\cdot}$. Small molecules produce not more than 6 charges, whereas macromolecules can produce not more than 25 charge states, which occur with different frequencies from one to a maximum of [M+25H]$^{25+\cdot}$. Some examples of radical cation formations are as follows:

$$M+ e^- \rightarrow M^{+\cdot} + 2e^-$$

$$M+ e^- \rightarrow [M+H]^{+\cdot} + 2e^-$$

$$M+ e^- \rightarrow [M-H]^{+\cdot} + 2e^-$$

There are several physical models of ESI ion sources in both micro–ESI and nano–ESI, where the flow rate is very low, causing increased sensitivity [18]. The principle of ESI techniques is illustrated in Figure 18–2 and summarized in Table 18–1.

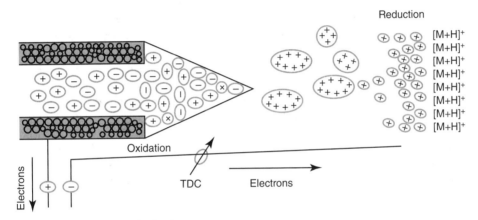

FIGURE 18-2 Electrospray ionization.

TABLE 18-1 Brief summary of MS ionization techniques (ESI and MALDI)				
Technique	Principle of Action	Charge of Ions	Mass Range	Applications
ESI	Uses an electric field to generate sprays of fine droplets; as the droplets evaporate, ions are formed	Multiply charged (the larger analyte molecule acquires multiple charges)	>100 kDa	10^{-15} mole, LC-MS of peptide mixtures; tandem MS; protein identification by comparing experimental MS/MS spectra with theoretical MS/MS spectra generated from protein databases
MALDI	Uses laser rays to desorb and ionize analyte molecules cocrystallized with a matrix on a metal surface	Mostly singly charged	>100 kDa	10^{-15} mole, determination of spots on two-dimensional polyacrylamide gel electrophoresis; identification of molecular weight; protein identification by "peptide mass fingerprinting"

MATRIX-ASSISTED LASER DESORPTION IONIZATION

The matrix-assisted laser desorption ionization (MALDI) MS technique enables visualization of the spatial delivery of protein and peptide compounds and their biomarkers within a tiny sample from an animal plant tissue. In MALDI analysis the compound is mixed with solvents such as water, ethanol, and acetonitrile containing small, crystallized organic compounds. Commonly used organic compounds are α-cyano-4-hydroxycinnamic acid, 3,5-dimethoxy-4-hydroxycinnamic acid, and 2,5-dihydroxybenzoic acid with a small portion of trifluoroacetic acid in a matrix that is mixed with the compound (e.g., protein sample). The solution is spotted onto a MALDI plate (a metal plate designed for this purpose) and uses ultraviolet lasers such as nitrogen lasers (337 nm) and frequency-tripled and -quadrupled neodymium-doped, yttrium, and aluminum garnet (Nd:YAG) lasers (355 nm and 266 nm, respectively) [19]. An infrared laser causes a softer mode of ionization and is rarely applied in MALDI. The compound must be well miscible, which spreads throughout the crystal matrix when a solvent is vaporized. Then, the matrix and the compound can be cocrystallized in a MALDI spot that is absorbed by a laser and ionized [20]. The matrix transfers part of the charges to the compound (e.g., protein) and ionizes these molecules while protecting them from the disruptive energy of the laser. Quasimolecular ions are observed after this process. It can cause neutral loss [5] by adding $[M+H]^+$ or removing $[M-H]^+$ of a proton [18,21], thereby generating singly-charged ions. However, multiply charged ions ($[M+nH]^{n+}$) can also be formed based on the function of the matrix laser intensity and/or the voltage applied. This technique requires several hundred laser shots to achieve an acceptable signal-to-noise ratio for ion detection. It is used in top-down analysis of high-molecular-weight proteins but generates a shot-to-shot inconsistent result that is strongly based on sample preparation methods [18, 21]. The principle of the MALDI technique is shown in Figure 18-3 and summarized in Table 18-1.

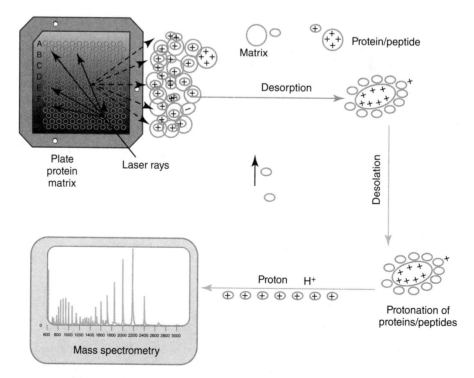

FIGURE 18-3 Matrix-assisted laser desorption ionization.

SAMPLE PURIFICATION AND ISOLATION TECHNIQUES

MS can determine certain mass ranges in proteomic analysis. Proteins are commonly digested by trypsin, chymotrypsin, pepsin, and thermolysin. In addition, proteins, can also be digested by urea, Tris-HCl, and tris(2-coboxymethyl) phosphine. A general approach for extracting and isolating a complex protein mixture is depicted in Figure 18-4a. The four major protein purification and isolation techniques in proteomics are tandem affinity purification (TAP), isotope-coded affinity tagging (ICAT), isobaric tags for relative and absolute quantitation (iTRAQ), and absolute quantitation of proteomics and SILAC [22–24].

TANDEM AFFINITY PURIFICATION

TAP is a simple two-step affinity purification method for the separation of TAP-tagged proteins mixed with other related proteins in a protein–protein interaction study. Identification of a single subunit of protein is important for understanding its function. This technique is used to purify protein complexes from various biological systems, including bacteria, yeasts, plants, and mammalian cells [25, 26]. The complex of TAP–tag is attached to the protein of interest that contains two different purification tag units separated by trypsin digestion. The original TAP–tag unit (domain A) of protein binds to IgG and calmodulin-binding peptide that is separated by highly specific tobacco etch virus protease [27]. TAP is modified into localization and purification tags that can be used for affinity purification of fusion proteins to study nuclear localization signals [28]; these signals can also be detected by TAP technique with the calmodulin-binding

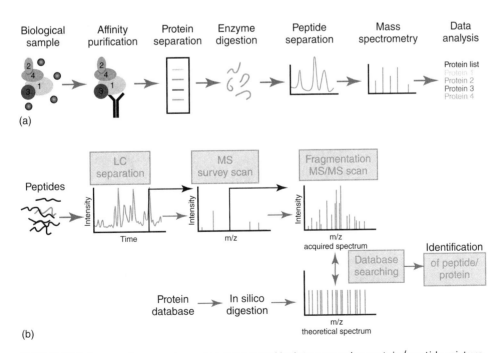

FIGURE 18-4 A general approach used to extract and isolate a complex protein/peptide mixture. (a) A biological sample is purified and separated into its constituents. (b) Peptide separation and optimization in MS and identification.

peptide domain that is separated by mutation [29]. The TAP–tag approach can be applied to subcellular localization through fusion of green fluorescent protein. It can also trace glucocorticoid steroidal dependent translocation to a DNA and/or transcriptional. The TAP-tagging approach has been successfully used in mammalian cells to measure many protein complexes [30], and data are further confirmed with a database [31]. It has limited application, however, for nonprotein moieties, including small molecular drugs, metabolites, or nucleic acids.

ISOTOPE-CODED AFFINITY TAGGING

Discovered in 1999, ICAT is designed to be a high-throughput screening technique for estimating the protein content of two different samples by a gel-free process. ICAT is a proteomic method designed to identify and quantify proteins in a two–cell population. The protein must contain a cysteine residue that can be measured. The principle of the ICAT strategy is based on the specificity of sulfhydryl groups of cysteine and its biotin affinity tag linkers. A selective subunit of protein purified by this technique is based on the stable isotope affinity tagging of the cysteine residues [32, 33]. Phosphate or sulfhydryl groups play a key role in this approach, which depends on chemical labeling reagent and mass tag linker. The chemical reagent contains three common reactive groups that allow a selective labeling of cysteine residue in the ICAT strategy. It can compare the difference in protein expression in the light ^{12}C (d0, no deuterium) and heavy ^{13}C (d8, deuterium) tagged cells. These cells are dissolved and proteins can be extracted to obtain heavy and light ICAT-tagged proteins. These samples can be mixed and enzymatically digested to break the proteins into smaller peptide fragments that can bind to ICAT reagents. ICAT-tagged proteins and ICAT-labeled peptides can bind to a magnet like molecule avidin and can be separated to identify heavy and light ICAT-tagged proteins. The heaviest ^{13}C and light ^{12}C fragments can be analyzed for quantity and mass, which is possible only with the MS method. Because their masses can differ by 8-Da units, sequencing can help to identify these fragments. Some proteins can also appear in one cell type that may not be identified [34] and separated by improving a peak resolution in liquid chromatography (LC) [35].

ICAT strategy can also be used for both gel-free and gel-based separations in which two–dimensional gel electrophoresis can be applied [36]. In this approach, labeled proteins are dissolved in a buffer solution and isolated by gel electrophoresis with the trichloroacetic acid precipitation method to obtain a clean sample. Both the buffer and ICAT reagent can also be mixed in a stoichiometric ratio to maintain 3-mM ICAT concentration in solution [37]. This strategy can improve the sensitivity of peptide abundance and is critical for peptide sequencing. LC/MS/MS analytical data are further confirmed by database search to identify ICAT-labeled proteins [38].

ISOBARIC TAGS FOR RELATIVE AND ABSOLUTE QUANTITATION

iTRAQ is also a non–gel-based separation technique like ICAT that is used to measure protein or peptide in a different environment. It is gaining importance over traditional proteomic methods for identifying biomarkers in various disease conditions [39–41]. This labeling technique involves stable incorporation of isotopes into an amine-tagging reagent to study comparative quantitation of various proteins in a complex cell matrix. In the iTRAQ approach, the labeling reagent consists of a quantification group (N-methylpiperazine), a balance group (carbonyl), and a hydroxyl succinimide ester group that reacts with the N-terminal amino groups of peptides and amino acids (i.e., lysine). The labeling reagents covalently react with the amino group of lysine. In iTRAQ up to four or eight labels can be introduced into multiplexing experiments for comparative studies. Eight iTRAQ reagents are usually selected in this technique and are exclusively distributed among the balance and reporter groups [39].

In MS/MS analysis, the signal intensity ratios of the reporter groups represent ratios of the peptide quantities and can be used to estimate relative quantities of the peptides. MS/MS spectra of the individual peptides can indicate signals replicating amino acid sequences and reporter ions that match the protein contents of the samples. A database search is then performed using fragmentation data to identify labeled peptides. Later, the corresponding proteins are quantified at the same time as the iTRAQ mass reporter ion used to relatively quantify the peptides. Quantitation of protein from multiple samples can be achieved in the same run when the iTRAQ-modified peptides are analyzed by MS/MS. The ratios of peptide quantities among different samples are expressed as signal intensity ratios of the reporter groups (m/z: 113, 114, 115, 116, 117, 118, 119, and 121). The iTRAQ-labeling peptides can be coeluted on a reverse-phase column chromatography [41, 42] but cannot be separated into a single state at a particular isoelectric point. It can be resolved, however, by changing the isoelectric point in a medium. With this strategy, a lower abundance of protein signal can be identified. This strategy has shown promising results in proteomic study.

STABLE ISOTOPE LABELING BY AMINO ACID IN CELL CULTURE

MS-based stable isotope quantitation is becoming extremely popular for simultaneous and automated identification and estimation of complex protein mixtures. SILAC is an easy, economical, and accurate method that can be applied as a quantitative proteomic approach in any cell culture system. SILAC stable isotope quantitation is based on labeling amino acids that can be introduced into a cell culture medium to encode cellular proteins. This MS-based technique measures differences in the protein abundance among samples with nonradioactive isotopic labeling. The stable isotopes can be identified within specific amino acid residues, including ^{13}C, ^{15}N labeling [7, 8, 43]. The technique is initially introduced for mammalian cell culture and later extended to bacteria and plants to study specific cellular functional activities. In SILAC, two or more cell cultures are grown in different media that contain amino acids with natural, heavy, or stable isotopes including arginine or lysine and all peptides can be tagged except C-terminal of each protein. Cells are cultured in a heavy medium to grow at least five doublings to allow sufficient time for incorporation of the stable amino acids [44]. After five cell doublings, approximately 97% of the protein may be present in a stable isotope form. Labeled proteins can be separated based on their residue mass differences that can correlate to a number of stabled isotopes and amino acids in the protein [45].

This technique is limited in that it cannot analyze patient samples directly. Before MS analysis, samples need to be purified by either one-dimensional or two-dimensional strong cation exchange chromatography. It can be applied to post-translational modifications (PTMs) with methylation that can occur on arginine and lysine residues [44]. SILAC strategy can also be adopted for identifying *in vivo* methylation of proteins including DNA, RNA, and other substrates. For example, methylated arginine peptide substitute can easily be separated by a mass difference of 4 Da and 8 Da for mono- and di-substituted, respectively [46, 47]. It can also be used to study PTMs of proteins including phosphorylation to identify a specific protein network.

INSTRUMENTATION

MS instrumentation can be divided into various categories, including triple quadrupole tandem mass spectrometers, MS/MS high-resolution spectrometers, ion cyclotron resonance, quadrupole ion trap, and tandem time of flight. In both the quadrupole and ion trap systems, radiofrequency (RF) and direct current (DC) voltages can be applied to separate ions. Tandem MS can have two quadrupole, two magnetic analyzer, or one magnetic and one quadrupole models that can be built as hybrid spectrometers [48]. The hybrid MS can be combined with two different mass analyzers to build an MS/MS system. In high resolution, a quadrupole ion trap and time of flight analyzer systems should be able to sort out fragmentation ions of interest. Such ions are further excited and induced to fragments within a certain period of time to generate signals.

MS ANALYZERS

MS analyzers can select ions based on the m/z ratio in magnetic or electric fields. The common MS analyzers in proteomics research are quadrupole, ion trap, time of flight, and Fourier transform ion cyclotron resonance based on instruments. Some can be designed with several analyzers of the same or different types that can be combined to obtain maximum response.

Quadrupole Analyzers

Quadrupole MS is highly stable and can have excellent mass resolution with high sensitivity because of the electron or proton multiplier detectors. Quadrupole refers to four parallel metal rods that operate together electronically. Their arrangement is depicted in **Figure 18-5**. Quadrupole MS works based on the m/z ratio. Some of the ions can travel through the X-direction between the rods by applying an RF voltage between a pair of opposite rods [49]. These ions can receive energy from the field and oscillate through it with increasingly large amplitude until they encounter one of the rods. If they discharge, certain ions will be transmitted to the other end of the quadrupole without hitting X-electrodes. Another range of ions can follow the Y-direction and become unstable because of the defocusing effect of DC. A fraction, however, can be stabilized by alternating current. Another fraction can follow the Y-direction based on mass to the other end of the quadrupole without colliding with Y-electrodes, thereby generating signals [50, 51]. By modifying the RF/DC ratios, a fraction of these ions can travel in an undesired Z-direction; however, these ions can be angled to the desired Y-direction to hit the detector and generate signals. The quadrupole system is equipped with convenient filters that can be tuned to obtain the required ions by adjusting the DC/RF ratios. With continuous adjustment, the DC amplitude and RF voltage (at fixed ω) may generate the entire mass spectrum expected to be scanned.

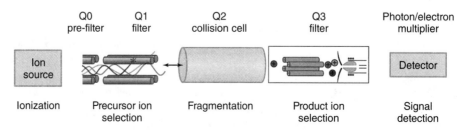

FIGURE 18-5 Schematic diagram of triple quadrupole mass spectrometer.

Time of Flight Analyzer

In time of flight, ions travel in a horizontal path and move vertically into a flight tube to produce a signal. Ions can descend due to gravitational force, however, based on their mass. As a result, ions can collide with the detector to generate a signal. By adjusting DC amplitude and RF, voltage ions can impact the detector and generate a spectrum that can be scanned. In time of flight, time is calculated as

$$t^2 = \frac{m}{z} \times \left(\frac{d^2}{2eVs} \right)$$

Where z refers to a charge of the electron ($e = 1.6 \times 10^{-19}$ coulombs). The charge is accelerated by potential V. Ions move a distance, d, through the chamber tube (field free) unit, before colliding with the detector. The m/z ion stands in a quadratic relationship to the flight time and the higher mass ions can reach faster than lighter ions to the detector [16, 50].

Detectors

Typically, two types of detectors used in MS are the electron and photon multipliers. These detectors can be used with various plates, including photographic plates, faraday cylinders, and array detector plates to amplify signals [18]. MS operating software can calculate a signal intensity based on m/z and measures values in either Thomson or Dalton (1 m/z = 1 Da = 1.665402×10^{-27} kg). Ion signals can be collected and combined to generate an MS spectrum. MS-based software like bioanalyst can convert MS scans into a stick spectrum by reconstruction or deconvulation mode. MS spectra may not correspond to an exacted molecular weight because the isotopes may be in a heavier or lighter state with different isotope distribution. For example, carbon has two isotopes C-12 with mass (m/z) 12.00000 Da with 98% of relative abundance and C-13 has mass 13.003355 Da (1.112%). Hydrogen has two H-1, 1.00782 Da (99.985%) and H-2, 2.014 Da (0.015); nitrogen has two N-14, 14.003074 Da (99.63%), N-15, 15.0000108 Da (0.37%); oxygen has three O-15, 15.994915 Da (99.76%), O-16, 16.999133 Da (0.04%), O-17, 17.999169 Da (0.20%); and sulfur has four isotopes S-31, 31.972970 Da (95.03%), S-32, 32.971456 Da (0.75%), S-33, 33.967866 Da (4.22%), and S-35, 35.967080 Da (0.02%). C-12 is the most common; C-13 is the second most common isotope of carbon, available roughly with probability of 1%. The C-13 isotope can shift the peak by 1 Da. The peptide mass can be calculated based on the number of isotopes and neutral loss. The full isotope pattern of a peptide can calculate as follows:

$$P(L, k) = \sum \times \sum_{}^{k} \times \left\{ n_1, \frac{i}{w_1}, p_1 \right\} \times P(L - \{I\}, \times k - i)$$

$$I \, \varepsilon \, L \quad i = 0,$$
$$I \, \% \, w_1 = 0$$

I is the peak of an isotope cluster (peak r_i) with I Da of additional mass compared with the mono-isotope peak. Supplied with C, N, O, and S atoms in a peptide, the relative heights of r_i can be calculated with binominal convolution. For example, a list L of isotope appears as ^{13}C, ^{15}N, ^{17}O, ^{18}O, because the effects of S and H isotopes are nominal. For each element $I \, \varepsilon \, L$, p_1 is the frequency of occurrence of an isotope, W_1 is the integer offset weight of the isotope (1 for ^{13}C, 2 for ^{18}O, etc.), and n_1 is the number of atoms. If P represents the joint isotope distribution, P (L, k) is the probability of seeing peak r_k, given a list L of isotopes available. Then, it keeps (2). This is not always true, but in practice we manipulate by looking at the peak difference k over a range (k− §, k + §).

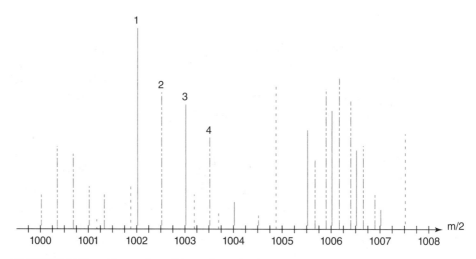

FIGURE 18-6 MS spectrum of peptide peaks and noise.

We can calculate the isotope pattern of a peptide if we know the expected chemi-cal composition, which depends on the mass, not on the m/z ratio. Such a pattern can measure the peptide content from nonpeptide content by deconvoluting the signals. An example of MS spectrum of a peptide along with the noise-to-signal ratio is shown in Figure 18-6. It explains peptide peak and noise. In this example, true peptide peaks are shown as solid bars or dashed lines and noise is shown as a dotted line. Peaks 1 to 4 belong to two alternative and regularly arranged peaks that show a charge 1 with molecular weights of peptide 1001 and 1001.5 Da, respectively.

METABOLOMICS ANALYSIS BY LC-MS

Nicotine is extensively metabolized by the liver CYP2A6 using C-oxidation to major metabolite cotinine and to other minor metabolites such as cotinine-N-oxide and nor-nicotine. Cotinine is further hydroxylated by CYP2A6 to *trans* 3'-hydroxycotinine and forms norcotinine upon N-methylation and other minor metabolites [1, 2, 52]. CYP2A6-mediated metabolism of nicotine produces metabolites, some of which are toxic and known to cause oxidative stress, leading to liver damage and pulmonary and pancreatic cancer. In addition, nicotine is known to be toxic to other cells, including brain [53]. To study nicotine metabolism, we developed a simple, fast, and sensitive ESI LC-MS/MS analytical method to simultaneously measure nicotine and four of its metabolites in HIV-1—positive and HIV-negative smokers' plasmas. Nicotine, cotinine, *trans* 3'-hydroxycotinine, nornicotine, and norcotinine were dissolved at a concentration of 1 mg/mL in 80% methanol (v/v). A working aqueous solution of these compounds was serially diluted to obtain at least eight standards. These solutions were used for MS optimization and the production of the calibration curve [52].

MS/MS CONDITIONS

The proton adduct m/z [M+H] + precursor ions of nicotine, cotinine, *trans*3'-hydroxyco-tinine, nornicotine, and norcotinine were selected in the positive mode. Precursor ions were fragmented by applying collisionally activated dissociation gas and collision energy to obtain their most abundant and stable product ions. The product ions for nicotine (177.1), cotinine (80.1), *trans* 3'-hydroxycotinine (80.1), nornicotine (132.0), norcotinine (80.1), nicotine-d4 (121.0), and cotinine-d3 (101.2) were optimized by adjusting collision energy, curtain gas, entrance potentials, and source gas 2. The MRM transitions (m/z) [M+H]+, (Q1→Q3) selected for quantitative analysis were 162.22→177.1 for nicotine, 177.17→80.1 for cotinine, 193.15→80.1 for *trans* 3'-hydroxycotinine, 149.22→132.0 for nornicotine, and 163.19→80.1 for norcotinine. The chromatographic separation was achieved by a reverse–phase MS 18 column (50 × 4.6 mm, inner diameter 5 μm) using isocratic mobile phase composed of 55% acetonitrile in water containing 0.05% formic acid at a flow rate of 0.4 mL/min [52].

SAMPLE PREPARATION AND EXTRACTION

A simple strong cation solid-phase extraction technique was used for sample extraction. The strong cation solid-phase extraction columns (strong cation exchange 30 mg, 1-mL cartridge) were preconditioned with 1 mL methanol and 0.6% formic acid in water. The analytes were eluted with 1 mL of a 7% ammonium hydroxide in methanol solution for LC-MS/MS analysis. In this technique, the use of formic acid and ammoniated methanolic solutions for solid-phase extraction cartridge conditioning and elution, respectively, enabled the generation of clear and reliable samples. We observed an increased ionization and peak response upon reconstituting in acetonitrile–water–formic acid mixture. In general, LC-MS/MS bioanalytical results are frequently inconsistent because of ineffective sample preparation and extraction methods. These problems can be eliminated, however, by modifying sample extraction techniques and MS parameters including MRM transitions. Liquid–liquid and solid-phase extractions are generally the most effective approach [54]. The nicotine is metabolized to cotinine by C-oxidation and nornicotine by N-demethylation followed by norcotinine by C-oxidation. The cotinine is further metabolized to cotinine N-oxide by N-oxidation, *trans* 3'-hydroxycotinine by hydroxylation, and norcotinine by N-demethylation (**Figure 18-7**).

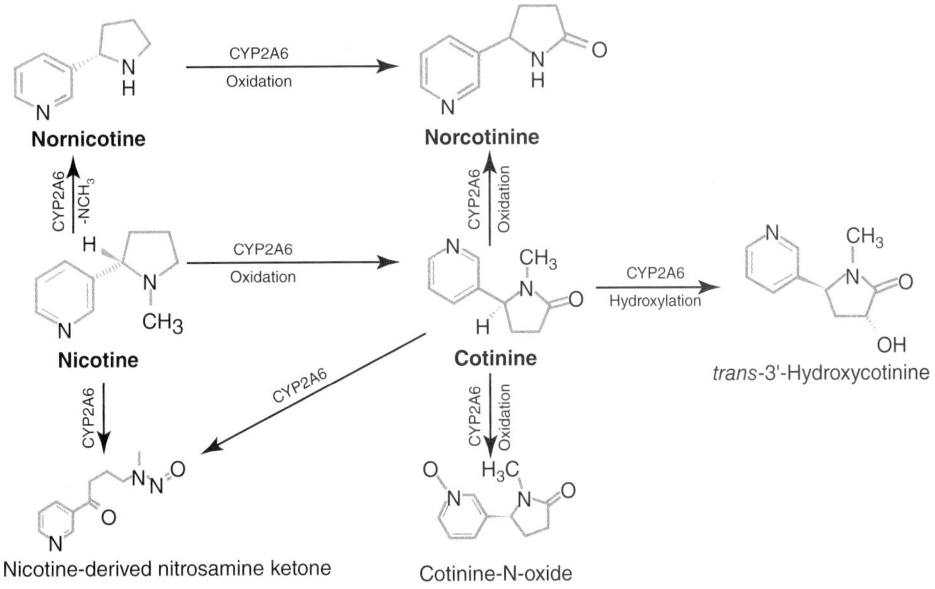

FIGURE 18-7 The metabolomics of nicotine in human plasma. Conversion of nicotine to cotinine, nornicotine, and cotinine conversion into cotinine N-oxide, norcotinine, and *trans* 3'-hydroxycotinine found in the plasma of HIV-1–positive smokers and HIV-negative smokers. (Reproduced from Earla R, Ande A, McArthur C, Kumar A, Kumar S. Enhanced nicotine metabolism in HIV-1-positive smokers compared to HIV-negative smokers: Simultaneous determination of nicotine and its four metabolites in their plasma using a simple and sensitive ESI-LC-MS/MS technique. *Drug Metab Dispos.* 2013; Dec 3.)

PROTEOMICS ANALYSIS

Proteomics intend to identify, characterize, and map gene functions at the protein level either in cells, tissues, or organisms. The object of proteomics is fractionation of a complex protein mixture by electrophoretic or chromatographic separation methods followed by identification of the components in the individual reactions by MS. MS can yield ion of proteins, peptides, and their fragments to provide the primary information regarding protein components, which can be further confirmed by a database searching. Four such database searching algorithms are available for peptide and protein analysis. *Descriptive approach* algorithms are based on a mechanistic prediction of fragmentation pattern of peptides in an MS/MS spectrometer. It is then quantified to determine the quality of the match between the expected and the experimental spectra. Mathematical methods such as correlation analysis have been applied to assess match quality. *Interpretative approaches* mainly depend on manual or automated interpretation of a partial sequence from an MS/MS mass spectrum and incorporation of that sequence into a database search. *Stochastic approaches* are based on probability approaches for the formation of MS/MS mass spectra and the fragmentation of peptides. Basic probabilities of fragment ions are acquired from a spectrum of known sequence. The stochastic approach uses statistical limits on the determination and fragmentation process to create possibility that the meet is correct. *Statistical and possibility approaches* estimate the connection among the MS/MS spectra and sequences. The probability of peptide identification and its significance are then derived from the model [55]. Proteomics are usually applied to large-scale analyses of proteins at the level of whole organism, tissue, cell, or subcellular compartments. MS-based approaches are currently the most popular techniques for proteome analysis.

A proteomics experiment starts with sample preparation, purification, and extraction, including cell lysis and protein digestion by chemical and enzymatic methods (Figure 18-4). Proteins can also be extracted by sample extraction procedures (i.e., liquid–liquid, protein precipitation, and solid-phase extractions).

BOTTOM-UP APPROACH

The term "shotgun" proteomics is derived from the genomics applied to identify protein sequencing in a mixture including cells, tissue, or subcellular components. The resulting peptide fragments are separated and identified by reverse-phase liquid chromatography, followed by MS/MS [56–58]. Most bottom-up applications need tandem data acquisition in which peptides undergo treatment with an inert gas such as nitrogen, helium, or argon. Types of treatments most frequently used are collision-activated dissociation or collision-induced dissociation. Alternative techniques, such as electron captured dissociation or electron transfer dissociation and surface-induced dissociation, have also been used. The gas-phase collision-activated or collision-induced dissociation is the most frequently applied method in commercial MS/MS application [55]. Electron fragmentation procedures in the bottom-up approach generally produce better fragmentation patterns and are able to find the sequences of large peptides that are multiply charged. These data may improve the characterization and PTMs of proteins.

Protein molecules are activated into unimolecular charged ions rather than multiply-charged ions in MS analysis. A peptide separation and optimization in MS is shown in Figure 18-4b. As the analyte collides with gases, the molecules gain energy and transform into ions, causing fragmentation. Fragmentation pattern of protein or peptide molecules varies, based on the sequence of amino acids and activation energy.

At a higher dissociation energy, fragmentation mainly generates amino acid side chains, and at low dissociation energies fragmentation mainly occurs along the peptide backbone [59, 60]. At low-energy collision-induced or collision-activated dissociation, conditions are normally used in triple quadrupole, quadrupole time of flight, and linear Paul trap mass spectrometers. In these cases B-ions, Y-ions, neutral losses of water, and ammoniated mass signals dominate the mass spectrum [61, 62].

Most algorithms assume that peptides fragment specially into Y- and B-ions. Scattering of intensities between Y- and B-ions can vary according to equipment (e.g., linear ion trap as compared with quadrupole time of flight). The data generated by these instruments, however, are insufficient to determine m/z ratio accuracy and resolve weight capacity. *m/z* ratio signals and noise may fluctuate based on electronic and chemical parameters and the concentrations of peptide at the ion source. Based on X-precursor (m/z) value, a list of fragment ions can be matched for amino acid sequence within the measurement and fragmentation of the mass spectrometer as shown in **Figure 18-8**. Although a high accuracy tandem mass spectra of multiply charged ions identify the precursor peptide, it is difficult to calculate an accurate molecular weight of a peptide because of poor reproducibility and inconsistent results. MS software determines the charge states of ions and performs deconvolution or reconstruction to determine the m/z ratio of the isotope peak. With low-resolution MS, variations in charge states (plus 2 or plus 3 charge intensities) that a peptide can assume may make it difficult to obtain the same results twice.

The N-terminal and C-terminal fragmentation approach may be used for molecular weight calculations and to correctly determine peptide ion charge states [63, 64]. In efficient tandem mass spectra, several molecular ion charge states exist. If precursor ion is expected to be doubly charged, the conclusive ions present in the spectrum should double the molecular weight. If the ion is triply charged, then the corresponding fragment ions will triple the molecular weight. The newer linear ion traps with higher scan speeds can arrange the high-resolution scan without reducing efficiency of data acquisition. Most large-scale MS/MS data are acquired by automated methods such as data-dependent data acquisition, which generates MS/MS based on ion abundance. When the ion abundance level is fixed just above the background noise of MS/MS data, it can continuously be acquired during mass scanning [65]. Important advantages of the bottom-up approach are that it produces better front-end separation of peptides compared with proteins and it is more sensitive than the top-down method.

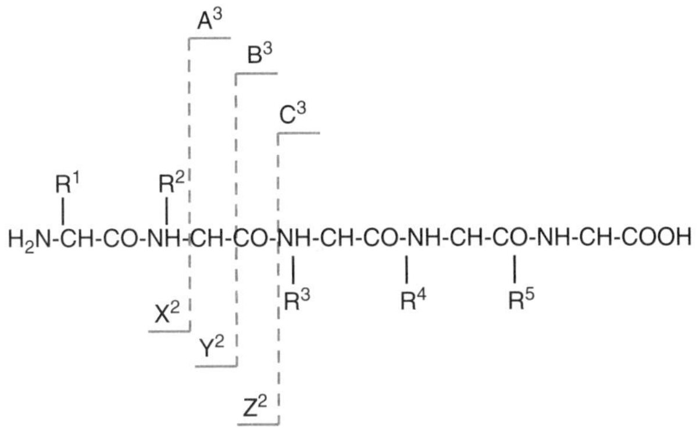

FIGURE 18-8 Graphical illustration of N-terminal X2, Y2, and Z2 ions and C-terminal A3, B3, and C3 ions for a five amino acid peptide.

Top-Down Approach

The top-down approach is an alternative to the more commonly used bottom-up sequencing. It involves direct determination of intact protein molecular ions and their fragment ion. In the top-down approach, protein samples are not supposed to be digested enzymatically. Subsequent measurement of the protein molecular weight and fragmentation of the intact protein are accomplished when various technologies are combined with database searching. This search leads to quantification and conformation of the source protein.

The main advantage of this method is its ability to find 100% sequence coverage that improves PTM evaluations [20, 43, 66]. Top-down proteomic analysis covers higher sequence coverage and reduces issues regarding peptide to protein mapping. The results obtained by top-down proteomic analysis help to identify specific protein isoforms [10, 67]. Another advantage of top-down proteomics is improved accuracy and reliability of protein quantification instead of peptide quantification [45, 68]. This type of protein analysis is performed by high-resolution instruments such as a FTMS and linrea triple quadrupole orbitrap, which resolve isotopic proteins. Such high-resolution mass spectral systems can detect small mass differences between proteins, thereby providing more detailed information of intact proteins (top-down proteomics). For example, the mass difference of trimethylation versus acetylation is 0.03639 Da, corresponding to 3 ppm for a 12,000-Da protein, both of which are commonly observed on core histones. Similarly, the mass difference between lysine and methionine residues is 2.94553 Da; for 12,000-, 100,000-, and 200,000-Da proteins this corresponds to 245, 29, and 15 ppm, respectively. For peptides, these differences in mass are detected with low-resolution instrumentation. For large-molecular-weight proteins, however, high mass accuracy is required to identify these potential isoforms.

In addition to accurate mass measurements, the mono-isotopic peak of a multiply charged protein is usually below signal to noise level, and its ability to distinguish between isotopic peaks for a single charge state is different. As a result, molecular weight and mass are accurately assigned. Our ability to interpret the accurate mass of an intact protein provides important information for PTMs of proteins. The mass accuracy especially provides improved form modification based on the stoichiometric ratio. Further challenges arise if multiple peptide sequences belonging to the same protein are identified as several isoforms with stoichiometric combinations. Knowing the intact masses, however, would provide information on how many modifications were present per protein molecule, greatly simplifying the analysis.

Top-down approaches can be broadly applied when analyzing degradome sequencing and provide a comprehensive means of analyzing patterns of RNA degradation using a peptidome, a comprehensive fact database for endogenous peptides present in the cell, tissue, organism, or system. Application of technologies developed for top-down MS to the degradome/peptidome analysis has a more trackable molecular weight range for MS analysis and has been shown to be very useful [69]. Degradomic/peptidomic profiling of blood plasma from cancer patients provides highly sensitive information to changes that are present in cells but not identifiable by traditional bottom-up proteomics analysis. The degradome/peptidome contains the changes between cancer and control cell samples and shows disease-associated markers with possible diagnostic utility of chemical modifications [70].

MS-Based Proteomics Applications

MS-based proteomics application has become an important area in drug discovery and delivery research. The biomarkers play a key role in discovery and development of protein and peptide analyses. These biomarkers correspond to specific biological or disease states for proteomics application. MS-based proteomics methods have developed a number of biomarkers that show marked improvement in diagnosis and handling of complex human diseases [71]. Target-based proteomics strategies with MS can provide adequate sensitivity that allows for the detection of lower signal intensity of peptides and proteins.

Biomarker identification is typically difficult for clinical application because it requires advanced analytical methods. Currently, the most commonly available procedure for biomarker identification is immunoassay. The sensitivity and specificity of immunoassays are based on antibody-based affinity proteins, but this procedure is costly and laborious [36]. An alternative to antibody-based assay is MS-based proteomics analysis. Such analysis does not need antibody-based affinity material for the application of targeted protein and peptide analyses. MS-based proteomics measurements mainly use two approaches: selected reaction monitoring and MRM. Targeted MS measurements generate data with high sensitivity and specificity data by triple quadrupole mass spectrometers, which generate consistent, reproducibile, and high-precision sensitivity data with dynamic range and reduce coefficient of variation between samples [72]. LC-selected reaction monitoring generates results that show potential information on proteins and peptides in various biological samples [25].

The selected reaction monitoring approach is based on precursor ions of proteins following a single stage of molecular ion selection, but the MRM approach measurements are based on preselected precursor ions of proteins following two stages with molecular ion selection of product ions. In the first stage of selection of both selected reaction monitoring and MRM, the precursor ion of an intact protein is selected in the quadrupole after ionization of molecular ion by applying declustering potential. In the second stage, product ion is selected in the second quadrupole after fragmentation of the precursor ion by applying collision-activated or collision-induced dissociation in the second quadrupole. These product ions are selected for the third quadrupole and the m/z ratio with their corresponding fragment ions are recorded, as shown in Figure 18-3. Results obtained by proteolysis of peptide targets can be confirmed from database or public repositories such as the Peptide Atlas and the Global Proteome Machine [72].

Additionally, computational methods have been developed for prediction of proteotypic peptides in amino acid sequences of a protein. In the MS method, sensitivity is improved and the expected therapeutic level is necessary for evaluation of disease-specific markers. The MRM strategy can dramatically enhance the sensitivity, dynamic range, and selectivity of MS analysis. The stable isotope standards by antipeptide antibodies [35] method demonstrated that enhanced sensitivity of analytical determinations ultimately improves detection and quantification of low intensity signal in plasma even with various endogenous interferences. A series of systems was used to analyze proteomics in animal serum samples spiked with various concentrations of proteolytic peptides to evaluate the detection sensitivity, reproducibility, and recovery. The MRM method with dual-ion funnel and multicapillary inlet interface method improved reproducibility, robustness, and sensitivity [40]. Another MS strategy, named high-pressure high-resolution isolation with specific selection and multiplexing, was also developed to further improve sensitivity and ruggedness for measuring of low protein concentrations (pg/mL) [73, 74].

PROTEIN PHOSPHORYLATION

A glycogen phosphorylase was first identified in 1955. Protein phosphorylation analysis is important in signaling studies. Multiple diseases may be the cause of about 30% phosphorylation of proteins in the human genome [75]. Phosphoproteomic analysis was used in the presence of titanium and zinc oxides by immobilized metal ion (Fe^{3+} or Ga^{3+}) affinity chromatography and metal oxide affinity chromatography [76]. The antibody-based arrays and fluorescence-based single-cell analysis are more sensitive techniques than metallic affinity chromatography techniques. Other techniques that offer high sensitivity and throughput include protein- and antibody-based arrays and fluorescence-based single-cell analysis. Usually, these methods need prior knowledge about targets. In phosphoproteomic analysis, addition of metaphosphoric acid or phosphoric acid increases molecular weight by 80 Da, and 98 Da, respectively, at the amino acid phosphorylation site on peptide fragment ions. Serine and threonine containing peptides undergo phosphorylation that cleaves the phosphoester bond with loss of phosphoric acid in the MS/MS spectrum.

PROTEIN GLYCOSYLATION

Characterization of glycoproteins or proteins by enzymatic process, in which sugar moieties (glycones) attached to the proteins, lipids, or other organic molecules, is applied extensively in proteomics analysis. Glycosylation is an important process for a wide range of biological applications, including cell attachment, protein–ligand interactions, protein function, localization, stability, and secretion [77]. Five types of glycosylation process are characterized by glycosidic linkages: N-linked, O-linked, C-linked glycosylation, glypiation (glycosylphosphatidylinositol anchor attachment), and phosphoglycosylation. MS technology is mainly used for identification of N-linked and O-linked proteins. Generally, N-linked glycans are linked to the nitrogen atom of asparagine or arginine side chains and O-linked glycans are mainly attached to the hydroxy oxygen atom of serine, threonine, and tyrosine; hydroxylysine; or hydroxyproline side chains. N-linked glycosylation sites can be localized and estimated to be present at the amino acid motif N-XS/T, where X represents any amino acid except cyclic ones.

Glycosylation studies are typically performed using three different approaches: characterization of the glycan in the intact glycoproteins, characterization of glycopeptides, and structural analysis of chemically or enzymatically released glycans. Here glycoproteins are purified by lectins such as concanavalin A or wheat-germ agglutinin. Alternatively, glycoproteins and peptides can be captured with hydrazide chemistry [78]. Intact N-linked glycans are enzymatically released with an amidase (peptide N-glycosidase F), which cleaves the linkage between the core GlcNAc (five different N-glycan linkages is the most common) and the asparagine residue. Two other enzymes, endoglycosidase D (which releases all classes of N-linked sugars) and endoglycosidase H (which releases oligomannose and hybrid N-glycans but not complex N-glycans), are also useful [79]. Denaturation of the glycoprotein does not appear to significantly enhance O-deglycosylation. There are few opportunities for enzymatic cleavage of O-linked glycans; O-glycanase, which cleaves at core structures of an O-linked glycan, is one of the only enzymatic means available. The most common modification of the core Gal-β(1-3)-GalNAc is a mono-, di-, or trisialylation [80, 81]. Because glycoproteomics is still an emerging field, MS-based analysis is just beginning to provide a means for characterizing this heterogeneous family of PTMs [80–82].

POST-TRANSLATIONAL MODIFICATIONS

PTM is the biochemical alteration of a protein at the amino acid side chain to extend functions of the protein. The process involves functional group conjugation of acetate, phosphate, lipids, and carbohydrates. PMT causes changes in chemical and biological properties of an amino acid (e.g., citrullination) or through structural changes (e.g., formation of disulfide bridges). PTMs include glycosylation, phosphorylation, ubiquitination, nitrosylation, methylation, acetylation, and lipidation. Identifying and understanding PTMs is a critical step in the study of disease treatment and prevention and cell biology. Biological functions of cells are mediated in part by protein PTMs. These modifications can be normal or active, altering the chemical and biological property of a protein in indirect ways. PTMs of protein changes are not easily discerned by standard protein profiling methods [83, 84]. Drug discovery and development studies report large-scale PTM profiling methods that have generated sufficient information on cells and cell biology [85]. Several issues, however, still need to be resolved. So far, most PTM studies have focused on common modifications, such as phosphorylation, glycosylation, ubiquitination, sumoylation, and acetylation, as discussed previously.

Protein modifications are involved in most signaling events that communicate with the nucleus through the cell membrane in response to external stimulation. The organization and rearrangement of modular domains in different signaling proteins due to PTMs creates complexity in signaling networks and pathways. In addition to changing catalytic roles, PTMs direct the assembly of multiprotein complexes and provide a means for crosstalk among convergent pathways in a transient and reversible manner. Proteins are not only modified by small chemical moieties but also through conjugation with other proteins. For example, ubiquitin, a small protein of 76 amino acids, is covalently attached to a specific lysine residue in substrate proteins by ubiquitin-ligase enzymes [86]. Polyubiquitylation can target proteins for proteasome-mediated degradation and generates important roles in the regulation of protein that are available in the cell. PTMs represent a central mechanism for signal transduction and regulation of proteins. These mechanisms provide key information on protein targets and modified amino acid sites. Such important information has a significant role in cell signaling and regulation of proteins. Simplification of sample preparation and extraction such as organelle isolation, subcellular fractionation, or plasma membrane preparations can also improve detection of substoichiometric PTMs. Selective changes, such as phosphorylation, can occur in a sample at any given time and often need selective modification before MS detection.

As with conventional bottom-up proteomics, targeted PTM analytical techniques are used to achieve higher sensitivity and a broad range of proteome coverage. Efficient cellular preparations and protein-extraction procedures are key to the success of PTM studies. There has been significant improvement in sample preparation and analytical techniques for large-scale PTM analysis (**Figure 18-9**). Chemical and affinity-based methods are commonly used to improve modified proteins or peptides [87]. Chemical strategies include the introduction of affinity tags onto modified proteins/peptides. These strategies are chemically tailor-made kinases and glycosyltransferases where affinity tags are introduced onto phosphorylated and glycosylated proteins, allowing selective estimation [88]. One PTM in phosphoserine and phosphothreonine converts to dehydroalanine and dehydroaminobutyric acid by β-elimination of the phosphate group, which allows detection of this modification. An alternative chemical strategy involves the selection of phosphorylated residues by coupling a solid phase support by phosphoramidate chemistry. Sometimes, however, chemical methodologies involve unwanted side reactions, which ultimately import sample complexity and complication in detection of *in vivo* modifications [87].

Advanced MS technologies are applied to identify both PTMs and complement antibody-based approaches. PTMs can either raise or lower the molecular weight of peptides, resulting in alteration of specific signals in the MS/MS analysis. For example, the addition or removal of phosphate groups (±80 Da) or aceytyl groups (±42 Da) produce mass differences, or, similarly, deamidation of asparagine and glutamine to aspartate and glutamate generates mass differences by +1 Da. Also, formation of cysteine-cysteine (Cys-Cys) disulfide bonds change masses by −2 Da. Although routinely studied in biological research, detection and differentiation of PTMs still do not solidify conventional

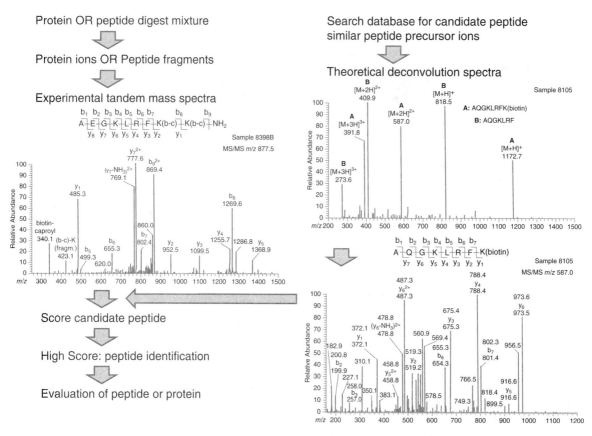

FIGURE 18-9 A protein mixture is digested, and the resulting peptides are analyzed by MS/MS to obtain experimental spectra. Search programs find database candidate sequences whose theoretical spectra are compared with the experimental spectrum. The best match (highest-scoring candidate sequence) defines the identified database peptide and the matching database protein. Evaluation software then determines whether the peptide and protein identifications are expected or not.

bottom-up proteomics strategies, because of low PTM stoichiometry and complicated MS spectrometry [85].

SUMMARY

MS/MS is one of the most important techniques in drug delivery and drug discovery research. Today, it is a commonly used method for drug metabolomics and proteomics analysis. The tandem MRM technique is mainly used for quantitative biomarker and to study drug metabolomics, including proteomics by using ESI. The ESI technique is used to study nicotine metabolomics in HIV-1–positive smokers and HIV-negative smokers' plasma and measures four major metabolites in the plasma. Another tandem mass spectrometry ionization technique, MALDI, is widely used for bottom-up and top-down proteomics analysis to study PTMs of proteins, such as phosphorylation and glycosylation. In addition to MALDI, proteomics involves various purification and isolation procedures such as TAP, ICAT, iTRAQ, and absolute quantitation of proteomics and SILAC.

ACKNOWLEDGMENT

This work was supported by a grant from the National Institutes of Health (R01EY009171).

REVIEW QUESTIONS

1. How do you define proteomics and explain its functions and applications?
2. What is the difference between peptides and proteins?
3. Discuss a strategy involving biological intermediate for *in vivo* methylation of proteins, DNA, RNA, and other cellular substrates.
4. What is the main reason for the use of MS techniques in protein and peptide drug delivery?
5. Explain MS analyzers used in proteomics analysis.
6. What are the most common available isotopic molecular weights for carbon (C), nitrogen (N), oxygen (O), sulfur (S), and hydrogen (H)?

REFERENCES

1. Benowitz NL Pharmacology of nicotine: addiction, smoking-induced disease, and therapeutics. *Annu Rev Pharmacol Toxicol.* 2009;49:57-71.
2. Hecht SS, Hochalter JB, Villalta PW, Murphy SE 2'-Hydroxylation of nicotine by cytochrome P450 2A6 and human liver microsomes: formation of a lung carcinogen precursor. *Proc Natl Acad Sci USA.* 2000;97:12493-12497
3. Gill SC, von Hippel PH. Calculation of protein extinction coefficients from amino acid sequence data. *Anal Biochem.* 1989;182 (2):319-326.
4. Theiss C, Trostmann I, Andree S, et al. Pigment-pigment and pigment-protein interactions in recombinant water-soluble chlorophyll proteins (WSCP) from cauliflower. *J Phys Chem B.* 2007;111 (46):13325-13335.
5. Ong SE, Blagoev B, Kratchmarova I, et al. Stable isotope labeling by amino acids in cell culture, SILAC, as a simple and accurate approach to expression proteomics. *Mol Cell Proteom.* 2002;1(5):376-386.
6. Zhu H, Pan S, Gu S, Bradbury EM, Chen X. Amino acid residue specific stable isotope labeling for quantitative proteomics. *Rapid Commun Mass Spectr.* 2002;16(22):2115-2123.
7. Vidal M, Chan DW, Gerstein M, et al. The human proteome—a scientific opportunity for transforming diagnostics, therapeutics, and healthcare. *Clin Proteom.* 2012;9(1):6.
8. Chandramouli K, Qian PY. Proteomics: challenges, techniques and possibilities to overcome biological sample complexity. *Hum Genom Proteom.* 10.4061/2009/239204.
9. Jiang H, English AM. Quantitative analysis of the yeast proteome by incorporation of isotopically labeled leucine. *J Proteom Res.* 2002;1(4):345-350.
10. Anderson NL. The clinical plasma proteome: a survey of clinical assays for proteins in plasma and serum. *Clin Chem.* 2010;56(2):177-185.
11. Peng M, Taouatas N, Cappadona S, et al. Protease bias in absolute protein quantitation. *Nat Methods.* 012;9(6):524-525.
12. Biemann K. Mass Spectrometry. *Annu Rev Biochem.* 1963; 32:755-780.
13. Schwahn AB, Wong JW, Downard KM. Signature peptides of influenza nucleoprotein for the typing and subtyping of the virus by high resolution mass spectrometry. *Analyst.* 2009;134(11):2253-2261.
14. Fenn JB. Electrospray ionization mass spectrometry: How it all began. *J Biomol Techn.* 2002; 13(3):101-118.
15. Miyazaki S, Takahashi M, Ohira M, et al. Monolithic silica rod columns for high-efficiency reversed-phase liquid chromatography. *J Chromatogr A.* 2011;1218(15):1988-1994.
16. Harvey DJ, Sobott F, Crispin M, et al. Ion mobility mass spectrometry for extracting spectra of N-glycans directly from incubation mixtures following glycan release: application to glycans from engineered glycoforms of intact, folded HIV gp120. *J Am Soc Mass Spectrom.* 2011;22(3):568-581.

17. Savitski MM, Fischer F, Mathieson T, Sweetman G, Lang M, Bantscheff M. Targeted data acquisition for improved reproducibility and robustness of proteomic mass spectrometry assays. *J Am Soc Mass Spectrom.* 2010;21(10):1668-1679.

18. Aebersold R, Mann M. Mass spectrometry-based proteomics. *Nature.* 2003;422(6928):198-207.

19. Tsarbopoulos A, Karas M, Strupat K, Pramanik BN, Nagabhushan TL, Hillenkamp F. Comparative mapping of recombinant proteins and glycoproteins by plasma desorption and matrix-assisted laser desorption/ionization mass spectrometry. *Anal Chem.* 1994;66(13):2062-2070.

20. Eckerskorn C, Strupat K, Karas M, Hillenkamp F, Lottspeich F. Mass spectrometric analysis of blotted proteins after gel electrophoretic separation by matrix-assisted laser desorption/ionization. *Electrophoresis.* 1992;13(9-10):664-665.

21. Yang HJ, Park KH, Kim HS, Kim J. Characterization of unknown compounds from stainless steel plates in matrix-assisted laser desorption/ionization mass spectrometry. *J Am Soc Mass Spectrom.* 2010;21(12):2000-2004.

22. Kukrer B, Barbu IM, Copps J, et al. Conformational isomers of calcineurin follow distinct dissociation pathways. *J Am Soc Mass Spectrom.* 2012;23(9):1534-1543.

23. Xiao Z, Veenstra TD. Comparison of protein expression by isotope-coded affinity tag labeling. *Methods Mol Biol.* 2008;428:181-192.

24. Sturm R, Sheynkman G, Booth C, Smith LM, Pedersen JA, Li L. Absolute quantification of prion protein (90-231) using stable isotope-labeled chymotryptic peptide standards in a LC-MRM AQUA workflow. *J Am Soc Mass Spectrom.* 2012;23(9):1522-1533.

25. Gregan J, Riedel CG, Petronczki M, et al. Tandem affinity purification of functional TAP-tagged proteins from human cells. *Nat Protoc.* 2007;2(5):1145-1151.

26. Angrand PO, Segura I, Volkel P, et al. Transgenic mouse proteomics identifies new 14-3-3-associated proteins involved in cytoskeletal rearrangements and cell signaling. *Mol Cell Proteom.* 2006;5(12):2211-2227.

27. Rigaut G, Shevchenko A, Rutz B, Wilm M, Mann M, Seraphin B. A generic protein purification method for protein complex characterization and proteome exploration. *Nat Biotechnol.* 1999;17(10):1030-1032.

28. Essex A, Dammermann A, Lewellyn L, Oegema K, Desai A. Systematic analysis in *Caenorhabditis elegans* reveals that the spindle checkpoint is composed of two largely independent branches. *Mol Biol Cell.* 2009;20(4):1252-1267.

29. Rohila JS, Chen M, Cerny R, Fromm ME. Improved tandem affinity purification tag and methods for isolation of protein heterocomplexes from plants. *Plant J Cell Mol Biol.* 2004;38(1):172-181.

30. Brajenovic M, Joberty G, Kuster B, Bouwmeester T, Drewes G. Comprehensive proteomic analysis of human Par protein complexes reveals an interconnected protein network. *J Biol Chem.* 2004;279(13):12804-12811.

31. Guerrero C, Tagwerker C, Kaiser P, Huang L. An integrated mass spectrometry-based proteomic approach: quantitative analysis of tandem affinity-purified in vivo cross-linked protein complexes (QTAX) to decipher the 26 S proteasome-interacting network. *Mol Cell Proteom.* 2006;5(2):366-378.

32. Bonzon-Kulichenko E, Perez-Hernandez D, Nunez E, et al. A robust method for quantitative high-throughput analysis of proteomes by ^{18}O labeling. *Mol Cell Proteom.* 2011;10(1):M110 003335.

33. Andersen CA, Gotta S, Magnoni L, Raggiaschi R, Kremer A, Terstappen GC. Robust MS quantification method for phospho-peptides using 18O/16O labeling. *BMC Bioinform.* 2009;10:141.

34. Leitner A, Lindner W. Applications of chemical tagging approaches in combination with 2DE and mass spectrometry. *Methods Mol Biol.* 2009;519: 83-101.

35. Yi EC, Li XJ, Cooke K, et al. Increased quantitative proteome coverage with (13)C/(12)C-based, acid-cleavable isotope-coded affinity tag reagent and modified data acquisition scheme. *Proteomics.* 2005;5(2):380-387.

36. Adam GC, Sorensen EJ, Cravatt BF. Chemical strategies for functional proteomics. *Mol Cell Proteom.* 2002;1(10):781-790.

37. Aebersold R, Goodlett DR. Mass spectrometry in proteomics. *Chem Rev.* 2001;101(2):269-295.

38. Gygi SP, Rist B, Gerber SA, Turecek F, Gelb MH, Aebersold R. Quantitative analysis of complex protein mixtures using isotope-coded affinity tags. *Nat Biotechnol.* 1999;17(10):994-999.

39. Aggarwal K, Choe LH, Lee KH. Shotgun proteomics using the iTRAQ isobaric tags. *Brief Funct Genom Proteom.* 2006;5(2):112-120.

40. Zieske LR. A perspective on the use of iTRAQ reagent technology for protein complex and profiling studies. *J Exp Bot.* 2006;57(7):1501-1508.

41. Abdallah C, Sergeant K, Guillier C, Dumas-Gaudot E, Leclercq CC, Renaut J. Optimization of iTRAQ labelling coupled to OFFGEL fractionation as a proteomic workflow to the analysis of microsomal proteins of *Medicago truncatula* roots. *Proteome Sci.* 2012;10(1):37.

42. Bantscheff M, Boesche M, Eberhard D, Matthieson T, Sweetman G, Kuster B. Robust and sensitive iTRAQ quantification on an LTQ Orbitrap mass spectrometer. *Mol Cell Proteom.* 2008;7(9):1702-1713.

43. Ong SE, Kratchmarova I, Mann M. Properties of ^{13}C-substituted arginine in stable isotope labeling by amino acids in cell culture (SILAC). *J Proteom Res.* 2003;2(2):173-181.

44. Ong SE, Mittler G, Mann M. Identifying and quantifying in vivo methylation sites by heavy methyl SILAC. *Nat Methods.* 2004;1(2):119-126.

45. Soufi B, Kumar C, Gnad F, Mann M, Mijakovic I, Macek B. Stable isotope labeling by amino acids in cell culture (SILAC) applied to quantitative proteomics of Bacillus subtilis. *J Proteom Res.* 2010;9(7):3638-3646.

46. Ong SE, Mann M. A practical recipe for stable isotope labeling by amino acids in cell culture (SILAC). *Nat Protoc.* 2006;1(6):2650-2660.

47. Gruhler S, Kratchmarova I. Stable isotope labeling by amino acids in cell culture (SILAC). *Methods Mol Biol.* 2008;424:101-111.

48. Lam H. Building and searching tandem mass spectral libraries for peptide identification. *Mol Cell Proteom.* 2011;10(12):R111 008565.

49. Ecker J. Profiling eicosanoids and phospholipids using LC-MS/MS: principles and recent applications. *J Separ Sci.* 2012;35(10-11):1227-1235.

50. Konn C, Charlou JL, Donval JP, Holm NG. Characterisation of dissolved organic compounds in hydrothermal fluids by stir bar sorptive extraction-gas chomatography-mass spectrometry. Case study: the Rainbow field (36 degrees N, Mid-Atlantic Ridge). *Geochem Trans.* 2012;13(1):8.

51. Huntscha S, Singer HP, McArdell CS, Frank CE, Hollender J. Multiresidue analysis of 88 polar organic micropollutants in ground, surface and wastewater using online mixed-bed multilayer solid-phase extraction coupled to high performance liquid chromatography-tandem mass spectrometry. *J Chromatogr A.* 2012;1268:74-83.

52. Earla R, Ande A, McArthur C, Kumar A, Kumar S. Enhanced nicotine metabolism in HIV-1-positive smokers compared to HIV-negative smokers: simultaneous determination of nicotine and its four metabolites in their plasma using a simple and sensitive ESI-LC-MS/MS technique. *Drug Metab Dispos.* 2013. 10.1124/dmd.113.055186.

53. Benowitz NL Clinical pharmacology of nicotine: implications for understanding, preventing, and treating tobacco addiction. *Clin Pharmacol Ther.* 2008;83:531-541.

54. Earla R, Cholkar K, Gunda S, Earla RL, Mitra AK. Bioanalytical method validation of rapamycin in ocular matrix by QTRAP LC-MS/MS: application to rabbit anterior tissue distribution by topical administration of rapamycin nanomicellar formulation. *J Chromatogr B Analyt Technol Biomed Life Sci.* 2012;908:76-86.

55. Sadygov RG, Cociorva D, Yates JR, 3rd. Large-scale database searching using tandem mass spectra: looking up the answer in the back of the book. *Nat Methods.* 2004;1(3):195-202.

56. Yates JR, 3rd. Mass spectral analysis in proteomics. *Annu Rev Biophys Biomol Struct.* 2004;33:297-316.

57. Link AJ, Eng J, Schieltz DM, et al. Direct analysis of protein complexes using mass spectrometry. *Nat Biotechnol.* 1999;17(7):676-682.

58. Wolters DA, Washburn MP, Yates JR, 3rd. An automated multidimensional protein identification technology for shotgun proteomics. *Anal Chem.* 2001;73(23):5683-5690.

59. Hunt DF, Yates JR, 3rd, Shabanowitz J, Winston S, Hauer CR. Protein sequencing by tandem mass spectrometry. *Proc Natl Acad Sci USA.* 1986;83(17):6233-6237.

60. Johnson RS, Martin SA, Biemann K, Stults JT, Watson JT. Novel fragmentation process of peptides by collision-induced decomposition in a tandem mass spectrometer: differentiation of leucine and isoleucine. *Anal Chem.* 1987;59(21):2621-2625.

61. Tabb DL, MacCoss MJ, Wu CC, Anderson SD, Yates JR, 3rd. Similarity among tandem mass spectra from proteomic experiments: detection, significance, and utility. *Anal Chem.* 2003;75(10):2470-2477.

62. Hampel G, Wortmann B, Blaickner M, et al. Irradiation facility at the TRIGA Mainz for treatment of liver metastases. *Appl Radiat Isotop.* 2009;67(7-8 Suppl):S238-S241.

63. Colinge J, Magnin J, Dessingy T, Giron M, Masselot A. Improved peptide charge state assignment. *Proteomics.* 2003;3(8):1434-1440.

64. Sadygov RG, Eng J, Durr E, et al. Code developments to improve the efficiency of automated MS/MS spectra interpretation. *J Proteom Res.* 2002;1(3):211-215.

65. Colinge J, Chiappe D, Lagache S, Moniatte M, Bougueleret L. Differential proteomics via probabilistic peptide identification scores. *Anal Chem.* 2005;77(2):596-606.

66. Schulze WX, Mann M. A novel proteomic screen for peptide-protein interactions. *J Biol Chem.* 2004;279(11):10756-10764.

67. MacCoss MJ, Wu CC, Yates JR, 3rd. Probability-based validation of protein identifications using a modified SEQUEST algorithm. *Anal Chem.* 2002;74(21):5593-5599.

68. Ibarrola N, Kalume DE, Gronborg M, Iwahori A, Pandey A. A proteomic approach for quantitation of phosphorylation using stable isotope labeling in cell culture. *Anal Chem.* 2003;75(22):6043-6049.

69. Fernandez RM, Bleda M, Nunez-Torres R, et al. Four new loci associations discovered by pathway-based and network analyses of the genome-wide variability profile of Hirschsprung's disease. *Orph J Rare Dis.* 2012;7(1):103.

70. Shen Y, Tolic N, Liu T, et al. Blood peptidome-degradome profile of breast cancer. *PloS One.* 2010;5(10):e13133.

71. Pernemalm M, Lewensohn R, Lehtio J. Affinity prefractionation for MS-based plasma proteomics. *Proteomics.* 2009;9(6):1420-1427.

72. Li J, Rix U, Fang B, et al. A chemical and phosphoproteomic characterization of dasatinib action in lung cancer. *Nat Chem Biol.* 2010;6(4):291-299.

73. Angel TE, Aryal UK, Hengel SM, et al. Mass spectrometry-based proteomics: existing capabilities and future directions. *Chem Soc Rev.* 2012;41(10):3912-3928.

74. Jonker N, Kool J, Irth H, Niessen WM. Recent developments in protein-ligand affinity mass spectrometry. *Anal Bioanal Chem.* 2011;399(8):2669-2681.

75. Cohen P. The origins of protein phosphorylation. *Nat Cell Biol.* 2002;4(5):E127-E130.

76. Aryal UK, Ross AR. Enrichment and analysis of phosphopeptides under different experimental conditions using titanium dioxide affinity chromatography and mass spectrometry. *Rapid Commun Mass Spectrom.* 2010;24(2):219-231.

77. Marino K, Bones J, Kattla JJ, Rudd PM. A systematic approach to protein glycosylation analysis: a path through the maze. *Nat Chem Biol.* 2010;6(10):713-723.

78. Bond MR, Kohler JJ. Chemical methods for glycoprotein discovery. *Curr Opin Chem Biol.* 2007;11(1):52-58.

79. Trimble RB, Tarentino AL. Identification of distinct endoglycosidase (endo) activities in *Flavobacterium meningosepticum*: endo F1, endo F2, and endo F3. Endo F1 and endo H hydrolyze only high mannose and hybrid glycans. *J Biol Chem.* 1991;266(3):1646-1651.

80. Fukuda M, Lauffenburger M, Sasaki H, Rogers ME, Dell A. Structures of novel sialylated O-linked oligosaccharides isolated from human erythrocyte glycophorins. *J Biol Chem.* 1987;262(25): 11952-11957.

81. Pahlsson P, Blackall DP, Ugorski M, Czerwinski M, Spitalnik SL. Biochemical characterization of the O-glycans on recombinant glycophorin A expressed in Chinese hamster ovary cells. *Glycoconj J.* 1994;11(1):43-50.

82. Iwase K, Mori K, Hoshikawa A, Ishigaki T. Synthesis of new compound Gd5Ni19 with a superlattice structure and hydrogen absorption properties. *Inorg Chem.* 2011;50(22):11631-11635.

83. Jensen ON. Modification-specific proteomics: characterization of post-translational modifications by mass spectrometry. *Curr Opin Chem Biol.* 2004;8(1):33-41.

84. Simon GM, Cravatt BF. Challenges for the "chemical-systems" biologist. *Nat Chem Biol.* 2008;4(11): 639-642.

85. Choudhary C, Mann M. Decoding signalling networks by mass spectrometry-based proteomics. *Nat Rev.* 2010;11(6):427-439.

86. Welchman RL, Gordon C, Mayer RJ. Ubiquitin and ubiquitin-like proteins as multifunctional signals. *Nat Rev.* 2005;6(8):599-609.

87. Nielsen ML, Vermeulen M, Bonaldi T, Cox J, Moroder L, Mann M. Iodoacetamide-induced artifact mimics ubiquitination in mass spectrometry. *Nat Methods.* 2008;5(6):459-460.

88. Jensen LJ, Kuhn M, Stark M, et al. STRING 8—a global view on proteins and their functional interactions in 630 organisms. *Nucleic Acids Res.* 2009;37(database issue):D412-D416.

GLOSSARY

2/4/A1 cells   A fetal-rat-intestine–derived cell line that displays a lot of morphological features similar to the cells of the small intestine and is used to study drug transport across the intestine.

ABC transporters   ABC family includes a superfamily of membrane-bound proteins involved in the translocation of various substances including sugars, amino acids, sterols, peptides, proteins, antibiotics, toxins, and xenobiotics in both prokaryotes and eukaryotes.

Active DPIs   See Active Inhalers

Active inhalers   Aerosol inhalers that impart self-containing electrical or mechanical energy to facilitate drug aerosolization.

Active transport   The movement of biochemicals across cell membranes against the concentration gradient with utilization of energy.

Adeno-associated viral vectors   Gene transfer vectors that offer sustained gene expression due to the lack of pathogenicity and minimal immunogenicity of the virus as well as efficient and sustained gene expression in dividing and non-dividing cells.

Adeno-associated virus   A nonpathogenic human parvovirus with no known disease association.

Adenoviruses   Unenveloped, double-stranded DNA viruses with an icosahedral protein capsid of 70–100 nm in diameter encasing a viral genome of 36 kb. Attributes include highly efficient gene transduction in dividing and non-dividing cells, high titer production (1012–1013 virus particles per ml) of recombinant viruses, accepting up to 8 kb of exogenous sequence, and lack of insertional oncogenesis associated with retroviruses.

Adherens junctions   These are protein complexes that occur at cell–cell junctions in epithelial and endothelial tissues; usually more basal than tight junctions.

Adsorptive endocytosis   A drug molecule that nonspecifically adsorbs to the surface of the cell and is generally absorbed by endolysosomal trafficking pathways.

Aerosol   A suspension of small particles or droplets in gas or vapor or a therapeutic substance dispensed from a pressurized container. Aerosols consist of drug or any chemical substance as dispersed phase and gas as the dispersion medium. Aerosols are the products containing therapeutic agents dissolved, suspended, or emulsified in a propellant mixture or a mixture of solvents and propellants.

Alginates   Alginic acid and its salts (e.g., sodium or calcium alginate); they are polysaccharides extracted from brown seaweed.

Alternate copolymer   A polymer in which monomers A and B are attached to one another in the form of ABAB.

Anterior segment of the eye   Front part of the eye comprising cornea, conjunctiva, iris, ciliary body, aqueous humor, and lens.

Appendageal route   A minor route of drug transport through the skin.

Aqueous humor   A fluid present in the anterior segment, secreted by the ciliary processes into the posterior segment at the rate of 2.0–2.5 µL/min. It supplies the majority of nutrition and oxygen to avascular tissues (lens and cornea).

Bidirectional inhalers   Bidirectional inhalers exploit the anatomy of the nasopharyngeal tract using the principle of blowing up a balloon. Exhaling against the balloon wall closes the soft palate and separates the nasal cavity from the mouth. This mechanism cuts the communication between the cranial surface of the soft palate and the posterior margin of the nasal septum. Thus, the air entering a nostril through the sealing nozzle takes a 180-degree turn and exits through the other nostril in the opposite direction.

Bioadhesion   The ability of a synthetic or a natural material to "stick" (adhere) to a biological tissue for extended time periods by interfacial forces; the interaction between the polymer and the epithelial surface.

Bioadhesive systems   Systems that provide intimate contact between a dosage form and the absorbing tissue, which may result in high concentration in a local area and, hence, high drug flux through the absorbing tissue.

Bioavailability   The fraction of an administered dose of unchanged drug that reaches the systemic circulation.

Biocompatibility   Concept that refers to a set of properties that a material must have to be used safely in a biological organism.

Biodegradable implants   Implants that employ inert polymer, which can be degraded within a biological system into nontoxic metabolites that are excreted by the body.

Biopharmaceutics classification system   A system to differentiate the drugs on the basis of their solubility and permeability.

Block copolymer   A polymer in which monomers A and B are attached to one another in the form of AABB.

Blood-aqueous barrier   A barrier formed by epithelium in the non-pigmented layer of the ciliary epithelium and in the posterior iridial epithelium and by the endothelium of the iridial vessels.

Blood-cerebrospinal fluid barrier   The second barrier that a systemically administered drug encounters before entering the central nervous system. Because the cerebrospinal fluid can exchange molecules with the interstitial fluid of the brain parenchyma, the transport of blood-borne molecules into the cerebrospinal fluid is carefully regulated by the blood-cerebrospinal fluid barrier. It is found in the epithelium of the choroid plexus, which is arranged in a manner that limits the passage of molecules and cells into the cerebrospinal fluid.

Blood-retinal barrier   Barrier formed by the vascular endothelium of the retinal vessels and the retinal pigment epithelium. The blood-retinal barrier forms an outer barrier in the retinal pigment epithelium and an inner barrier in the endothelial membrane of the retinal vessels.

Blood–brain barrier   A highly selective permeability barrier that separates the circulating blood from the brain extracellular fluid in the central nervous system. This barrier has a unique anatomical structure compared to other blood vessels and restricts the passive diffusion of hydrophilic and charged compounds from inside the capillary into brain.

Branched polymers   Polymers with side-branch chains that extend out from the central structure reducing the ability of the polymer chains to pack together.

Breast cancer resistant protein (BCRP/ABCG2)   The *ABCG2* gene was discovered in cell lines selected for high-level resistance for mitoxantrone and is responsible for efflux of multiple anticancer and other categories of drugs.

Buccal drug delivery   Administration of drug via buccal mucosa or lining of the cheek.

Bulk erosion   A system of polymer matrix erosion in which water rapidly penetrates the entire dosage form and polymer degradation occurs throughout the matrix.

Burst phase   The phase of drug release in an erosion-controlled system undergoing bulk erosion in which the polymer matrix forms pores and the surface-bound and encapsulated drug molecules that have access to these water-filled pores are quickly released into the surrounding medium.

Caco-2 cells   Cultured cell line originally derived from colon carcinoma that displays a lot of morphological features similar to the cells of the small intestine and is used to study drug transport across the intestine.

Capsules   A dosage form in which drugs are usually enclosed in a soft or hard soluble gelatin shell.

Carbomer   The general name given to any of a specific group of high-molecular-weight, crosslinked polymers of acrylic acid; known commercially as Carbopol.

Carboxymethyl cellulose   Formed by carboxymethylating cellulose and is typically found as a sodium or calcium salt.

Carrageenan   A natural ingredient obtained from red seaweed.

Carrier-limited transport   A mechanism responsible for moving compounds, like neurotransmitters, toxic substances, and antibiotics out of the cell.

Carrier-mediated transport   Movement of nutrients, drugs, or substances across biological barriers with the help of transmembrane proteins resulting in facilitated diffusion or active transport.

Caucasian colon adenocarcinoma cells   See Caco-2 cells.

Cellulose   An abundant natural polymer present in plants composed of glucose monomers attached together to form long and tightly packed chains.

Central nervous system   The part of the nervous system consisting of the brain and spinal cord.

Chewable tablets   Tablets that disintegrate rapidly when chewed in the mouth. They usually contain flavoring agents to improve taste and are especially useful for pediatric and geriatric patients.

Chitosan   A cationic polymer obtained from the very abundant natural source of chitin. Chitin is isolated from the exoskeleton of crustaceans such as crabs and shrimps and is turned into chitosan through a partial deacetylation process.

Chlorofluorocarbons (CFCs)   It is a liquefied compressed gas usually used as a propellant in pressurized, metered dose inhalers.

Choroid   A highly vascularized tissue located between retina and sclera. Its major function is to provide nourishment to the photoreceptor cells in the retina.

Ciliary body   A ring-shaped muscle attached to the iris; formed by ciliary muscles and the ciliary processes.

Clearance   The amount of liquid filtered out of the blood by the kidneys or the amount of blood cleaned per time. It has the units of a volumetric flow rate (volume/time).

Coated tablet   A tablet in which the uncoated core tablet is covered with one or more layer of additional excipient substances, often for a defined purpose.

Colloidal drug delivery systems   Particulate or vesicular dosage forms essentially required for effective transportation of loaded drug to the target site.

Compensatory mechanism   Presence of overlapping biological pathways that perform the same function as a more prevalent pathway in the cell.

Conjunctiva   A vascularized mucous membrane lining the inner surface of eyelids and the anterior surface of sclera up to the limbus. It facilitates lubrication in the eye by generating mucus and helps with tear film adhesion.

Contact lens   A thin, curve-shaped plastic disk that is designed to be placed over the cornea. The lens adheres to surface of the cornea by interfacial tension.

Controlled drug delivery   The use of dosage forms that release the total dose of drug into available biological fluids at a slower rate or more constant rate after administration or only at the targeted site of administration.

Copolymer   A polymer chain containing two different monomer units.

Cornea   An avascular, transparent structure (forming the front part of the eye) continuous with the sclera at the limbus. The cornea is devoid of blood vessels and receives it nourishment and oxygen supply from the aqueous humor and the tear film while the corneal periphery receives nourishment from the limbal capillaries.

Cross-linked polymers   Polymers in which adjacent chains are bonded to one another at various locations and in all directions along their length forming a three-dimensional network.

Cytochrome P450   A large familiy of enzymes responsible for metabolizing multiple targets through monooxygenase reaction.

Depletion zone   The drug-free region created within a formulation particle once the drug diffuses out of it.

Desmosome   A cell structure specialized for cell-to-cell adhesion.

Developability criteria   A set of parameters defined and tested during the drug discovery process to assure the eventual therapeutic and financial success of the lead molecule. This includes the druggability criteria that includes the parameters tested to assure therapeutic success of the lead molecule.

Diffusing chamber   Ussing chamber or diffusion chamber consisting of two hollow halves clamped together with the epithelial tissue between them to study permeability of drug across the tissue.

Diffusion-controlled systems   The formulation in which the net movement of the drug substance across its encapsulating material is driven by the concentration gradient.

Disintegrating tablets   Tablets that can disintegrate within approximately 30 seconds in the oral cavity without the need for chewing or drinking liquids.

Dispersible tablets   There are two types: one is an immediately released dosage form that instantaneously disintegrates in the mouth when it is in contact with the saliva, and the other one is a uncoated or film-coated tablets that produce a uniformly dispersed liquid before administration.

DMPK   The study of **d**rug **m**etabolism and **p**harmaco**k**inetics together.

Douching   The irrigation of vagina with a liquid possessing either cosmetic or medicinal actions. This is a cleaning technique that has been practiced for some time mainly for the treatment of inadequate vaginal hygiene, restoring the normal vaginal pH after vaginal infections or simply cleaning.

Drug delivery   The method or process of administering a pharmaceutical compound to achieve a therapeutic effect in human or animals.

Drug metabolism   The biochemical modification of pharmaceutical substances or xenobiotics respectively by living organisms, usually through specialized enzymatic systems. Drug metabolism often converts lipophilic chemical compounds into more readily excreted hydrophilic products.

Drug-in-adhesive (DIA) patches   Patches that contain a drug dispersed in an adhesive polymer and sandwiched between a backing membrane and release liner.

Druggability criteria   See Developability criteria.

Dry powder inhalers   Pulmonary drug delivery devices containing solid drug suspended in a dry powder mix that can be fluidized when the patient inhales.

Effervescent tablet   A tablet intended to be dissolved in the mouth or dispersed in water before administration. The uncoated tablet contains acidic and base substances that react rapidly in water to release carbon dioxide.

Efflux transporters   Transport proteins responsible for moving compounds, like neurotransmitters, toxic substances, and antibiotics out of the cell. They belong to the ABC transporter family.

Efflux trasnport   See Carrier-limited transport.

Electroporation   One of the physical methods involving the application of a pulsed electrical field into living cells enhances the permeability of cell membranes by creating transient pores across the membrane resulting in cellular uptake of genes, proteins, and drug molecules, etc.

Electrospray ionization   A soft ionization technique that is typically used to determine the molecular weights of proteins, peptides, and other macromolecules. Soft ionization is a useful technique when considering biological molecules of large molecular mass, such as the aforementioned, because this process does not fragment the macromolecules into smaller charged particles, rather it turns the macromolecule being ionized into small droplets. These droplets will then be further desolvated into even smaller droplets, which creates molecules with attached protons. These protonated and desolvated molecular ions will then be passed through the mass analyzer to the detector, and the mass of the sample can be determined.

Endocytosis   An energy utilizing process by which cells absorb molecules by engulfing them.

Endothelium   The endothelium is the thin layer of cells that lines the interior surface of blood vessels and lymphatic vessels.

Enhanced permeability and retention effect   A phenomenon in which tumor endothelium possess leaky and discontinuous vasculature structure, impaired lymphatic drainage/recovery system, allowing easier extravasation in the tumor region.

Enteric coatings   Coatings of polymers designed to remain intact in the acidic environment of the stomach and then dissolve after passing into the alkaline environment of the small intestine.

Enterocytes   Also known as intestinal absorptive cells are simple columnar epithelial cells found in the small intestines, colon, and appendix. They have a surface coating of a glycoprotein matrix containing digestive enzymes and have microvilli on the apical surface to increase surface area for the digestion and transport of molecules from the intestinal lumen.

Epithelium   The layers of cells that line hollow organs and glands. It also makes up the outer surface of organs and the body.

Erosion front   In a swelling controlled system. the outermost layer that separates the polymer matrix from the aqueous media.

Erosion-controlled systems   A delivery system in which drug molecules are either entrapped or encapsulated within the polymeric matrix and the rate of drug release is controlled by polymer matrix erosion.

Erythropoietin   An endogenous protein produced by the body to induce erythropoiesis, the production of red blood cells.

Ethyl cellulose   A water insoluble cellulose derivative having ethyl group substitutions attached on the cellulose backbone structure.

Everted sacs   A technique in which a segment of the intestine is inverted inside out using a cylindrical object such as a glass rod. The two ends of the intestinal segment are tied, and the inside of the resulting sac is filled with an oxygenated buffer to be placed in solution of drug for which permeability is being measured.

Excised intestinal tissue   A technique involving removal of the intestinal tissue from an animal (usually rat or mouse) to study intestinal permeation.

Extemporaneous compounding   The mixing of the ingredients of a prescription or drug formula; generally referring to a manual process performed for individual orders by a dispenser or pharmacist.

Extravascular route   Drug administration by any other route than the intravenous route.

Fickian kinetics   Drug movement that follows Fick's laws of diffusion.

Films/strips   Thin, flexible strips composed of a drug dissolved/dispersed/distributed in a water-dissolving polymer, which hydrates, adheres and quickly dissolves within few seconds when placed in the oral cavity.

First pass metabolism   A phenomenon by which a drug or substance taken by mouth, after absorption, is altered or degraded by the intestine and liver, whereby the concentration of a drug or active substance is greatly reduced before it reaches the general systemic circulation.

Gastrointestinal tract   An organ system located between the mouth and the anus responsible for consuming and digesting foodstuffs, absorbing nutrients, and expelling waste.

Gene delivery   Application of principles of cell biology, chemistry, and physics to facilitate gene transfer from the site of administration to the nuclei of intended cells.

Gene gun   Also called ballistic DNA transfer or DNA-coated particle bombardment, is a device for injecting cells with genetic information. The payload is an elemental particle of a heavy metal (gold or tungsten) coated with plasmid DNA. The DNA-coated particles are propelled against tissues and cells by accelerating forces such as pressurized inert gas (helium) or high-voltage electronic discharge.

Gene therapy   Therapy that uses a gene-coding sequence as a pharmaceutical agent in providing a gene product missing in patients because of genetic mutation. Gene therapy requires a method effective in delivering a therapeutic gene into cells where treatment is needed.

Glycosylation   The attachment of sugar moieties to proteins.

Half-life   The time it takes for the plasma concentration or the amount of drug in the body to be reduced by 50%. The half-life of a drug depends on its clearance and volume of distribution. The elimination half-life is considered to be independent of the amount of drug in the body.

Half-life of elimination   See Half-life.

Hard shell capsule   A capsule usually made of two pieces, a telescoping cap and a body. The length of the cap is usually slightly shorter than that of the body. When the cap is pressed on the body, the two pieces fit firmly and form a closed space inside for the drug load.

High-throughput screening   A method for scientific experimentation especially used in drug discovery and relevant to the fields of biology and chemistry. Using robotics, data processing and control software, liquid handling devices, and sensitive detectors high-throughput screening allows a researcher to quickly conduct millions of chemical, genetic, or pharmacological tests.

HT-29 cells   Cultured cell line originally derived from human colonic carcinoma that displays a lot of morphological features similar to the cells of the small intestine especially expression of mucin and is used to study drug transport across intestine.

Hybrid systems   A monolithic polymer matrix that contains drug surrounded by a rate controlling membrane.

Hydrocolloids   Hydrocolloids are high-molecular-weight polysaccharides from natural origins. They are extracts from seaweeds and plants or can be polysaccharides produced by bacteria.

Hydrodynamic gene delivery   The application of controlled hydrodynamic pressure using a tail vein injection of plasmid DNA for effective gene transfer.

Hydrofluoroalkane (HFA)   A liquefied compressed gas usually used as a propellant in pressurized metered dose inhalers.

Hydrophobic drugs   Drugs with high octanol/water partition coefficients.

Immobilized artificial membrane (IAM) columns   Hollow columns filled with lipid material and used to simulate drug transport across biological membranes.

Implants   Drug eluting devices specially designed for local sustained drug release over long periods.

In silico   An expression used to mean performed on computer or via computer simulation.

In situ forming systems   Implant systems made of biodegradable products, which can be injected via a syringe into the body, and once injected congeal to form a solid biodegradable implant.

In situ gelling systems   Polymeric aqueous solutions that undergo a sol-to-gel transition in response to environmental or physiological stimuli; also called hydrogels.

In vitro   Studies that are performed with cells or biological molecules studied outside their normal biological context; for example, proteins are examined in solution or cells in artificial culture medium.

In vivo   Studies in which the effects of various biological entities are tested on whole, living organisms, usually animals including humans and plants as opposed to a partial or dead organism or those done in vitro.

Influx trasnsport   See Carrier-mediated transport.

Inhalation route   Administration of drugs that are mainly directed to the lungs through the nasal cavity.

Intra-arterial route   Administration of drugs directly into the artery.

Intra-dermal injection   Administration of drugs in a small quantity just beneath the skin.

Intra-articular injection   Administration of drugs directly inject into joints.

Intra-cavernous injection   Administration of drugs into the base of the penis. It is mainly used for treatment of erectile dysfunction in men.

Intramedullary Injection   It involves administration of drugs directly inject into bone marrow.

Intramuscular route   Administration of drugs into muscle mass (upper arm, thigh, or buttock).

Intraoral mucoadhesive patches   Patches that contains a bioadhesive agent such as polyacrylic polmers, povidone, cellulose derivatives (sodium carboxymethyl cellulose) that retains the formulation onto the oral mucosa (buccal, palatal, or gingival mucosa) and is intended for sustained or prolonged release of drug the oral cavity and/or systemically.

Intraoral transmucosal drug delivery   Delivery of drug candidates across the mucosa of oral cavity.

Intraperitoneal injection   The injection of drugs directly into peritoneal cavity. This route is generally preferred for veterinary medicines and systemic administration of drugs in animal testing because of the ease of administration compared to other parenteral methods.

Intrathecal injection   The administration of drugs directly into the subarachnoid space of the spine or the cerebrospinal fluid to avoid the blood–brain barrier.

Intravenous route   The administration of drugs directly into the vein using a syringe attached to a hollow needle or by perfusion.

Intravitreal injections   The injection of the drug solution directly into the vitreous via pars plana using a 30-G needle. This route provides higher drug concentrations in the vitreous and retina.

Ion exchange resins (IERs)   Insoluble high-molecular-weight polymers that have the ability to reversibly interchange ions in an aqueous environment.

Iontophoresis   A non-invasive technique that involves the application of a small current to drive charged and neutral drug molecules across the skin.

Iris   The pigmented portion of the eye (most anterior portion of the uveal tract) consisting of pigmented epithelial cells and circular muscles (constrictor iridial sphincter muscles).

Isobaric tags for relative and absolute quantitation   A non-gel based separation technique that is used to measure protein or peptide in a different environment. This labeling technique involves stable incorporation of isotopes into an amine-tagging reagent to study comparative quantitation of various proteins in a complex cell matrix.

Isoelectric point   The pH at which a particular molecule or surface carries no net electrical charge.

Isotope-coded affinity tagging   A high-throughput screening technique for estimating protein content of two different samples by a gel-free process. It is designed to identify and quantify proteins in a two-cell population.

Lag phase   The phase of drug release in an erosion-controlled systems undergoing bulk erosion in which the drug release slows down after burst phase due to self-healing.

Laser ablation   A technique in which a laser is applied on top of the skin. The skin surface is heated and water molecules begin to evaporate, forming microchannels for drug to travel through.

Lead molecule   In drug discovery, a chemical compound that has pharmacological or biological activity likely to be therapeutically useful but may still have suboptimal structure that requires modification to fit better to the target. Also called a lead compound.

Lens   A crystalline and flexible structure enclosed in a capsule. It is suspended from the eye's ciliary muscles by very thin fibers called the zonules. It is very important for vision and offers protection to retina from UV radiation in conjunction with ciliary muscles.

Lentivirus   A subset of retroviruses with the ability to integrate into host chromosomes and to infect non-dividing cells. These viruses can cause severe immunologic and neurologic disease in their natural hosts.

Linear polymers   Polymers in which the monomers are joined together end-to-end making single chains that are flexible and can easily interact with each other.

Lipinski's rule   A rule that aims to correlate a drug candidate's physicochemical parameters with its absorption, permeability, and pharmacologic efficacy.

Lipinski's rule of five   For a drug molecule to be well absorbed via passive diffusion, the drug molecule should have no more than 5 hydrogen bond donors, no more than 10 hydrogen-bond acceptors, a molecular mass less than 500 daltons, and an octanol-water partition coefficient log P not greater than 5.

Liposomes   Artificial vesicles composed of phospholipids with the drug entrapped in their core or attached to the membrane.

Lozenges   Tablets that are dissolved in the mouth and active ingredients have immediately local or systemic effect by direct absorption through mucosa to avoid first-pass metabolism.

Lysosomes   A membrane-bound cell organelle found in animal cells that are structurally and chemically spherical vesicles containing metabolizing enzymes capable of breaking down most biomolecules.

Madin-Darby canine kidney cells   See MDCK cells.

Magnetofection   A transfection technique that employs magnetic nanoparticles made of iron oxide with or without coupling with non-viral or viral vectors to enhance gene transfer into target cells or tissues in the presence of an external magnetic field.

Mass median aerodynamic diameter   Diameter of a sphere of unit density that has the same settling velocity in air as the aerosol particle in question. The mass median aerodynamic diameter divides the aerosol size distribution in half. In other words, it is the diameter at which 50% of the particles of an aerosol by mass are larger and 50% are smaller.

Mass spectrometer   The mass spectrometer is essentially an instrument that can be used to measure the mass, or more correctly the mass/charge ratio, of ionized atoms or other electrically charged particles. It makes use of the basic magnetic force on a moving charged particle.

Mass spectrometry   Mass spectrometry is an analytical technique that can provide both qualitative (structure) and quantitative (molecular mass or concentration) information on analyte molecules after their conversion to ions.

Matrix-assisted laser desorption ionization (MALDI)   In MALDI analysis, the analyte is first co-crystallized with a large molar excess of a matrix compound, usually an ultraviolet (UV)-absorbing weak organic acid, after which laser radiation of this analyte-matrix mixture results in the vaporization of the matrix which carries the analyte with it. The matrix therefore plays a key role by strongly absorbing the laser light energy and causing, indirectly, the analyte to vaporize. The matrix also serves as a proton donor and receptor, acting to ionize the analyte in both positive and negative ionization modes, respectively.

Matrix-type system   A system in which drug is dispersed in a polymer matrix with the adhesive spread along its circumference.

MDCK cell   A cell line derived from dog renal epithelium that displays a lot of morphological features similar to the cells of the small intestine and is used to study drug transport across the intestine.

Medicated chewing gum   Solid or semi-solid, single-dose preparations that have to be chewed but not swallowed. They containing masticatory gum base with one or more pharmacologically active substances that are released by chewing.

Membrane vesicle   A small organelle within a cell, consisting of fluid enclosed by a lipid bilayer membrane.

Methylcellulose   Methyl substitutions on the cellulose structure produce methylcellulose, a water-soluble cellulose derivative.

Microemulsions   These are isotropic, thermodynamically stable transparent (or translucent) systems of oil, water, and surfactant, frequently in combination with a co-surfactant with particles of droplets size usually in the range of 20–200 nm.

Microencapsulation   A process in which tiny particles or droplets are surrounded by a coating to give small capsules many useful properties.

Microneedles   Minimally invasive technique that temporarily disrupts the stratum corneum by creation of microchannels through which the drug can be delivered. This strategy involves use of micron-sized needles fabricated of different materials and geometries to create transient aqueous conduits across the skin.

Microparticles   See Microspheres.

Microspheres   Small spherical particles, with diameters in the micrometer range (typically $1\,\mu m$ to $1,000\,\mu m$ [1 mm]). These are often referred to as microparticles.

Monolithic system   A formulation in which drugs are uniformly dispersed and completely or partially dissolved in a water-insoluble polymer matrix and released from the system through simple diffusion.

Monomers   The building blocks of polymers.

Morphology   A branch of life science dealing with the study of gross structure of an organism or taxon and its component parts.

Mucoadhesive polymers   When polymer interacts with the mucus layer covering a tissue, it is generally referred to as a mucoadhesion. Polymers that facilitate the mucoadhesion by their specific properties.

Mucociliary clearance   The body's defense mechanisms that work by entrapping potentially hazardous substances such as dust and microorganisms within the viscoelastic mucus lining the nasal passages.

Multidrug resistance   Alteration in the expression of some critical proteins in cancer cells resulting in the cells becoming resistant to chemotherapy is called as multidrug resistance. It is a term broadly used for aquired resistance by cells to multiple types of drugs upon exposure to certain types of drugs.

Multidrug resistance proteins (MRPs/ABCC)   A family of 13 members, 9 of which are transporters referred to as the multidrug resistance proteins. They are known to be involved in ion transport, toxin secretion, and signal transduction.

Multilayered tablets   A multilayer tablet usually consists of a hydrophilic matrix core containing the active ingredient and impermeable or semi-permeable polymeric coatings that function as the barrier layers to adjust the hydration or swelling rate of core.

Nanomedicine   The application of nanotechnology to medicine, in particular, in diagnostic testing and drug delivery systems.

Nanomicelles   Micellar delivery systems that have particle size smaller than 1 micron.

Nanoparticles   See Polymeric nanoparticles.

Narrow therapeutic index drugs   Drugs in which small differences in dose or blood concentration may lead to dose and blood concentration-dependent, serious therapeutic failures or adverse drug reactions.

Nasal drug delivery   Administration via the nasal route involving transport across the nasal membrane.

Nebulizer   A drug delivery device used to administer medication in the form of a mist inhaled into the lungs.

Non-biodegradable implants   Implants that require surgery for implantation and removal.

Ocular drug delivery   Drug administration to the eye.

Oligopeptide   A protein fragment or molecule that usually consists of less than 25 amino acid residues linked in a polypeptide chain.

Oral route   Administration through the mouth.

Osmosis   The diffusion of solvent molecules from a region of low solute concentration to a region of high solute concentration that are separated by a semipermeable membrane.

Osmosis-Controlled Systems Delivery   Systems in which the osmotic pressure between the dosage form and the surrounding environment is the rate-determining factor and which can be controlled by using different types of semipermeable membranes and pharmaceutical excipients.

Otologic administration   Administration of drugs to the ear canal mainly in the form of drops. This route is generally administered for removal of wax and treatment of outer ear and ear canal infections.

P-glycoprotein   Also known as multidrug resistance protein 1 (MDR1) or ATP-binding cassette sub-family B member 1 (ABCB1) or cluster of differentiation 243 (CD243); an important protein of the cell membrane that pumps many foreign substances out of cells.

Palatal, gingival, periodontal drug delivery   Administration of drug via soft palate, gingival membrane, and around a tooth, respectively.

PAMPA   See Parallel artificial membrane permeation assay.

Paracellular pathway   The transfer of substances across an epithelium by passing through the intercellular space between the cells.

Parallel artificial membrane permeation assay   A method that determines the permeability of substances from a donor compartment, through a lipid-infused artificial membrane, and into an acceptor compartment.

Parenteral route   In Greek and Latin, *par* means beyond and *enteral* means intestinal. In the parenteral route, drugs are directly introduced to the systemic circulation.

Passive diffusion   The movement of biochemicals across cell membranes. It does not require an input of chemical energy and is driven by the growth of entropy of the system.

Patches   Intraoral mucoadhesive patches can be designed to deliver drugs locally in the oral cavity and/or systemically.

Pectin   A natural anionic heteropolysaccharide prevalently found in fruit cell walls. It is largely made up of galacturonic acid residues.

Pegylation   The process of covalent attachment of different lengths of polyethylene glycol chains to another molecule, normally a drug or a therapeutic protein. This addition allows the therapeutic drugs to reduce clearance by the kidneys because of an increase in size.

PEGylation   Covalent attachment of polyethylene glycol to a small molecule proteins or other polymeric material. In biological processes, it is generally used to alleviate metabolic degradation and plasma clearance.

Peptide and protein drugs   A group of drugs that includes monoclonal antibodies, hormones, recombinant proteins, small and large oligopeptide–based agents, and related compounds.

Percutaneous absorption   A passive process in which drugs or therapeutic molecules pass through the skin into the body.

Peribulbar route   Injection into the extracellular spaces of the rectus muscles and their intramuscular septa.

Periocular route   Administration to the periphery of the eye or the region surrounding the eye. This route includes peribulbar, posterior juxtascleral, retrobulbar, subtenon and subconjunctival routes.

Permeability   Measurement of the ability of a drug molecule to traverse a biomembrane barrier.

pH   A measure of the acidity or basicity of an aqueous solution. Solutions with a pH less than 7 are said to be acidic and solutions with a pH greater than 7 are basic or alkaline.

Pharmacodynamics   The study of the biochemical and physiological effects of drugs on the body or on microorganisms or parasites within or on the body and the mechanisms of drug action and the relationship between drug concentration and effect. In simple terms, it is the science of what the drug does to the body.

Pharmacokinetics   A branch of pharmacology dedicated to determining the fate of substances administered into a living organism. In simple terms it is the science of what the body does to the drug.

Pharmacotherapy   It is the use of drugs that produce effects on or within the body that are beneficial in the treatment of a given medical condition.

Phosphorylation   The addition of a phosphate group to a protein or other organic molecule.

Photoporation   A laser-assisted method of gene delivery resembling that of electroporation and sonoporation mechanistically. Laser pulses serve as a physical force to create transient pores in cell membranes, allowing DNA to enter.

pKa   An acid dissociation constant and a quantitative measure of the strength of an acid in solution.

Polaxamers   Triblock copolymers based on ethylene oxide (EO) and propylene oxide (PO); also called Pluronics©.

Poly(vinyl alcohol)   A synthetic polymer produced from polyvinyl acetate, in which the acetate groups are partially hydrolyzed and replaced with hydroxyl group.

Polyethylene glycols (PEGs)   Synthetic polymers formed by an addition reaction of ethylene oxide and water.

Polymeric nanoparticulate systems   Polymeric systems of sub 1 micron size that act as carriers and protect the drug from degradation and control its release.

Polymers Large, high-molecular-weight substances composed of a large number of repeating units. These macromolecules are synthesized as smaller repeating units (or monomers) become attached covalently into a chain-like structure.

Polymersomes Membrane enclosed spherical vesicular structures composed of macromolecular aggregates of amphiphilic block copolymers.

Polyvinylpyrrolidone A synthetic neutral homopolymer that comes in many different solubility grades.

Post-translational modification An enzymatic processing of the newly synthesized polypeptide chain post-translation completion. They are known to be essential mechanisms used by eukaryotic cells to diversify their protein functions and dynamically coordinate their signaling networks.

Posterior juxtascleral injection A method of delivering the drug directly onto the outer surface of sclera employing a blunt tipped curved cannula.

Posterior segment of the eye Back of the eye including sclera, choroid, retina and vitreous body.

Powder A mixture of finely divided drugs and/or chemicals in dry form for internal or external use.

Pressurized metered dose inhalers Inhalers in which drug is dispersed in propellants, and the device facilitates aerosolization of the drug. These devices allow multiple dosing utilizing metering valves in conjunction with propellants.

Prodrugs Bioreversible derivatives of drug molecules that are enzymatically or chemically transformed *in vivo* to release the active parent drug, which can then elicit the desired pharmacodynamic response.

Propellant A liquefied gas with a vapor pressure greater than atmospheric pressure at a temperature of 40°C. The propellant is the driving force or the "heart" of aerosols.

Protein and peptide Typically, a peptide consists of a chain of amino acids with amide bonds. When the peptide chain folds into a three-dimensional configuration, it is called as protein. Proteins and peptides are biochemical compounds made up of amino acid residues that are chemically formed by the formation of an amide link between the α-carboxyl groups of one amino acid attached to the α-amino group of an adjacent amino acids.

Proteolysis The breakdown of proteins into smaller polypeptides or amino acids.

Proteomics The study of proteins and their fragments including peptides and free amino acids. It is an essential aspect of biological research to be able to detect post-translational protein modifications such as phosphorylation and glycosylation.

Pulmonary drug delivery Administration in which medication is inhaled through the lungs and enters the bloodstream through the alveolar epithelium.

Pulsatile capsules Capsules in which the release consists of predetermined lag time without any release before a rapid and complete release occurs at a particular time.

Quadrupole mass spectrometer Spectrometer consisting of an ionizer (bombardment by electrons from a hot filament), an ion accelerator, and a mass filter with four parallel metal rods that operate together electronically.

Quick dissolving dosage forms Forms that disintegrate or undergo dissolution within a few seconds to a minute upon coming into contact with saliva in the oral cavity thereby releasing the drug.

Radiofrequency ablation Minimally invasive technique used to disrupt the barrier properties of the stratum corneum and enhance drug permeation.

Random copolymer A polymer in which monomers A and B are attached to one another in random form ABBA.

Receptor mediated endocytosis A highly specific process in which the drug molecule is designed to interact with a cell surface protein and then is absorbed by endolysosomal trafficking pathways.

Rectal drug delivery The administration of drugs into the rectum or colon via the anus in the form of suppositories and enemas.

Reservoir system   A type of diffusion controlled system in which the drug is present as a reservoir surrounded by a rate-controlling polymer membrane.

Residence time   The amount of time in which the drugsremain in the gastrointestinal tract.

Retina   A multi-layered, light sensitive tissue that lines the back of the eye. It consists of neural layer, pigment epithelium, and millions of photoreceptors (rods and cones) that capture and subsequently convert light rays into electrical impulses. Such impulses are transferred by optic nerve to brain where images are formed.

Retrobulbar injection   The injection in the conical compartment within the rectus muscles and intramuscular septa.

Retroviruses   Enveloped viruses with capsid encapsulating a viral genome and two key enzymes: reverse transcriptase, which generates DNA from viral RNA and integrase, which incorporates DNA into the host genome. These are infectious viruses that can integrate into transduced cells with high frequency and that may have oncogenic potential in their natural hosts.

Rheology   The study of the flow of matter, primarily in the liquid state, but also as "soft solids" or solids under conditions in which they respond with plastic flow rather than deforming elastically in response to an applied force.

Route of administration   The method or path by which a drug substance enters the body.

Sclera   The whitish outermost layer surrounding the globe and is called the "white of the eye." It is composed of collagen bundles, mucopolysaccharides, and elastic fibers. This tissue acts as a principal shield to protect the intraocular contents.

Self-healing   Polymer chain relaxation and rearrangement that occurs as a result of degradation products formed in the presence of water in systems undergoing bulk erosion. This eventually leads to the closing of pores that had originally allowed the influx of water.

Slow dissolving dosage forms   Forms that dissolve slower in the oral cavity compared to quick dissolving dosage forms, i.e., within 1 to 10 mins.

Soft-shell capsules   Also known as softgels, a continuous and closed soft shell often surrounds the contents. Sometimes softgels are called one-piece capsules.

Solid lipid nanoparticles   Sub-micron sized lipid matrices that are solid at body temperature.

Solutions   A homogeneous mixture composed of only one phase. Most drugs are administered as solutions.

Sonophoresis   Also known as phonophoresis, the application of low-frequency ultrasound (20–100 kHz) to deliver drugs into the skin.

Sonoporation   Application of ultrasound to cells for gene delivery by modifying the permeability of the cell plasma membrane. This technique is usually used in molecular biology and nonviral gene therapy to facilitate uptake of large molecules such as DNA into the cell.

Stable isotope labeling by amino acid   A mass spectrometry–based stable isotope quantitation technique for simultaneous and automated identification and estimation of complex protein mixtures. This method is based on labeling amino acids that can be introduced into a cell culture medium to encode cellular proteins and measure differences in the protein abundance among samples with non-radioactive isotopic labeling.

Structural-activity relationship   The relationship between the chemical or 3D structure of a molecule and its biological activity.

Sub-labial route   Administration of drugs between the lip and the gingiva.

Subconjunctival injections   The introduction of an active ingredient beneath the conjunctiva.

Subcutaneous route   Administration of drugs into the fatty tissue below the skin.

Sublingual drug delivery   Administration of drugs in the area beneath the tongue.

Subtenon injection   Administration of drug into the tenon's capsule located around the upper portion of the eye and into the belly of the superior rectus muscle.

Suppository   A drug delivery system that is inserted into the rectum (rectal suppository), vagina (vaginal suppository), or urethra (urethral suppository) where it dissolves or melts and is absorbed into the blood stream. They are used to deliver both systemically and locally acting medications.

Surface erosion   A system of polymer matrix erosion in which the erosion begins at the outer surface of the dosage form and gradually moves inwards resulting in drug release and a decrease in the device dimensions.

Suspensions   A heterogeneous mixture of drugs and excipients containing solid particles sufficiently large for sedimentation.

Swelling   The increase in the volume of a formulation system caused by the absorption of a liquid or vapor.

Swelling-controlled systems polymeric delivery   Systems that release the drug upon exposure to water caused by swelling of the system.

Tablets   A compressed form of powder that consists of drug along with other inactive ingredients that allow proper disintegration, dissolution, and absorption of the dosage form.

Tandem affinity purification   A simple two-step affinity purification method for the separation of TAP-tagged proteins, which is mixed with other related proteins in a protein-protein interaction study.

TC-7 cells   Cells derived from Caco-2 cells that express more metabolizing enzymes than the parent cells.

TEER value   The transendothelial electrical resistance or the transepethelial electrical resistance value is a measurement used to estimate the permeability through endothelial cells or epithelial cells, respectively, *in vitro*.

Therapeutic window   The range of drug dosages that can treat disease effectively while staying within the safety range.

Tight junctions   Also known as occluding junctions or zonulae occludentes (singular, zonula occludens), the closely associated areas of two cells whose membranes join together forming a virtually impermeable barrier to fluid.

Time-of-flight analyzer   Secondary ion mass spectrometry using a pulsed primary ion beam to desorb and ionize species from a sample surface. The resulting secondary ions are accelerated into a mass spectrometer, where they are mass analyzed by measuring their time-of-flight from the sample surface to the detector.

Topical delivery   Delivery of drugs into skin layers.

Topology   The study of shapes, dimensions, and transformation.

Transcellular pathway   The transport of molecules in which the substances travel through the cell, passing through both the apical membrane and basolateral membrane.

Transcytosis   When the contents of an endocytosed vesicle by-pass lysosomes and are released across the basolateral membrane resulting in transports of the contents of the vesicle across the cell layer.

Transdermal drug delivery   Administration of drugs through the skin into the systemic circulation.

Transdermal patches   Transdermal drug delivery systems consisting of medicated adhesive patches that deliver drugs systemically when placed on the skin.

Transfected MDCK cell lines   MDCK cell lines in which certain genes are overexpressed to study their effects on intestinal transport of certain drugs.

Transmucosal drug delivery   Administration of a substance, such as a drug, through the mucous membranes.

Transmucosal hydrogels   Flexible formulations composed of swellable hydrophilic matrices that swell on coming in contact with saliva in the oral cavity and release drug through the spaces in the network of hydrogels.

Ultrasonic nebulizers   Nebulizers that use a transducer of piezo-electric crystal to produce high frequency sound waves in the nebulizer solution.

Ussing chambers   See Diffusion chambers.

Vaginal drug delivery   Administration of drugs via the vagina or the vaginal route.

Vaginal rings Flexible, thin, and circular-shaped devices that are capable of releasing pharmacologically active agents into systemic circulation in a controlled manner over an extended period of time.

Vesicular transport Transport of drugs or cellular matter through vesicles that are small organelles within a cell, consisting of fluid enclosed by a lipid bilayer membrane.

Viral vector Genetic tool that is commonly used by molecular biologists to deliver genetic material into cells. This process can be performed inside a living organism (*in vivo*) or in cell culture (*in vitro*). Delivery of genes by a virus is termed *transduction* and the infected cells are described as *transduced*.

Vitreous humor A jelly-like substance between the retina and lens of the eye. This hydrogel matrix consists of hyaluronic acid, proteoglycans, and collagen fibrils. Separated from the anterior segment by the hyaloid membrane, the vitreous is joined to the retina via ligaments.

Volume of distribution A pharmacological, theoretical volume that the total amount of administered drug would have to occupy (if it were uniformly distributed) to provide the same concentration as it currently is in blood plasma.

Wafers Thin porous wafer-like tablets or strips formulated by lyophilization of polymer containing an active pharmaceutical ingredient. The formulation instantaneously disintegrates when placed in the oral cavity releasing the drug subsequently.

Xanthan gum A high-molecular-weight natural polymer produced by microbial fermentation. It is a heteropolysaccharide that can be used as a thickening agent and as a suspending and emulsifying agent for water-based products.

INDEX

Note: Page numbers followed by *f* and *t* indicate material in figures and tables respectively.